Total Knee Arthroplasty

Alfred J. Tria Jr. • Giles R. Scuderi
Editors

Total Knee Arthroplasty

A Curated AI Literature Review

Springer

Editors
Alfred J. Tria Jr.
Department of Orthopedics
Rutgers-Robert Wood Johnson
Medical School
New Brunswick, NJ, USA

Giles R. Scuderi
Department of Orthopedic Surgery
Northwell Health
Garden City, NY, USA

ISBN 978-3-032-00174-0 ISBN 978-3-032-00175-7 (eBook)
https://doi.org/10.1007/978-3-032-00175-7

This Springer imprint is published by the registered company Springer Nature Switzerland AG
The registered company address is: Gewerbestrasse 11, 6330 Cham, Switzerland

Preface

> Love the discipline you know, and let it support you.
> Marcus Aurelius (Meditations, Book 4, Article 31)

Total knee arthroplasty (TKA) has become one of the most common surgical procedures around the world. As demand has increased, supportive science and literature have both expanded exponentially.

Artificial intelligence (AI) has become part of everyday living and supportive in its nature. The purpose of this book is to search the current Springer Nature published literature and develop a small compendium of the most significant articles relevant to TKA. The key words were selected by the editors and submitted to the machines for further key word development and subsequent references. The generated references were then reviewed by the editors for relevance to the individual chapters. The references were returned to the machines for generated summaries, which are once again reviewed by the editors.

As we come to realize, the introduction of AI-generated medical textbooks is transformative and complements rather than supplants current traditional medical textbooks. While upholding the foundational principles of medical education, this technology has the potential to enhance the accessibility and relevance of educational resources. The editors hope that this textbook will illustrate the value of AI for literature searches and support of medical academic literature.

New Brunswick, NJ, USA — Alfred J. Tria Jr.
New York, NY, USA — Giles R. Scuderi

Total Knee Arthroplasty: An AI Literature Review

Auto-summaries can be generated by either an abstractive or an extractive auto-summarization:

- An extraction-based summarizer identifies the most important sentences of a text and uses the original sentences to create the summary.
- An abstraction-based summarizer creates new text based on deep learning. New phrases are created to summarize the content.

The auto-summaries you will find in this book have been generated via an abstractive summarization approach.

Each chapter was carefully edited by Dr. Alfred Tria and Dr. Giles Scuderi. The editors selected the papers, which were then auto summarized. The editors have edited the auto-summaries to support the understanding of the original content. You will find the editors' reviews and guidance on the auto-summaries in their chapter introductions. In machine-generated books, editors are defined as those who curate the content for the book by selecting the papers to be auto-summarized and by organizing the output into a meaningful order. Next to the thoughtful curation of the papers, editors should guide the readers through the auto-summaries and make transparent why they selected the papers. The ultimate goal is to provide a current literature review of Springer Nature publications on a given topic in order to support readers in overcoming information overload and to help them dive into a topic faster; to identify interdisciplinary overlaps; and to present papers that might not have been on the readers' radar.

Please note that the selected papers are not used to train an LLM while the auto-summaries are created.

Contents

Chapter 1
Evolution of Total Knee Arthroplasty Design

Alfred J. Tria Jr. and Giles R. Scuderi

Introduction by the Editors

The evolution of modern total knee arthroplasty (TKA) began over 50 years ago. Seeking alternatives for arthrodesis and fascial arthroplasty for the treatment of knee arthritis, surgeons and engineers were developing various implants such as the Polycentric, the ICLH, and the Freeman Swanson prostheses. In 1970, the Duocondylar Prosthesis was designed as a modification of the Polycentric Knee Prosthesis. Further refinements lead to the Duopatellar Prosthesis that was designed by Insall and Walker. This implant was the precursor of the Total Condylar Prosthesis that was a cruciate sacrificing design with a conforming articular surface, an anterior femoral flange and a dome shaped patellar component. While first implanted in 1974, this prothesis was the first real modern TKA design that became the foundation for future implants. With the growing number of implants and surgical experience, there was debate about the utility of posterior cruciate ligament (PCL) retention. By 1978, Insall and Burstein introduced the Insall Burstein posterior stabilized knee prothesis. This innovative design substituted the PCL with a spine- cam mechanism that provided greater stability with better kinematics and range of motion. Over time, there became two camps of knee arthroplasty surgeons, those who retained the PCL and those who preferred PCL substitution. While this debate continued, further refinements in implants designs continued with more shapes and sizes to better accommodate the individual anatomy, along with improvements accommodate higher range of motion and normal knee kinematics. To reduce the stresses and possible polyethylene wear, mobile bearing designs with a more conforming articulation were introduced. The mobile bearing designs reduced the

A. J. Tria Jr. (✉)
Department of Orthopedics, Rutgers-Robert Wood Johnson Medical School, New Brunswick, NJ, USA

G. R. Scuderi
Department of Orthopedic Surgery, Northwell Health, Garden City, NY, USA

A. J. Tria Jr., G. R. Scuderi (eds.), *Total Knee Arthroplasty*,
https://doi.org/10.1007/978-3-032-00175-7_1

kinematic conflict of a conforming surface by decoupling the flexion-extension and rotation with a rotating tibial platform. More recently, there has been a move toward more guided motion knee designs with the medial pivot and medial congruent prosthesis, that provide rollback and motion based upon the differential conformity of the articular surface. These newer designs have features that accommodate both sacrificing or retention of the PCL. With the vast number of current implant designs on the international market, it is apparent that there is an effort, realistic or not, to find the "holy grail" and provide patients with a durable knee prothesis that will restore normal function without residual symptoms.

This chapter reviews five references that highlights the development of TKA. With our editorial prerogative, we reviewed each of the referenced articles and summarized our own conclusions, as detailed below. As you read each of the computer-generated summaries that follow in this chapter you can draw your own conclusions.

Slamin et al. favor the development of patient specific designs. The article reviews the importance of the use of both MRI studies and CT examinations to obtain appropriate data for customization. The computer assisted software allows the information to be imported to produce a solid model. While the precision of the implant is certainly improved, there are two major problems with this approach. The implant itself must be taken to the operating room where it must be coordinated with the soft tissues and the existing deformity of the knee. The surgical manipulations often result in a mismatch between the remaining bone surfaces and the custom implant. The second issue is the underlying cost of the manufacturing process. In an age where the costs of medical care continue to increase there is less and less room for an increase in the implant budgeted amounts.

Zanasi et al. Reviewed newer perioperative protocols. The mini-midvastus surgical approach certainly is valuable for the acceptable visualization with less dissection. However, the technique is more demanding and involves a learning curve for the surgeon. The article goes on to discuss implant choices and emphasizes the value of the UKA over the TKA. The authors did report that the UKA does have a higher revision rate than the TKA. The UKA revision rate is secondary to standard complications, such as loosening or malpositioning), and progression of disease. Therefore, it is critical for the surgeon to fully evaluate the knee for the extent of the presenting disease and the possible advancement in the future. Bicompartmental prostheses are quite unusual and are probably not an effective alternative between UKA and TKA.

Zhao et al. evaluated the value of a multimodal approach to decrease the use of opioids following TKA. Local infiltration, nerve blocks, and oral medications certainly form the basis for such protocols; however, implementation of these methodologies requires an organized team approach with collaboration of all the specialties.

Conteduca et al. reviewed patient specific instrumentation and observed that there is a problem with sagittal plane accuracy. The technology does require preoperative CT and MRI scans to create disposable instruments. With this additional cost and the sagittal plane problems, the approach does not seem to be valuable.

The authors favor the accuracy of computer assisted surgery but does not give good data to support this alternative.

Bozic et al. use the new ICD-10-CM coding to show that Infection was the primary reason for revision, followed by mechanical loosening in TKA. The data is more detailed with this coding and may lead to more insight into the unexplained 15 percent dissatisfaction rate for the replacements.

This chapter shows that there is still room for improvement in implant designs, surgical techniques, and perioperative management to address the 15 percent of patients who are not entirely pleased with their implants. Infection and mechanical loosening remain the major issues leading to revision. While these factors need to be considered, it is often difficult to explain the patient dissatisfaction when the implant itself appears to be functioning in a perfectly normal manner. These discrepancies may be secondary to a multitude of factors that have not yet been thoroughly researched. It is a known fact that younger patients are less satisfied, and this may be due to functional demands that are not achievable with the present designs. Expectations may need to be better counseled with the understanding that the implant can relieve symptoms of pain better than it can support return to "normal" functional demands. Anterior knee pain is often difficult to understand even in the non-operated knee. Thus, the entire TKA picture continues to evolve with all aspects requiring investigation and modification.

Machine Generated Summaries

Disclaimer: The summaries in this chapter were generated from Springer Nature publications using abstractive AI auto-summarization: An abstraction-based summarizer creates new text based on deep learning. New phrases are created to summarize the content. As the constituted sentences are machine selected, they may not fully reflect the body of the work, so we strongly advise that the original content is read and cited. The auto-generated summaries were curated by the editor to meet Springer Nature publication standards.

1.1 Evolution of Customization Design for Total Knee Arthroplasty [71]

This is a machine-generated summary of:

Slamin, John; Parsley, Brian Evolution of customization design for total knee arthroplasty [71].

Published in: Current Reviews in Musculoskeletal Medicine (2012).

Link to original: https://doi.org/10.1007/s12178-012-9141-z

If you want to cite the papers, please refer to the original.

For technical reasons we could not place the page where the original quote is coming from.

1.1.1 Research Highlights

Traditionally, custom implants have been utilized in orthopedic surgery for cases where standard implants do not suffice, such as in patients with juvenile rheumatoid arthritis or unusual bone geometry. These custom solutions have been particularly valuable in revision surgeries where bone erosion is present, requiring additional fixation features. However, the process of creating these implants has evolved significantly over the years. Now a new study by John Slamin et al. explores the advancements in patient-specific instrumentation and implants, highlighting the potential benefits of these innovations in improving surgical outcomes and patient satisfaction.

The study delves into the methods used to create patient-specific implants, which involve advanced imaging techniques like MRI and CT scans to capture detailed anatomical data. This data is then processed through segmentation to create a point cloud representing the joint's outer surface. The point cloud is imported into computer-assisted design (CAD) software to develop a solid model for designing customized implants. The research emphasizes the advantages of using MRI for soft tissue analysis and CT for hard tissue imaging, allowing for precise customization of implants that better fit individual patients' anatomy. The study also reviews various approaches by different manufacturers, including complete patient-specific systems that incorporate both custom instrumentation and implants.

The main advances highlighted by Slamin includes the potential for improved surgical precision and reduced operative time with patient-specific systems. These systems can lead to better postoperative alignment and potentially restore near-normal joint kinematics, addressing common issues like implant overhang that contribute to patient dissatisfaction. Future study directions could focus on further refining these technologies to enhance their cost-effectiveness and accessibility, ensuring broader adoption in clinical practice. By continuing to innovate in this field, there is potential to significantly improve outcomes for patients undergoing joint replacement surgeries.

1.2 Innovations in Total Knee Replacement: New Trends in Operative Treatment and Changes in Peri-Operative Management [72]

This is a machine-generated summary of:

Zanasi, Stefano Innovations in total knee replacement: new trends in operative treatment and changes in peri-operative management [72].

Published in: European Orthopaedics and Traumatology (2011).

Link to original: https://doi.org/10.1007/s12570-011-0066-6

1.2.1 Research Highlights

The knee joint, being the largest in the human body, plays a crucial role in weight-bearing and is often susceptible to injuries and osteoarthritis. Osteoarthritis can affect one or more of the knee's three compartments, leading to pain and functional impairment. When non-surgical interventions fail to alleviate pain, knee replacement surgery becomes a viable option. Orthopaedic surgeons can choose between total knee replacement (TKR) and partial knee replacement, also known as unicompartmental knee replacement (UKR), depending on the extent of joint damage. Now, a new study by Stefano Zanasi et al. explores various surgical techniques and prosthetic options for knee replacement, emphasizing minimally invasive surgery (MIS) approaches.

The study reviews multiple cases to illustrate the effectiveness of MIS techniques in both TKR and UKR procedures. MIS involves smaller incisions, less muscle dissection, and specialized instruments that allow for precise surgical interventions with minimal tissue damage. The mini-midvastus approach is highlighted as a gold standard technique that provides excellent visibility of the knee joint while preserving soft tissue integrity. The authors discuss the advantages of UKR over TKR, such as shorter hospital stays, reduced pain, better post-operative range of motion, and easier revision surgeries if needed. They also examine bi-unicompartmental replacements for cases involving two compartments and emphasize the importance of careful patient selection to achieve optimal outcomes.

The study suggests that future advancements in knee replacement surgery may focus on improving prosthetic designs and surgical techniques to better mimic natural knee kinematics. The use of computer-assisted surgical navigation systems is highlighted as a promising tool for enhancing implant positioning accuracy and limb alignment during TKR procedures. Additionally, the authors note that high-flex TKA designs and gender-specific solutions are being developed to address the unique anatomical needs of different patient populations. Overall, this research underscores the potential benefits of MIS techniques in achieving faster recovery times and improved functional outcomes for patients undergoing knee replacement surgery.

1.3 Advances in Perioperative Pain Management for Total Knee Arthroplasty: A Review of Multimodal Analgesic Approaches [73]

This is a machine-generated summary of:

Zhao, Chengcheng; Liao, Qimeng; Yang, Dinglong; Yang, Mingyi; Xu, Peng Advances in perioperative pain management for total knee arthroplasty: a review of multimodal analgesic approaches [73].

Published in: Journal of Orthopaedic Surgery and Research (2024).

Link to original: https://doi.org/10.1186/s13018-024-05324-4

If you want to cite the papers, please refer to the original.

For technical reasons we could not place the page where the original quote is coming from.

1.3.1 Research Highlights

Total knee arthroplasty (TKA) is a prevalent orthopedic procedure aimed at improving joint function and alleviating pain by replacing damaged knee joints with artificial implants. It is considered the most effective treatment for end-stage knee disease, with primary knee osteoarthritis being the leading indication for TKA. Despite advancements in surgical techniques, managing postoperative pain remains a significant challenge, as many patients experience moderate to severe pain following surgery. This pain can lead to prolonged hospital stays, increased opioid use, and higher risks of adverse events. Now, a new study by Chengcheng Zhao et al. reviews current research on perioperative pain control in TKA and evaluates the effectiveness of various analgesic interventions.

The study conducted by Zhao involved a systematic review of randomized controlled trials focusing on different pain management strategies for TKA patients. The authors analyzed several analgesic methods through individual meta-analyses, highlighting the benefits of local infiltration analgesia and peripheral nerve blocks in reducing postoperative pain intensity and morphine use while improving functional outcomes. The study emphasizes the importance of multimodal analgesia, which integrates preoperative, intraoperative, and postoperative strategies to minimize opioid consumption and enhance analgesic efficacy. This approach includes preemptive analgesia, neuraxial anesthesia, peripheral nerve blocks, local infiltration analgesia, and oral or intravenous medications targeting various pain pathways.

The findings from Zhao study underscores the complexity of managing postoperative pain in TKA patients and highlight the need for individualized perioperative analgesic plans. While multimodal analgesia has become the standard approach for perioperative pain management in TKA, there is no universally agreed-upon protocol for its implementation. Future study should focus on identifying and standardizing the most effective multimodal strategies to optimize patient outcomes. Additionally, exploring nonpharmacological methods such as cryotherapy and physical therapy could further enhance recovery experiences and long-term outcomes for TKA patients.

1.4 Patient-Specific Instruments in Total Knee Arthroplasty [74]

This is a machine-generated summary of:

Conteduca, Fabio; Iorio, Raffaele; Mazza, Daniele; Ferretti, Andrea Patient-specific instruments in total knee arthroplasty [74].

Published in: International Orthopaedics (2014).

Link to original: https://doi.org/10.1007/s00264-013-2230-9

If you want to cite the papers, please refer to the original.

For technical reasons we could not place the page where the original quote is coming from.

1.4.1 Research Highlights

Total knee arthroplasty (TKA) is a widely successful orthopedic procedure that significantly restores function in arthritic knees. However, surgical technique errors and improper component placement can compromise long-term outcomes, with deviations in the mechanical axis leading to poor implant survivorship due to abnormal stress. Computer-assisted surgery (CAS) has been shown to improve coronal alignment compared to standard techniques, but it is often associated with longer surgery times and increased complexity. Now, a new study by Fabio Conteduca et al. explores the reliability of patient-specific instruments (PSI) in TKA, aiming to address these challenges by reducing costs and surgical time while maintaining accuracy.

The study involved a comprehensive review of existing literature and an evaluation of the authors' own experiences with PSI in TKA. PSI technology uses preoperative CT or MRI scans to create disposable cutting jigs tailored to a patient's unique anatomy, potentially simplifying the procedure compared to CAS. The authors assessed the accuracy of PSI by using intra-operative knee navigation software during surgeries. Their findings indicated satisfactory alignment on the tibial coronal plane but highlighted challenges in achieving correct alignment on the tibial sagittal plane. The study also compared PSI with extra-medullary tibial instrumentation, revealing that while PSI showed promise, it did not consistently achieve the same degree of accuracy as CAS techniques.

The study concludes that while PSI offers potential benefits such as reduced surgical time and cost, its accuracy does not yet match that of CAS systems, particularly in the sagittal plane. Future study could focus on improving PSI technology to enhance its reliability and effectiveness. The authors recommend careful verification of alignment during procedures involving PSI to prevent malalignment. Despite its promise, further advancements are needed for PSI to become a more reliable alternative in TKA procedures.

1.5 The Epidemiology of Revision Total Knee Arthroplasty in the United States [75]

This is a machine-generated summary of:

Bozic, Kevin J.; Kurtz, Steven M.; Lau, Edmund; Ong, Kevin; Chiu, Vanessa; Vail, Thomas P.; Rubash, Harry E.; Berry, Daniel J. The Epidemiology of Revision Total Knee Arthroplasty in the United States [75].

Published in: Clinical Orthopaedics and Related Research® (2009).

Link to original: https://doi.org/10.1007/s11999-009-0945-0

If you want to cite the papers, please refer to the original.

For technical reasons we could not place the page where the original quote is coming from.

1.5.1 Research Highlights

Total knee arthroplasty (TKA) is a widely successful and cost-effective procedure for alleviating pain and improving function in patients with advanced knee arthritis. However, the number of revision TKA procedures has been increasing in the United States, driven by factors such as higher primary TKA volumes, changes in surgical techniques, and expanding indications to younger patients. Despite this trend, most existing data on TKA failures come from limited sources like single-center studies, leaving a gap in understanding the broader epidemiology of revision TKA across diverse healthcare settings. Now, a new study by Kevin J. Bozic et al. addresses this gap by utilizing newly implemented ICD-10-CM diagnosis and procedure codes to analyze revision TKA procedures using a large administrative database.

The study employed the Nationwide Inpatient Sample (NIS) to identify revision TKA procedures performed in the U.S. from October 2015 to December 2016. The NIS is a comprehensive survey of hospitals that provides a representative sample of discharges across various hospital types and regions. The researchers analyzed data from 30,000 revision TKA procedures, examining factors such as patient demographics, causes of failure, length of hospital stay, and total charges. They found that infection was the most common cause for revision TKA, particularly for arthrotomy/removal of prosthesis procedures. Mechanical loosening was frequently cited for component revisions. The study also highlighted variations in procedure types and outcomes based on age groups, hospital settings, and geographic regions.

The implementation of new ICD-10-CM codes has enabled more detailed tracking of revision TKA causes and procedures across the U.S., offering insights previously unavailable from smaller studies. While the study provides valuable data on current trends in revision TKA, it also underscores the need for improved clinical documentation and coding accuracy to enhance data reliability. Future study could focus on refining these codes and expanding research into prevention strategies for common failure causes like infection. As primary TKA volumes are expected to rise significantly, understanding failure mechanisms will be crucial for improving patient outcomes and guiding future research efforts in knee arthroplasty.

Bibliography

1. Howell SM, Kuznik K, Hull ML, Siston RA. Results of an initial experience with custom-fit positioning total knee arthroplasty in a series of 48 patients. Orthopedics. 2008;31:857–63.
2. Laskin RS. Minimally invasive total knee replacement using a mini-mid vastus incision technique and results. Surg Technol Int. 2004;13:231–8.

3. Bonutti P. Suspended leg approach and arthroscopic-assisted techniques. In: Scuderi GR, Tria AJ, editors. Minimally invasive surgery in orthopaedics. New York: Springer; 2009. p. 301–7.
4. Schroer WC, Diesfeld PJ, Reedy ME, LeMarr AR. Mini-subvastus approach for total knee arthroplasty. J Arthroplast. 2008;23:9–25.
5. Leopold SS. Minimally invasive total knee arthroplasty for osteoarthritis. N Engl J Med. 2009;360(17):1749–58.
6. King J, Stamper DL, Schaad DC, Leopold SS. Minimally invasive total knee arthroplasty compared with traditional total knee arthroplasty. Assessment of the learning curve and the postoperative recuperative period. J Bone Joint Surg Am. 2007;89:1497–503.
7. Cheng T, Liu T, Zhang G, Peng X, Zhang X. Does minimally invasive surgery improve short-term recovery in total knee arthroplasty? Clin Orthop Relat Res. 2010;468:1635–48.
8. Banks SA, Frely BJ, Boniforti F, Reischmidt C, Romagnoli S. Comparing in vivo kinematics of unicondylar and bi-unicondylar knee replacement. Knee Surg Sports Traumatol Arthrosc. 2005;13:551–6.
9. Andriacchi TP, Andersson GB, Fermier RW, Stern D, Galante JO. A study of lower-limb mechanics during stair-climbing. J Bone Joint Surg Am. 1980;62:749–57.
10. Patil S, Colwell CW, Ezet KA, D'Lima DD. Can normal knee kinematics be restored with unicompartmental knee replacement? J Bone Joint Surg Am. 2005;87:332–8.
11. McAlindon TE, Snow S, Cooper C, Dieppe PA. Radiographic patterns of osteoarthritis of the knee joint in the community: the importance of the patellofemoral joint. Ann Rheum Dis. 1992;51:844–9.
12. Witvoet J. Should patellofemoral prostheses still be used for the treatment of isolated patellofemoral osteoarthritis? Eur Instruc Course Lect. 2005;7:174–83.
13. Berger RA, Meneghini RM, Jacobs JJ, Sheinkop MB, Della Valle CJ, Rosenberg AG, Galante JO. Results of unicompartmental knee arthroplasty at a minimum of ten years of follow-up. J Bone Joint Surg Am. 2005;87:999–1006.
14. Confalonieri N, Manzotti A, Cerveri P, De Momi E. Bi-unicompartmental versus total knee arthroplasty: a matched paired study with early clinical results. Arch Orthop Trauma Surg. 2009;129:1157–63.
15. Fuchs S, Frisse D, Tibesku CO, Genkinger M, Laaß H, Rosenbaum D. Proprioceptive function, clinical results and quality of life after unicondylar sledge prostheses. Am J Phys Med Rehab. 2002;81:478–82.
16. Romagnoli S, Camera A, Bertolotti M, Arnaldi E. La protesi Bimonocompartimentale con rispetto ricostruzione del LCA. Anno XIV: Il Ginocchio; 1998.
17. Levitan D. Patellofemoral knee replacement effective when following strict indication criteria. Orthop Today Int. 2006;9:8.
18. Tria AJ Jr. Bicompartmental arthroplasty of the knee. Instr Course Lect. 2010;59:61–73.
19. Rolston L, Bresh J, Engh GA, Alois F, Kreuzer S, Nadaudad M, Puri L, Wood D. Bicompartmental knee arthroplasty: a bone-sparing, ligament sparing, and minimally invasive alternative for active patients. Orthopedics. 2007;30(8 Suppl):70–3.
20. Callahan CM, Drake BG, Heck DA, Dittus RS. Patient outcomes following tricompartmental total knee replacement. A meta-analysis JAMA. 1994;271:1349–57.
21. Li G, Most E, Sultan PG, Schule S, Zayontz S, Park SE, Rubash HE. Knee kinematics with a high-flexion posterior stabilized total knee prosthesis: an *in vitro* robotic experimental investigation. J Bone Joint Surg Am. 2004;86:1721–9.
22. Munzinger UK, Maffiuletti NA, Guggi T, Bizzini M, Preiss S, Drobny T. Five-year results of the Innex total knee arthroplasty system. Int Orthop. 2010;34:1159–65.
23. Siston RA, Giori NJ, Goodman SB, Delp SL. Surgical navigation for total knee arthroplasty: a perspective. J Biomech. 2007;40:728–35.
24. Stulberg SD, Loan P, Sarin V. Computer-assisted navigation in total knee replacement: results of an initial experience in thirty-five patients. J Bone Joint Surg Am. 2002;84(Suppl 2):90–8.
25. Delp SL, Stulberg SD, Davies B, Picard F, Leitner F. Computer assisted knee replacement. Clin Orthop Relat Res. 1998;354:49–56.

26. Hirsh J, Hoak J. Management of deep vein thrombosis and pulmonary embolism. A statement for healthcare professionals. Council on thrombosis (in consultation with the council on cardiovascular radiology). American Heart Association Circulation. 1996;93:2212–45.
27. Pineo GF, Hull RD. Prophylaxis of venous thromboembolism following orthopedic surgery: mechanical and pharmacological approaches and the need for extended prophylaxis. Thromb Haemost. 1999;82:918–24.
28. Borris LC. Rivaroxaban and dabigatran etexilate: two new oral anticoagulants for extended postoperative prevention of venous thromboembolism after elective total hip arthroplasty. Arch Orthop Trauma Surg. 2010;130:583–9.
29. Karam JA, Schwenk ES, Parvizi J. An update on multimodal pain management after total joint arthroplasty. J Bone Joint Surg Am. 2021;103(17):1652–62.
30. Albrecht E, Guyen O, Jacot-Guillarmod A, Kirkham KR. The analgesic efficacy of local infiltration analgesia vs femoral nerve block after total knee arthroplasty: a systematic review and meta-analysis. Br J Anaesth. 2016;116(5):597–609.
31. Bourne RB, Chesworth BM, Davis AM, Mahomed NN, Charron KD. Patient satisfaction after total knee arthroplasty: who is satisfied and who is not? Clin Orthop Relat Res. 2010;468(1):57–63.
32. Runge C, Jensen JM, Clemmesen L, Knudsen HB, Holm C, Børglum J, et al. Analgesia of combined femoral triangle and obturator nerve blockade is superior to local infiltration analgesia after total knee arthroplasty with high-dose intravenous dexamethasone. Reg Anesth Pain Med. 2018;43(4):352–6.
33. Chan EY, Fransen M, Sathappan S, Chua NH, Chan YH, Chua N. Comparing the analgesia effects of single-injection and continuous femoral nerve blocks with patient controlled analgesia after total knee arthroplasty. J Arthroplast. 2013;28(4):608–13.
34. Kim K, Elbuluk A, Yu S, Iorio R. Cost-effective peri-operative pain management: assuring a happy patient after total knee arthroplasty. Bone Joint J. 2018;100-b(1 Supple A):55–61:55–61.
35. Sato K, Adachi T, Shirai N, Naoi N. Continuous versus single-injection sciatic nerve block added to continuous femoral nerve block for analgesia after total knee arthroplasty: a prospective, randomized, double-blind study. Reg Anesth Pain Med. 2014;39(3):225–9.
36. Reddi D, Curran N, Stephens R. An introduction to pain pathways and mechanisms. Br J Hosp Med (Lond). 2013;74(Suppl 12):C188–91.
37. Li D, Alqwbani M, Wang Q, Liao R, Yang J, Kang P. Efficacy of adductor canal block combined with additional analgesic methods for postoperative analgesia in total knee arthroplasty: a prospective, double-blind, randomized controlled study. J Arthroplast. 2020;35(12):3554–62.
38. Wang Y, Feng W, Zang J, Gao H. Effect of patellar denervation on anterior knee pain and knee function in total knee arthroplasty without patellar resurfacing: a meta-analysis of randomized controlled trials. Orthop Surg. 2020;12(6):1859–69.
39. Pepper AM, Mercuri JJ, Behery OA, Vigdorchik JM. Total hip and knee arthroplasty perioperative pain management: what should be in the cocktail. JBJS Rev. 2018;6(12):e5.
40. Kehlet H, Dahl JB. The value of "multimodal" or "balanced analgesia" in postoperative pain treatment. Anesth Analg. 1993;77(5):1048–56.
41. Qin L, You D, Zhao G, Li L, Zhao S. A comparison of analgesic techniques for total knee arthroplasty: a network meta-analysis. J Clin Anesth. 2021;71:110257.
42. Gaffney CJ, Pelt CE, Gililland JM, Peters CL. Perioperative pain management in hip and knee arthroplasty. Orthop Clin North Am. 2017;48(4):407–19.
43. Andersen KV, Nikolajsen L, Haraldsted V, Odgaard A, Søballe K. Local infiltration analgesia for total knee arthroplasty: should ketorolac be added? Br J Anaesth. 2013;111(2):242–8.
44. Kissin I. Preemptive analgesia. Anesthesiology. 2000;93(4):1138–43.
45. Grape S, Tramèr MR. Do we need preemptive analgesia for the treatment of postoperative pain? Best Pract Res Clin Anaesthesiol. 2007;21(1):51–63.
46. Price AJ, Alvand A, Troelsen A, Katz JN, Hooper G, Gray A, et al. Knee replacement. Lancet. 2018;392(10158):1672–82.

47. Liu J, Wang F. Preoperative celecoxib analgesia is more efficient and equally tolerated compared to postoperative celecoxib analgesia in knee osteoarthritis patients undergoing total knee arthroplasty: a randomized, controlled study. Medicine (Baltimore). 2018;97(51):e13663.
48. Xu B, Wang Y, Zeng C, Wei J, Li J, Wu Z, et al. Analgesic efficacy and safety of ketamine after total knee or hip arthroplasty: a meta-analysis of randomised placebo-controlled studies. BMJ Open. 2019;9(9):e028337.
49. Busch CA, Shore BJ, Bhandari R, Ganapathy S, MacDonald SJ, Bourne RB, et al. Efficacy of periarticular multimodal drug injection in total knee arthroplasty: a randomized trial. J Bone Jt Surg Am. 2006;88(5):959–63.
50. Liu Y, Zeng Y, Zeng J, Li M, Wei W, Shen B. The efficacy of liposomal bupivacaine compared with traditional peri-articular injection for pain control following total knee arthroplasty: an updated meta-analysis of randomized controlled trials. BMC Musculoskelet Disord. 2019;20(1):306.
51. Wang Q, Sun J, Hu Y, Zeng Y, Hu J, Yang J, et al. Effects of morphine on peri-articular infiltration analgesia in total knee arthroplasty: a prospective, double-blind, randomized controlled trial. Int Orthop. 2020;44(12):2587–95.
52. Li Z, Li Z, Cheng K, Weng X. The efficacy and safety of glucocorticoid on periarticular infiltration analgesia in total knee arthroplasty: a systematic review and meta-analysis of randomized controlled trials. J Arthroplast. 2021;36(9):3340–50.
53. Wang Q, Zhao C, Hu J, Ma T, Yang J, Kang P. Efficacy of a modified cocktail for periarticular local infiltration analgesia in total knee arthroplasty: a prospective, double-blinded, randomized controlled trial. J Bone Joint Surg Am. 2023;105(5):354–62.
54. Paul JE, Arya A, Hurlburt L, Cheng J, Thabane L, Tidy A, et al. Femoral nerve block improves analgesia outcomes after total knee arthroplasty: a meta-analysis of randomized controlled trials. Anesthesiology. 2010;113(5):1144–62.
55. Jaeger P, Baggesgaard J, Sørensen JK, Ilfeld BM, Gottschau B, Graungaard B, et al. Adductor Canal block with continuous infusion versus intermittent boluses and morphine consumption: a randomized, blinded controlled clinical trial. Anesth Analg. 2018;126(6):2069–77.
56. Shah NA, Jain NP, Panchal KA. Adductor canal blockade following total knee arthroplasty-continuous or single shot technique? Role in postoperative analgesia, ambulation ability and early functional recovery: a randomized controlled trial. J Arthroplast. 2015;30(8):1476–81.
57. Cheah JW, Sing DC, Hansen EN, Aleshi P, Vail TP. Does intrathecal morphine in spinal anesthesia have a role in modern multimodal analgesia for primary total joint arthroplasty? J Arthroplast. 2018;33(6):1693–8.
58. Jia XF, Ji Y, Huang GP, Zhou Y, Long M. Comparison of intrathecal and local infiltration analgesia by morphine for pain management in total knee and hip arthroplasty: a meta-analysis of randomized controlled trial. Int J Surg. 2017;40:97–108.
59. Kayupov E, Okroj K, Young AC, Moric M, Luchetti TJ, Zisman G, et al. Continuous adductor canal blocks provide superior ambulation and pain control compared to epidural analgesia for primary knee arthroplasty: a randomized controlled trial. J Arthroplast. 2018;33(4):1040–4.e1.
60. Rantasalo MT, Palanne R, Juutilainen K, Kairaluoma P, Linko R, Reponen E, et al. Randomised controlled study comparing general and spinal anaesthesia with and without a tourniquet on the outcomes of total knee arthroplasty: study protocol. BMJ Open. 2018;8(12):e025546.
61. Ryu JH, Jeon YT, Min B, Hwang JY, Sohn HM. Effects of palonosetron for prophylaxis of postoperative nausea and vomiting in high-risk patients undergoing total knee arthroplasty: a prospective, randomized, double-blind, placebo-controlled study. PLoS One. 2018;13(5):e0196388.
62. Song MH, Kim BH, Ahn SJ, Yoo SH, Kang SW, Kim YJ, et al. Peri-articular injections of local anaesthesia can replace patient-controlled analgesia after total knee arthroplasty: a randomised controlled study. Int Orthop. 2016;40(2):295–9.
63. Brouwers HFG, de Vries AJ, van Zuilen M, van Kouswijk HW, Brouwer RW. The role of computer-assisted cryotherapy in the postoperative treatment after total knee arthroplasty:

positive effects on pain and opioid consumption. Knee Surg Sports Traumatol Arthrosc. 2022;30(8):2698–706.
64. Liu Y, Si H, Zeng Y, Li M, Xie H, Shen B. More pain and slower functional recovery when a tourniquet is used during total knee arthroplasty. Knee Surg Sports Traumatol Arthrosc. 2020;28(6):1842–60.
65. Lützner J, Dexel J, Kirschner S. No difference between computer-assisted and conventional total knee arthroplasty: five-year results of a prospective randomised study. Knee Surg Sports Traumatol Arthrosc. 2013;21(10):2241–7.
66. Hoffart HE, Langenstein E, Vasak N. A prospective study comparing the functional outcome of computer-assisted and conventional total knee replacement. J Bone Joint Surg Br. 2012;94(2):194–9.
67. Thienpont E, Bellemans J, Delport H, Van Overschelde P, Stuyts B, Brabants K, Victor J. Patient-specific instruments: industry's innovation with a surgeon's interest. Knee Surg Sports Traumatol Arthrosc. 2013;21(10):2227–33.
68. Ng VY, DeClaire JH, Berend KR, Gulick BC, Lombardi AV Jr. Improved accuracy of alignment with patient-specific positioning guides compared with manual instrumentation in TKA. Clin Orthop Relat Res. 2012;470(1):99–107.
69. Heck DA, Melfi CA, Mamlin LA, Katz BP, Arthur DS, Dittus RS, Freund DA. Revision rates after knee replacement in the United States. Med Care. 1998;36:661–9.
70. Mahomed NN, Barrett J, Katz JN, Baron JA, Wright J, Losina E. Epidemiology of total knee replacement in the United States Medicare population. J Bone Joint Surg Am. 2005;87:1222–8.
71. Slamin J, Parsley. Brian evolution of customization design for total knee arthroplasty. Curr Rev Musculoskelet Med. 2012;5:290–5. https://doi.org/10.1007/s12178-012-9141-z.
72. Zanasi. Stefano innovations in total knee replacement: new trends in operative treatment and changes in peri-operative management. European. Orthop Traumatol. 2011;2:21–31. https://doi.org/10.1007/s12570-011-0066-6.
73. Zhao C, Liao Q, Yang D, Yang M, Xu. Peng advances in perioperative pain management for total knee arthroplasty: a review of multimodal analgesic approaches. J Orthop Surg Res. 2024;19:843. https://doi.org/10.1186/s13018-024-05324-4.
74. Conteduca F, Iorio R, Mazza D, Ferretti. Andrea patient-specific instruments in total knee arthroplasty. Int Orthop. 2014;38:259–65. https://doi.org/10.1007/s00264-013-2230-9.
75. Bozic KJ, Kurtz SM, Lau E, Ong K, Chiu V, Vail TP, Rubash HE, Berry DJ. The epidemiology of revision Total knee arthroplasty in the United States. Clin Orthop Relat Res. 2009;468:45–51. https://doi.org/10.1007/s11999-009-0945-0.

Chapter 2
Kinematics of Total Knee Arthroplasty

Alfred J. Tria Jr. and Giles R. Scuderi

Introduction by the Editors

Knee kinematics is an analysis of motion patterns and understanding knee kinematics is essential for successful total knee arthroplasty (TKA). There is a wide variety of TKA designs available today with various geometries and kinematic profiles. Despite improvements in TKA design, there is still approximately 10–15% dissatisfied patients. It may be that variations in the knee kinematics between the native knee and replaced knee may impact patient satisfaction, as it has been reported that kinematic patterns have correlated with patient satisfaction, outcome score and overall survivorship. While there is no established consensus, variations from normal knee kinematics in TKA design will impact the functional outcome with limited range of motion, paradoxical sagittal femorotibial translation and loss of axial rotation.

Normal knee kinematics is complex with a combination of differential rolling, gliding and rotation as the femoral condyle flexes on the tibial articular surface. This is further impacted by the interaction of the anterior cruciate (ACL) and posterior cruciate ligaments (PCL). Various designs have attempted to restore knee kinematic by either retaining or substituting the PCL. This has been a topic of debate, as advocates of PCL retention claim more normal kinematics. Yet proponents of PCL sacrificing and substitution report improved functional outcomes. Each of these philosophies of implant design necessitate specific design features. PCL retaining

A. J. Tria Jr. (✉)
Department of Orthopedics, Rutgers-Robert Wood Johnson Medical School, New Brunswick, NJ, USA

G. R. Scuderi
Department of Orthopedic Surgery, Northwell Health, Garden City, NY, USA

A. J. Tria Jr., G. R. Scuderi (eds.), *Total Knee Arthroplasty*,
https://doi.org/10.1007/978-3-032-00175-7_2

designs have a less conforming tibial articulation, relying on the PCL balance to control the differential femorotibial rollback in flexion. PCL substituting designs have a more congruent tibial articulation with a central tibial post that engages a transverse femoral cam as the knee flexes. More recently, there has been greater interest in the medial stabilized TKA, medial pivot and medial congruent designs that are PCL sacrificing and provide a more guided femorotibial motion with a more conforming medial tibial articulation and limited conformity on the lateral side, permitting a more guided differential rollback with flexion.

TKA kinematics does not rely on implant design alone. Recently a great deal of attention has been given to the surgical technique and alignment. Although a neutral mechanical alignment has been a preferred target, it has been challenged as not restoring normal knee kinematics. The drive to preserve native knee kinematics has spurred the development of more individualized alignment strategies. While these alternative alignment techniques have shown comparable or even supposedly superior clinical outcomes compared to mechanical alignment, the full potential, effectiveness, and safety of kinematic alignment and its derivative variations remain to be conclusively determined.

With our editorial prerogative, we reviewed each of the referenced articles and summarized our own conclusions, as detailed below. As you read each of the computer-generated summaries that follow in this chapter you can draw your own conclusions.

Mengyuan et al. favor the single radius total knee over the multi-radius design because of increased stability documented using a portable optical marker-based motion analysis system. The single radius also had higher functional scores; however, longer term follow up is necessary to document that the increased stability does not lead to increased loosening.

Fujimoto et al**.** evaluated the flexion gap width in a cruciate retaining TKA. This study concludes that a wide gap affects rollback, but the tight gap hinders function. Laxity of 1–2 millimeters appears to be best but this article does not correlate with the actual patient outcomes.

Kiyohara et al. investigated the kinematic changes after TKA using a bicruciate substituting knee. The study showed that the knee kinematics are significantly altered after TKA. This finding is not particularly unexpected. The authors found that greater than 10 degrees of rotational mismatch leads to loss of femoral rotation and documented the importance of surgical technique.

Planckaert et al. looked at gait patterns in three groups: healthy patients, asymptomatic TKA patients, and TKA patients with anterior knee pain. The painful knees had distinct gait patterns. This information showed that kinematic patterns do correlate with symptoms; however, it does not give a guideline for the surgical procedure to avoid the painful result.

Onitsuka et al.used a markerless motion capture system to classify patients based on their movement patterns. The system may have application in the future but has not yet been fully tested in the clinical setting.

Digennaro et al. compared two TKA designs using fluoroscopic analysis. The bicruciate substituting knee design did have more pronounced rollback and screw home mechanism that correlated with higher KOOS scores for pain and function. The reference does support that improved kinematics correlates with a better clinical result.

Kesmiri et al. investigated patellar kinematics and showed that the femoral component rotation correlates best. However, it is not clear that the ligament balanced surgical technique improves this any more than other approaches.

Yamazaki et al. used x-ray fluoroscopy to estimate the three-dimensional position of the knee implants that did have tantalum beads in the tibial polyethylene insert. While this data is important, it is not clear that this technique can be used with similar accuracy without the beads for markers.

Yamada et al. evaluated the joint line inclination and limb alignment in a single prosthetic design and concluded that neither element correlated with short term PROMs. The information is not that reliable because of the short-term analysis and goes against many other publications.

Nakajima et al. investigated a single implant design and showed that a kinematically aligned knee had better clinical results. It should be noted that half of the implants did not achieve kinematic alignment thus questioning whether this was due to difficulty with the surgical technique or directly related to the implanted prosthesis.

Kim et al. used a musculoskeletal model to illustrate the change in kinematics related to MCL tension. He showed that both femoral rollback and rotation were affected. This study illustrates that kinematics is a result of both prosthetic design and surgical technique.

Yao et al. reported that the bicompartmental knee had the best kinematics. However, other literature shows that the implant is difficult to design and implant routinely.

Minoda et al. in their study concluded that the restoring the joint line closer to normal did not necessarily correlate with improved kinematics. Kinematics is certainly multifactorial, but the conclusion is somewhat at odds with other publications.

Ishida et al. studied a single TKA design and concluded that the medial pivot knee affected patellofemoral contact points. This is interesting data but really needs to be applied to other designs to see if there is a similar finding.

Assessing knee kinematics following surgery and proof of concept for each design can be a laborious task. Many methods of analysis have been utilized including radiographs with skin markers, roentgen stereophotogrammetry, in vivo fluoroscopy, magnetic resonance imaging, computerized tomography, and computerized simulation. While each technology has provided insight into knee kinematics, each one has its limitations and shortcomings. These articles show that the kinematic pattern of the TKA after surgery is affected by many different factors including the method of analysis, the surgical technique, and the implant design. Correlating the kinematics with the clinical result is another variable in the equation and all these factors have to be included before a final conclusion can be generated.

Machine Generated Summaries

Disclaimer: The summaries in this chapter were generated from Springer Nature publications using abstractive AI auto-summarization: An abstraction-based summarizer creates new text based on deep learning. New phrases are created to summarize the content. As the constituted sentences are machine selected, they may not fully reflect the body of the work, so we strongly advise that the original content is read and cited. The auto-generated summaries were curated by the editor to meet Springer Nature publication standards.

2.1 Alterations of Kinematics in Knees after Single Versus Multiple Radius Femoral Prostheses Total Knee Arthroplasty: A Retrospective Study [82]

This is a machine-generated summary of:

Li, Mengyuan; Fu, Guangtao; Huang, Wenhan; Lin, Bofu; Zhang, Ruiying; Zhang, Yu; Ma, Yuanchen; Zheng, Qiujian Alterations of kinematics in knees after single versus multiple radius femoral prostheses total knee arthroplasty: a retrospective study [82].

Published in: BMC Musculoskeletal Disorders (2020).

Link to original: https://doi.org/10.1186/s12891-020-03425-9

If you want to cite the papers, please refer to the original.

For technical reasons we could not place the page where the original quote is coming from.

2.1.1 Research Highlights

Total knee arthroplasty (TKA) is a common procedure for alleviating pain and improving function in patients with end-stage osteoarthritis of the knee. Despite its effectiveness, a significant percentage of patients remain dissatisfied due to issues such as limited range of motion and instability. These postoperative complaints are thought to be linked to altered in vivo kinematics of the knee following TKA. Recent attention has focused on the importance of prosthetic designs that mimic natural knee kinematics, particularly concerning the femoral component's curvature. Now, a new study by Mengyuan Li et al. investigates how different femoral prosthesis designs—single-radius (SR) versus multi-radius (MR)—affect knee kinematics during walking.

The study employed a retrospective, comparative design approved by an institutional review board, involving patients who underwent unilateral TKA with either SR or MR femoral components. Gait analysis was conducted using a portable optical marker-based motion analysis system to measure degrees of freedom (DOF) kinematics during treadmill walking. The study included patients with primary symptomatic osteoarthritis and excluded those with inflammatory arthritis or significant lower extremity conditions. Healthy individuals were also recruited as controls. The surgeries were performed by an experienced surgeon using standardized procedures, and post-operative rehabilitation included full-weight bearing and various exercises. Kinematic data were collected and analyzed using statistical methods to compare the SR and MR groups against each other and healthy controls.

The findings revealed that SR knees demonstrated better stability in internal/external rotation, valgus/varus rotation, and proximal/distal translation compared to MR knees, which may explain the higher functional scores observed in the SR group. The study suggests that SR designs may offer advantages in performing activities requiring stability, such as jumping or jogging. However, limitations include the small sample size and retrospective design, which could introduce selection bias. Future studies could explore larger sample sizes and different prosthetic designs to further understand the impact on gait kinematics and patient outcomes after TKA.

2.2 Intra-Operative Gaps Affect Outcome and Postoperative Kinematics In Vivo Following Cruciate-Retaining Total Knee Arthroplasty [83]

This is a machine-generated summary of:

Fujimoto, Eisaku; Sasashige, Yoshiaki; Tomita, Tetsuya; Sasaki, Hirofumi; Touten, Yoriko; Fujiwara, Yuusuke; Ochi, Mitsuo Intra-operative gaps affect outcome and postoperative kinematics in vivo following cruciate-retaining total knee arthroplasty [83].

Published in: International Orthopaedics (2015).
Link to original: https://doi.org/10.1007/s00264-015-2847-y

If you want to cite the papers, please refer to the original.
For technical reasons we could not place the page where the original quote is coming from.

2.2.1 Research Highlights

Total knee arthroplasty (TKA) aims to relieve pain and restore knee function, requiring a stable range of motion and proper soft-tissue balance. Achieving accurate intra-operative gap and soft-tissue balance is challenging, prompting the development of an offset-type tensor for TKA procedures. This device allows for gap and soft-tissue balance assessments under physiological conditions. While cruciate retaining (CR) TKA designs control both posterior cruciate and collateral ligaments, the influence of posterior cruciate ligament (PCL) tension on postoperative kinematics remains unclear. Now, a new study by Eisaku Fujimoto et al. investigates how intra-operative component gaps affect in vivo kinematics and outcomes in CR TKA.

The study utilized a two-dimensional/three-dimensional registration technique to analyze anterior-posterior translation and axial rotation kinematics between narrow and wide component gaps in CR TKA under weight-bearing and non-weight-bearing conditions. Thirty patients with primary varus osteoarthritis underwent implantation of the scorpio a Non Restrictive Geometry Cruciate Retaining implant (Stryker Orthopaedics) CR cementless TKA. The surgeries employed a modified gap-balance technique with the Stryker Joint Dependent Kinematics system to ensure ligament balance and satisfactory alignment. The offset tensor device measured ligament balance and joint gaps by applying a constant distraction force. Patients performed deep knee bends under fluoroscopic monitoring to assess kinematic differences between narrow and wide gap groups. Significant differences were observed in medial condyle positions during non-weight-bearing conditions, while no significant differences were found under weight-bearing conditions.

The study advances understanding of how intra-operative joint gaps influence postoperative kinematics in CR TKA. It suggests that a wide flexion gap may lead to late rollback under non-weight-bearing conditions, while a tight flexion gap could hinder daily activities. The findings indicate that 1–2 mm laxity at 0°–90° component gaps may be necessary for comfortable daily activities. Future study could explore increasing the sample size to include patients with poor clinical outcomes, providing further insights into in vivo kinematics after TKA. Additionally, evaluating other daily motions such as gait or stair navigation could offer a more comprehensive understanding of functional outcomes post-TKA.

2.3 Comparison of In Vivo Knee Kinematics Before and After Bicruciate-Stabilized Total Knee Arthroplasty During Squatting [84]

This is a machine-generated summary of:

Kiyohara, Masato; Hamai, Satoshi; Gondo, Hirotaka; Higaki, Hidehiko; Ikebe, Satoru; Okazaki, Ken; Nakashima, Yasuharu Comparison of in vivo knee kinematics before and after bicruciate-stabilized total knee arthroplasty during squatting [84].

Published in: BMC Musculoskeletal Disorders (2021).

Link to original: https://doi.org/10.1186/s12891-021-04669-9

If you want to cite the papers, please refer to the original.

For technical reasons we could not place the page where the original quote is coming from.

2.3.1 Research Highlights

Total knee arthroplasty (TKA) is a widely used procedure to alleviate pain and restore function in patients with advanced knee osteoarthritis. Despite advancements in surgical techniques and implant designs, patient satisfaction post-TKA remains suboptimal, with physiological knee kinematics playing a crucial role in functional outcomes. Bicruciate-stabilized TKA (BCS-TKA) aims to replicate natural knee kinematics through its unique design, yet its impact on kinematic changes during activities like squatting has not been thoroughly investigated. Now, a new study by Masato Kiyohara et al. explores the effects of BCS-TKA on skeletal kinematics during squatting, focusing on femoral anterior-posterior (AP) translation and axial rotation relative to the tibia.

The study involved a cohort of patients undergoing primary BCS-TKA for advanced medial knee osteoarthritis. Using a prospective design, the researchers assessed pre- and postoperative skeletal kinematics through continuous radiographic imaging during squatting. The surgical procedure followed a standardized technique with precise alignment of femoral and tibial components. Radiographic measurements were meticulously conducted using computed tomography to evaluate component rotational alignment. The primary outcomes included changes in total femoral AP translation and rotation angles relative to the tibia. Statistical analyses were performed to compare pre- operative and postoperative kinematic parameters, revealing significant changes in tibiofemoral functional flexion angles and femoral AP positions post-surgery.

The study highlights that BCS-TKA significantly alters knee kinematics, with increased posterior femoral AP position and greater total AP translation during squatting compared to preoperative states. These findings suggest that both preoperative skeletal kinematics and surgical techniques influence postoperative outcomes. A notable observation was that a total component rotational mismatch angle over 10° significantly reduced postoperative femoral rotation relative to the tibia. Future studies could explore how these kinematic changes impact clinical outcomes such as muscle strength and balance function, providing further insights into optimizing TKA procedures for improved patient satisfaction and functional performance.

2.4 Total Knee Arthroplasty with Unexplained Pain: New Insights from Kinematics [85]

This is a machine-generated summary of:

Planckaert, Célia; Larose, Gabriel; Ranger, Pierre; Lacelle, Marc; Fuentes, Alexandre; Hagemeister, Nicola Total knee arthroplasty with unexplained pain: new insights from kinematics [85].

Published in: Archives of Orthopaedic and Trauma Surgery (2018).

Link to original: https://doi.org/10.1007/s00402-018-2873-5

If you want to cite the papers, please refer to the original.

For technical reasons we could not place the page where the original quote is coming from.

2.4.1 Research Highlights

Total knee arthroplasty (TKA) is a widely accepted treatment for end-stage knee osteoarthritis, yet a significant percentage of patients report dissatisfaction post-surgery, often due to persistent anterior knee pain. This pain persists even when common causes such as prosthesis placement issues, infections, or surgical errors are ruled out. Previous studies have linked similar pain in patellofemoral syndrome to altered tibiofemoral kinematics, but no research has specifically analyzed the kinematics of painful TKA. Now, a new study by Célia Planckaert et a. investigates the kinematic characteristics of TKA patients with unexplained anterior knee pain, comparing them to asymptomatic TKA patients and healthy controls.

The study involved three groups: healthy subjects, asymptomatic TKA patients, and TKA patients with unexplained anterior knee pain. Participants underwent various assessments including radiological evaluations, subjective patient-reported outcomes, musculoskeletal assessments by physiotherapists, and kinematic analysis during gait using a specialized knee harness with reflective markers. The study focused on analyzing flexion/extension rotation, varus/valgus rotation, and internal/external tibial rotation during walking. Statistical analyses were conducted to compare the kinematic data across the groups while accounting for demographic differences such as age and BMI. The results indicated that painful TKA patients exhibited distinct gait patterns characterized by dynamic flexion contracture and valgus movement during certain phases of walking.

The findings suggest that painful TKA patients display gait kinematics similar to those observed in patellofemoral syndrome, potentially contributing to their anterior knee pain. The study highlights the importance of considering muscle flexibility and component rotational alignment in managing post-TKA pain. Future study could explore personalized conservative treatments targeting these kinematic factors to alleviate symptoms in painful TKA patients. Additionally, further research could benefit from assessing pre-surgical conditions and employing multiple evaluators for radiological assessments to enhance the robustness of the findings.

2.5 Clinical Utility of Markerless Motion Capture for Kinematic Evaluation of Sit-to-Stand During 30 S-CST at One Year Post Total Knee Arthroplasty: A Retrospective Study [86]

This is a machine-generated summary of:

Onitsuka, Katsuya; Kubota, Keisuke; Yokoyama, Moeka; Miyazawa, Taku; Hamaguchi, Toyohiro; Taniguchi, Hiroto; Usuki, Naohiro; Miyamoto, Satoshi; Okazaki, Ken; Murata, Kenji; Kanemura, Naohiko Clinical utility of markerless motion capture for kinematic evaluation of sit-to-stand during 30 s-CST at 1 year post total knee arthroplasty: a retrospective study [86].

Published in: BMC Musculoskeletal Disorders (2023).
Link to original: https://doi.org/10.1186/s12891-023-06364-3

2.5.1 Research Highlights

Osteoarthritis of the knee is a prevalent condition among older adults, often necessitating total knee arthroplasty (TKA) to restore physical function and improve quality of life. Evaluating physical function post-surgery is crucial, typically involving performance-based tests and patient-reported outcome measures (PROMs). However, these assessments often lack detailed insights into the kinematic changes that occur during movements like the sit-to-stand (STS) test. Now, a new study by Katsuya Onitsuka et al. explores the use of markerless motion capture technology to analyze STS kinematics in TKA patients, aiming to provide a novel indicator of postoperative functional recovery.

The study involved patients who underwent unilateral TKA at Tokyo Women's Medical University Yachiyo Medical Center. Using a markerless motion capture system called Pose-Cap, researchers captured and analyzed STS movements during the 30-second chair stand test (s-CST) 1 year post-surgery. The system automatically extracted joint positions from video footage, allowing for detailed kinematic analysis without the need for markers or complex equipment. Principal component analysis was employed to reduce the dimensionality of kinematic data, followed by cluster analysis to classify patients based on their movement patterns. The study identified five principal components related to joint angular velocities and movement timing, which were used to classify patients into three subgroups with distinct kinematic characteristics.

The findings suggest that different STS strategies are associated with varying levels of functional recovery and patient satisfaction post-TKA. Patients employing a momentum transfer strategy demonstrated better outcomes in PROMs, including achieving a "forgotten joint" state where they are less aware of their operated joint in daily activities. This research highlights the potential of markerless motion capture as a clinical tool for assessing functional recovery and guiding physical therapy interventions. Future study could focus on integrating dynamic muscular variables into the analysis for more comprehensive assessments and exploring how these kinematic insights can inform personalized rehabilitation strategies for TKA patients.

2.6 Design and Kinematics in Total Knee Arthroplasty [87]

This is a machine-generated summary of:

Digennaro, Vitantonio; Zambianchi, Francesco; Marcovigi, Andrea; Mugnai, Raffaele; Fiacchi, Francesco; Catani, Fabio Design and kinematics in total knee arthroplasty [87].

Published in: International Orthopaedics (2014).

Link to original: https://doi.org/10.1007/s00264-013-2245-2

If you want to cite the papers, please refer to the original.

For technical reasons we could not place the page where the original quote is coming from.

2.6.1 Research Highlights

Total knee arthroplasty (TKA) is widely recognized as the gold standard for treating symptomatic, late-stage knee osteoarthritis. Despite advancements in surgical techniques and implant designs, patient satisfaction post-TKA remains suboptimal. Traditional implant designs assumed a changing center of rotation during knee flexion, leading to multiradius femoral components. However, recent studies suggest that a single-radius design might better replicate natural knee kinematics. Now, a new study by Vitantonio Digennaro et al. investigates the clinical outcomes and in vivo kinematics of two different guided-motion TKA designs in a large cohort of patients to understand how kinematic patterns influence clinical results and patient satisfaction.

The study involved a retrospective analysis of patients who underwent primary navigated TKA using either the Scorpio Non-Restrictive Geometry (NRG) or the Journey Bi-Cruciate Stabilised (BCS) prosthetic designs. All procedures were performed by experienced surgeons using a computer-assisted surgical navigation system. The researchers evaluated clinical outcomes using the Knee Injury and Osteoarthritis Outcome Score (KOOS) and conducted fluoroscopic assessments to analyze kinematic patterns during various activities. The study found that the Journey BCS group had significantly higher KOOS scores in pain and quality of life subscales compared to the Scorpio NRG group. Fluoroscopic analysis revealed distinct differences in kinematic patterns between the two designs, with the BCS design showing more pronounced rollback and screw-home mechanisms.

The findings suggest that prosthetic design significantly impacts clinical outcomes and complications in TKA. The Journey BCS design's asymmetric spine-cam mechanism and anatomically shaped tibial insert may contribute to improved kinematics, potentially leading to better patient satisfaction. However, complications such as stiffness were more common in the BCS group, possibly due to excessive femoral rollback causing mechanical stress on soft tissues. Future study could focus on optimizing prosthetic designs to balance improved kinematics with reduced complication rates, enhancing overall patient outcomes after TKA.

2.7 Is it Possible to Re-Establish Pre-Operative Patellar Kinematics Using a Ligament-Balanced Technique in Total Knee Arthroplasty? A Cadaveric Investigation [88]

This is a machine-generated summary of:

Keshmiri, Armin; Springorum, Hans; Baier, Clemens; Zeman, Florian; Grifka, Joachim; Maderbacher, Günther Is it possible to re-establish pre-operative patellar kinematics using a ligament-balanced technique in total knee arthroplasty? A cadaveric investigation [88].

Published in: International Orthopaedics (2014).

Link to original: https://doi.org/10.1007/s00264-014-2507-7

If you want to cite the papers, please refer to the original.

For technical reasons we could not place the page where the original quote is coming from.

2.7.1 *Research Highlights*

Total knee arthroplasty (TKA) is widely recognized as a highly successful procedure in orthopedic surgery, yet anterior knee pain remains a significant postoperative complication, often attributed to patellar maltracking. Recent studies suggest that rotational malalignment of the femoral and tibial components, particularly the internal rotation of the femoral component, may contribute to altered patellofemoral kinematics and subsequent anterior knee pain. Now, a new study by Armin Keshmiri et al. investigates the influence of ligament-balanced femoral component rotation on patellar kinematics in TKA using a commercial imageless computer navigation system.

The study utilized ten lower limbs from five cadavers, ensuring they were free from arthritic deterioration or previous surgical interventions that could affect patellar tracking. Patellar kinematics were analyzed before and after standard TKA with various femoral and tibial component alignments using an optical imageless computer navigation system. The researchers performed a standard surgical procedure with precise anatomical closure and used passive motion machines to simulate movement between 0° and 90° of flexion. Different rotational alignments were tested, including ligament-balanced, external, and internal rotations of the femoral component relative to the posterior condylar line. The study employed linear mixed models for statistical analysis to compare pre-operative natural knee kinematics with those post-TKA under different alignment conditions.

The findings indicate that ligament-balanced femoral component rotation most closely re-establishes natural patellofemoral kinematics compared to other alignment techniques. While femoral component rotation significantly impacts patellar mediolateral shift, tilt, and epicondylar distance, tibial component rotation appears to have negligible influence on these parameters. Future study could explore the clinical relevance of these findings in live patients and assess whether new prosthetic designs might further enhance the restoration of natural patellofemoral kinematics in TKA.

2.8 3D Kinematics of Mobile-Bearing Total Knee Arthroplasty Using X-Ray Fluoroscopy [89]

This is a machine-generated summary of:

Yamazaki, Takaharu; Futai, Kazuma; Tomita, Tetsuya; Sato, Yoshinobu; Yoshikawa, Hideki; Tamura, Shinichi; Sugamoto, Kazuomi 3D kinematics of mobile-bearing total knee arthroplasty using X-ray fluoroscopy [89].

Published in: International Journal of Computer Assisted Radiology and Surgery (2014).

Link to original: https://doi.org/10.1007/s11548-014-1093-x

Copyright of the summarized publication:

If you want to cite the papers, please refer to the original.

For technical reasons we could not place the page where the original quote is coming from.

2.8.1 Research Highlights

In the field of orthopedics, total knee arthroplasty (TKA) is a widely used treatment for patients with functional disabilities and arthritic knees, where the articular cartilage is damaged. TKA implants typically consist of metallic femoral and tibial components with a polyethylene-bearing insert in between, which replaces the damaged cartilage and provides a low-friction surface. The success of TKA depends on the design of the joint surface and surgical technique, as improper movement can lead to implant wear and postoperative pain. Accurate assessment of TKA kinematics is crucial for evaluating surgical outcomes and improving implant designs. However, current imaging techniques like CT and MRI face limitations in capturing dynamic knee motion due to metal artifacts and environmental restrictions. Now, a new study by Takaharu Yamazaki et al. proposes a novel technique using X-ray fluoroscopy to analyze the kinematics of mobile-bearing inserts in TKA, addressing these challenges.

The study utilized X-ray fluoroscopy combined with computer-aided design (CAD) models to estimate the three-dimensional pose of knee implants. The researchers inserted tantalum beads into the polyethylene insert during surgery to track its movement, as these beads are visible in X-ray images unlike the radiolucent insert itself. A contour-based registration technique was employed to estimate the pose of femoral and tibial components by matching their silhouettes in X-ray images with CAD models. For the mobile-bearing insert, a feature-based registration technique was used to determine its pose based on the positions of the tantalum beads. The accuracy of this method was validated through experiments involving synthetic images and clinical application on nine TKA patients during dynamic motion.

The study demonstrated that this new technique allows for accurate kinematic analysis of mobile-bearing inserts in TKA, even when only three bead projections are visible in fluoroscopic images. This advancement provides valuable insights into implant performance during activities such as deep knee bending. Future study could focus on integrating preoperative and intraoperative data with postoperative kinematic analysis to further enhance implant design and surgical techniques. Additionally, automating certain manual processes involved in image analysis could improve efficiency and reduce labor-intensive tasks. This research contributes significantly to understanding TKA kinematics and optimizing patient outcomes through improved implant designs.

2.9 The Impact of Postoperative Inclination of the Joint Line on Clinical Outcomes in Total Knee Arthroplasty Using a Prosthesis with Anatomical Geometry [90]

This is a machine-generated summary of:

Yamada, Manabu; Nakajima, Arata; Sonobe, Masato; Akatsu, Yorikazu; Yamamoto, Keiichiro; Saito, Junya; Norimoto, Masaki; Koyama, Keita; Taniguchi, Shinji; Aoki, Yasuchika; Suguro, Toru; Nakagawa, Koichi The impact of postoperative inclination of the joint line on clinical outcomes in total knee arthroplasty using a prosthesis with anatomical geometry [90].

Published in: Scientific Reports (2023).

Link to original: https://doi.org/10.1038/s41598-023-28182-2

2.9.1 Research Highlights

Total knee arthroplasty (TKA) is a common surgical procedure aimed at alleviating pain and restoring function in patients with knee osteoarthritis. Despite generally acceptable outcomes, a significant percentage of patients report dissatisfaction and poor patient-reported outcomes (PROs) post-surgery. One hypothesized reason for this dissatisfaction is the failure to restore the physiological joint line during surgery. Kinematically aligned TKA (KA-TKA) was introduced to address this by replicating the natural joint line, but concerns about the longevity of components remain. Now, a new study by Manabu Yamada et al. investigates whether restoring the physiological joint line using a prosthesis with anatomical geometry through mechanically aligned TKA (MA-TKA) can improve PROs while maintaining long-term implant survival.

The study involved primary TKAs in patients with osteoarthritis who received the FINE knee prosthesis (Teijin Nakashima Medical Co, Okayama, Japan), which features an oblique femorotibial joint line designed to mimic anatomical geometry. The surgeries were performed by a single senior orthopedic surgeon using conventional instruments to achieve mechanically neutral alignment. Clinical outcomes were assessed preoperatively and 3 years postoperatively using various measures, including the Knee Society Score (KSS) and Japanese Knee Osteoarthritis Outcome Score (KOOS). Radiographic evaluations were conducted to assess limb alignment and joint line inclination. Statistical analyses, including multivariate logistic regression, were used to identify factors associated with postoperative outcomes.

The study found that neither postoperative limb alignment nor joint line inclination significantly impacted short-term PROs. Age at operation was identified as a significant factor associated with higher postoperative knee function scores. These findings suggest that targeting a specific joint line inclination may not be necessary for improving clinical outcomes in TKA. Future studies should focus on individualized approaches that consider each patient's unique anatomical characteristics and investigate the long-term effects of restoring physiological joint line inclination on clinical outcomes after TKA. Additionally, further research is needed to explore the impact of patellar replacement and femoral rotational alignment on postoperative results.

2.10 Association Between Limb Alignment and Patient-Reported Outcomes after Total Knee Arthroplasty Using an Implant That Reproduces Anatomical Geometry [91]

This is a machine-generated summary of:

Nakajima, Arata; Sonobe, Masato; Akatsu, Yorikazu; Aoki, Yasuchika; Takahashi, Hiroshi; Suguro, Toru; Nakagawa, Koichi Association between limb alignment and patient-reported outcomes after total knee arthroplasty using an implant that reproduces anatomical geometry [91].

Published in: Journal of Orthopaedic Surgery and Research (2018).

Link to original: https://doi.org/10.1186/s13018-018-1030-8

If you want to cite the papers, please refer to the original.

For technical reasons we could not place the page where the original quote is coming from.

2.10.1 Research Highlights

Over the past two decades, conventional total knee arthroplasty (TKA) has focused on restoring neutral limb alignment to enhance knee function and longevity. While these procedures have effectively alleviated pain and corrected deformities, patient satisfaction with TKAs remains lower compared to total hip arthroplasties, highlighting the need for improved surgical techniques. Recently, kinematically aligned (KA) TKAs were introduced by Bellemans, aiming to restore the physiological joint line by implanting components with mild varus alignment. However, the superiority of KA TKAs over mechanically aligned (MA) TKAs in terms of patient satisfaction is still debated, and there is limited information on the postoperative relationship between limb alignment and patient-reported outcomes in KA TKAs. Now, a new study by Arata Nakajima et al. investigates whether different alignment categories in patients undergoing TKAs with the FINE (Teijin Nakashima Medical Co, Okayama, Japan) knee influence postoperative outcomes.

The study retrospectively analyzed patients who underwent TKA using the FINE total knee system, which features a unique design intended to facilitate kinematic alignment through conventional osteotomy techniques. The researchers categorized patients based on their postoperative alignment using various radiographic parameters, including the angle between the joint line and mechanical axis (AJLMA). Patients were divided into two groups: those with an AJLMA of $\geq 3°$ (kinematic alignment) and those with $<3°$. The study assessed outcomes using the Knee Society Score (KSS) and Japanese Knee Injury and Osteoarthritis Outcome Score (J-KOOS). Statistical analyses revealed no significant differences in KSS scores across different alignment categories. However, patients with kinematic alignment demonstrated significantly higher scores in the J-KOOS Activities of Daily Living (ADL) subscale compared to those without it.

The findings suggest that reproducing the physiological joint line through kinematic alignment may enhance ADL outcomes for TKA patients. Although approximately half of the implants did not achieve kinematic alignment due to potential osteotomy inaccuracies or soft tissue balancing issues, this study highlights the potential benefits of using anatomically designed implants like the FINE total knee. Future studies should focus on mid- to long-term follow-up to determine if kinematic alignment can consistently improve patient-reported outcomes and contribute to implant longevity. Additionally, exploring alternative measurement methods for evaluating kinematic alignment could further refine surgical techniques and improve patient satisfaction.

2.11 Impacts of Medial Collateral Ligament (MCL) Stiffness Adjustment on Knee Joint Mechanics in Mechanically Aligned Posterior-Substituting (PS) Total Knee Arthroplasty (TKA) [92]

This is a machine-generated summary of:

Kim, Junseo; Jung, Tae-Gon; Shin, Taejin; Kim, SeongHun; Kwak, Dai-Soon; Koh, In Jun; Lim, Dohyung Impacts of medial collateral ligament (MCL) stiffness adjustment on knee joint mechanics in mechanically aligned posterior-substituting (PS) total knee arthroplasty (TKA) [92].

Published in: Biomedical Engineering Letters (2025).

Link to original: https://doi.org/10.1007/s13534-025-00463-x

If you want to cite the papers, please refer to the original.

For technical reasons we could not place the page where the original quote is coming from.

2.11.1 Research Highlights

In total knee arthroplasty (TKA) for varus knee deformities, managing medial collateral ligament (MCL) tension is crucial for achieving optimal knee alignment and joint stability. Proper MCL tension prevents postoperative complications such as midflexion instability and uneven load distribution, which can lead to accelerated wear of prosthetic components. Despite its importance, there is a lack of standardized guidelines for MCL tension management during varus knee TKA. Now, a new study by Junseo Kim et al. addresses this gap by analyzing the influence of MCL adjustment on knee biomechanics during a squat motion using a musculoskeletal model.

The study utilized a musculoskeletal model with TKA to simulate squat motions and assess the effects of varying MCL stiffness on femoral rollback, internal-external rotation, varus-valgus rotation, joint contact forces, and muscle activities. Five distinct models were developed by modifying the stiffness of the MCL to represent different tension states. The researchers validated their model by comparing predicted joint contact forces and kinematic characteristics with existing literature. The results showed that variations in MCL stiffness significantly affected femoral rollback and rotation, as well as joint contact forces, particularly in models with increased stiffness. However, muscle activity remained largely unchanged across different models due to the equilibrium of internal and external forces in the simulation.

The findings highlight the importance of achieving balanced MCL tension to optimize knee kinematics while avoiding excessive joint loading. Adjusting MCL stiffness within a physiologically appropriate range can minimize complications such as instability and prosthetic wear. Future study should focus on developing standardized intraoperative protocols that incorporate real-time kinematic assessments and consider patient-specific factors like preoperative ligament laxity. By refining ligament tensioning strategies during TKA, surgeons can improve long-term outcomes and patient satisfaction, ultimately enhancing surgical precision and implant longevity.

2.12 Bicompartmental, Medial and Patellofemoral Knee Replacement Might Be Able to Maintain Unloaded Knee Kinematics [93]

This is a machine-generated summary of:

Yao, Daiwei; Akram, Imran; Daniilidis, Kiriakos; Labey, Luc; Innocenti, Bernardo; Tibesku, Carsten Bicompartmental, medial and patellofemoral knee replacement might be able to maintain unloaded knee kinematics [93].

Published in: Archives of Orthopaedic and Trauma Surgery (2021).

Link to original: https://doi.org/10.1007/s00402-021-03816-0

If you want to cite the papers, please refer to the original.

For technical reasons we could not place the page where the original quote is coming from.

2.12.1 *Research Highlights*

Total knee arthroplasty (TKA) is a widely used procedure for treating symptomatic knee osteoarthritis, significantly enhancing patients' quality of life. Various TKA procedures, such as cruciate ligament-retaining and cruciate ligament-resecting TKA, are employed based on the patient's age and the functionality of their cruciate ligaments. However, these procedures often rely on the capsule-ligament apparatus for stabilization, which can lead to complications if ligament balancing is not achieved. A notable issue arises when only one cruciate ligament is resected, potentially compromising joint stability. Now, a new study by Daiwei Yao et al. investigates the biomechanical effects of bicompartmental knee arthroplasty (BKA) compared to partial and full cruciate ligament-resecting TKA on femorotibial and patellofemoral joints.

The study utilized six freshly frozen human cadavers to compare the kinematics of BKA with those of different TKA models and native knees. The experimental setup involved a knee kinematics rig similar to the Oxford rig, where various loading conditions were applied to simulate passive and active movements. The researchers measured kinematic parameters such as inferior-superior and anterior-posterior translations of femoral condyles during flexion. Infrared cameras tracked motion patterns, which were digitally reconstructed alongside computed tomography images for precise analysis. Statistical comparisons were made using paired Student's t-tests at 5° increments across different configurations: native knee, BKA, partial cruciate-retaining TKA, and cruciate ligament-resecting TKA.

The study found that BKA demonstrated kinematics more closely resembling a native knee than other TKA models, particularly in terms of external femoral rotation under active conditions. However, no significant differences were observed between BKA and TKA models in passive or active test conditions across all movement sequences. Future study could focus on improving prosthesis design to better replicate natural knee kinematics and address limitations such as small sample sizes in cadaveric studies. Further research is needed to explore anatomical and design factors influencing physiologic kinematics for enhanced treatment outcomes in knee arthroplasty patients.

2.13 The Modification of Bone Cut Angle and Joint Line Obliquity Did Not Change the Tibiofemoral Kinematics and Stability of Knee Joint After Total Knee Arthroplasty [94]

This is a machine-generated summary of:

Minoda, Yukihide; Sugama, Ryo; Ohta, Yoichi; Ohyama, Yohei; Masuda, Sho; Ikebuchi, Mitsuhiko; Nakamura, Hiroaki The modification of bone cut angle and joint line obliquity did not change the tibiofemoral kinematics and stability of knee joint after total knee arthroplasty [94].

Published in: Archives of Orthopaedic and Trauma Surgery (2023).
Link to original: https://doi.org/10.1007/s00402-023-04899-7

If you want to cite the papers, please refer to the original.

For technical reasons we could not place the page where the original quote is coming from.

2.13.1 Research Highlights

Total knee arthroplasty (TKA) is a widely used procedure to alleviate pain and enhance function in patients with end-stage knee osteoarthritis. Despite its success, patient satisfaction rates for TKA are lower compared to total hip arthroplasty, potentially due to the mechanical alignment technique used in TKA, which alters the natural joint line angle. This alteration may lead to abnormal tibiofemoral kinematics and reduced patient satisfaction. Now, a new study by Yukihide Minoda et al. colleagues investigates whether kinematically aligned (KA) TKA, which aims to restore the natural joint line angle, improves tibiofemoral kinematics in patients with varus knee osteoarthritis.

In this prospective cohort study, patients undergoing TKA for varus knee osteoarthritis were included, while those with valgus deformity or other conditions were excluded. The study utilized a navigation system to perform surgeries and measure intraoperative tibiofemoral kinematics. Two types of trial components were used: one following the usual mechanical alignment (MA) and another specifically designed for KA TKA. The primary outcome was tibiofemoral rotational kinematics, while the secondary outcome was varus-valgus laxity of the knee joint. Measurements were taken using a navigation system across various degrees of knee flexion. Statistical analyses were conducted to compare the outcomes between KA and MA TKA.

The study found no significant differences in tibiofemoral rotational kinematics or varus-valgus laxity between KA and MA TKA in patients with varus osteoarthritis. This suggests that restoring the joint line angle closer to normal does not necessarily improve knee kinematics or stability. Future study could explore other factors such as ligament balance, articulation surface design, and hip-knee-ankle angle to enhance postoperative outcomes. Additionally, further research is needed to assess these findings in different prosthesis designs and in patients with valgus knees.

2.14 In Vivo Comparisons of Patellofemoral Kinematics Before and After ADVANCE® Medial-Pivot Total Knee Arthroplasty [95]

This is a machine-generated summary of:

Ishida, Kazunari; Matsumoto, Tomoyuki; Tsumura, Nobuhiro; Chinzei, Nobuaki; Kitagawa, Atsushi; Kubo, Seiji; Chin, Takaaki; Iguchi, Tetsuhiro; Akisue, Toshihiro; Nishida, Kotaro; Kurosaka, Masahiro; Kuroda, Ryosuke In vivo comparisons of patellofemoral kinematics before and after ADVANCE® Medial-Pivot total knee arthroplasty [95].

Published in: International Orthopaedics (2012).

Link to original: https://doi.org/10.1007/s00264-012-1634-2

If you want to cite the papers, please refer to the original.

For technical reasons we could not place the page where the original quote is coming from.

2.14.1 Research Highlights

Total knee arthroplasty (TKA) is a widely accepted procedure that typically results in high patient satisfaction. However, the kinematics of the knee joint post-TKA often differ from normal knee kinematics, which can lead to issues such as wear and malalignment. Understanding the kinematics of artificial knee joints is crucial for improving TKA outcomes. Although the patellofemoral joint significantly impacts prosthetic knee function, its kinematics are less understood than those of the tibiofemoral joint. Now, a new study by Kazunari Ishida et al. investigates the in vivo patellofemoral kinematics of the ADVANCE® Medial-Pivot (MP) TKA (Microport Orthopedics, Arlington, Tenn, USA), comparing pre- and postoperative conditions to assess potential effects on patients.

The study involved ten subjects with varus deformity due to osteoarthritis who underwent ADVANCE® MP TKA. The surgeries were performed by an experienced surgeon using a conventional manual technique, with specific attention to rotational alignment and tibial osteotomy. Pre- and postoperative patellofemoral kinematics were evaluated using lateral radiographs taken during deep knee bending exercises. Key measurements included patella flexion angle and patellofemoral contact point (PC), analyzed using imaging software by blinded authors. The study found that while TP and PF angles showed no significant differences pre- and post-surgery, PC translated proximally with increased flexion postoperatively, differing from preoperative conditions.

The study provides novel insights into the patellofemoral joint kinematics of ADVANCE® MP TKA (, highlighting differences from other prosthetic designs like posterior-stabilized (PS) and cruciate-retaining (CR) TKAs. The findings suggest that the medial-pivot design influences patellofemoral contact dynamics, potentially affecting patient outcomes. Future study could explore long-term effects on implant survival and wear, as well as comparisons with other prosthetic designs to better understand these kinematic changes' clinical implications. Comprehensive evaluations including both objective measures and patient-reported outcomes are necessary to fully assess the benefits of this design approach in TKA.

Bibliography

1. Frankel VH, Burstein AH, Brooks DB. Biomechanics of internal derangement of the knee. Pathomechanics as determined by analysis of the instant centers of motion. J Bone Joint Surg Am. 1971;53(5):945–62.
2. Hollister AM, Jatana S, Singh AK, et al. The axes of rotation of the knee. Clin Orthop Relat Res. 1993;290:259–68.
3. Hamilton DF, Lane JV, Gaston P, et al. What determines patient satisfaction with surgery? A prospective cohort study of 4709 patients following total joint replacement. BMJ Open. 2013;3(4):e002525.
4. Li M, Deng Z, Jiang H, et al. Single radius versus multiple radius femoral prostheses in total knee arthroplasty: a meta-analysis. Int J Clin Exp Med. 2019;12(8):9508–21.
5. Larsen B, Jacofsky MC, Jacofsky DJ. Quantitative, comparative assessment of gait between single-radius and multi-radius Total knee arthroplasty designs. J Arthroplast. 2015;30(6):1062–7.
6. Cook LE, Klika AK, Szubski CR, et al. Functional outcomes used to compare single radius and multiradius of curvature designs in total knee arthroplasty. J Knee Surg. 2012;25(3):249–53.
7. Gomez-Barrena E, Fernandez-Garcia C, Fernandez-Bravo A, et al. Functional performance with a single-radius femoral design total knee arthroplasty. Clin Orthop Relat Res. 2010;468(5):1214–20.
8. Collados-Maestre I, Lizaur-Utrilla A, Gonzalez-Navarro B, et al. Better functional outcome after single-radius TKA compared with multi-radius TKA. Knee Surg Sports Traumatol Arthrosc. 2017;25(11):3508–14.
9. Tamaki M, Tomita T, Yamazaki T, et al. Factors in high-flex posterior stabilized fixed-bearing total knee arthroplasty affecting in vivo kinematics and anterior tibial post impingement during gait. J Arthroplast. 2013;28(10):1722–7.
10. Sumner B, McCamley J, Jacofsky DJ, et al. Comparison of knee kinematics and kinetics during stair descent in single- and multi-radius Total KneeArthroplasty. J Knee Surg. 2019;33:1020–8. https://doi.org/10.1055/s-0039-1692652.
11. Komistek RD, Mahfouz MR, Bertin KC, Rosenberg A, Kennedy W. In vivo determination of total knee arthroplasty kinematics: a multicenter analysis of an asymmetrical posterior cruciate retaining total knee arthroplasty. J Arthroplast. 2008;23(1):41–50.
12. Murakami K, Hamai S, Okazaki K, Ikebe S, Shimoto T, Hara D, Mizu-uchi H, Higaki H, Iwamoto Y. In vivo kinematics of healthy male knees during squat and golf swing using image-matching techniques. Knee. 2016;23(2):221–6. https://doi.org/10.1016/j.knee.2015.08.004.
13. Dennis DA, Komistek RD, Scuderi GR, Zingde S. Factors affecting flexion after total knee arthroplasty. Clin Orthop Relat Res. 2007;464:53–60. https://doi.org/10.1097/BLO.0b013e31812f785d.

14. Moro-oka TA, Muenchinger M, Canciani JP, Banks SA. Comparing in vivo kinematics of anterior cruciate-retaining and posterior cruciate-retaining total knee arthroplasty. Knee Surg Sports Traumatol Arthrosc. 2007;15(1):93–9. https://doi.org/10.1007/s00167-006-0134-6.
15. Broberg JS, Ndoja S, MacDonald SJ, Lanting BA, Teeter MG. Comparison of contact kinematics in posterior-stabilized and cruciate-retaining total knee arthroplasty at long-term follow-up. J Arthroplast. 2020;35(1):272–7. https://doi.org/10.1016/j.arth.2019.07.046.
16. Yue B, Varadarajan KM, Moynihan AL, Liu F, Rubash HE, Li G. Kinematics of medial osteoarthritic knees before and after posterior cruciate ligament retaining total knee arthroplasty. J Orthop Res. 2011;29(1):40–6. https://doi.org/10.1002/jor.21203.
17. Grieco TF, Sharma A, Dessinger GM, Cates HE, Komistek RD. In vivo kinematic comparison of a bicruciate stabilized total knee arthroplasty and the normal knee using fluoroscopy. J Arthroplast. 2018;33(2):565–71. https://doi.org/10.1016/j.arth.2017.09.035.
18. Kono K, Inui H, Tomita T, Yamazaki T, Taketomi S, Sugamoto K, Tanaka S. Bicruciate-stabilised total knee arthroplasty provides good functional stability during high-flexion weight-bearing activities. Knee Surg Sports Traumatol Arthrosc. 2019;27(7):2096–103. https://doi.org/10.1007/s00167-019-05375-9.
19. Kitagawa A, Tsumura N, Chin T, Gamada K, Banks SA, Kurosaka M. In vivo comparison of knee kinematics before and after high-flexion posterior cruciate-retaining total knee arthroplasty. J Arthroplast. 2010;25(6):964–9.
20. Hamai S, Moro-oka TA, Miura H, Shimoto T, Higaki H, Fregly BJ, Iwamoto Y, Banks SA. Knee kinematics in medial osteoarthritis during in vivo weight-bearing activities. J Orthop Res. 2009;27(12):1555–61. https://doi.org/10.1002/jor.20928.
21. Kiyohara M, Hamai S, Gondo H, Higaki H, Ikebe S, Ushio T, Murakami K, Nakashima Y. Tibiofemoral kinematics in healthy and osteoarthritic knees during twisting. J Orthop. 2020;21:213–7. https://doi.org/10.1016/j.jor.2020.03.051.
22. Harman MK, Banks SA, Kirschner S, Lutzner J. Prosthesis alignment affects axial rotation motion after total knee replacement: a prospective in vivo study combining computed tomography and fluoroscopic evaluations. BMC Musculoskelet Disord. 2012;13(1):206. https://doi.org/10.1186/1471-2474-13-206.
23. Powers CM. The influence of altered lower-extremity kinematics on patellofemoral joint dysfunction: a theoretical perspective. J Orthop Sports Phys Ther. 2003;33(11):639–46.
24. Smith AJ, Lloyd DG, Wood DJ. Pre-surgery knee joint loading patterns during walking predict the presence and severity of anterior knee pain after total knee arthroplasty. J Orthop Res. 2004;22(2):260–6.
25. Bourne RB, Chesworth BM, Davis AM, et al. Patient satisfaction after total knee arthroplasty: who is satisfied and who is not? Clin Orthop Relat Res. 2010;468(1):57–63.
26. Yu B, Holly-Crichlow N, Brichta P, Reeves GR, Zablotny CM, Nawoczenski DA. The effects of the lower extremity joint motions on the total body motion in sit-to-stand movement. Clin Biomech (Bristol, Avon). 2000;15:449–55.
27. van der Kruk E, Silverman AK, Reilly P, Bull AMJ. Compensation due to age-related decline in sit-to-stand and sit-to-walk. J Biomech. 2021;122:110411.
28. Gunston FH. Polycentric knee arthroplasty. Prosthetic simulation of normal knee movement. J Bone Joint Surg Br. 1971;53:272–7.
29. Hollister AM, Jatana S, Singh AK, Sullivan WW, Lupichuk AG. The axes of rotation of the knee. Clin Orthop Relat Res. 1993;290:259–68.
30. Nogler M, Hozack W, Collopy D, Mayr E, Deirmengian G, Sekyra K. Alignment for total knee replacement: a comparison of kinematic axis versus mechanical axis techniques. A cadaver study. Int Orthop. 2012;2249–2253:2249–53. https://doi.org/10.1007/s00264-012-1642-2.
31. Victor J, Mueller JK, Komistek RD, Sharma A, Nadaud MC, Bellemans J. In vivo kinematics after a cruciate-substituting TKA. Clin Orthop Relat Res. 2010;468(3):807–14. https://doi.org/10.1007/s11999-009-1072-7.
32. Catani F, Ensini A, Belvedere C, Feliciangeli A, Benedetti MG, Leardini A, Giannini S. In vivo kinematics and kinetics of a bi-cruciate substituting total knee arthroplasty: a combined fluoroscopic andgait analysis study. J Orthop Res. 2009;27(12):1569–75.

33. Dennis DA, Komistek RD, Mahfouz MR, Haas BD, Stiehl JB. Multicenter determination of in vivo kinematics after total knee arthroplasty. Clin Orthop Relat Res. 2003;416:37–57.
34. Dennis DA, Komistek RD, Mahfouz MR, Walker SA, Tucker A. A multicenter analysis of axial femorotibial rotation after total knee arthroplasty. Clin Orthop Relat Res. 2004;428:180–9.
35. Catani F, Innocenti B, Belvedere C, Labey L, Ensini A, Leardini A. The mark Coventry award: articular contact estimation in TKA using in vivo kinematics and finite element analysis. Clin Orthop Relat Res. 2010;468:19–28.
36. Miller MC, Berger RA, Petrella AJ, et al. Optimizing femoral component rotation in total knee arthroplasty. Clin Orthop. 2001;392:38–45.
37. Heesterbeek PC, Jacobs WH, Wymenga A. Effects of the balanced gap technique on femoral component rotation in TKA. Clin Orthop. 2009;467:1015–22. https://doi.org/10.1007/s11999-008-0539-2.
38. Kienapfel H, Springorum H-P, Ziegler A, et al. Der Einfluss der Femur- und Tibiakomponentenrotation auf das patellofemorale Versagen beim künstlichen Kniegelenkersatz. Orthopade. 2003;32:312–8. https://doi.org/10.1007/s00132-002-0441-7.
39. Belvedere C, Catani F, Ensini A, et al. Patellar tracking during total knee arthroplasty: an in vitro feasibility study. Knee Surg Sports Traumatol Arthrosc. 2007;15:985–93. https://doi.org/10.1007/s00167-007-0320-1.
40. Banks SA, Hodge WA. Accurate measurement of three-dimensional knee replacement kinematics using single-plane fluoroscopy. IEEE Trans Biomed Eng. 1996;43:638–49.
41. Hirokawa S, Abrar Hossain M. A 3D kinematic estimation of knee prosthesis using X-ray projection images: clinical assessment of the improved algorithm for fluoroscopy images. Med Biol Eng Comput. 2008;46:1253–62.
42. Fantozzi S, Leardini A, Banks SA, Marcacci M, Giannini S, Cantani F. Dynamic in-vivo tibiofemoral and bearing motions in mobile bearing knee arthroplasty. Knee Surg Sports Traumatol Arthrosc. 2004;12:144–51.
43. Wolterbeek N, Garling EH, Mertens B, Valstar ER, Nelissen RGHH. Mobile bearing knee kinematics change over time. A fluoroscopic study in rheumatoid arthritis patients. Clin Biomech. 2009;24:441–5.
44. Canny J. A computational approach to edge detection. IEEE Trans Pattern Anal Mach Intell. 1986;8:679–98.
45. Grood ES, Suntay WJ. A joint coordinate system for the clinical description of three-dimensional motions: application to the knee. J Biomech Eng. 1983;105:136–44.
46. Nakajima A, et al. Association between limb alignment and patient-reported outcomes after total knee arthroplasty using an implant that reproduces anatomical geometry. J Orthop Surg Res. 2018;13(1):320. https://doi.org/10.1186/s13018-018-1030-8.
47. Dossett HG, Estrada NA, Swartz GJ, LeFevre GW, Kwasman BG. A randomised controlled trial of kinematically and mechanically aligned total knee replacements: two-year clinical results. Bone Joint J. 2014;96-B:907–13.
48. Waterson HB, Clement ND, Eyres KS, Mandalia VI, Toms AD. The early outcome of kinematic versus mechanical alignment in total knee arthroplasty: a prospective randomized control trial. Bone Joint J. 2016;98-B:1360–8.
49. Young SW, et al. The Chitranjan S. Ranawat award: no difference in 2-year functional outcomes using kinematic versus mechanical alignment in TKA: a randomized controlled clinical trial. Clin Orthop Relat Res. 2017;475(1):9–20.
50. Hommel H, Perka C, Pfitzner T. Preliminary results of a new surgical technique in total knee arthroplasty (TKA) using the native ligament tension for femoral implant positioning in varus osteoarthritis. Arch Orthop Trauma Surg. 2016;136(7):991–7.
51. Delport H, Labey L, de Corte R, Innocenti B, Sloten JV, Bellemans J. Collateral ligament strains during knee joint laxity evaluation before and after TKA. Clin Biomech. 2013;28(7):777–82.
52. Berube EE, Xiang W, Manzi J, Mayman D, Westrich G, Wright T, Chalmers B, Imhauser C, Sculco P, Kahlenberg C. Anterior-posterior laxity in midflexion after posterior-stabilized TKA is sensitive to MCL tension in passive flexion: an in vitro biomechanical study. J Bone Joint Surg Am. 2024;106(16):1486–92.

53. Lee S, Yang J, Lee Y, Yoon J. A novel medial soft tissue release method for varus deformity during total knee arthroplasty: femoral origin release of the medial collateral ligament. Knee Surg Relat Res. 2016;28(2):153–60.
54. Müller J, Zakaria T, van der Merwe W, D'Angelo F. Computational modelling of mobile bearing TKA anterior-posterior dislocation. Comput Methods Biomech Biomed Engin. 2016;19(5):549–62.
55. Reynolds R, Walker P, Buza J. Mechanisms of anterior-posterior stability of the knee joint under load bearing. J Biomech. 2017;57:39–45.
56. Athwal K, Daou HE, Kittl C, Davies A, Deehan D, Amis A. The superficial medial collateral ligament is the primary medial restraint to knee laxity after cruciate-retaining or posterior-stabilised total knee arthroplasty: effects of implant type and partial release. Knee Surg Sports Traumatol Arthrosc. 2016;24(8):2646–55.
57. Kia M, Wright T, Cross M, Mayman D, Pearle A, Sculco P, Westrich G, Imhauser C. Femoral component external rotation affects knee biomechanics: a computational model of posterior-stabilized TKA. Clin Orthop Relat Res. 2018;476(1):113–23.
58. Escamilla RF, et al. Effects of technique variations on knee biomechanics during the squat and leg press. Med Sci Sports Exerc. 2001;33(9):1552–66.
59. Mason JJ, et al. Patellofemoral joint forces. J Biomech. 2008;41(11):2337–48.
60. Booth RE Jr. The posterior stabilized: a knee for all seasons. Orthopedics. 2001;24:887–8.
61. Clark CR, Rorabeck CH, MacDonald S, MacDonald D, Swafford J, Cleland D. Posterior-stabilized and cruciate-retaining total knee replacement: a randomized study. Clin Orthop Relat Res. 2001;392:208–12. https://doi.org/10.1097/00003086-200111000-00025.
62. Victor J, Banks S, Bellemans J. Kinematics of posterior cruciate ligament-retaining and -substituting total knee arthroplasty: a prospective randomised outcome study. J Bone Joint Surg Br. 2005;87:646–55. https://doi.org/10.1302/0301-620X.87B5.15602.
63. Insall JN, Ranawat CS, Aglietti P, Shine J. A comparison of four models of total knee-replacement prostheses. J Bone Joint Surg Am. 1976;58:754–65. https://doi.org/10.2106/00004623-197658060-00003.
64. Walker PS, Sathasivam S. Design forms of total knee replacement. Proc Inst Mech Eng H. 2000;214:101–19. https://doi.org/10.1243/0954411001535282.
65. Gemayel AC, Varacallo M. Total knee replacement (TKR) techniques (updated 24 Feb 2019). In: StatPearls [internet]. Treasure Island: StatPearls Publishing; 2019. https://www.ncbi.nlm.nih.gov/books/NBK538208/.
66. Daniel DM, Stone ML, Barnett P, Sachs R. Use of the quadriceps active test to diagnose posterior cruciate-ligament disruption and measure posterior laxity of the knee. J Bone Joint Surg Am. 1988;70:386–91. https://doi.org/10.2106/00004623-198870030-00010.
67. Mu S, Moro-Oka T, Johal P, Hamai S, Freeman MA, Banks SA. Comparison of static and dynamic knee kinematics during squatting. Clin Biomech. 2011;26:106–8.
68. Daniilidis K, Skwara A, Vieth V, Fuchs-Winkelmann S, Heindel W, Stuckmann V, Tibesku CO. Highly conforming polyethylene inlays reduce the in vivo variability of knee joint kinematics after total knee arthroplasty. Knee. 2012;19:260–5.
69. Dennis DA, Komistek RD, Mahfouz MR. In vivo fluoroscopic analysis of fixed-bearing total knee replacements. Clin Orthop Relat Res. 2003;410:114–30.
70. Maderbacher G, Keshmiri A, Krieg B, Greimel F, Grifka J, Baier C. Kinematic component alignment in total knee arthroplasty leads to better restoration of natural tibiofemoral kinematics compared to mechanic alignment. Knee Surg Sports Traumatol Arthrosc. 2019;27(5):1427–33.
71. Ishikawa M, Kuriyama S, Ito H, Furu M, Nakamura S, Matsuda S. Kinematic alignment produces near-normal knee motion but increases contact stress after total knee arthroplasty: a case study on a single implant design. Knee. 2015;22:206–12.
72. Nakamura S, Tian Y, Tanaka Y, et al. The effects of kinematically aligned total knee arthroplasty on stress at the medial tibia: a case study for varus knee. Bone Joint Res. 2017;6(1):43–51.
73. Ishida K, Shibanuma N, Matsumoto T, et al. Factors affecting intraoperative kinematic patterns and flexion angles in navigated total knee arthroplasty. Knee Surg Sports Traumatol Arthrosc. 2015;23(6):1741–7.

74. Tsubosaka M, Ishida K, Kodato K, et al. Mid-flexion stability in the anteroposterior plane is achieved with a medial congruent insert in cruciate-retaining total knee arthroplasty for varus osteoarthritis. Knee Surg Sports Traumatol Arthrosc. 2021;29(2):467–73.
75. Lustig S, Sappey-Marinier E, Fary C, Servien E, Parratte S, Batailler C. Personalized alignment in total knee arthroplasty: current concepts. SICOT J. 2021;7:19.
76. Chew JT, Stewart NJ, Hanssen AD, Luo ZP, Rand JA, An KN. Differences in patellar tracking and knee kinematics among three different total knee designs. Clin Orthop Relat Res. 1997;345:87–98.
77. Dalury DF, Dennis DA. Extensor mechanism problems following total knee replacement. J Knee Surg. 2003;16:118–22.
78. Barnes CL, Sharma A, Blaha JD, Nambu SN, Carroll ME. Kneeling is safe for patients implanted with medial-pivot total knee arthroplasty designs. J Arthroplast. 2011;26:549–54.
79. Omori G, Onda N, Shimura M, Hayashi T, Sato T, Koga Y. The effect of geometry of the tibial polyethylene insert on the tibiofemoral contact kinematics in Advance medial pivot total knee arthroplasty. J Orthop Sci. 2009;14:754–60.
80. Leszko F, Sharma A, Komistek RD, Mahfouz MR, Cates HE, Scuderi GR. Comparison of in vivo patellofemoral kinematics for subjects having high-flexion total knee arthroplasty implant with patients having normal knees. J Arthroplast. 2010;25:398–404.
81. Stiehl JB, Komistek RD, Dennis DA, Keblish PA. Kinematics of the patellofemoral joint in total knee arthroplasty. J Arthroplast. 2001;16:706–14.
82. Li M, Fu G, Huang W, Lin B, Zhang R, Zhang Y, Ma Y, Zheng Q. Alterations of kinematics in knees after single versus multiple radius femoral prostheses total knee arthroplasty: a retrospective study. BMC Musculoskelet Disord. 2020;21 https://doi.org/10.1186/s12891-020-03425-9.
83. Fujimoto E, Sasashige Y, Tomita T, Sasaki H, Touten Y, Fujiwara Y, Ochi M. Intra-operative gaps affect outcome and postoperative kinematics in vivo following cruciate-retaining total knee arthroplasty. Int Orthop. 2015;40:41–9. https://doi.org/10.1007/s00264-015-2847-y.
84. Kiyohara M, Hamai S, Gondo H, Higaki H, Ikebe S, Okazaki K, Nakashima Y. Comparison of in vivo knee kinematics before and after bicruciate-stabilized total knee arthroplasty during squatting. BMC Musculoskelet Disord. 2021;22:772. https://doi.org/10.1186/s12891-021-04669-9.
85. Planckaert C, Larose G, Ranger P, Lacelle M, Fuentes A, Hagemeister N. Total knee arthroplasty with unexplained pain: new insights from kinematics. Arch Orthop Trauma Surg. 2018;138:553–61. https://doi.org/10.1007/s00402-018-2873-5.
86. Onitsuka K, Kubota K, Yokoyama M, Miyazawa T, Hamaguchi T, Taniguchi H, Usuki N, Miyamoto S, Okazaki K, Murata K, Kanemura N. Clinical utility of markerless motion capture for kinematic evaluation of sit-to-stand during 30 s-CST at one year post total knee arthroplasty: a retrospective study. BMC Musculoskelet Disord. 2023;24 https://doi.org/10.1186/s12891-023-06364-3.
87. Digennaro V, Zambianchi F, Marcovigi A, Mugnai R, Fiacchi F, Catani F. Design and kinematics in total knee arthroplasty. Int Orthop. 2014;38:227–33. https://doi.org/10.1007/s00264-013-2245-2.
88. Keshmiri A, Springorum H, Baier C, Zeman F, Grifka J, Maderbacher G. Is it possible to reestablish pre-operative patellar kinematics using a ligament-balanced technique in total knee arthroplasty? A cadaveric investigation. Int Orthop. 2014;39:441–8. https://doi.org/10.1007/s00264-014-2507-7.
89. Yamazaki T, Futai K, Tomita T, Sato Y, Yoshikawa H, Tamura S, Sugamoto K. 3D kinematics of mobile-bearing total knee arthroplasty using X-ray fluoroscopy. Int J Comput Assist Radiol Surg. 2014;10:487–95. https://doi.org/10.1007/s11548-014-1093-x.
90. Yamada M, Nakajima A, Sonobe M, Akatsu Y, Yamamoto K, Saito J, Norimoto M, Koyama K, Taniguchi S, Aoki Y, Suguro T, Nakagawa K. The impact of postoperative inclination of the joint line on clinical outcomes in total knee arthroplasty using a prosthesis with anatomical geometry. Sci Rep. 2023;13 https://doi.org/10.1038/s41598-023-28182-2.

91. Nakajima A, Sonobe M, Akatsu Y, Aoki Y, Takahashi H, Suguro T, Nakagawa K. Association between limb alignment and patient-reported outcomes after total knee arthroplasty using an implant that reproduces anatomical geometry. J Orthop Surg Res. 2018;13 https://doi.org/10.1186/s13018-018-1030-8.
92. Kim J, Jung T-G, Shin T, Kim SH, Kwak D-S, Koh IJ, Lim D. Impacts of medial collateral ligament (MCL) stiffness adjustment on knee joint mechanics in mechanically aligned posterior-substituting (PS) total knee arthroplasty (TKA). Biomedical. Eng Lett. 2025;15:455–65. https://doi.org/10.1007/s13534-025-00463-x.
93. Yao D, Akram I, Daniilidis K, Labey L, Innocenti B, Tibesku C. Bicompartmental, medial and patellofemoral knee replacement might be able to maintain unloaded knee kinematics. Arch Orthop Trauma Surg. 2021;142:501–9. https://doi.org/10.1007/s00402-021-03816-0.
94. Minoda Y, Sugama R, Ohta Y, Ohyama Y, Masuda S, Ikebuchi M, Nakamura H. The modification of bone cut angle and joint line obliquity did not change the tibiofemoral kinematics and stability of knee joint after total knee arthroplasty. Arch Orthop Trauma Surg. 2023;143:6345–51. https://doi.org/10.1007/s00402-023-04899-7.
95. Ishida K, Matsumoto T, Tsumura N, Chinzei N, Kitagawa A, Kubo S, Chin T, Iguchi T, Akisue T, Nishida K, Kurosaka M, Kuroda R. In vivo comparisons of patellofemoral kinematics before and after ADVANCE® medial-pivot total knee arthroplasty. International Orthopaedics. 2012;36:2073–7. https://doi.org/10.1007/s00264-012-1634-2.

Chapter 3
Imaging Modalities for Total Knee Arthroplasty

Alfred J. Tria Jr. and Giles R. Scuderi

Introduction by the Editors

Imaging the knee prior to and following total knee arthroplasty (TKA) play a crucial role in the indication for surgery, surgical planning and post-operative management. While there are several modalities to image and evaluate the knee, each has its own merits. Preoperative radiographs provide the overall impression of the knee demonstrating the degree of arthritis, alignment, and deformity. The utility may also be integrated into surgical planning with a personalized approach to the correction of the deformity and implant selection. The postoperative radiographs are valuable in routine surveillance, assessing the ultimate outcome and diagnosing complications such as loosening, wear, instability and infection. Computerized tomography (CT) scans provide a 3-D assessment of the knee and have been helpful in the preoperative planning for component size and position, as well as the postoperative evaluation of component position and rotation. Data collected from CT based surgical plans have been used in creating the virtual bone models in robotic surgery. The CT scan has also been helpful following surgery, in diagnosing osteolysis or loosening that is not evident on standard radiographs. Magnetic resonance imaging (MRI) provides a great deal of information about the bone and surrounding soft tissue and when coupled with specific software has been used for establishing the preoperative plan in robotic surgery. Fluroscopy allows for the assessment of real-time joint motion and evaluation of the knee kinematics. It allows observation of the movement of femoral and tibial components following TKA. With the introduction of advanced technology with a personalized approach to TKA, we have seen the

A. J. Tria Jr. (✉)
Department of Orthopedics, Rutgers-Robert Wood Johnson Medical School, New Brunswick, NJ, USA

G. R. Scuderi
Department of Orthopedic Surgery, Northwell Health, Garden City, NY, USA

A. J. Tria Jr., G. R. Scuderi (eds.), *Total Knee Arthroplasty*,
https://doi.org/10.1007/978-3-032-00175-7_3

increased use of advanced imaging to provide a 3-D modeling of the knee that is incorporated into the surgical planning.

This chapter focuses on numerous references that highlights imaging of TKA and its impact on evaluation, surgical planning and postoperative evaluation. This chapter is divided into separate sections on plain radiographs, magnetic resonance imaging (MRI), computerized tomography (CT), fluoroscopy, and advanced imaging. Using our editorial prerogative, we reviewed each of the referenced articles and summarized our own conclusions, as detailed below. As you read each of the computer-generated summaries that follow in this chapter you can draw your own conclusions.

The section on plain radiographs cover the topics of bone density, alignment, implant sizing and knee modeling. Almhdie-Imjabbar et al. evaluated the trabecular bone density along with Kellgren-Lawrence grades to develop a TKA risk profile. This appears to be a sound approach but still requires further validation. Kazemi et al. looked at the correlation between short and full-length x-rays for alignment. This has been an ongoing problem with the added difficulty in some clinical settings to obtain the full-length films. However, this study does indicate that the full-length views are the most accurate for measuring knee alignment. Zheng et al. developed a calibration cage to use radiographs to derive patient specific models of the femur and tibia for accurate preoperative planning. While the models are derived from less expensive imaging, it is not clear about the expense and availability of the cage. Lutz et al., and Shetty et al. both explored the utility of creating lower limb bone models with CT scans and radiographs for TKA planning. It appears within each of the modeling soft ware programs, radiographs provide comparable data to the CT scans. Yu et al. showed that models generated with imaging and artificial intelligence (AI) could be used for TKA component sizing. This may have some application in the future. Soda et al. studied the posterior condylar offset ratio and showed its relationship to flexion. The article confirms published information. Concerned about bone quality, Windisch et al. used DXA scans to look at bone density after surgery. It remains to be seen if these findings will be of clinical value. Shetty et al. utilizing a radiograph based approach to create a virtual knee model developed a technique to manufacture patient specific instruments. While they did improve the accuracy measurements, there is a significant cost increase and long-term clinical benefits remain to be seen.

There has been a great deal of research on the utility of MRI imaging on patient selection and surgical planning. Kang et al., Violeti et al., Theeuwen et al., and Sgroiet et al. look at various parameters of CT scans versus MRI images on a patient specific surgical approach to TKA and show equal benefits to both with less exposure to the patient with the MRI. Heilmeier et al. used MRI to predict the odds risk for TKA in the future. The study is well based but validation and application in the future remains to be seen. Pathak et al. used MRI to show that the flexion gap is asymmetric in the normal knee. While this is not particularly new information, it does show an MRI application. Zhao et al. developed a muscle area ratio using MRI as a novel indicator to evaluate obesity that may show promise in the future versus using BMI. Lung et al. reviewed an institutional database and noticed that primary care physicians tended to order MRIs on patients who would ultimately be indicated for TKA, increasing the cost of care. While the figures are interesting, the authors do not offer a clear education solution that would not in itself increase expenses. Bourdon et al. explored a novel method to improve the accuracy of positron emission tomography/ magnetic resonance imaging (PET/MRI) in detecting early inflammatory processes around TKA implants by addressing the challenges posed by metal-induced signal attenuation. This may have application in the future but there is still inter-observer variability. Balcarek's et al. showed the sensitivity of posterior condylar offset (PCO) measurements to minor changes in MRI scan orientation, suggesting that even small degrees of femur rotation can introduce systematic errors. This underscores the need for standardized imaging protocols to ensure accurate PCO assessment, which is vital for TKA planning and prosthesis design.

CT scans have commonly been used in knee evaluation. Watanabe et al., Reilly et al., and Konigsberg et al., each looked at aspects of observer reliability when addressing CT scans. Each article found good reliability but emphasized the importance of interpreting the reference points that are used. Awengen et al., Rasch et al., Hirschmann et al., and Verschueren et al. showed that SPECT/CT results may correlate with symptomatic knees and may be used as a biomarker for biomechanics. These findings are valuable but require considerable x-ray exposure and cost. Mhaskar et al. looked at supine CT that could be used in the early post operative period when standing x-rays may be more difficult to obtain. At this point the application is not as accurate and may have use in the future but at a significant cost and exposure. Lei et al. used CT data to show that the surgical epicondylar axis reproducibility is inconsistent and should be supported with multiple other references. Adkar et al. and Schotanus et al., used CT templating for prosthesis sizing and/or digital models. This may be helpful in planning and may save time in the operating room but requires further validation. Lei et al. used full length CT data for intraoperative positioning and showed its value especially with respect to the tibial component position. Still, the time saved may not be a significant component for the clinical result. Sharma et al. optimized the femoral component rotation using CT to determine the condylar twist angle. The accuracy appears to be excellent, but no comparisons are offered in the study. Figueroa et al. showed that CT can be used to measure component rotation but a good deal of further study is required. Du et al. classified the trochlear groove into 4 types based upon 3D computed tomography and noted an association with the shape and alignment of the femur but not with the size. This may help in the future with prosthetic design. Verburg et al. showed that CT imaging can measure the extent of cement penetration. This may have some application for surgical techniques. Tian et al. used CT scans to extract radiomic data and used this to develop a nomogram to predict patient satisfaction. The model did show superior predictive performance to models that use only clinical or radiomic data. The future of this model remains to be seen.

Fluoroscopy has been shown to provide assessment of real time knee motion and the interaction of the femur and tibia. Yamazai et al. used fluoroscopy to evaluate the kinematics of a mobile bearing prosthesis. This technique does require tantalum bead insertion into the polyethylene which may limit its application. Hirokowa et al.

proposes a 2-step algorithm for prosthetic position that requires further development in the future.

To complete the imaging portfolio, Hill et al. illustrated the limited application of three phase bone scans for painful TKAs. This study agrees with other publications. Barnsley et al. conducted a systematic review and meta-analysis to look at various nuclear modalities to evaluate prosthetic loosening and showed that SPECT/CT arthrography may have promise in the future. While Bao et al. demonstrated a high specificity and sensitivity for SPECT/CT arthrography for suspected joint loosening. This technology may be useful in complex cases but is not a first line test.

This chapter does provide insights into the current and advancing image technologies that are being investigated to improve patient evaluation and surgical technique. More advanced imaging provides greater detail to a patient specific approach to TKA.

3.1 Plain X-Rays

Machine Generated Summaries

Disclaimer: The summaries in this chapter were generated from Springer Nature publications using abstractive AI auto-summarization: An abstraction-based summarizer creates new text based on deep learning. New phrases are created to summarize the content. As the constituted sentences are machine selected, they may not fully reflect the body of the work, so we strongly advise that the original content is read and cited. The auto-generated summaries were curated by the editor to meet Springer Nature publication standards.

3.1.1 Subchondral Tibial Bone Texture of Conventional X-Rays Predicts Total Knee Arthroplasty [80]

This is a machine-generated summary of:

Almhdie-Imjabbar, Ahmad; Toumi, Hechmi; Harrar, Khaled; Pinti, Antonio; Lespessailles, Eric Subchondral tibial bone texture of conventional X-rays predicts total knee arthroplasty [80].

Published in: Scientific Reports (2022).

Link to original: https://doi.org/10.1038/s41598-022-12083-x

If you want to cite the papers, please refer to the original.

For technical reasons we could not place the page where the original quote is coming from.

3.1.1.1 Research Highlights

Osteoarthritis (OA) is a prevalent condition, particularly affecting the knee, and is a leading cause of disability among older adults. Despite advancements in understanding its pathophysiology, particularly the role of subchondral bone, effective disease-modifying treatments remain elusive, often leaving joint replacement surgery as the primary option for severe cases. A significant challenge in OA management is identifying patients at high risk for total knee arthroplasty (TKA). The study by Almhdie-Imjabbar et al. explores the potential of trabecular bone texture (TBT) analysis from baseline knee radiographs to predict TKA risk in patients with knee osteoarthritis (KOA).

The study utilized data from the Osteoarthritis Initiative (OAI) cohort, focusing on individuals with or at risk of symptomatic KOA. Researchers applied TBT analysis to baseline knee radiographs to assess its predictive power for TKA. The study involved logistic regression models incorporating clinical covariates, radiological scores, and TBT parameters. The dataset was divided into two scenarios based on different inclusion criteria related to Kellgren-Lawrence (KL) grades. The models were evaluated using tenfold cross-validation to ensure robustness. Results indicated that combining TBT parameters with KL grades significantly improved the prediction of TKA risk compared to models using only clinical covariates or KL grades alone.

The study highlights the potential of integrating TBT analysis into clinical practice for better risk stratification in KOA patients. Future study could explore combining MRI-based parameters with radiographic TBT analysis to enhance predictive accuracy further. Additionally, considering time-dependent outcomes and incorporating patient-reported outcomes could refine prediction models. While the current model shows promise, especially in identifying high-risk individuals for targeted interventions, further research is needed to validate these findings across diverse populations and imaging protocols. This approach could ultimately aid in developing more personalized treatment strategies and delaying or preventing the need for joint replacement surgery.

3.1.2 Correlation of Short Knee and Full-Length X-Rays in Evaluating Coronal Plane Alignment in Total Knee Arthroplasty [81]

This is a machine-generated summary of:

Kazemi, Seyyed-Morteza; Qoreishi, Seyyed-Mohammad; Maleki, Arash; Minaei-Noshahr, Reza; Hosseininejad, Seyyed-Mohsen Correlation of short knee and full-length X-rays in evaluating coronal plane alignment in total knee arthroplasty [81].

Published in: Journal of Orthopaedic Surgery and Research (2022).

Link to original: https://doi.org/10.1186/s13018-022-03246-7

3.1.2.1 Research Highlights

Postoperative coronal plane limb alignment is crucial for the longevity of total knee arthroplasty (TKA). Traditionally, surgeons have used the femorotibial angle (FTA) from short knee anteroposterior (AP) radiographs to assess alignment due to its simplicity and reduced radiation exposure compared to full-length hip-knee-ankle (HKA) radiographs. However, discrepancies in alignment measurements between short and full-length radiographs have been reported, raising questions about the reliability of using short knee radiographs alone. The study by Kazemi et al. investigates whether short knee radiographs can adequately replace full-length radiographs for assessing coronal alignment in TKA patients without extra-articular deformities.

The study involved a retrospective cross-sectional analysis of Iranian patients who underwent TKA by the same surgeon. Exclusion criteria included congenital limb anomalies and other conditions affecting limb alignment. Preoperative tibial and femoral bowing angles were assessed using full-length radiographs to exclude knees with extra-articular deformities. Postoperative alignment was evaluated using both short knee AP and full-length radiographs at 6 weeks. The researchers measured anatomical and mechanical angles, including MPTA (Medial Proximal Tibial Angle).

, LDFA (Lateral Distal Femoral Angle), FTA-short, FTA-long, and HKA. Correlation coefficients were calculated to assess the relationship between these measurements. The study found that while there was a good correlation between some measurements, such as postoperative FTA-short and HKA, others showed only fair or low correlation.

The findings suggest that short knee radiographs may not be sufficient for accurately assessing coronal alignment in TKA patients, as significant discrepancies were observed when compared to full-length radiographs. This has implications for clinical practice, as relying solely on short knee radiographs could lead to misclassification of limb alignment. Future study could explore personalized approaches to distal femur cutting angles during surgery or investigate alternative imaging techniques that balance accuracy with reduced radiation exposure. The study highlights the need for careful consideration of imaging protocols in TKA to ensure optimal patient outcomes.

3.1.3 A Novel Technology for 3D Knee Prosthesis Planning and Treatment Evaluation Using 2D X-Ray Radiographs: A Clinical Evaluation [82]

This is a machine-generated summary of:

Zheng, Guoyan; Hommel, Hagen; Akcoltekin, Alper; Thelen, Benedikt; Stifter, Jan; Peersman, Geert A novel technology for 3D knee prosthesis planning and treatment evaluation using 2D X-ray radiographs: a clinical evaluation [82].

Published in: International Journal of Computer Assisted Radiology and Surgery (2018).

Link to original: https://doi.org/10.1007/s11548-018-1789-4

If you want to cite the papers, please refer to the original.

For technical reasons we could not place the page where the original quote is coming from.

3.1.3.1 Research Highlights

Total knee arthroplasty (TKA) is a widely successful orthopedic procedure, with survival rates exceeding 90% after 10 years. Despite these outcomes, the number of TKA failures remains significant due to factors such as improper sizing and positioning of femoral and tibial components. Accurate preoperative planning is crucial to mitigate these issues, traditionally relying on radiographs and CT-based approaches. However, these methods have limitations, including inaccuracies due to patient positioning and increased radiation exposure. The study by Zheng et al. introduces a novel technology that uses conventional X-ray radiographs for TKA planning and evaluation, offering a potentially more accessible and cost-effective solution.

The study employs an innovative method that integrates an X-ray image calibration cage with a statistical shape model-based reconstruction program. This approach allows for the derivation of patient-specific models of the femur and tibia from weight-bearing X-ray images without requiring specialized imaging devices. The process involves calibrating X-ray images using embedded fiducials in the calibration cage, followed by iterative scaled registration to match statistical shape models to the X-ray scene. The technology was validated on 50 cases, comparing its accuracy against CT-based measurements considered as the ground truth. The results demonstrated that this method could accurately predict implant sizes and assess postoperative prosthesis alignment with minimal deviation from CT-based evaluations.

The main advancement of this study is the development of a low-cost, low-radiation alternative to CT-based TKA planning and evaluation methods. This technology enables accurate preoperative planning and postoperative assessment using only conventional X-ray machines, making it more accessible for widespread clinical use. Future study could focus on automating certain aspects of the process to reduce user interaction and further refine landmark definition accuracy. Additionally, addressing limitations such as knee joint immobilization during image acquisition could enhance the robustness of this approach. Overall, this technology represents a significant step forward in improving TKA outcomes through more precise planning and evaluation techniques.

3.1.4 The Epicondylar Ratio Can Be Reliably Determined in both Computed Tomography and X-Ray [83]

This is a machine-generated summary of:

Lutz, Bernd; Polcikova, Lucia; Faschingbauer, Martin; Reichel, Heiko; Bieger, Ralf The epicondylar ratio can be reliably determined in both computed tomography and X-ray [83].

Published in: Archives of Orthopaedic and Trauma Surgery (2021).

3.1.4.1 Research Highlights

In revision total knee arthroplasty (rTKA), surgeons often face challenges due to femoral or tibial bone loss, complicating the reconstruction of the joint line (JL). An anatomically accurate JL position is crucial, as deviations can lead to complications such as increased patellofemoral compression forces, anterior knee pain, and decreased implant survival rates. Current methods for estimating the JL position include relative techniques like the adductor tubercle and epicondylar ratio (ER). However, the ideal imaging modality for measuring ER remains unclear. The study by Lutz et al. evaluates the use of computed tomography (CT) for measuring ER in rTKA, hypothesizing that CT may offer more reliable measurements than X-ray.

The study involved a retrospective analysis of patients who underwent rTKA, with inclusion criteria requiring high-quality CT and X-ray images. The researchers defined landmarks on both imaging modalities, aligning the JL tangentially to the femoral component's condyles and using specific anatomical points for measurement. Two blinded observers measured all images, with one observer repeating measurements after a two-week interval to assess intra- and interobserver agreement using the intraclass correlation coefficient (ICC). The results showed good to excellent agreement between observers and an excellent correlation between CT and X-ray measurements for both lateral epicondylar ratio (LER) and medial epicondylar ratio (MER).

While the study demonstrated comparable reliability between CT and X-ray for measuring ER, it did not confirm the hypothesized superiority of CT. The selection of slices in CT may introduce variability, particularly affecting LER measurements. Despite these findings, CT may still be preferred in cases with extension lag or rotational issues affecting X-ray validity. Future study could explore whether analysis with correct plain alignment enhances measurement accuracy in CT. The study suggests that while ER measurement is reliable in both modalities, it should be used alongside other methods like the Figgie distance in cases of extensive femoral bone loss.

3.1.5 CT-Based 3D Reconstruction of Lower Limb Versus X-Ray-Based 3D Reconstruction: A Comparative Analysis and Application for a Safe and Cost-Effective Modality in TKA [84]

This is a machine-generated summary of:

Shetty, Vivek; Wagh, Yash; Karade, Vikas; Maurya, Amit; Parihar, Mangal; Shekhar, Sajeev; Tandel, Jignesh CT-Based 3D Reconstruction of Lower Limb Versus X-Ray-Based 3D Reconstruction: A Comparative Analysis and Application for a Safe and Cost-Effective Modality in TKA [84].

Published in: Indian Journal of Orthopaedics (2021).

Link to original: https://doi.org/10.1007/s43465-021-00456-9

If you want to cite the papers, please refer to the original.

For technical reasons we could not place the page where the original quote is coming from.

3.1.5.1 Research Highlights

Total knee arthroplasty (TKA) has seen significant advancements in pre-operative and intra-operative planning using patient-specific instrumentation, computer navigation, and robotic techniques. These methods rely on virtual models of the lower limb constructed from CT or MRI scans to improve surgical alignment accuracy and patient outcomes. However, CT-based reconstructions are costly and expose patients to higher radiation levels. The study by Shetty et al. evaluates an X-ray-based bone reconstruction method as a cost-effective and safer alternative for TKA planning.

The study involved collecting data from patients who underwent TKA, using both pre-operative CT scans and weight-bearing long-leg X-rays. The researchers developed lower limb bone models from both imaging modalities, using MIMICs software for CT reconstructions and a specialized technology for X-ray reconstructions. The models were exported as STL (Stereolithography) files, which included surface mesh details. Anatomical parameters were measured by importing these models into cloud-based software designed for surgical planning. The study focused on comparing the accuracy of anatomical measurements and surface reconstruction between the two methods. Statistical analyses, including Pearson's correlation coefficient and intraclass correlation coefficient (ICC), were performed to assess the correlation and reproducibility of measurements between the groups.

The results demonstrated that the anatomical parameters measured using the X-ray-based method were comparable to those obtained from CT scans, with high Pearson's correlation coefficients indicating strong agreement. The ICC values showed excellent reproducibility within both groups. The study suggests that this X-ray-based technology could serve as a cost-effective alternative to CT for computer-assisted TKA methods, offering advantages such as weight-bearing imaging that reveals true deformities of the lower limb. Future study could focus on validating this technology in practical applications like robotic surgeries, although further evaluation is needed to confirm its efficacy in such settings.

3.1.6 The Epicondylar Ratio Can Be Reliably Used on X-Ray of the Knee to Determine the Joint Line [85]

This is a machine-generated summary of:

Lutz, Bernd; Trubrich, Angela; Kappe, Thomas; Reichel, Heiko; Bieger, Ralf The epicondylar ratio can be reliably used on X-ray of the knee to determine the joint line [85].

Published in: Archives of Orthopaedic and Trauma Surgery (2018).

Link to original: https://doi.org/10.1007/s00402-018-3003-0

If you want to cite the papers, please refer to the original.

For technical reasons we could not place the page where the original quote is coming from.

3.1.6.1 Research Highlights

Total knee arthroplasty (TKA) is a common surgical procedure, and its success largely depends on the accurate restoration of the joint line (JL). An elevated JL can lead to complications such as patellar tendon impingement, increased patellofemoral compression forces, and altered knee kinematics, potentially resulting in anterior knee pain and reduced implant survival. Despite various methods proposed for calculating the JL, there remains controversy over the best approach. The study by Lutz et al. investigates the correlation between epicondylar ratios (ER) measured on MRI and anterior posterior (AP) X-rays to improve preoperative planning in revision TKA.

The study involved a series of patients who underwent arthroscopic knee surgery, with specific inclusion criteria ensuring correct leg rotation on X-rays and high-quality MRI scans. The researchers defined reliable bony landmarks for measuring ER on both MRI and X-ray images. They calculated the lateral epicondylar ratio (LER) and medial epicondylar ratio (MER) using these landmarks. The study found good to excellent intramethod intraobserver and interobserver agreement for ER measurements on both imaging modalities. However, the correlation between ERs obtained from MRI and X-ray was only fair, likely due to inherent differences between three-dimensional MRI and two-dimensional X-ray imaging techniques.

The main advance of this study is the demonstration of reliable ER measurements on both MRI and X-ray, which can aid in preoperative planning for revision TKA when limited imaging history is available. The fair correlation between MRI and X-ray suggests that MRI could serve as a fallback option when preoperative X-rays are insufficient. Future study could focus on assessing the impact of rotational differences in X-ray images on ER measurements. Additionally, further research might explore optimizing imaging techniques to enhance intermethod correlation, potentially improving surgical outcomes in TKA revisions.

3.1.7 Development of an Artificial Intelligence Model for Predicting Implant Size in Total Knee Arthroplasty Using Simple X-Ray Images [86]

This is a machine-generated summary of:

Yu, Yeuni; Cho, Yoon Jae; Park, Sohee; Kim, Yun Hak; Goh, Tae Sik Development of an artificial intelligence model for predicting implant size in total knee arthroplasty using simple X-ray images [86].

Published in: Journal of Orthopaedic Surgery and Research (2024).

Link to original: https://doi.org/10.1186/s13018-024-05013-2

If you want to cite the papers, please refer to the original.

For technical reasons we could not place the page where the original quote is coming from.

3.1.7.1 Research Highlights

Preoperative templating in total knee arthroplasty (TKA) is crucial for ensuring optimal surgical outcomes, as it helps in accurately predicting implant sizes to avoid mismatches and manage inventory efficiently. Despite its importance, traditional templating methods are labor-intensive and can vary in accuracy depending on the practitioner. The study by Yu et al. explores the potential of using artificial intelligence (AI) to predict implant sizes using only radiographs, without relying on demographic data, thereby addressing a significant gap in current methodologies.

The study involved 200 patients with knee osteoarthritis who underwent TKA, with surgeries performed by a single surgeon using the NexGen® implant (Zimmer Biomet, Warsaw, IN, USA). The researchers collected lateral view X-ray images of the patients' knees and retrospectively analyzed the inserted implant sizes. They developed a convolutional neural network model using the ResNet-50 architecture to predict implant sizes based solely on these X-rays. The images were pre-processed into grayscale and resized to fit the model's requirements. Data augmentation techniques were employed to enhance the training dataset, which was divided into training and test sets. The model's performance was evaluated using cross-validation, achieving high accuracy rates for predicting both femur and tibia implant sizes.

The study demonstrated that AI models could effectively predict TKA component sizes using only simple radiographs, achieving micro F1-scores of 0.92 for femur and 0.89 for tibia predictions within ± one size margin. This approach offers a promising alternative to traditional methods by reducing labor and time required for preoperative planning. However, the study's limitations include its single institution setting and reliance on data from a specific demographic group, which may affect generalizability. Future studies could focus on expanding the dataset across multiple centers and diverse populations to enhance the model's applicability and accuracy in different clinical settings.

3.1.8 New Parameter of Flexion after Posterior Stabilized Total Knee Arthroplasty: Posterior Condylar Offset Ratio on X-Ray Photographs [87]

This is a machine-generated summary of:

Soda, Yoshinori; Oishi, Jiro; Nakasa, Tomoyuki; Nishikawa, Koichiro; Ochi, Mitsuo New parameter of flexion after posterior stabilized total knee arthroplasty: posterior condylar offset ratio on X-ray photographs [87].

Published in: Archives of Orthopaedic and Trauma Surgery (2007).
Link to original: https://doi.org/10.1007/s00402-007-0295-x

If you want to cite the papers, please refer to the original.

For technical reasons we could not place the page where the original quote is coming from.

3.1.8.1 Research Highlights

In recent years, the development of artificial knee joints has focused on achieving deep flexion, particularly in Japan, where lifestyle demands high degrees of knee flexion. Previous studies have linked postoperative flexion angles to various factors, emphasizing the importance of maintaining posterior clearance to prevent flexion limitations. However, the significance of posterior condylar offset (PCO) may vary depending on patient body type and knee joint size. The study by Soda et al. investigates the role of the posterior condylar offset ratio (PCOR) in predicting postoperative flexion outcomes in posterior-stabilized (PS) type total knee arthroplasty (TKA).

The study involved patients who underwent NexGen PS type TKA for osteoarthritis and were evaluated at least 1 year postoperatively. Researchers calculated PCOR from postoperative lateral view radiographs and assessed its relationship with flexion angle and achievement rate. Patients were categorized into groups based on their postoperative flexion angles and achievement rates: Group L (lower flexion) and Group H (higher flexion), as well as Group P (lower achievement rate) and Group G (higher achievement rate). Statistical analysis using the Mann–Whitney U test revealed significant differences in PCOR between these groups. The findings suggest that a lower PCOR is associated with reduced postoperative flexion, potentially due to factors such as smaller femoral component size or anterior placement during surgery.

The study advances our understanding of how femoral component size and placement affect postoperative knee flexion in PS type TKA. While PCOR provides a simple parameter for assessing postoperative flexion status using plain radiographs, the authors acknowledge limitations, including the influence of numerous other factors on flexion outcomes. Future study could explore these additional factors to enhance surgical techniques further. Nonetheless, this research highlights the potential of PCOR as a useful tool for predicting knee function after TKA, emphasizing the importance of appropriate component sizing and placement during surgery.

3.1.9 Osteodensitometry Measurements of Periprosthetic Bone Using Dual Energy X-Ray Absorptiometry Following Total Knee Arthroplasty [88]

This is a machine-generated summary of:

Windisch, C.; Windisch, B.; Kolb, W.; Kolb, K.; Grützner, P.; Roth, A. Osteodensitometry measurements of periprosthetic bone using dual energy X-ray absorptiometry following total knee arthroplasty [88].

Published in: Archives of Orthopaedic and Trauma Surgery (2012).

Link to original: https://doi.org/10.1007/s00402-012-1601-9

If you want to cite the papers, please refer to the original.

For technical reasons we could not place the page where the original quote is coming from.

3.1.9.1 Research Highlights

Total knee arthroplasty (TKA) is a common surgical procedure aimed at alleviating pain and restoring function in patients with severe knee arthritis. However, changes in load distribution following TKA can lead to alterations in bone structure, particularly around the prosthesis. Understanding these changes is crucial for improving patient outcomes and prosthesis longevity. The study by Windisch et al. investigates the changes in bone density over time following cement-free TKA, focusing on specific regions of interest (ROIs) and examining associations with factors such as age, sex, severity of arthrosis, and axis alignment.

The study involved a prospective cohort of patients with primary varus gonarthrosis undergoing cement-free TKA. Participants were divided into two groups based on the number of postoperative osteodensitometry examinations they underwent using dual-energy X-ray absorptiometry (DXA). Bone density measurements were taken preoperatively and at several intervals postoperatively across seven defined ROIs around the knee joint. Statistical analyses, including correlation, variance, and regression analyses, were conducted to assess the significance of changes in bone density and their associations with preoperative parameters. The results indicated significant changes in bone density within the first 12 months postoperatively, with notable gender-specific differences observed in certain ROIs.

The study advances our understanding of periprosthetic bone density changes following TKA by highlighting significant early postoperative alterations and gender-specific differences. The findings suggest that initial high bone density values may be protective against postoperative loss. Future study could focus on long-term monitoring of bone density changes beyond 12 months to better understand the stabilization process and its implications for prosthesis integration. Additionally, exploring interventions to mitigate early bone loss could enhance patient outcomes and prosthesis longevity.

3.1.10 A Study of Surgical Accuracy with X-Ray-Based Patient-Specific Instrument (X3DPSI®) Vs Conventional Instrument in Total Knee Arthroplasty Surgeries [89]

This is a machine-generated summary of:

Shetty, Vivek; Shekhar, Sajeev; Karade, Vikas; Maurya, Amit; Sankar, Manu; Wagh, Yash A Study of Surgical Accuracy with X-Ray-Based Patient-Specific Instrument (X3DPSI®) vs Conventional Instrument in Total Knee Arthroplasty Surgeries [89].

Published in: Indian Journal of Orthopaedics (2022).

Link to original: https://doi.org/10.1007/s43465-022-00623-6

If you want to cite the papers, please refer to the original.

For technical reasons we could not place the page where the original quote is coming from.

3.1.10.1 Research Highlights

Total knee arthroplasty (TKA) is a common surgical procedure aimed at alleviating pain and improving the quality of life for patients with severe knee joint issues. The success of TKA largely depends on the precise alignment and positioning of implant components, which can significantly affect the longevity of the implant and patient outcomes. Traditional methods using conventional instrumentation (CI) for bone cuts, such as intramedullary femoral referencing and extramedullary tibial referencing, have limitations, especially in cases involving extra-articular deformities or obese patients. The study by Shetty et al. explores an innovative X-ray-based method for designing patient-specific instruments (PSIs) to improve postoperative alignment in TKA.

The study conducted by Shetty et al. involved a prospective analysis of ten patients undergoing TKA at a tertiary medical care center. The researchers utilized a novel X-ray-based approach to create virtual bone models using specialized software developed by AlgoSurg Inc. This method involved taking standard preoperative scanograms with calibration markers, reconstructing bone models, and designing PSIs for both femur and tibia without the need for CT or MRI scans. Intraoperatively, guide pins were placed using these PSIs, followed by conventional instrumentation for comparison. The study focused on measuring the mechanical axis alignments virtually achieved through this new method versus those obtained using CI.

The findings suggest that the X-ray-based PSI method offers significant advantages over traditional CI techniques in achieving accurate postoperative alignment. The study reported statistically significant improvements in the hip-knee-ankle (HKA) angle and mechanical axis deviation (MAD) with the PSI approach. Future study phases will involve actual bone cuts using this novel method in a larger sample size to further validate these results. This innovative approach could potentially offer a cost-effective, less invasive alternative to CT/MRI-based PSIs, reducing radiation exposure and improving surgical outcomes in TKA procedures.

Bibliography

1. Brandt, K. D., Dieppe, P.; Radin, E. Etiopathogenesis of osteoarthritis. *Med. Clin. N. Am. 93*, 1–24 (2009).
2. Janvier, T. *et al.* Subchondral tibial bone texture analysis predicts knee osteoarthritis progression: data from the osteoarthritis initiative: Tibial bone texture and knee OA progression. *Osteoarthr. Cartil. 25*, 259–266 (2017).
3. Kraus, V. B. *et al.* Predictive Validity of Radiographic Trabecular Bone Texture in Knee Osteoarthritis: The Osteoarthritis Research Society International/Foundation for the National Institutes of Health Osteoarthritis Biomarkers Consortium. *Arthritis & Rheumatology (Hoboken, N.J.) 70*, 80–87 (2018).
4. Kraus, V. B. *et al.* Subchondral bone trabecular integrity predicts and changes concurrently with radiographic and magnetic resonance imaging-determined knee osteoarthritis progression. *Arthritis Rheum. 65*, 1812–1821 (2013).
5. Woloszynski, T. *et al.* Prediction of progression of radiographic knee osteoarthritis using tibial trabecular bone texture. *Arthritis Rheum. 64*, 688–695 (2012).
6. Woloszynski, T., Podsiadlo, P., Stachowiak, G. W. and Kurzynski, M. A dissimilarity-based multiple classifier system for trabecular bone texture in detection and prediction of progression of knee osteoarthritis. *Proc. Inst. Mech. Eng. H 226*, 887–894 (2012).
7. MacKay, J. W. *et al.* Association of subchondral bone texture on magnetic resonance imaging with radiographic knee osteoarthritis progression: Data from the osteoarthritis initiative bone ancillary study. *Eur. Radiol. 28*, 4687–4695 (2018).
8. Nguyen, K. L. *et al.* Interest of texture analysis and neural networks for the characterization of knee osteoarthritis radiographic progression in OAI and MOST cohorts. *Bone Rep. 13*, 100696 (2020).
9. Leung, K. *et al.* Prediction of total knee replacement and diagnosis of osteoarthritis by using deep learning on knee radiographs: Data from the osteoarthritis initiative. *Radiology 296*, 584–593 (2020).
10. Podsiadlo, P., Cicuttini, F. M., Wolski, M., Stachowiak, G. W. and Wluka, A. E. Trabecular bone texture detected by plain radiography is associated with an increased risk of knee replacement in patients with osteoarthritis: A 6 year prospective follow up study. *Osteoarthr. Cartil. 22*, 71–75 (2014).

11. McAlindon, T. *Biomarker Qualification Letter of Intent (LOI) Template by Tufts Medical Center*. (Food and Drug Administration (FDA), 2019). https://www.fda.gov/media/135989/download.
12. Leptak, C. and Seymour, S. *Letter of Intent: Determination Letter*. (Food and Drug Administration (FDA), 2019). https://www.fda.gov/media/135988/download.
13. Skou, S. T. *et al.* Criteria used when deciding on eligibility for total knee arthroplasty: Between thinking and doing. *Knee 23*, 300–305 (2016).
14. Glasser J, Mariorenzi M, Blood T, O'Donnell S, Garcia D, Antoci V. Distal femoral valgus cut angles unreliable in total knee arthroplasty. J Orthop. 2021;24:29–33.
15. Yau W, Chiu K, Tang W, Ng T. Coronal bowing of the femur and tibia in Chinese: its incidence and effects on total knee arthroplasty planning. J Orthop Surg. 2007;15(1):32–6.
16. Kim J-M, Hong S-H, Lee B-S, Kim D-E, Kim K-A, Bin S-I. Femoral shaft bowing in the coronal plane has more significant effect on the coronal alignment of TKA than proximal or distal variations of femoral shape. Knee Surg Sports Traumatol Arthrosc. 2015;23(7):1936–42.
17. Munro BH. Correlation. Statistical methods for health care research. 1997:224–45.
18. Lombardi AV Jr, Berend KR, Ng VY. Neutral mechanical alignment: a requirement for successful TKA: affirms. Orthopedics. 2011;34(9):e504–6.
19. Kniesel B, Konstantinidis L, Hirschmüller A, Südkamp N, Helwig P. Digital templating in total knee and hip replacement: an analysis of planning accuracy. Int Orthop. 2014;38(4):733–9.
20. Alzahrani MM, Wood TJ, Somerville LE, Howard JL, Lanting BA, Vasarhelyi EM. Correlation of short knee radiographs and full-length radiographs in patients undergoing total knee arthroplasty. JAAOS-J Am Acad Orthopaedic Surg. 2019;27(11):e516–21.
21. Tanzer M, Makhdom AM. Preoperative planning in primary total knee arthroplasty. J Am Acad Orthop Surg. 2016;24(4):220–30.
22. Werner FW, Ayers DC, Maletsky LP, Rullkoetter PJ. The effect of valgus/varus malalignment on load distribution in total knee replacements. J Biomech. 2005;38(2):349–55.
23. D'Lima DD, Hermida JC, Chen PC, Colwell CW Jr. Polyethylene wear and variations in knee kinematics. Clin Orthopaedics Relat Res. 2001;392:124–30.
24. D'Lima DD, Chen PC, Colwell CW Jr. Polyethylene contact stresses, articular congruity, and knee alignment. Clin Orthopaedics Relat Res. 2001;392:232–8.
25. Vanlommel L, Vanlommel J, Claes S, Bellemans J. Slight undercorrection following total knee arthroplasty results in superior clinical outcomes in varus knees. Knee Surg Sports Traumatol Arthrosc. 2013;21(10):2325–30.
26. Fang DM, Ritter MA, Davis KE. Coronal alignment in total knee arthroplasty: just how important is it? J Arthroplasty. 2009;24(6):39–43.

27. Ritter MA, Davis KE, Meding JB, Pierson JL, Berend ME, Malinzak RA. The effect of alignment and BMI on failure of total knee replacement. JBJS. 2011;93(17):1588–96.
28. Abu-Rajab RB, Deakin AH, Kandasami M, McGlynn J, Picard F, Kinninmonth AW. Hip–knee–ankle radiographs are more appropriate for assessment of post-operative mechanical alignment of total knee arthroplasties than standard AP knee radiographs. J Arthroplasty. 2015;30(4):695–700.
29. Kraus VB, Vail TP, Worrell T, McDaniel G. A comparative assessment of alignment angle of the knee by radiographic and physical examination methods. Arthritis Rheum. 2005;52(6):1730–5.
30. Okamoto S, Mizu-uchi H, Okazaki K, Hamai S, Tashiro Y, Nakahara H, Iwamoto Y (2016) Two-dimensional planning can result in internal rotation of the femoral component in total knee arthroplasty. Knee Surg Sports Traumatol Arthrosc 24:229–235
31. De Valk E, Noorduyn J, Mutsaerts E (2016) How to assess femoral and tibial component rotation after total knee arthroplasty with computed tomography: a systematic review. Knee Surg Sports Traumatol Arthrosc 24:3517–3528
32. Ettinger M, Claassen L, Paes P, Calliess T (2016) 2D versus 3D templating in total knee arthroplasty. Knee 23:149–151
33. Kobayashi A, Ishii Y, Takeda M, Noguchi H, Higuchi H, Toyabe S (2012) Comparison of analog 2D and digital 3D preoperative templating for predicting implant size in total knee arthroplasty. Comput Aided Surg 17:96–101
34. Meijer M, Velleman T, Boerboom A, Bulstra S, Otten E, Stevens M, Reininga I (2016) The validity of a new low-dose stereoradiography system to perform 2D and 3D knee prosthetic alignment measurements. PLoS One 11:e0146187
35. Servien E, Viskontas D, Giuffrè BM, Coolican MRJ, Parker DA (2007) Reliability of bony landmarks for restoration of the joint line in revision knee arthroplasty. Knee Surg Sports TraumatolArthrosc 16:263–269
36. Talbot BS, Weinberg EP (2016) MR imaging with metal-suppression sequences for evaluation of total joint arthroplasty. Radiographics 36:209–225
37. König C, Sharenkov A, Matziolis G, Taylor WR, Perka C, Duda GN, Heller MO (2010) Joint line elevation in revision TKA leads to increased patellofemoral contact forces. J Orthop Res 28:1–5
38. Yoshii I, Whiteside LA, White SE, Milliano MT (1991) Influence of prosthetic joint line position on knee kinematics and patellar position. J Arthroplasty 6:169–177
39. Bieger R, Huch K, Kocak S, Jung S, Reichel H, Kappe T (2014) The influence of joint line restoration on the results of revision total knee arthroplasty: comparison between distance and ratio-methods. Arch Orthop Trauma Surg 134:537–541
40. Lutz B, Trubrich A, Kappe T, Reichel H, Bieger R (2018) The epicondylar ratio can be reliably used on X-ray of the knee to determine the joint line. Arch Orthop Trauma Surg 93:1–6
41. Kim AD, Scott RD (2016) Can the visibility of both prosthetic posterior femoral condyles on a postoperative radiograph assure that limb rotation is

appropriate to allow accurate measurement of the anatomic knee axis? J Arthroplasty 31:2593–2596
42. Lonner JH, Laird MT, Stuchin SA (1996) Effect of rotation and knee flexion on radiographic alignment in total knee arthroplasties. Clin Orthop Relat Res 331:102–106
43. Radtke K, Becher C, Noll Y, Ostermeier S (2009) Effect of limb rotation on radiographic alignment in total knee arthroplasties. Arch Orthop Trauma Surg 130:451–457
44. Van der List, J. P., Chawla, H., Joskowicz, L., and Pearle, A. (2016). Current state of computer navigation and robotics in unicompartmental and total knee arthroplasty: A systematic review with meta-analysis. *Knee Surgery, Sports Traumatology, Arthroscopy, 24*, 3482–3495. https://doi.org/10.1007/s00167-016-4305-9
45. Waddell, B. S., Carroll, K., and Jerabek, S. (2017). Technology in arthroplasty: Are we improving value? *Current Reviews in Musculoskeletal Medicine, 10*(3), 378–387. https://doi.org/10.1007/s12178-017-9415-6
46. Kayani, B., Konan, S., Ayuob, A., Onochie, E., Al-Jabri, T., and Haddad, F. S. (2019). Robotic technology in total knee arthroplasty: A systematic review. *EFORT Open Reviews, 4*, 611–617. https://doi.org/10.1302/2058-5241.4.190022
47. Battenberg, A. K., Netravali, N. A., and Lonner, J. H. (2020). A novel handheld robotic-assisted system for unicompartmental knee arthroplasty: Surgical technique and early survivorship. *Journal of Robotic Surgery, 14*, 55–60. https://doi.org/10.1007/s11701-018-00907-w
48. Parratte, S., Price, A. J., Jeys, L., Jackson, W. F., and Clarke, H. D. (2019). Accuracy of a new robotically assisted technique for total knee arthroplasty: A cadaveric study. *Journal of Arthroplasty, 34*, 2799–2803. https://doi.org/10.1016/j.arth.2019.06.040
49. Chytas, D., Malahias, M. A., and Nikolaou, V. S. (2019). Augmented reality in orthopedics: current state and future directions. *Frontiers in Surgery, 6*, 38. https://doi.org/10.3389/fsurg.2019.00038
50. Walbron, P., Common, H., Thomazeau, H., Hosseini, K., Peduzzi, L., Bulaid, Y., et al. (2020). Virtual reality simulator improves the acquisition of basic arthroscopy skills in first-year orthopedic surgery residents. *Orthopaedics and Traumatology, Surgery and Research, 106*(717), 724. https://doi.org/10.1016/j.otsr.2020.03.009
51. Karade, V., and Ravi, B. (2015). 3D femur model reconstruction from biplane X-ray images: A novel method based on Laplacian surface deformation. *International Journal of CARS, 10*, 473–485. https://doi.org/10.1007/s11548-014-1097-6
52. Karade, V., Maurya, A., inventors; Karade, V., assignee. Systems and methods for obtaining 3-d images from x-ray information for deformed elongate bones. WIPO(PCT)-WO2019180745. https://patents.google.com/patent/WO2019180745/en. Accessed 26 Sep 2019

53. Raluca, M., Comaneanu, T., Mihai, V., Daniel, C., and Mihai, C. (2012). Virtual 3D reconstruction, diagnosis and surgical planning with Mimics software. *International Journal of Nano and Biomaterials, 4*, 69–77. https://doi.org/10.1504/IJNBM.2012.048212
54. Folinais, D., Thelen, P., Delin, C., Radier, C., Catonne, Y., and Lazennec, J. Y. (2013). Measuring femoral and rotational alignment: EOS system versus computed tomography. *Orthopaedics and Traumatology, Surgery and Research, 99*, 509–516. https://doi.org/10.1016/j.otsr.2012.12.023
55. Zheng, G., Hommel, H., Akcoltekin, A., Thelen, B., Stifter, J., and Peersman, G. (2018). A novel technology for 3D knee prosthesis planning and treatment evaluation using 2D X-ray radiographs: A clinical evaluation. *International Journal of CARS, 13*, 1151–1158. https://doi.org/10.1007/s11548-018-1789-4
56. Kim, H., Lee, K., Lee, D., and Baek, N. (2019). 3D reconstruction of leg bones from X-ray images using CNN-based feature analysis. *International Conference on Information and Communication Technology Convergence*. https://doi.org/10.1109/ictc46691.2019.8939984
57. Kasten, Y., Doktofsky, D., and Kovler, I. (2020). End-to-end convolutional neural network for 3D reconstruction of knee bones from bi-planar X-ray images. *Electrical Engineering and Systems Science*. https://arxiv.org/abs/2004.00871.
58. Schlatterer B, Suedhoff I, Bonnet X, Catonne Y, Maestro M, Skalli W (2009) Skeletal landmarks for TKR implantations: evaluation of their accuracy using EOS imaging acquisition system. Orthop Traumatol Surg Res 95:2–11
59. Bellemans J (2004) Restoring the joint line in revision TKA: does it matter? Knee 11:3–5
60. Hofmann AA, Kurtin SM, Lyons S, Tanner AM, Bolognesi MP (2006) Clinical and radiographic analysis of accurate restoration of the joint line in revision total knee arthroplasty. J Arthroplasty 21:1154–1162
61. König C, Sharenkov A, Matziolis G, Taylor WR, Perka C, Duda GN, Heller MO (2010) Joint line elevation in revision TKA leads to increased patellofemoral contact forces. J Orthop Res 28:1–5
62. Martin JW, Whiteside LA (1990) The influence of joint line position on knee stability after condylar knee arthroplasty. Clin Orthop Relat Res 259:146–156
63. Seil R, Pape D (2011) Causes of failure and etiology of painful primary total knee arthroplasty. Knee Surg Sports Traumatol Arthrosc 19:1418–1432
64. Pietrini SD, LaPrade RF, Griffith CJ, Wijdicks CA, Ziegler CG (2009) Radiographic identification of the primary posterolateral knee structures. Am J Sports Med 37:542–551
65. Griffin FM, Math K, Scuderi GR, Insall JN, Poilvache PL (2000) Anatomy of the epicondyles of the distal femur: MRI analysis of normal knees. J Arthroplasty 15:354–359
66. Blackley HR, Howell GE, Rorabeck CH. Planning and management of the difficult primary hip replacement: preoperative planning and technical considerations. Instr Course Lect. 2000;49:3–11.

67. Kunze KN, Polce EM, Patel A, Courtney PM, Levine BR. Validation and performance of a machine-learning derived prediction guide for total knee arthroplasty component sizing. Arch Orthop Trauma Surg. 2021;141:2235–44.
68. Kunze KN, Polce EM, Patel A, Courtney PM, Sporer SM, Levine BR. Machine learning algorithms predict within one size of the final implant ultimately used in total knee arthroplasty with good-to-excellent accuracy. Knee Surg Sports Traumatol Arthrosc. 2022;30:2565–72.
69. Sershon RA, Li J, Calkins TE, Courtney PM, Nam D, Gerlinger TL, Sporer SM, Levine BR. Prospective validation of a demographically based primary total knee arthroplasty size calculator. J Arthroplasty. 2019;34:1369–73.
70. Bellemans J, Banks S, Victor J, Vandenneucker H, Moemans A (2002) Fluoroscopic analysys of the kinematics of deep flexion in total knee arthroplasty. J Bone Joint Surg Br 84:50–53
71. Walker P, Garg A (1991) Range of motion in total knee arthroplasty. Clin Orthop 262:227–235
72. Daniilidis, K., and Tibesku, C. O. (2014). A comparison of conventional and patient-specific instruments in total knee arthroplasty. *International Orthopaedics, 38*(3), 503–508. https://doi.org/10.1007/s00264-013-2028-9
73. Hafez, M. A., and Moholkar, K. (2017). Patient-specific instruments: Advantages and pitfalls. *SICOT-J, 3*, 66. https://doi.org/10.1051/sicotj/2017054
74. Abdel-Aziz, Y., and Karara, H. (2014). Direct linear transformation from comparator coordinates into object space coordinates in close-range photogrammetry. *Photogrammetric Engineering and Remote Sensing*. https://doi.org/10.14358/PERS.81.2.103
75. Howell, S. M., Kuznik, K., Hull, M. L., and Siston, R. A. (2008). Results of an initial experience with custom-fit positioning total knee arthroplasty in a series of 48 patients. *Orthopedics, 31*(9), 857–864. https://doi.org/10.3928/01477447-20080901-15
76. Noble, J. W., Moore, C. A., and Liu, N. (2012). The value of patient-matched instrumentation in total knee arthroplasty. *Journal of Arthroplasty, 27*(1), 153–155. https://doi.org/10.1016/j.arth.2011.07.006
77. Spencer, B. A., Mont, M. A., McGrath, M. S., Boyd, B., and Mitrick, M. F. (2009). Initial experience with custom-fit total knee replacement: Intra-operative events and long-leg coronal alignment. *International Orthopaedics, 33*(6), 1571–1575. https://doi.org/10.1007/s00264-008-0693-x
78. Thienpont, E., Paternostre, F., Pietsch, M., Hafez, M., and Howell, S. (2013). Total knee arthroplasty with patient-specific instruments improves function and restores limb alignment in patients with extra-articular deformity. *The Knee, 20*(6), 407–411. https://doi.org/10.1016/j.knee.2013.07.001
79. Lin, Y., et al. (2020). Patient-specific or conventional instrumentations: A meta-analysis of randomized controlled trials. *BioMed Research International*. https://doi.org/10.1155/2020/2164371
80. Almhdie-Imjabbar, Ahmad; Toumi, Hechmi; Harrar, Khaled; Pinti, Antonio; Lespessailles, Eric Subchondral tibial bone texture of conventional X-rays pre-

dicts total knee arthroplasty. Scientific Reports (2022). https://doi.org/10.1038/s41598-022-12083-x
81. Kazemi, Seyyed-Morteza; Qoreishi, Seyyed-Mohammad; Maleki, Arash; Minaei-Noshahr, Reza; Hosseininejad, Seyyed-Mohsen Correlation of short knee and full-length X-rays in evaluating coronal plane alignment in total knee arthroplasty. Journal of Orthopaedic Surgery and Research (2022). https://doi.org/10.1186/s13018-022-03246-7
82. Zheng, Guoyan; Hommel, Hagen; Akcoltekin, Alper; Thelen, Benedikt; Stifter, Jan; Peersman, Geert A novel technology for 3D knee prosthesis planning and treatment evaluation using 2D X-ray radiographs: a clinical evaluation. International Journal of Computer Assisted Radiology and Surgery (2018). https://doi.org/10.1007/s11548-018-1789-4
83. Lutz, Bernd; Polcikova, Lucia; Faschingbauer, Martin; Reichel, Heiko; Bieger, Ralf The epicondylar ratio can be reliably determined in both computed tomography and X-ray. Archives of Orthopaedic and Trauma Surgery (2021). https://doi.org/10.1007/s00402-021-03888-y
84. Shetty, Vivek; Wagh, Yash; Karade, Vikas; Maurya, Amit; Parihar, Mangal; Shekhar, Sajeev; Tandel, Jignesh CT-Based 3D Reconstruction of Lower Limb Versus X-Ray-Based 3D Reconstruction: A Comparative Analysis and Application for a Safe and Cost-Effective Modality in TKA. Indian Journal of Orthopaedics (2021). https://doi.org/10.1007/s43465-021-00456-9
85. Lutz, Bernd; Trubrich, Angela; Kappe, Thomas; Reichel, Heiko; Bieger, Ralf The epicondylar ratio can be reliably used on X-ray of the knee to determine the joint line. Archives of Orthopaedic and Trauma Surgery (2018). https://doi.org/10.1007/s00402-018-3003-0
86. Yu, Yeuni; Cho, Yoon Jae; Park, Sohee; Kim, Yun Hak; Goh, Tae Sik Development of an artificial intelligence model for predicting implant size in total knee arthroplasty using simple X-ray images. Journal of Orthopaedic Surgery and Research (2024). https://doi.org/10.1186/s13018-024-05013-2
87. Soda, Yoshinori; Oishi, Jiro; Nakasa, Tomoyuki; Nishikawa, Koichiro; Ochi, Mitsuo New parameter of flexion after posterior stabilized total knee arthroplasty: posterior condylar offset ratio on X-ray photographs. Archives of Orthopaedic and Trauma Surgery (2007). https://doi.org/10.1007/s00402-007-0295-x
88. Windisch, C.; Windisch, B.; Kolb, W.; Kolb, K.; Grützner, P.; Roth, A. Osteodensitometry measurements of periprosthetic bone using dual energy X-ray absorptiometry following total knee arthroplasty. Archives of Orthopaedic and Trauma Surgery (2012). https://doi.org/10.1007/s00402-012-1601-9
89. Shetty, Vivek; Shekhar, Sajeev; Karade, Vikas; Maurya, Amit; Sankar, Manu; Wagh, Yash A Study of Surgical Accuracy with X-Ray-Based Patient-Specific Instrument (X3DPSI®) vs Conventional Instrument in Total Knee Arthroplasty Surgeries. Indian Journal of Orthopaedics (2022). https://doi.org/10.1007/s43465-022-00623-6

3.2 MRI

Machine Generated Summaries
Disclaimer: The summaries in this chapter were generated from Springer Nature publications using abstractive AI auto-summarization: An abstraction-based summarizer creates new text based on deep learning. New phrases are created to summarize the content. As the constituted sentences are machine selected, they may not fully reflect the body of the work, so we strongly advise that the original content is read and cited. The auto-generated summaries were curated by the editor to meet Springer Nature publication standards.

3.2.1 MRI-Based or CT-Based Patient-Specific Instrumentation in Total Knee Arthroplasty: How Do the Two Systems Compare? [69]

This is a machine-generated summary of:

Kang, Dong-Geun; Kim, Kang-Il; Bae, Jung-Kwon MRI-based or CT-based patient-specific instrumentation in Total knee Arthroplasty: How do the two systems compare? [69].

Published in: Arthroplasty (2020).

Link to original: https://doi.org/10.1186/s42836-019-0020-6

If you want to cite the papers, please refer to the original.

For technical reasons we could not place the page where the original quote is coming from.

3.2.1.1 Research Highlights

Patient-specific instrumentation (PSI) is a novel technology aimed at enhancing the accuracy of alignment and biomechanics restoration in total knee arthroplasty (TKA). PSI systems, which are based on preoperative imaging, utilize custom-made cutting jigs tailored to a patient's anatomy. While MRI-based PSI offers detailed visualization of articular cartilage without radiation exposure, it is costly and time-consuming. Conversely, CT-based PSI provides quicker scans but lacks cartilage detail and involves radiation. Despite numerous studies on PSI's efficacy compared to conventional methods, few have directly compared MRI- and CT-based systems. The study by Kang et al. investigates the accuracy of bone resection using MRI-versus CT-based PSI systems in TKA.

The study was a prospective analysis involving patients with primary osteoarthritis and varus deformity undergoing TKA with either MRI- or CT-based PSI systems. Participants were randomly assigned to receive preoperative imaging via MRI or CT, followed by the creation of patient-specific cutting jigs using Materialise® software. The surgical procedures were performed by a single surgeon using a minimally invasive approach, with bone resection thickness measured intraoperatively and compared to preoperative plans. Radiographic assessments of mechanical axis (MA) and component alignments were conducted preoperatively and years post-surgery. Clinical outcomes were evaluated using the Knee Society knee score among other metrics. Statistical analyses were performed to compare differences between the two groups.

The study found no significant differences between MRI- and CT-based PSI systems in terms of planned versus actual bone resection thickness, postoperative MA, or component alignments. Both systems demonstrated high accuracy in bone resection, with minimal mean absolute differences observed. The findings suggest that while MRI provides detailed cartilage visualization, it does not confer superior accuracy over CT in predicting resection thickness for TKA. Future study could explore cost-effectiveness and resource implications of each modality to guide clinical decision-making regarding imaging choices for PSI in TKA.

3.2.2 Baseline Knee Joint Effusion and Medial Femoral Bone Marrow Edema, in Addition to MRI-Based T2 Relaxation Time and Texture Measurements of Knee Cartilage, Can Help Predict Incident Total Knee Arthroplasty 4–7 Years Later: Data from the Osteoarthritis Initiative [70]

This is a machine-generated summary of:

Heilmeier, Ursula; Wamba, John Mbapte; Joseph, Gabby B.; Darakananda, Karin; Callan, Jennifer; Neumann, Jan; Link, Thomas M. Baseline knee joint effusion and medial femoral bone marrow edema, in addition to MRI-based T2 relaxation time and texture measurements of knee cartilage, can help predict incident total knee arthroplasty 4–7 years later: data from the Osteoarthritis Initiative [70].

Published in: Skeletal Radiology (2018).
Link to original: https://doi.org/10.1007/s00256-018-2995-4

If you want to cite the papers, please refer to the original.
For technical reasons we could not place the page where the original quote is coming from.

3.2.2.1 Research Highlights

Total knee arthroplasty (TKA) is a common surgical intervention for end-stage knee osteoarthritis (OA), providing pain relief and improved function for many patients. However, TKA carries risks such as prosthesis failure and infection, and the number of revision surgeries is expected to rise with increasing longevity. Current research focuses on delaying the need for TKA by identifying early prognostic markers of knee OA progression. Despite the potential of MRI in predicting TKA, existing studies have been limited by small sample sizes and high-risk populations. The study by Heilmeier et al. investigates whether advanced MRI-based techniques can serve as long-term predictors of TKA.

The study utilized data from the Osteoarthritis Initiative, a large multi-center cohort study in the United States, to assess whether baseline MRI features could predict TKA incidence 7–10 years later. Researchers selected subjects aged 45–79 with available baseline MRI scans and no history of inflammatory arthritis. The study included 99 TKA cases matched with controls based on gender, body mass index (BMI), race, and baseline osteoarthritis severity. MRI assessments included modified Whole-Organ Magnetic Resonance Imaging Scoring (WORMS), standard relaxation time measurements, and gray-level co-occurrence matrix (GLCM) texture analysis. Statistical analyses evaluated the association between these imaging features and subsequent TKA occurrence.

The study found that advanced MR-based cartilage imaging techniques, such as relaxation time measurements in the lateral femoral compartment and GLCM texture analysis, were associated with increased odds of incident TKA 7–10 years later. Specifically, a one-standard deviation increase in relaxation time values was linked to a 32% higher risk of undergoing knee replacement. Additionally, joint effusion and bone marrow edema patterns were significant predictors of future TKA. The findings suggest that these imaging markers could help identify patients at risk for TKA earlier in the disease course when interventions might delay surgery. Future studies should focus on validating these results in larger cohorts with longer follow-up periods to fully explore their predictive potential.

3.2.3 Is Flexion Gap Rectangular in Native Indian Knees? Results of an MRI Study [71]

This is a machine-generated summary of:

Pathak, Subodh Kumar; Sethi, Manish; Salunke, Abhijeet Ashok; Thivari, Praveen; Gautam, Rakesh Kumar; Anjum, Rashid; Chawla, Jasneet; Sharma, Aryan Is Flexion Gap Rectangular in Native Indian Knees? Results of an MRI Study [71].

Published in: Indian Journal of Orthopaedics (2021).

Link to original: https://doi.org/10.1007/s43465-021-00418-1

If you want to cite the papers, please refer to the original.

For technical reasons we could not place the page where the original quote is coming from.

3.2.3.1 Research Highlights

Total knee arthroplasty (TKA) is widely recognized as the preferred treatment for degenerative knee joint diseases, primarily due to its ability to restore the normal femorotibial mechanical axis. A critical factor in the success of TKA is achieving a well-balanced knee from flexion to full extension, which involves creating balanced and symmetrical flexion-extension gaps. However, recent reports suggest that the shape of the flexion gap may be influenced by the natural laxity of ligaments, potentially leading to asymmetry. This asymmetry could affect the durability of prosthetic components under cyclical loading. The study by Pathak et al. investigates these concerns by examining the normal flexion gap in the knees of the Indian population and exploring gender differences in ligament laxity.

The study involved 50 asymptomatic volunteers with normal knee radiographs and no history of knee injury or surgery. Using magnetic resonance imaging (MRI), researchers assessed joint characteristics and quantified anatomical variations in medial and lateral joint openings under valgus or varus stresses at 0° of flexion. Participants were positioned on a specially fabricated board to ensure consistent imaging conditions, with varus or valgus stress applied using custom-made blocks. The MRI scans were analyzed using specialized software to measure the shape and width of the flexion gap based on specific reference lines. Statistical analysis revealed significant differences in ligament laxity between genders, with females exhibiting greater lateral joint gaps compared to males.

The findings indicate that the lateral flexion gap is generally larger than the medial gap, suggesting a natural asymmetry that challenges traditional concepts of maintaining a rectangular flexion gap during TKA. This study highlights the need for reconsidering surgical approaches to accommodate physiological variations in ligament laxity, particularly given cultural practices such as squatting and sitting cross-legged prevalent in certain populations. Future study should focus on understanding how these asymmetrical flexion gaps impact implant longevity and patient outcomes post-TKA, especially considering lifestyle factors unique to different demographic groups. The research underscores the importance of tailoring TKA procedures to individual anatomical and cultural needs for improved surgical success.

3.2.4 Plain Radiographs Underestimate the Asymmetry of the Posterior Condylar Offset of the Knee Compared with MRI [72]

This is a machine-generated summary of:

Voleti, Pramod B.; Stephenson, Jason W.; Lotke, Paul A.; Lee, Gwo-Chin Plain Radiographs Underestimate the Asymmetry of the Posterior Condylar Offset of the Knee Compared With MRI [72].

Published in: Clinical Orthopaedics and Related Research® (2013).

Link to original: https://doi.org/10.1007/s11999-013-2946-2

If you want to cite the papers, please refer to the original.

For technical reasons we could not place the page where the original quote is coming from.

3.2.4.1 Research Highlights

The restoration of the posterior condylar offset (PCO) during total knee arthroplasty (TKA) is crucial for optimizing knee kinematics and preventing complications such as impingement and instability. Traditionally, PCO has been measured using lateral radiographs, but these do not account for variations in cartilage thickness or potential inaccuracies in imaging technique. The study by Voleti et al. explores the use of MRI to measure PCO more accurately, comparing it with traditional radiographic methods to better understand the anatomical differences between the medial and lateral femoral condyles.

The study involved a cohort of patients aged 18–40 years who underwent both MRI and plain radiography of the knee. Excluding those with any history of knee pathology, the researchers measured PCO using both imaging modalities. For MRI, a novel three-dimensional protocol was developed to assess the true PCO of each femoral condyle and, considering the cartilage thickness. The results showed significant variability in PCO among individuals and highlighted an asymmetry between the medial and lateral condyles, with MRI measurements consistently larger than those obtained from radiographs. Statistical analysis confirmed that radiographs underestimated PCO compared to MRI, particularly at the medial femoral condyle.

This study advances our understanding of knee anatomy by demonstrating that MRI provides a more accurate assessment of PCO than traditional radiography. The findings suggest that future TKA designs could benefit from incorporating these precise measurements to better replicate natural knee kinematics. Future study could focus on validating this MRI technique in diverse populations and exploring its application in arthritic knees requiring TKA. Additionally, further research might investigate how these anatomical insights can inform prosthesis design to improve surgical outcomes and patient satisfaction.

3.2.5 Predictive Value of Adipose to Muscle Area Ratio Based on MRI at Knee Joint for Postoperative Functional Outcomes in Elderly Osteoarthritis Patients Following Total Knee Arthroplasty [73]

This is a machine-generated summary of:

Zhao, Guanglei; Liu, Changquan; Chen, Kangming; Chen, Feiyan; Lyu, Jinyang; Chen, Jie; Shi, Jingsheng; Huang, Gangyong; Wei, Yibing; Wang, Siqun; Xia, Jun Predictive value of adipose to muscle area ratio based on MRI at knee joint for postoperative functional outcomes in elderly osteoarthritis patients following total knee arthroplasty [73].

Published in: Journal of Orthopaedic Surgery and Research (2020).

Link to original: https://doi.org/10.1186/s13018-020-02014-9

For technical reasons we could not place the page where the original quote is coming from.

3.2.5.1 Research Highlights

Obesity is a significant global health issue, particularly prevalent among the elderly, and is associated with various diseases, including osteoarthritis (OA). Total knee arthroplasty (TKA) is a common treatment for end-stage OA, but obesity can negatively impact surgical outcomes. Traditionally, body mass index (BMI) has been used to assess obesity; however, it does not account for body composition variations such as muscle and fat distribution. The study by Zhao et al. introduces the adipose to muscle area ratio (AMR) as a novel indicator to evaluate obesity and predict postoperative outcomes in elderly OA patients undergoing TKA.

The study retrospectively analyzed TKA cases from Huashan Hospital, Fudan University, focusing on patients with knee magnetic resonance imaging (MRI). The researchers measured AMR at three levels of the knee joint using MRI images and calculated an average AMR value. They assessed functional outcomes using the Knee Society Score (KSS) and Hospital for Special Surgery (HSS) score before surgery and at follow-up. Statistical analyses were conducted to explore correlations between AMR, BMI, and postoperative outcomes. The study found that AMR had stronger correlations with patient-reported outcome measures (PROMS) than BMI did, suggesting that AMR might be a better predictor of functional outcomes in this patient population.

The introduction of AMR as an obesity assessment tool marks a potential advancement in predicting surgical outcomes for elderly OA patients undergoing TKA. Unlike BMI, AMR provides insights into local muscle and fat distribution at the knee joint, which may influence recovery and complication rates. Future study could focus on larger sample sizes to validate these findings further and explore the relationship between AMR and postoperative complications more comprehensively. As MRI becomes more common in clinical practice, AMR could aid in developing personalized treatment plans to improve patient outcomes after TKA.

3.2.6 No Differences in Mid-Term Survival and Clinical Outcome Between CT- and MRI-Based Patient-Specific Instrumentation for Total Knee Arthroplasty, a Randomized Controlled Trial [74]

This is a machine-generated summary of:

Theeuwen, D. M. J.; Haveman, I.; Boonen, B.; van Haaren, E. H.; Hendrickx, R. P. M.; Schotanus, M. G. M. No differences in mid-term survival and clinical outcome between CT- and MRI-based patient-specific instrumentation for total knee arthroplasty, a randomized controlled trial [74].

Published in: European Journal of Orthopaedic Surgery & Traumatology (2023).
Link to original: https://doi.org/10.1007/s00590-023-03680-1

If you want to cite the papers, please refer to the original.

For technical reasons we could not place the page where the original quote is coming from.

3.2.6.1 Research Highlights

Total knee arthroplasty (TKA) is a prevalent treatment for advanced osteoarthritis of the knee joint, with patient-specific instrumentation (PSI) being one method to optimize pre-operative planning. PSI involves creating custom jigs using computed tomography (CT) or magnetic resonance imaging (MRI) to ensure precise surgical alignment. However, the standardization of image acquisition methods among PSI manufacturers remains inconsistent. Previous studies have indicated that MRI-based PSI may result in fewer radiological outliers, but no significant differences in clinical outcomes or prosthesis survival have been observed. The study by Theeuwen et al. addresses this knowledge gap by conducting a randomized controlled trial (RCT) to compare the mid-term clinical outcomes and survival rates of CT- and MRI-based PSI in TKA.

The study was a single-center, prospective, randomized, single-blind controlled trial involving patients who underwent TKA with either CT- or MRI-based PSI. Participants were followed up for an average of 5 years postoperatively. Due to the COVID-19 pandemic, data collection was adapted; patients were contacted by phone and completed patient-reported outcome measures (PROMs) via mail instead of attending in-person clinic visits. The study utilized various PROMs, including the Oxford Knee Score and the EuroQol EQ-5D, to assess clinical outcomes over time. Statistical analysis was performed using a generalized linear mixed model to evaluate differences between the two groups.

At mid-term follow-up, no significant difference in prosthesis survival rates was found between CT- and MRI-based PSI groups, although the EQ-5D Visual Analog Scale showed a statistically significant difference favoring the MRI group. The study suggests that both imaging modalities are reliable for use in TKA surgery, providing satisfactory outcomes for patients. Future study could explore long-term prosthesis survival using radio stereometric analysis to detect early component migration and further validate PROMs as effective tools for assessing clinical outcomes post-TKA. Additionally, integrating wearable motion sensors may enhance understanding of recovery trajectories following surgery.

3.2.7 MRI Use Leading Up to Total Knee Arthroplasty: A Retrospective Cohort Study [75]

This is a machine-generated summary of:

Lung, Tiffany; Lex, Johnathan R.; Pincus, Daniel; Gatley, Jodi; Wasserstein, David; Paterson, J. Michael; Ravi, Bheeshma MRI use leading up to total knee arthroplasty: a retrospective cohort study [75].

Published in: European Journal of Orthopaedic Surgery & Traumatology (2024).

Link to original: https://doi.org/10.1007/s00590-024-03940-8

If you want to cite the papers, please refer to the original.

For technical reasons we could not place the page where the original quote is coming from.

3.2.7.1 Research Highlights

Total knee arthroplasty (TKA) is a common procedure for treating end-stage knee osteoarthritis (OA) when conservative management fails. The standard diagnostic tool for OA is radiography, which is accessible and often sufficient without additional imaging. However, magnetic resonance imaging (MRI) can provide detailed soft tissue assessment but adds significant costs and is not typically necessary for diagnosing OA. Despite guidelines advising against routine MRI use in confirmed OA cases, some studies indicate that MRIs are still ordered pre-operatively, contributing to increased healthcare costs and longer wait times for patients. The study by Lung et al. evaluates the prevalence of MRI use in patients undergoing TKA and identifies factors associated with increased MRI utilization.

The study was a retrospective cohort analysis of older adults in Ontario, Canada who received their first primary elective TKA between April 2011 and March 2020.

Researchers used data from the Canadian Institute for Health Information Discharge Abstract Database and the Ontario Health Insurance Plan to identify patients who had an MRI within 2 years before their surgery. The study examined patient demographics, comorbidities, socioeconomic status, and physician characteristics to understand MRI usage patterns. Statistical analyses were conducted to determine trends over time and assess the impact of reducing unnecessary MRIs on healthcare costs. The findings revealed that 9.5% of TKA patients had an MRI ordered primarily by primary care physicians, with younger, healthier, and more affluent patients being more likely to receive an MRI.

The study highlights the potential for significant cost savings by reducing unnecessary MRIs before TKA, estimating millions of dollars could be saved annually in Ontario alone. It suggests that interventions such as educating primary care providers or restricting MRI ordering privileges could help optimize resource use. Future study could focus on quality improvement initiatives to further reduce unnecessary imaging and improve access to timely orthopedic care. By aligning practice with existing guidelines that recommend against routine MRI use in confirmed OA cases, healthcare systems can enhance efficiency and reduce wait times for joint replacement surgeries.

3.2.8 Attenuation Correction for PET/MRI to Measure Tracer Activity Surrounding Total Knee Arthroplasty [76]

This is a machine-generated summary of:

Bourdon, Caleigh E.; Koudys, Zachary J.; Lanting, Brent A.; Appleton, C. Thomas; Thiessen, Jonathan D.; Teeter, Matthew G. Attenuation correction for PET/MRI to measure tracer activity surrounding total knee arthroplasty [76].

Published in: European Journal of Hybrid Imaging (2022).

Link to original: https://doi.org/10.1186/s41824-022-00152-3

If you want to cite the papers, please refer to the original.

For technical reasons we could not place the page where the original quote is coming from.

3.2.8.1 Research Highlights

Total knee arthroplasty (TKA) is a common surgical procedure for treating severe osteoarthritis by replacing the knee joint with a metallic implant. While TKA often alleviates pain and enhances mobility, some patients experience complications such as inflammation, osteolysis, and infections, which are typically detected at advanced stages using conventional imaging techniques. These late-stage identifications complicate treatment and often necessitate revision surgeries. The study by Bourdon et al. explores a novel method to improve the accuracy of positron emission tomography/ magnetic resonance imaging (PET/MRI) in detecting early inflammatory processes around TKA implants by addressing the challenges posed by metal-induced signal attenuation.

The study utilized a segmentation-based attenuation correction (AC) approach that incorporates computer-aided design (CAD) models of TKA implants to enhance PET/MRI imaging accuracy. A cadaver knee with a cruciate-retaining TKA implant was used, and fluorodeoxyglucose (FDG) tracer vials were strategically placed around the implant. The researchers employed metal artifact reduction techniques during MRI acquisition and manually registered CAD models to the MR data to correct for signal voids caused by metal implants. By filling these voids with appropriate linear attenuation coefficients (LAC) based on implant materials, they generated accurate MR-based μ maps for PET data reconstruction. This method was compared against simpler AC approaches, demonstrating reduced errors in activity measurements near metal components.

The study's findings suggest that using implant CAD models significantly improves the reliability of PET/MRI measurements of cellular activity in knee joints post-TKA. The approach effectively reduces errors associated with metal-induced signal attenuation, offering potential for earlier detection and treatment of complications without revision surgeries. Future study could focus on automating the CAD model registration process to minimize inter-observer variability and enhance clinical applicability. Additionally, exploring alternative methods for cases where exact CAD models are unavailable could further refine this promising technique for broader clinical use.

3.2.9 Sagittal Magnetic Resonance Imaging-Scan Orientation Significantly Influences Accuracy of Femoral Posterior Condylar Offset Measurement [77]

This is a machine-generated summary of:

Balcarek, Peter; Hosseini, Ali Seif Amir; Streit, Ulrike; Brodkorb, Tobias Franz; Walde, Tim Alexander Sagittal magnetic resonance imaging-scan orientation significantly influences accuracy of femoral posterior condylar offset measurement [77].

Published in: Archives of Orthopaedic and Trauma Surgery (2017).

Link to original: https://doi.org/10.1007/s00402-017-2838-0

If you want to cite the papers, please refer to the original.

For technical reasons we could not place the page where the original quote is coming from.

3.2.9.1 Research Highlights

The concept of femoral posterior condylar offset (PCO) restoration has gained importance in recent years for its role in improving knee joint kinematics and range of motion following total knee arthroplasty (TKA). Accurate measurement of PCO is crucial, as it can influence femoral component positioning and potentially reduce complications such as flexion instability. Traditional methods using plain radiographs have limitations, prompting the use of magnetic resonance imaging for more precise measurements. However, the impact of sagittal scan orientation on PCO measurement accuracy has not been thoroughly investigated. The study by Balcarek et al. explores how simulated femur rotation affects the accuracy of medial and lateral PCO measurements.

The study involved MRI investigations of ten asymptomatic knee joints, using a proton density-weighted fat-suppressed MRI. The researchers defined a true-sagittal plane perpendicular to the transepicondylar axis and simulated mild femoral internal and external rotations by angulating sagittal images by ±3°. Each knee underwent three scans with different axial localizer scan angulations. Medial and lateral PCO sizes were measured independently by two blinded investigators using open-source PACS workstation software. The study assessed measurement accuracy through intra- and interrater reliability tests. Results indicated that simulated external rotation decreased medial PCO size, while internal rotation increased it, with lateral PCO size showing similar changes. The study found significant intra- and interrater reliability, although interrater reliability was less robust.

The findings highlight the sensitivity of PCO measurements to minor changes in MRI scan orientation, suggesting that even small degrees of femur rotation can introduce systematic errors. This underscores the need for standardized imaging protocols to ensure accurate PCO assessment, which is vital for TKA planning and prosthesis design. Future studies could explore the clinical relevance of these measurement variations and further investigate the relationship between PCO differences and knee joint kinematics. Additionally, expanding the sample size could provide more comprehensive insights into normative PCO values across diverse populations.

3.2.10 Can Rotational Alignment of Total Knee Arthroplasty Be Measured on MRI? [78]

This is a machine-generated summary of:

Sgroi, Mirco; Faschingbauer, M.; Javaheripour-Otto, K.; Reichel, H.; Kappe, T. Can rotational alignment of total knee arthroplasty be measured on MRI? [78].

Published in: Archives of Orthopaedic and Trauma Surgery (2015).

Link to original: https://doi.org/10.1007/s00402-015-2289-4

If you want to cite the papers, please refer to the original.

For technical reasons we could not place the page where the original quote is coming from.

3.2.10.1 Research Highlights

Total knee arthroplasty (TKA) aims to restore pain-free knee function, with correct rotational alignment being crucial for the prosthesis's function and longevity. Malrotation can lead to complications such as poor patellar tracking and flexion instability. Traditionally, computed tomography (CT) is the gold standard for assessing rotational alignment post-TKA, but it can be limited by artefacts from metallic components. Magnetic resonance imaging (MRI) has been considered as an alternative, though its accuracy compared to CT has not been fully validated. The study by Sgroi et al. investigates the accuracy and reliability of MRI versus CT in determining rotational alignment after TKA.

The study involved a cohort of patients scheduled for revision TKA, excluding those with cardiac pacemakers. Each patient underwent both CT and MRI scans using an artefact-reducing protocol. The femoral and tibial component orientations were measured on transverse slices from both imaging modalities. Two orthopaedic surgeons independently assessed the images to determine intraobserver and interobserver reliability. Statistical analysis was conducted using Pearson's correlation coefficient and the t-test to compare the measurements from CT and MRI. The results demonstrated a strong correlation between the two methods, particularly for tibial component measurements, with nearly perfect intrarater reliability.

The study suggests that MRI, when using an artefact-reduced protocol, can be a viable alternative to CT for evaluating rotational alignment after TKA. While the reliability of MRI was excellent for tibial components, it was only sufficient for femoral components, potentially due to sample size limitations and challenges in identifying anatomical landmarks. Future study could focus on larger patient cohorts or include asymptomatic controls to further validate these findings. Despite some limitations, this research indicates that MRI could offer a non-radiative option for assessing postoperative outcomes in TKA patients.

Bibliography

1. Papaioannou G, Nianios G, Mitrogiannis C, Fyhrie D, Tashman S, Yang KH. Patient-specific knee joint finite element model validation with high-accuracy kinematics from biplane dynamic roentgen stereogrammetric analysis. J Biomech. 2008;41(12):2633–8.
2. Nunley RM, Ellison BS, Zhu J, Ruh EL, Howell SM, Barrack RL. Do patient-specific guides improve coronal alignment in total knee arthroplasty? Clin Orthop Relat Res. 2012;470(3):895–902.
3. Nunley RM, Ellison BS, Ruh EL, Williams BM, Foreman K, Ford AD, et al. Are patient-specific cutting blocks cost-effective for total knee arthroplasty? Clin Orthop Relat Res. 2012;470(3):889–94.
4. Lombardi AV Jr, Berend KR, Adams JB. Patient-specific approach in total knee arthroplasty. Orthop. 2008;31(9):927–30.
5. Klatt, B. A., Goyal, N., Austin, M. S., and Hozack, W. J. (2008). Custom-fit total knee arthroplasty (otisknee) results in malalignment. *Journal of Arthroplasty, 23*(1), 26–29. https://doi.org/10.1016/j.arth.2007.10.001
6. Ng, V. Y., Declaire, J. H., Berend, K. R., Gulick, B. C., and Lombardi, A. V. (2012). Improved accuracy of alignment with patient-specific positioning guides compared with manual instrumentation in TKA. *Clinical Orthopaedics and Related Research*. https://doi.org/10.1007/s11999-011-1996-6
7. Spencer, B. A., Mont, M. A., McGrath, M. S., Boyd, B., and Mitrick, M. F. (2009). Initial experience with custom-fit total knee replacement: Intra-operative events and long-leg coronal alignment. *International Orthopaedics, 33*(6), 1571–1575. https://doi.org/10.1007/s00264-008-0693-x
8. White D, Chelule KL, Seedhom BB. Accuracy of MRI vs CT imaging with particular reference to patient specific templates for total knee replacement surgery. Int J Med Robot. 2008;4(3):224–31.
9. Pfitzner T, Abdel MP, von Roth P, Perka C, Hommel H. Small improvements in mechanical axis alignment achieved with MRI versus CT-based patient-specific instruments in TKA: a randomized clinical trial. Clin Orthop Relat Res. 2014;472(10):2913–22.
10. Silva A, Pinto E, Sampaio R. Rotational alignment in patient-specific instrumentation in TKA: MRI or CT? Knee Surg, Sports Traumatol, Arthrosc : Official J ESSKA. 2016;24(11):3648–52.

11. Asada S, Mori S, Matsushita T, Nakagawa K, Tsukamoto I, Akagi M. Comparison of MRI- and CT-based patient-specific guides for total knee arthroplasty. Knee. 2014;21(6):1238–43.
12. Cicuttini FM, Jones G, Forbes A, Wluka AE. Rate of cartilage loss at two years predicts subsequent total knee arthroplasty: a prospective study. Ann Rheum Dis. 2004;63(9):1124–7.
13. Yu A, Heilmeier U, Kretzschmar M, Joseph GB, Liu F, Liebl H, et al. Racial differences in biochemical knee cartilage composition between African-American and Caucasian-American women with 3 T MR-based T2 relaxation time measurements—data from the Osteoarthritis Initiative. Osteoarthritis Cartilage. 2015;23(9):1595–604.
14. Mosher TJ, Dardzinski BJ, Cartilage MRI. T2 relaxation time mapping: overview and applications. Semin Musculoskelet Radiol. 2004;8(4):355–68.
15. Haralick RM. Statistical and structured approaches to texture. Proc IEEE. 1979;67(5):786–804.
16. Eitner A, Hofmann GO, Schaible HG. Mechanisms of osteoarthritic pain. Studies in humans and experimental models. Front Mol Neurosci. 2017;10:349.
17. Kellgren JH, Lawrence JS. Radiological assessment of osteoarthrosis. Ann Rheum Dis. 1957;16(4):494–502.
18. Gersing AS, Schwaiger BJ, Nevitt MC, Joseph GB, Chanchek N, Guimaraes JB, et al. Is weight loss associated with less progression of changes in knee articular cartilage among obese and overweight patients as assessed with MR imaging over 48 months? Data from the Osteoarthritis Initiative. Radiology. 2017;284(2):508–20.
19. Willcox, N. M. J., Clarke, J. V., Smith, B. R. K., Deakin, A. H., and Deep, K. (2012). A comparison of radiological and computer navigation measurements of lower limb coronal alignment before and after total knee replacement. *The Journal of Bone and Joint Surgery Series B, 94*, 1234–1240. https://doi.org/10.1302/0301-620X.94B9.28250
20. Scott, W. N. (2017). *Insall and Scott surgery of the knee*. (6th ed.). Churchill Livingstone/Elsevier.
21. Tokuhara, Y., Kadoya, Y., Kanekasu, K., Kondo, M., Kobayashi, A., and Takaoka, K. (2006). Evaluation of the flexion gap by axial radiography of the distal femur. *The Journal of Bone and Joint Surgery Series B, 88*, 1327–1330. https://doi.org/10.1302/0301-620X.88B1017793
22. Tokuhara, Y., Kadoya, Y., Nakagawa, S., Kobayashi, A., Takaoka, K., and Surgeon, O. (2004). The flexion gap in normal knees AN MRI STUDY. *The Journal of Bone and Joint Surgery [British Volume], 86*, 1133–1139. https://doi.org/10.1302/0301-620X.86B8
23. Deep, K. (2014). Collateral ligament laxity in knees: what is normal? *Clinical Orthopaedics and Related Research, 472*, 3426–3431. https://doi.org/10.1007/s11999-014-3865-6
24. Okazaki, K., Miura, H., Matsuda, S., Takeuchi, N., Mawatari, T., Hashizume, M., et al. (2006). Asymmetry of mediolateral laxity of the normal knee. *Journal*

of Orthopaedic Science, 11, 264–266. https://doi.org/10.1007/s00776-006-1009-x
25. Yoo, J. C., Ahn, J. H., Sung, K. S., Wang, J. H., Lee, S. H., Bae, S. W., et al. (2006). Measurement and comparison of the difference in normal medial and lateral knee joint opening. *Knee Surgery, Sport Traumatology, Arthroscopy, 14*, 1238–1244. https://doi.org/10.1007/s00167-006-0095-9
26. Bellemans J, Banks S, Victor J, Vandenneucker H, Moemans A (2002) Fluoroscopic analysys of the kinematics of deep flexion in total knee arthroplasty. J Bone Joint Surg Br 84:50–53
27. Arabori M, Matsui N, Kuroda R, Mizuno K, Doita M, Kurosaka M, Yoshiya S. Posterior condylar offset and flexion in posterior cruciate-retaining and posterior stabilized TKA. *J Orthop Sci.* 2008;13:46–50.
28. Malviya A, Lingard EA, Weir DJ, Deehan DJ. Predicting range of movement after knee replacement: the importance of posterior condylar offset and tibial slope. *Knee Surg Sports Traumatol Arthrosc*. 2009;17:491–498.
29. Onodera T, Majima T, Nishiike O, Kasahara Y, Takahashi D. Posterior femoral condylar offset after total knee replacement in the risk of knee flexion contracture. *J Arthroplasty*. 2012 Nov 1 pii: S0883-5403(12)00557-8. https://doi.org/10.1016/j.arth.2012.07.029 [Epub ahead of print].
30. Seo SS, Ha DJ, Kim CW, Choi JS. Effect of posterior condylar offset on cruciate-retaining mobile TKA. *Orthopedics*. 2009;32:44–48.
31. Soda Y, Oishi J, Nakasa T, Nishikawa K, Ochi M. New parameter of flexion after posterior stabilized total knee arthroplasty: posterior condylar offset ratio on X-ray photographs. *Arch Orthop Trauma Surg*. 2007;127:167–170.
32. Kessler O, Patil S, Colwell CW Jr, D'Lima DD. The effect of femoral component malrotation on patellar biomechanics. *J Biomech*. 2008;41:3332–3339.
33. Rhoads DD, Noble PC, Reuben JD, Tullos HS. The effect of femoral component position on the kinematics of total knee arthroplasty. *Clin Orthop Relat Res*. 1993;286:122–129.
34. Kerkhoffs GM, Servien E, Dunn W, et al. The influence of obesity on the complication rate and outcome of total knee arthroplasty: a meta-analysis and systematic literature review. J Bone Joint Surg Am. 2012;94(20):1839–44. https://doi.org/10.2106/JBJS.K.00820.
35. Si HB, Zeng Y, Shen B, et al. The influence of body mass index on the outcomes of primary total knee arthroplasty. Knee Surg Sports Traumatol Arthrosc. 2015;23(6):1824–32. https://doi.org/10.1007/s00167-014-3301-1.
36. Sun K, Li H. Body mass index as a predictor of outcome in total knee replace: a systemic review and meta-analysis. Knee. 2017;24(5):917–24. https://doi.org/10.1016/j.knee.2017.05.022.
37. Giesinger JM, Loth FL, MacDonald DJ, et al. Patient-reported outcome metrics following total knee arthroplasty are influenced differently by patients' body mass index. Knee Surg Sports Traumatol Arthrosc. 2018;26(11):3257–64. https://doi.org/10.1007/s00167-018-4853-2.

38. Girardi FM, Liu J, Guo Z, et al. The impact of obesity on resource utilization among patients undergoing total joint arthroplasty. Int Orthop. 2019;43(2):269–74. https://doi.org/10.1007/s00264-018-4059-8.
39. Brown, M. J. C., Vella-Baldacchino, M., O'Flaherty, E. and Jenkins, P. J. Predicting patient reported outcome in total knee arthroplasty using body mass index and limb measurements. *Knee 25*, 915–922 (2018).
40. Visser AW, de Mutsert R, Loef M, et al. The role of fat mass and skeletal muscle mass in knee osteoarthritis is different for men and women: the NEO study. Osteoarthritis Cartilage. 2014;22(2):197–202. https://doi.org/10.1016/j.joca.2013.12.002.
41. Watts CD, Houdek MT, Wagner ER, et al. Subcutaneous fat thickness is associated with early reoperation and infection after total knee arthroplasty in morbidly obese patients. J Arthroplasty. 2016;31(8):1788–91. https://doi.org/10.1016/j.arth.2016.02.008.
42. Xu S, Chen JY, Lo NN, et al. The influence of obesity on functional outcome and quality of life after total knee arthroplasty: a ten-year follow-up study. Bone Joint J. 2018;100-B(5):579–83. https://doi.org/10.1302/0301-620X.100B5.BJJ-2017-1263.R1.
43. Overgaard A, Lidgren L, Sundberg M, et al. Patient-reported 1-year outcome not affected by body mass index in 3,327 total knee arthroplasty patients. Acta Orthop. 2019;90(4):360–5. https://doi.org/10.1080/17453674.2019.1604940.
44. Sveikata T, Porvaneckas N, Kanopa P, et al. Age, sex, body mass index, education, and social support influence functional results after total knee arthroplasty. Geriatr Orthop Surg Rehabil. 2017;8(2):71–7. https://doi.org/10.1177/2151458516687809.
45. Thijs E, Theeuwen D, Boonen B, van Haaren E, Hendrickx R, Vos R et al (2020) Comparable clinical outcome and implant longevity after CT- or MRI-based patient-specific instruments for total knee arthroplasty: a 2-year follow-up of a RCT. Knee Surg Sports Traumatol Arthrosc 28(6):1821–1826. https://doi.org/10.1007/s00167-019-05616-x
46. Schotanus MGM, Sollie R, van Haaren EH, Hendrickx RPM, Jansen EJP, Kort NP (2016) A radiological analysis of the difference between MRI- and CT-based patient-specific matched guides for total knee arthroplasty from the same manufacturer: a randomized controlled trial. Bone Jt J 98-B(6):786–92. https://doi.org/10.1302/0301-620X.98B6.36633
47. Kang Dong-Geun, Bae Jung-Kwon, Kim Kang-II (2021) MRI-based or CT-based patient-specific instrumentation in total knee arthroplasty: how do the two systems compare? Arthroplasty. https://doi.org/10.1186/s42836-019-0020-6
48. Newman S, Ahmed H, Rehmatullah N (2022) Radiographic vs. MRI vs. arthroscopic assessment and grading of knee osteoarthritis-are we using appropriate imaging? J Exp Orthop 9:1–6
49. Stanley AL, Edwards TC, Jaere MD, Lex JR, Jones GG (2023) An automated, web-based triage tool may optimise referral pathways in elective orthopaedic surgery: a proof-of-concept study. Digit Health 9:20552076231152176

50. Weiner JP, Abrams C (2011) The Johns Hopkins ACG® System: Technical Reference Guide Version 10.0
51. Korbin S et al (2020) PET/MRI reveals ongoing metabolic activity in ACL grafts one year post-ACL reconstruction. J Exp Orthop. https://doi.org/10.1186/s40634-020-00258-2
52. Vignal N, Cisternino S, Rizzo-Padoin N, San C, Hontonnou F, Gelé T et al (2018) [18F]FEPPA a TSPO radioligand: optimized radiosynthesis and evaluation as a PET radiotracer for brain inflammation in a peripheral LPS-injected mouse model. Molecules 23(6):1375
53. Wagenknecht G, Kaiser HJ, Mottaghy FM, Herzog H (2013) MRI for attenuation correction in PET: methods and challenges. Magn Reson Mater Phy 26:99–113
54. Ladefoged CN, Andersen FL, Keller SH, Löfgren J, Hansen AE, Holm S, Højgaard L, Beyer T (2013) PET/MR imaging of the pelvis in the presence of endoprostheses: reducing image artifacts and increasing accuracy through inpainting. Eur J Nucl Med Mol Imaging 40(4):594–601
55. Schramm G, Maus J, Hofheinz F, Petr J, Lougovski A, Beuthien-Baumann B, Platzek I, van den Hoff J (2014) Evaluation and automatic correction of metal-implant-induced artifacts in MR-based attenuation correction in whole-body PET/MR imaging. Phys Med Biol 59:2713
56. Voleti PB, Stephenson JW, Lotke PA, Lee GC (2014) Plain radiographs underestimate the asymmetry of the posterior condylar offset of the knee compared with MRI. Clin Orthop Relat Res 472:155–161
57. Voleti PB, Stephenson JW, Lotke PA, Lee GC (2015) No sex differences exist in posterior condylar offsets of the knee. Clin Orthop Relat Res 473:1425–1431
58. Cinotti G, Sessa P, Ripani FR, Postacchini R, Masciangelo R, Giannicola G (2012) Correlation between posterior offset of femoral condyles and sagittal slope of the tibial plateau. J Anat 221:452–458
59. Frosch S, Brodkorb T, Schüttrumpf JP, Wachowski MM, Walde TA, Stürmer KM, Balcarek P (2014) Characteristics of femorotibial joint geometry in the trochlear dysplastic femur. J Anat 225:367–373
60. Wernecke GC, Seeto BG, Chen DB, MacDessi SJ (2016) Posterior condylar cartilage thickness and posterior condylar offset of the femur: a magnetic resonance imaging study. J Orthop Surg (Hong Kong) 24:12–15
61. Weinberg DS, Streit JJ, Gebhart JJ, Williamson DF, Goldberg VM (2015) Important differences exist in posterior condylar offsets in an osteological collection of 1058 femurs. J Arthroplasty 30:1434–1438
62. Gungor HR, Ok N, Agladioglu K, Akkaya S, Kiter E (2014) Significance of asymmetrical posteromedial and posterolateral femoral condylar chamfer cuts in total knee arthroplasty. Knee Surg Sports Traumatol Arthrosc 22:2989–2994
63. Bell SW, Young P, Drury C, Smith J, Anthony I, Jones B, Blyth M, McLean A (2014) Component rotational alignment in unexplained painful primary total knee arthroplasty. Knee 21(1):272–277
64. Victor J (2009) Rotational alignment of the distal femur: a literature review. Orthop Traumatol Surg Res 95:365–372

65. Hung CLW, Pan YW, Yuen CK, Bong LH, Sha LWL, Man SWH (2009) Interobserver and intraobserver error in distal femur transepicondylar axis measurement with computed tomography. J Arthroplasty 24:96–100
66. Heyse TJ, le Chong R, Davis J, Boettner F, Haas SB, Potter HG (2012) MRI analysis for rotation of total knee components. Knee 19:571–575
67. Murakami AM, Hash TW, Hepinstall MS, Lyman S, Nestor BJ, Potter HG (2012) MRI evaluation of rotational alignment and synovitis in patients with pain after total knee replacement. J Bone Joint Surg Br 94:1209–1215
68. Berger RA, Rubash HE, Seel MJ, Thompson WH, Crossett LS (1993) Determining the rotational alignment of the femoral component in total knee arthroplasty using the epicondylar axis. Clin Orthop Relat Res 286:40–47
69. Kang, Dong-Geun; Kim, Kang-Il; Bae, Jung-Kwon MRI-based or CT-based patient-specific instrumentation in Total knee Arthroplasty: How do the two systems compare?. Arthroplasty (2020). https://doi.org/10.1186/s42836-019-0020-6
70. Heilmeier, Ursula; Wamba, John Mbapte; Joseph, Gabby B.; Darakananda, Karin; Callan, Jennifer; Neumann, Jan; Link, Thomas M. Baseline knee joint effusion and medial femoral bone marrow edema, in addition to MRI-based T2 relaxation time and texture measurements of knee cartilage, can help predict incident total knee arthroplasty 4–7 years later: data from the Osteoarthritis Initiative. Skeletal Radiology (2018). https://doi.org/10.1007/s00256-018-2995-4
71. Pathak, Subodh Kumar; Sethi, Manish; Salunke, Abhijeet Ashok; Thivari, Praveen; Gautam, Rakesh Kumar; Anjum, Rashid; Chawla, Jasneet; Sharma, Aryan Is Flexion Gap Rectangular in Native Indian Knees? Results of an MRI Study. Indian Journal of Orthopaedics (2021). https://doi.org/10.1007/s43465-021-00418-1
72. Voleti, Pramod B.; Stephenson, Jason W.; Lotke, Paul A.; Lee, Gwo-Chin Plain Radiographs Underestimate the Asymmetry of the Posterior Condylar Offset of the Knee Compared With MRI. Clinical Orthopaedics and Related Research® (2013). https://doi.org/10.1007/s11999-013-2946-2
73. Zhao, Guanglei; Liu, Changquan; Chen, Kangming; Chen, Feiyan; Lyu, Jinyang; Chen, Jie; Shi, Jingsheng; Huang, Gangyong; Wei, Yibing; Wang, Siqun; Xia, Jun Predictive value of adipose to muscle area ratio based on MRI at knee joint for postoperative functional outcomes in elderly osteoarthritis patients following total knee arthroplasty. Journal of Orthopaedic Surgery and Research (2020). https://doi.org/10.1186/s13018-020-02014-9
74. Theeuwen, D. M. J.; Haveman, I.; Boonen, B.; van Haaren, E. H.; Hendrickx, R. P. M.; Schotanus, M. G. M. No differences in mid-term survival and clinical outcome between CT- and MRI-based patient-specific instrumentation for total knee arthroplasty, a randomized controlled trial. European Journal of Orthopaedic Surgery & Traumatology (2023). https://doi.org/10.1007/s00590-023-03680-1
75. Lung, Tiffany; Lex, Johnathan R.; Pincus, Daniel; Gatley, Jodi; Wasserstein, David; Paterson, J. Michael; Ravi, Bheeshma MRI use leading up to total knee

arthroplasty: a retrospective cohort study. European Journal of Orthopaedic Surgery & Traumatology (2024). https://doi.org/10.1007/s00590-024-03940-8
76. Bourdon, Caleigh E.; Koudys, Zachary J.; Lanting, Brent A.; Appleton, C. Thomas; Thiessen, Jonathan D.; Teeter, Matthew G. Attenuation correction for PET/MRI to measure tracer activity surrounding total knee arthroplasty. European Journal of Hybrid Imaging (2022). https://doi.org/10.1186/s41824-022-00152-3
77. Balcarek, Peter; Hosseini, Ali Seif Amir; Streit, Ulrike; Brodkorb, Tobias Franz; Walde, Tim Alexander Sagittal magnetic resonance imaging-scan orientation significantly influences accuracy of femoral posterior condylar offset measurement. Archives of Orthopaedic and Trauma Surgery (2017). https://doi.org/10.1007/s00402-017-2838-0
78. Sgroi, Mirco; Faschingbauer, M.; Javaheripour-Otto, K.; Reichel, H.; Kappe, T. Can rotational alignment of total knee arthroplasty be measured on MRI?. Archives of Orthopaedic and Trauma Surgery (2015). https://doi.org/10.1007/s00402-015-2289-4

3.3 CT

Machine Generated Summaries

Disclaimer: The summaries in this chapter were generated from Springer Nature publications using abstractive AI auto-summarization: An abstraction-based summarizer creates new text based on deep learning. New phrases are created to summarize the content. As the constituted sentences are machine selected, they may not fully reflect the body of the work, so we strongly advise that the original content is read and cited. The auto-generated summaries were curated by the editor to meet Springer Nature publication standards.

3.3.1 Intra- and Inter-Observer Reliability of Implant Positioning Evaluation on a CT-Based Three-Dimensional Postoperative Matching System for Total Knee Arthroplasty [85]

This is a machine-generated summary of:

Watanabe, Shotaro; Akagi, Ryuichiro; Shiko, Yuki; Ono, Yoshimasa; Kawasaki, Yohei; Ohdera, Toshihiro; Ohtori, Seiji; Sasho, Takahisa Intra- and inter-observer reliability of implant positioning evaluation on a CT-based three-dimensional postoperative matching system for total knee arthroplasty [85].

Published in: BMC Musculoskeletal Disorders (2021).

Link to original: https://doi.org/10.1186/s12891-021-04228-2

If you want to cite the papers, please refer to the original.

For technical reasons we could not place the page where the original quote is coming from.

3.3.1.1 Research Highlights

Malposition of prostheses in total knee arthroplasty (TKA) can adversely affect clinical outcomes and the longevity of the implant. Traditional surgical techniques using intra- and extra-medullary guides often achieve accurate prosthesis positioning, but anatomical variations and surgical factors can lead to errors. Computer-assisted intraoperative navigation has shown promise in improving implant positioning accuracy. However, the reproducibility of postoperative alignment evaluation methods remains a concern, as many rely on plain radiographs, which may not provide sufficient accuracy. The study by Watanabe et al. explores the reliability of a CT-based evaluation system for assessing TKA component positioning post-surgery.

The study involved analyzing anonymized CT images from patients who underwent primary TKA, using a CT-based preoperative planning and postoperative evaluation system. Three experienced orthopedic surgeons independently evaluated the images, focusing on two reference axes: the traditional mechanical axis and an implant-based axis. The study aimed to measure intra- and inter-observer reliabilities in evaluating TKA component positioning using these axes. The researchers found that while both axes provided very good reliability for most measurements, the sagittal alignment assessment of the femoral component was less reliable due to difficulties in image matching caused by implant halation.

The study highlights that CT-based imaging techniques offer better accuracy for evaluating postoperative implant alignment compared to traditional radiography methods. By minimizing implant halation, the implant-based axis provides reliable reference points for evaluation when anatomical landmarks are difficult to identify. Future study could focus on refining image acquisition protocols to further reduce radiation exposure and improve measurement accuracy. Additionally, exploring rotational alignment assessment could enhance the comprehensive evaluation of TKA components post-surgery. The findings suggest that while both traditional and implant-based axes are useful, slight differences between them should be considered when interpreting results.

3.3.2 Symptomatic Versus Asymptomatic Knees after Bilateral Total Knee Arthroplasty: What Is the Difference in SPECT/CT? [86]

This is a machine-generated summary of:

Awengen, R.; Rasch, H.; Amsler, F.; Hirschmann, M. T. Symptomatic versus asymptomatic knees after bilateral total knee arthroplasty: what is the difference in SPECT/CT? [86].

Published in: European Journal of Nuclear Medicine and Molecular Imaging (2015).

Link to original: https://doi.org/10.1007/s00259-015-3278-0

If you want to cite the papers, please refer to the original.

For technical reasons we could not place the page where the original quote is coming from.

3.3.2.1 Research Highlights

Total knee arthroplasty (TKA) is a widely used treatment for end-stage osteoarthritis, yet many patients experience persistent pain post-surgery, with a significant percentage remaining dissatisfied. Diagnosing the cause of this pain can be challenging, often requiring advanced imaging techniques beyond standard radiographs. Single photon emission computed tomography combined with computed tomography (SPECT/CT) has emerged as a valuable tool in this context, offering enhanced sensitivity and specificity. The study by Awengen et al. investigates the differences in bone tracer uptake (BTU) between symptomatic and asymptomatic knees following bilateral TKA, aiming to identify patterns related to component position and alignment.

The study retrospectively analyzed data from patients who underwent staged bilateral primary TKA and reported unilateral knee pain. A standardized diagnostic algorithm was employed, including clinical examinations and SPECT/CT imaging. The researchers assessed mechanical alignment and TKA component position using validated software, mapping BTU across various anatomical zones. Statistical analyses were conducted to compare BTU patterns between symptomatic and asymptomatic knees. The findings revealed that symptomatic knees exhibited higher BTU across all regions compared to asymptomatic ones, with significant differences in component positioning noted, particularly in sagittal and rotational orientations.

This study advances our understanding of post-TKA pain by establishing BTU intensity thresholds that may indicate pathology. It highlights the importance of optimal prosthesis positioning to minimize postoperative complications. Future study could focus on larger patient cohorts to validate these findings further and explore the potential for quantitative BTU analysis in clinical practice. The insights gained could refine diagnostic algorithms and improve patient outcomes by tailoring interventions based on specific BTU patterns associated with mechanical alignment issues.

3.3.3 Inter-Observer Validation Study of Quantitative CT-Osteodensitometry in Total Knee Arthroplasty [87]

This is a machine-generated summary of:

Reilly, Keryn; Munro, Jacob; Pandit, Salil; Kress, Alexander; Walker, Cameron; Pitto, Rocco Paolo Inter-observer validation study of quantitative CT-osteodensitometry in total knee arthroplasty [87].

Published in: Archives of Orthopaedic and Trauma Surgery (2007).

Link to original: https://doi.org/10.1007/s00402-007-0351-6

If you want to cite the papers, please refer to the original.

For technical reasons we could not place the page where the original quote is coming from.

3.3.3.1 Research Highlights

Proximal tibial bone quality and bone mineral density (BMD) are crucial factors influencing the migration of implants following total knee arthroplasty (TKA). While dual-energy X-ray absorptiometry (DXA) has been widely used to measure BMD post-operatively, it is limited to two-dimensional analysis and cannot differentiate between cortical and cancellous bone. The study by Reilly et al. explores the use of quantitative computerized tomography (CT) osteodensitometry, a method that provides three-dimensional, volumetric analysis of both cortical and cancellous regions, to evaluate its reproducibility in measuring BMD in the proximal tibia.

The study involved an in vitro assessment using four cadaveric lower limbs fitted with PFC Sigma implants. Each limb underwent CT scanning at specific intervals both with and without the prosthesis. This process was repeated to ensure consistency, resulting in scans that were analyzed using specialized software to measure BMD in Hounsfield units. An inter-observer validation study was conducted where two observers independently measured cortical and cancellous BMD from selected slices. The results demonstrated a high correlation coefficient greater than 0.9 for all slices, indicating strong agreement between observers. Bland–Altman analysis further confirmed an acceptable level of inter-observer variability, supporting the method's reliability.

The study advances the understanding of BMD measurement techniques by demonstrating that quantitative CT osteodensitometry is a reproducible method for assessing bone density changes around the knee with minimal observer variation. This approach allows for independent analysis of cortical and cancellous BMD, which could enhance post-operative assessments following TKA. Future study could focus on clinical applications of this technology to assess bone density changes over time in patients receiving different types of tibial components. Additionally, further research may address the impact of metal scatter from implants on BMD measurements to refine this promising technique for broader clinical use.

3.3.4 4D-SPECT/CT in Orthopaedics: A New Method of Combined Quantitative Volumetric 3D Analysis of SPECT/CT Tracer Uptake and Component Position Measurements in Patients after Total Knee Arthroplasty [88]

This is a machine-generated summary of:

Rasch, Helmut; Falkowski, Anna L.; Forrer, Flavio; Henckel, Johann; Hirschmann, Michael T. 4D-SPECT/CT in orthopaedics: a new method of combined quantitative volumetric 3D analysis of SPECT/CT tracer uptake and component position measurements in patients after total knee arthroplasty [88].

Published in: Skeletal Radiology (2013).

Link to original: https://doi.org/10.1007/s00256-013-1643-2

If you want to cite the papers, please refer to the original.

For technical reasons we could not place the page where the original quote is coming from.

3.3.4.1 Research Highlights

Single-photon emission computed tomography (SPECT/CT) is increasingly utilized in diagnostic imaging, particularly for orthopedic patients experiencing complications after total knee arthroplasty (TKA). This imaging modality combines functional, structural, and mechanical information, offering significant clinical benefits. However, conventional analysis techniques often focus solely on areas of increased tracer intensity, neglecting regions of decreased intensity that may also be clinically relevant. The study by Rasch et al. introduces a novel method for volumetric quantification, normalization, and thresholding of SPECT data to enhance diagnostic accuracy in patients with painful TKA.

The study involved a prospective collection of SPECT/CT data from patients experiencing persistent pain after TKA. Excluding those who had undergone revision TKA, the researchers employed a hybrid system combining dual-head camera technology with integrated diagnostic CT. The analysis focused on the delayed phase SPECT/CT images using a validated anatomical localization scheme to measure tracer uptake in tibial, femoral, and patellar regions. The study assessed inter- and intra-observer reliability through intraclass correlation coefficients (ICCs) and Kappa statistics. Results demonstrated very good reliability for tracer uptake intensity measurements across most regions, with the femoral shaft serving as an ideal reference for normalizing SPECT data.

The study's findings suggest that this combined quantitative approach to analyzing SPECT tracer uptake and TKA component positioning offers a reliable method for assessing biomechanics in post-TKA patients. The method's high reproducibility and ease of application make it suitable for clinical use, potentially serving as both a screening tool and an outcome measure in clinical trials. Future study could explore its application in identifying specific pathological conditions such as component loosening or misalignment. The authors recommend further investigation into its clinical value through prospective studies to establish typical SPECT/CT tracer uptake patterns associated with various pathologies.

3.3.5 Inter- and Intra-Observer Reliability of Two-Dimensional CT Scan for Total Knee Rrthroplasty Component Malrotation [89]

This is a machine-generated summary of:

Konigsberg, Beau; Hess, Ryan; Hartman, Curtis; Smith, Lynette; Garvin, Kevin L. Inter- and Intraobserver Reliability of Two-dimensional CT Scan for Total Knee Arthroplasty Component Malrotation [89].

Published in: Clinical Orthopaedics and Related Research® (2013).

Link to original: https://doi.org/10.1007/s11999-013-3111-7

If you want to cite the papers, please refer to the original.

For technical reasons we could not place the page where the original quote is coming from.

3.3.5.1 Research Highlights

Total knee arthroplasty (TKA) is a common procedure with generally excellent outcomes, but a subset of patients experience complications such as knee pain, stiffness, and patellar instability. These issues are often attributed to rotational malalignment of the femoral and tibial components, which can lead to revision surgeries. Accurate measurement of component rotation is crucial for diagnosing malrotation before recommending revision surgery. Traditional methods like clinical assessment and plain radiography have limitations in detecting subtle malrotations. The study by Konigsberg et al. investigates the reliability of three-dimensional (3D) computerized tomography (CT) scans in measuring TKA component rotation, addressing a significant gap in the literature regarding intra- and interobserver reliability.

The study involved 50 patients who underwent 3D CT scans to evaluate potential revision surgery due to suspected malrotation-related complications. The researchers used an established protocol to measure femoral and tibial component rotations at specific anatomical landmarks. Two observers—a reconstruction surgeon and a musculoskeletal radiologist—assessed interobserver reliability, while intraobserver reliability was determined by repeated measurements from an orthopedic resident and attending surgeon. The study employed intraclass correlation coefficients (ICCs) to quantify reliability, finding that interobserver reliability ranged from fair to good, with better results for the tibial component than the femoral. Intraobserver reliability was generally good to very good, though variability in measurements was noted.

The findings suggest that while 3D CT scans provide a reliable method for assessing TKA component rotation, there is still notable variability that could impact clinical decision-making. The study highlights the need for careful consideration when using CT measurements to attribute symptoms or recommend revision surgery. Future study could explore larger sample sizes or different practice settings to validate these findings further. Additionally, integrating known control values might help identify potential biases in measurement accuracy. Despite its limitations, this research underscores the importance of precise measurement techniques in improving patient outcomes following TKA.

3.3.6 Clinical Value of SPECT/CT in the Painful Total Knee Arthroplasty (TKA): A Prospective Study in a Consecutive Series of 100 TKA [90]

This is a machine-generated summary of:

Hirschmann, Michael T.; Amsler, Felix; Rasch, Helmut Clinical value of SPECT/CT in the painful total knee arthroplasty (TKA): a prospective study in a consecutive series of 100 TKA [90].

Published in: European Journal of Nuclear Medicine and Molecular Imaging (2015).

Link to original: https://doi.org/10.1007/s00259-015-3095-5

If you want to cite the papers, please refer to the original.

For technical reasons we could not place the page where the original quote is coming from.

3.3.6.1 Research Highlights

Total knee arthroplasty (TKA) is a common procedure for alleviating knee pain and restoring function, yet a significant percentage of patients remain dissatisfied post-surgery, often experiencing persistent pain. Traditional diagnostic methods such as radiographs, computerized tomography (CT), and magnetic resonance imaging (MRI) frequently fail to pinpoint the exact cause of these issues due to the complex interplay of potential factors like infection, loosening, or malposition. The study by Hirschmann et al. explores the efficacy of a standardized diagnostic algorithm incorporating SPECT/CT imaging to improve diagnosis and treatment outcomes for patients with unresolved issues following TKA.

The study involved a prospective analysis of knees from patients experiencing persistent pain after primary TKA. Excluding those with prior revision surgeries or infections, each patient underwent clinical evaluations and SPECT/CT imaging as part of a routine diagnostic protocol. The SPECT/CT method utilized Tc-HDP injections and advanced imaging techniques to assess bone tracer uptake patterns and TKA component positioning in three dimensions. The researchers meticulously analyzed these images to identify correlations between component malposition, bone tracer uptake, and specific pathologies such as loosening or patellofemoral osteoarthritis. Statistical analyses confirmed that SPECT/CT significantly altered the clinical diagnosis and treatment plan in a substantial number of cases.

The study's findings underscore the potential of SPECT/CT to enhance diagnostic accuracy for post-TKA complications by providing detailed insights into bone remodeling processes and component alignment. Typical patterns of bone tracer uptake were identified for various conditions, offering a foundation for developing guidelines for interpreting SPECT/CT results in this context. Future study could focus on establishing specific bone tracer uptake thresholds indicative of pathologies, which would require larger patient samples. Additionally, improved collaboration between orthopedic surgeons and nuclear medicine specialists is essential for optimizing the use of SPECT/CT in clinical practice.

3.3.7 Comparing Supine CT Scanogram and Standing Long-Leg Radiograph for Postoperative Alignment in Total Knee Arthroplasty: A Prospective Study [91]

This is a machine-generated summary of:

Mhaskar, Vikram Arun; Saggar, Rachit; Karan, Satyabrat; Maheshwari, Jitendra Comparing supine CT scanogram and standing long-leg radiograph for postoperative alignment in total knee arthroplasty: a prospective study [91].

Published in: Archives of Orthopaedic and Trauma Surgery (2024).

Link to original: https://doi.org/10.1007/s00402-024-05743-2

If you want to cite the papers, please refer to the original.

For technical reasons we could not place the page where the original quote is coming from.

3.3.7.1 Research Highlights

Total knee arthroplasty (TKA) success heavily depends on precise postoperative alignment, as even minor deviations can lead to early implant failure and reduced patient satisfaction. Achieving mechanical alignment within ±3° of the 'Zero' axis in the coronal plane is a well-accepted surgical target, with malalignment potentially causing imbalanced loading and accelerated wear. Traditional methods like long leg standing radiographs (LLR) are considered the gold standard for assessing alignment but have limitations, especially in the immediate postoperative period. The study by Mhaskar et al. explores the use of supine computed tomography scanogram (CTS) as an alternative to LLR for evaluating coronal alignment post-TKA.

In this prospective comparative study, patients undergoing primary patient-specific TKA were assessed using both CTS on postoperative day 2 and LLR at 6 weeks postoperatively. The study included patients over 18 years with no prior surgery on the involved limb. Surgeries were performed using a medial parapatellar approach, with distal femoral cuts adjusted based on patient-specific valgus correction angles measured preoperatively. Postoperative coronal alignment was measured using standardized reconstructions from CTS and compared to LLR measurements. The study found that CTS provided similar coronal alignment measurements to LLR, with a mean difference of only 0.3°, which was not statistically significant. Inter-observer reliability was excellent for both modalities, although CTS showed slightly higher intraclass correlation coefficients.

While CTS offers practical benefits such as avoiding weight-bearing requirements and allowing immediate postoperative assessment, its variability suggests it should be used cautiously when precise alignment is critical. The study highlights that while CTS can be a useful tool for early decision-making or in non-ambulatory patients, LLR remains more reliable for ensuring accurate alignment due to its standardized protocols and ability to account for dynamic loading. Future studies could focus on improving CTS protocols and exploring its role in complex cases requiring immediate intervention.

3.3.8 Could Surgical Transepicondylar Axis Be Identified Accurately in Preoperative 3D Planning for Total Knee Arthroplasty? A Reproducibility Study Based on 3D-CT [92]

This is a machine-generated summary of:

Lei, Kai; Liu, Li Ming; Luo, Jiang Ming; Ma, Chao; Feng, Qing; Yang, Liu; Guo, Lin Could surgical transepicondylar axis be identified accurately in preoperative 3D planning for total knee arthroplasty? A reproducibility study based on 3D-CT [92].

Published in: Arthroplasty (2022).

Link to original: https://doi.org/10.1186/s42836-022-00147-2

If you want to cite the papers, please refer to the original.

For technical reasons we could not place the page where the original quote is coming from.

3.3.8.1 Research Highlights

Total knee arthroplasty (TKA) is a widely used procedure for managing late-stage knee osteoarthritis, with the goal of achieving balanced extension and flexion gaps to ensure satisfactory soft tissue balance. A key factor in achieving this balance is the accurate rotation of the femoral component, as malrotation can lead to complications such as pain and reduced implant longevity. The surgical transepicondylar axis (sTEA) is considered the best reference for determining femoral component rotation, but its identification during surgery can be challenging due to factors like poor visibility and individual differences among surgeons. The study by Lei et al. investigates the reproducibility of sTEA identification using preoperative CT images, aiming to address these challenges.

The study retrospectively analyzed preoperative femoral CT data from a series of TKA patients, excluding those with bony deformities that could affect sTEA identification. Six experienced TKA surgeons independently identified the sTEA on reconstructed CT models multiple times to assess intra- and inter-observer reproducibility. The study employed statistical methods, including intra-class correlation coefficients (ICCs), to evaluate reproducibility. Results showed moderate intra-observer reproducibility with ICCs ranging between 0.4 and 0.6, while inter-observer reproducibility was lower with an ICC of 0.3. These findings suggest that even with advanced imaging techniques, identifying sTEA remains challenging due to variability among observers.

The study highlights that the poor reproducibility of sTEA identification may contribute to inconsistencies in femoral component rotation during TKA, despite advancements in computer-assisted surgical techniques. Future study could explore alternative methods or reference axes for improving rotational alignment accuracy. Additionally, the research suggests that surgeon experience and clear anatomical landmarks are crucial for reliable sTEA identification. The authors recommend caution when using sTEA as a reference in TKA and suggest considering multiple reference axes or gap balancing techniques to achieve optimal outcomes. Further research is needed to validate these findings across different centers and explore correlations between observer experience and reproducibility.

3.3.9 Clinical Value of SPECT/CT for Evaluation of Patients with Painful Knees after Total Knee Arthroplasty- a New Dimension of Diagnostics? [93]

This is a machine-generated summary of:

Hirschmann, Michael T; Konala, Praveen; Iranpour, Farhad; Kerner, Anna; Rasch, Helmut; Friederich, Niklaus F Clinical value of SPECT/CT for evaluation of patients with painful knees after total knee arthroplasty- a new dimension of diagnostics? [93].

Published in: BMC Musculoskeletal Disorders (2011).

Link to original: https://doi.org/10.1186/1471-2474-12-36

If you want to cite the papers, please refer to the original.

For technical reasons we could not place the page where the original quote is coming from.

3.3.9.1 Research Highlights

Total knee arthroplasty (TKA) is a widely used surgical procedure for patients with severe osteoarthritis of the knee, often resulting in satisfactory long-term outcomes. However, a significant number of patients experience persistent or recurrent knee pain post-surgery, with common causes including infection, loosening, instability, and prosthetic malposition. Differentiating between these causes is crucial for determining the appropriate treatment approach. Currently, no single diagnostic imaging modality effectively integrates mechanical and metabolic data to address this issue. The study by Hirschmann et al. explores the clinical value of Single Photon Emission Computed Tomogaphy/CT(SPECT/CT) imaging in diagnosing and managing knee pain after primary TKA.

The study involved a prospective analysis of patients who had undergone primary TKA and subsequently reported knee pain. Excluding those with prior revision surgeries, all participants underwent clinical evaluations and radiological examinations, including standardized radiographs and Tc-99 m HDP SPECT/CT imaging. The research aimed to assess whether SPECT/CT could alter diagnoses or treatment plans compared to initial assessments. Data were analyzed using statistical methods to identify correlations between component positioning, tracer uptake, and diagnosis. The study found that SPECT/CT significantly changed the diagnosis and treatment plan in a substantial number of cases, with intraoperative findings confirming the post-SPECT/CT diagnoses in all revised patients.

The study highlights several advances in using SPECT/CT for evaluating painful knees post-TKA. It demonstrated that SPECT/CT could accurately localize pathological tracer uptake, particularly in complex anatomical areas like the patellofemoral joint. This capability allows for better differentiation between various causes of knee pain and offers insights into knee biomechanics by correlating metabolic changes with mechanical issues. Future studies could focus on establishing diagnostic thresholds for tracer activity and further exploring the relationship between component positioning and tracer uptake to enhance clinical decision-making in managing post-TKA complications.

3.3.10 Bloodpool SPECT as Part of Bone SPECT/CT in Painful Total Knee Arthroplasty (TKA): Validation and Potential Biomarker of Prosthesis Biomechanics [94]

This is a machine-generated summary of:

Verschueren, Jolien; Albert, Adrien; Carp, Laurens; Ceyssens, Sarah; Huyghe, Ivan; Stroobants, Sigrid; Paycha, Frédéric; Gnanasegaran, Gopinath; Van den Wyngaert, Tim Bloodpool SPECT as part of bone SPECT/CT in painful total knee arthroplasty (TKA): validation and potential biomarker of prosthesis biomechanics [94].

Published in: European Journal of Nuclear Medicine and Molecular Imaging (2019).

Link to original: https://doi.org/10.1007/s00259-018-4244-4

If you want to cite the papers, please refer to the original.

For technical reasons we could not place the page where the original quote is coming from.

3.3.10.1 Research Highlights

As the population ages, the demand for total knee arthroplasty (TKA) is expected to rise significantly in the United States and Europe. Despite TKA being a widely accepted treatment for end-stage osteoarthritis, a notable percentage of patients continue to experience pain or dissatisfaction post-surgery. Diagnosing the causes of recurrent pain can be challenging, often requiring advanced imaging techniques. Radionuclide bone scintigraphy with technetium-99 m labeled bisphosphonates, particularly when combined with hybrid Single Photon Emission Computed Tomogaphy/CT(SPECT/CT), has emerged as a valuable tool in orthopedic decision-making. The study by Verschueren et al. explores the potential benefits of incorporating early-phase blood pool SPECT imaging into this diagnostic process.

The study aimed to assess whether blood pool SPECT imaging could enhance inter-rater agreement and provide additional clinically relevant information compared to traditional planar imaging. The researchers conducted bone scintigraphy on patients with painful TKA, acquiring both blood pool and late-phase SPECT/CT images. Four nuclear medicine physicians evaluated tracer uptake using a standardized localization method. The study found that blood pool SPECT improved inter-rater agreement in most assessed areas and significantly increased rater confidence. Additionally, distinct patterns of tracer uptake were identified that correlated with prosthesis survival and biomechanical functioning, suggesting that blood pool SPECT could offer independent prognostic information.

The findings indicate that blood pool SPECT imaging provides incremental value over planar imaging by improving spatial localization and identifying unique uptake patterns associated with prosthesis failure. This technique may help differentiate between local stress and loosening of the tibial component, offering insights into prosthetic biomechanics. Future study could focus on linking specific uptake patterns with clinical or surgical diagnoses during follow-up or revision surgery. The integration of blood pool SPECT findings with late-phase SPECT/CT results could further enhance the diagnostic accuracy and management of patients experiencing pain after TKA.

3.3.11 The Accuracy of CT-Based Three-Dimensional Templating in Predicting Implant Sizes in Patients Undergoing Robot-Assisted Total Knee Arthroplasty [95]

This is a machine-generated summary of:

Adkar, Neeraj; Patil, Mangesh; Vaidya, Swapnil; Kumbar, Rajendra; Kerhalkar, Ravi; Mote, Girish; Thareja, Satwik; Sadalagi, Prajwal; Bajwa, Supreet The Accuracy of CT-Based Three-Dimensional Templating in Predicting Implant Sizes in Patients Undergoing Robot-Assisted Total Knee Arthroplasty [95].

Published in: Indian Journal of Orthopaedics (2024).

Link to original: https://doi.org/10.1007/s43465-024-01244-x

If you want to cite the papers, please refer to the original.

For technical reasons we could not place the page where the original quote is coming from.

3.3.11.1 Research Highlights

Total knee arthroplasty (TKA) is a widely accepted treatment for end-stage knee disease, with its demand expected to rise significantly in the coming years. Despite its success, a notable percentage of patients experience dissatisfaction post-surgery, often due to early failure from component malalignment. Accurate preoperative prediction of implant size is crucial for improving surgical outcomes and reducing costs. Traditional X-ray templating has shown limited accuracy in predicting implant sizes, particularly for the tibial component. The study by Adkar et al. explores the efficacy of CT-based preoperative planning in robot-assisted TKA (RA-TKA) to predict actual implant sizes used during surgery.

The study was conducted as a single-center retrospective observational analysis involving consecutive RA-TKA surgeries performed by the same surgical team. Preoperative planning involved acquiring axial CT scans of the hip, knee, and ankle regions, which were then processed using the Cuvis robotic system to create a virtual operative plan. This plan was used to predict necessary bone resections and implant sizes for both femoral and tibial components. During surgery, a fully automatic robotic arm system was employed to execute bone cuts based on the preoperative plan while allowing real-time adjustments for optimal gap balancing. The predicted implant sizes were compared with those used intraoperatively, and statistical analyses were performed to assess concordance.

The study found moderate agreement between predicted and actual tibial implant sizes and almost perfect agreement for femoral components. The use of CT-based planning in RA-TKA demonstrated potential benefits in reducing operating room setup time and resource requirements by accurately predicting implant sizes preoperatively. However, limitations such as its single-center design and lack of functional outcome data suggest that further research is needed. Future study could focus on prospective designs with longer follow-up periods to validate these findings and explore real-time intraoperative predictions using robotic systems for enhanced accuracy in TKA procedures.

3.3.12 Accuracy of CT-Based Patient-Specific Guides for Total Knee Arthroplasty in Patients with Post-Traumatic Osteoarthritis [96]

This is a machine-generated summary of:

Schotanus, M. G. M.; van Haaren, E. H.; Hendrickx, R. P. M.; Jansen, E. J. P.; Kort, N. P. Accuracy of CT-based patient-specific guides for total knee arthroplasty in patients with post-traumatic osteoarthritis [96].

Published in: European Journal of Orthopaedic Surgery & Traumatology (2015).

Link to original: https://doi.org/10.1007/s00590-015-1677-3

If you want to cite the papers, please refer to the original.

For technical reasons we could not place the page where the original quote is coming from.

3.3.12.1 Research Highlights

Total knee arthroplasty (TKA) has seen significant advancements in implant technology and surgical techniques, leading to improved patient outcomes. A critical factor in the longevity of TKA is the correct alignment of implant components, which can be enhanced through computer-assisted surgery (CAS) and patient-specific guides (PSG). While CAS has been effective, especially in complex cases, PSG offers a cost-effective and less complicated alternative. The study by Schotanus et al. investigates the efficacy of computerized tomography (CT)-based PSG in restoring biomechanical limb alignment and prosthetic component positioning in patients with post-traumatic knee osteoarthritis, particularly those with retained metal hardware.

The study reviewed a cohort of patients who underwent cemented TKA using CT-based PSG due to contraindications for MRI, such as retained metal hardware from previous surgeries. Thirty patients were included after excluding those with claustrophobia or implanted electronic devices. Pre-operative planning involved detailed CT scans to create digital models for optimal implant alignment. Disposable pin guides were manufactured based on these models and used during surgery to ensure precise component placement. Post-operative outcomes were assessed through radiographic measurements and clinical evaluations using the Oxford Knee Score and EuroQol-5D. The study found that CT-based PSG effectively restored limb alignment with minimal outliers, even in challenging cases involving retained metal hardware.

The findings suggest that CT-based PSG is a viable alternative to traditional methods and surgical navigation for TKA in patients with post-traumatic osteoarthritis. The study highlights the importance of detailed pre-operative planning, especially when dealing with retained metal hardware, as it allows for accurate alignment without necessitating hardware removal in most cases. Future studies could focus on larger patient cohorts to validate these preliminary results further and explore the potential benefits of PSG for less experienced surgeons or complex cases where traditional methods may fall short.

3.3.13 Clinical Value of CT-Based Patient-Specific 3D Preoperative Design Combined with Conventional Instruments in Primary Total Knee Arthroplasty: A Propensity Score-Matched Analysis [97]

This is a machine-generated summary of:

Lei, Kai; Liu, Li Ming; Xiang, Yi; Chen, Xin; Fan, Hua Quan; Peng, Yang; Luo, Jiang Ming; Guo, Lin Clinical value of CT-based patient-specific 3D preoperative design combined with conventional instruments in primary total knee arthroplasty: a propensity score-matched analysis [97].

Published in: Journal of Orthopaedic Surgery and Research (2020).

Link to original: https://doi.org/10.1186/s13018-020-02123-5

If you want to cite the papers, please refer to the original.

For technical reasons we could not place the page where the original quote is coming from.

3.3.13.1 Research Highlights

Restoring neutral mechanical alignment is crucial for successful total knee arthroplasty (TKA), as malalignment can lead to complications such as polyethylene wear and aseptic loosening. Despite advancements in surgical techniques, conventional TKA still results in a high incidence of lower limb malalignment. The study by Lei et al. introduces a novel technique combining computerized tomography (CT)-based patient-specific preoperative design with conventional osteotomy instruments, aiming to improve surgical precision without the drawbacks of high-tech methods like computer navigation and robotics.

The study involved a retrospective analysis of patients who underwent TKA using either the novel technique or the conventional method. Patients were matched using propensity score matching to minimize selection bias. The novel technique utilized full-length CT data for precise preoperative planning, allowing for accurate intraoperative positioning without the need for additional equipment. The surgeries were performed by the same senior surgeon, ensuring consistency in procedure and postoperative care. Key outcome measures included operation time, tourniquet time, hospital stay, intraoperative bleeding, and postoperative component positioning and alignment.

The findings suggest that the novel technique offers significant advantages over the conventional method. It resulted in better control of tibial component positioning and reduced lower limb alignment outliers, with shorter operation and tourniquet times. Although both groups showed significant improvements in functional outcomes at 6 months post-operation, the novel technique group reported better early pain scores. Future study could focus on comparing this approach with other advanced technologies like computer navigation or robotics and assessing long-term functional outcomes across multiple centers to validate these promising results further.

3.3.14 Role of Preoperative Calculation of Condylar Twist Angle (CTA) by CT Scan in Optimizing Femoral Component Rotation during TKA [98]

This is a machine-generated summary of:

Sharma, D.; Shukla, A.; Kumar, K. Role of preoperative calculation of condylar twist angle (CTA) by CT scan in optimizing femoral component rotation during TKA [98].

Published in: MUSCULOSKELETAL SURGERY (2017).

Link to original: https://doi.org/10.1007/s12306-017-0466-z

If you want to cite the papers, please refer to the original.

For technical reasons we could not place the page where the original quote is coming from.

3.3.14.1 Research Highlights

Total knee replacement (TKA) outcomes can be significantly affected by the rotational alignment of the femoral component, with internal rotation being a major cause of early revision due to complications such as postoperative pain and patellofemoral dislocation. Traditional methods for setting the external rotation of the femoral component often rely on arbitrary angles or bony landmarks, which can lead to inaccuracies. The study by Sharma et al. investigates the use of the condylar twist angle (CTA), measured via preoperative CT scans, to improve the accuracy of femoral component alignment during TKA.

The study was conducted prospectively on 53 knees with grade IV osteoarthritis at Dr. RML Hospital in New Delhi, India. Preoperative CT scans were used to measure the CTA, defined as the angle between the anatomical transepicondylar axis (aTEA) and the posterior condylar axis (PCA). During surgery, this angle was reproduced to align the femoral component parallel to aTEA. Postoperative CT scans were then used to assess the accuracy of this alignment. The results showed that using CTA allowed for precise alignment of the femoral component, with a mean error of only 0.8° ± 0.6° SD from parallel alignment with aTEA.

This study demonstrates that preoperative determination of CTA via CT scan is an effective method for achieving accurate rotational alignment of the femoral component in TKA. By individualizing external rotation based on CTA rather than using a fixed angle, surgeons can reduce errors associated with traditional methods. Future study could explore larger sample sizes and standardized implant use to further validate these findings. Additionally, while CT scans provide valuable data for this approach, considerations regarding radiation exposure and cost should be addressed in future research.

3.3.15 Is Computed Tomography an Accurate and Reliable Method for Measuring Total Knee Arthroplasty Component Rotation? [99]

This is a machine-generated summary of:

Figueroa, José; Guarachi, Juan Pablo; Matas, José; Arnander, Magnus; Orrego, Mario Is computed tomography an accurate and reliable method for measuring total knee arthroplasty component rotation? [99].

Published in: International Orthopaedics (2015).

Link to original: https://doi.org/10.1007/s00264-015-2917-1

If you want to cite the papers, please refer to the original.

For technical reasons we could not place the page where the original quote is coming from.

3.3.15.1 Research Highlights

Total knee arthroplasty (TKA) is a common surgical procedure, yet a significant percentage of patients remain unsatisfied post-operatively, with some requiring revision surgery due to complications such as patellofemoral maltracking. This maltracking is often linked to component malrotation, which can be assessed using computed tomography (CT) scans. However, the accuracy and reliability of CT scans in measuring TKA component rotation have not been thoroughly evaluated. The study by Figueroa et al. aims to simultaneously determine the accuracy and reliability of CT in assessing TKA component rotation.

In this study, TKA components were implanted in dry bone adult knee models by an experienced orthopedic knee surgeon. The models were divided into two groups: one with variable femoral component rotations and another with variable tibial tray rotations. CT scans with 0.5-mm cuts were performed on all models, and four blinded orthopedic knee surgeons independently measured the component rotations using an established technique based on Berger's protocol. The accuracy was determined by comparing the true component rotation with the CT-measured values, while intraobserver and interobserver reliability were assessed using intraclass correlation coefficients (ICC). The study found that the mean difference between true and CT-measured values was 1.5° ± 0.9° for femoral components and 2.3° ± 1.2° for tibial trays, indicating good intraobserver reliability for both components.

The study advances our understanding of CT scan utility in assessing TKA component rotation by demonstrating good inter- and intra-observer reliability, although it highlights potential discrepancies in accuracy, particularly for tibial trays. Future study could focus on validating these findings in clinical settings with real patients to enhance external validity. Additionally, increasing the number of observers and measurements could further strengthen the study's conclusions. These insights are crucial for surgeons evaluating patients with potential patellofemoral maltracking due to component malrotation, emphasizing the need for cautious interpretation of CT scan results in clinical practice.

Bibliography

1. Yoshino K, Hagiwara S, Nakamura J, Tsukeoka T, Tsuneizumi Y, Ohtori S. Intra- and interobserver reliability and agreement in three-dimensional computed tomography measurements of component positions after total knee arthroplasty. Knee. 2019;26:1102–10.

2. Saffarini M, Nover L, Tandogan R, Becker R, Moser LB, Hirschmann MT, et al. The original Akagi line is the most reliable: a systematic review of landmarks for rotational alignment of the tibial component in TKA. Knee Surg Sport Traumatol Arthrosc. 2019;27:1018–27.
3. Hirschmann MT, Iranpour F, Konala P, Kerner A, Rasch H, Cobb JP, et al. A novel standardized algorithm for evaluating patients with painful total knee arthroplasty using combined single photon emission tomography and conventional computerized tomography. Knee Surg Sport Traumatol Arthrosc. 2010;18:939–44.
4. Hirschmann MT, Konala P, Iranpour F, Kerner A, Rasch H, Friederich NF. Clinical value of 99mTc-HDP-SPECT-CT for assessment of patients with painful knees after total knee arthroplasty - a new dimension of diagnostics. BMC Musculoskelet Disord. 2011;4:12–36.
5. Hirschmann MT, Amsler F, Rasch H. Clinical value of SPECT/CT in the painful total knee arthroplasty (TKA): a prospective study in a consecutive series of 100 TKA. Eur J Nucl Med Mol Imaging. 2015. https://doi.org/10.1007/s00259-015-3095-5.
6. Rasch H, Falkowski AL, Forrer F, Henckel J, Hirschmann MT. 4D-SPECT/CT in orthopaedics: A new method of combined quantitative volumetric 3D analysis of SPECT/CT tracer uptake and component position measurements in patients after total knee arthroplasty. Skeletal Radiol. 2013;42:1215–23.
7. Hirschmann MT, Wagner CR, Rasch H, Henckel J. Standardized volumetric 3D-analysis of SPECT/CT imaging in orthopaedics: overcoming the limitations of qualitative 2D analysis. BMC Med Imaging. 2012;12(1):5.
8. Ming GL, Nilsson KG (2000) The effect of the preoperative bone quality on the fixation of the tibial component in total knee arthroplasty. J Arthroplasty 115(6):744–753
9. Peterson MM, Nielson PT, Lebech A, Toksvig-Larsen S, Lund B (1999) Preoperative bone mineral density of the proximal tibia and migration of thetibial component after uncemented total knee arthroplasty. J Arthroplasty 14(1):77–81
10. Trevisan C, Bigoni M, Denti M, Marinoni EC, Ortolani S (1998) Bone assessment after total knee arthroplasty by dual energy X-ray absorptiometry: analysis protocol and reproducibility. Calcif Tissue Int 62:359–361
11. Schmidt R, Pitto RP, Kress A et al (2005) Inter- and intraobserver assessment of periacetabular osteodensitometry after cemented and uncemented total hip arthroplasty using computed tomography. Arch Orthop Trauma Surg 125:291–297
12. Bland JM, Altman DG (1986) Statistical methods for assessing agreement between two methods of clinical measurement. Lancet Feb:307–310
13. Zannoni C, Viceconti M, Pierotti L, Cappello A (1998) Analysis of titanium induced CT artifacts in the development of biomechanical finite element models. Med Eng Phys 20:653–659

14. Pitto RP, Pandit S, Munro J. (2005) Bone remodelling of the proximal tibia after fixed versus rotating platform total knee arthroplasty. Proceedings of the 23rd world congress of SIROT, Istanbul, Turkey, pp 245
15. Hirschmann MT, Konala P, Iranpour F, Kerner A, Rasch H, Friederich NF. Clinical value of SPECT/CT for evaluation of patients with painful knees after total knee arthroplasty–a new dimension of diagnostics? BMC Musculoskelet Disord. 2011;12:36.
16. Berger RA, Crossett LS, Jacobs JJ, Rubash HE (1998) Malrotation causing patellofemoral complications after total knee arthroplasty. Clin Orthop Relat Res 356:144–153
17. Vince KG, Insall JN, Kelly MA. The total condylar prosthesis. 10- to 12-year results of a cemented knee replacement. *J Bone Joint Surg Br.* 1989;5:793–797.
18. Jazrawi LM, Birdzell L, Kummer FJ, Di Cesare PE (2000) The accuracy of computed tomography for determining femoral and tibial total knee arthroplasty component rotation. J Arthroplasty 15:761–766
19. Hirschmann M, Konala P, Amsler F, Iranpour F, Friederich N, Cobb J (2011) The position and orientation of total knee replacement components: a comparison of conventional radiographs, transverse 2D-CT slices and 3D-CT reconstruction. J Bone Joint Surg Br 93:629–633
20. Hirschmann MT, Henckel J, Rasch H. SPECT/CT in patients with painful knee arthroplasty-what is the evidence? Skelet Radiol. 2013;42(9):1201–7.
21. Hirschmann MT, Schon S, Afifi FK, Amsler F, Rasch H, Friederich NF, et al. Assessment of loading history of compartments in the knee using bone SPECT/CT: a study combining alignment and 99mTc-HDP tracer uptake/distribution patterns. J Orthop Res. 2013;31(2):268–74.
22. Hirschmann MT, Khan ZA, Sava MP et al (2024) Definition of normal, neutral, deviant and aberrant coronal knee alignment for total knee arthroplasty. Knee Surg Sports Traumatol Arthrosc 32(2):473–489. https://doi.org/10.1002/ksa.12066
23. Deakin AH, Sarungi M (2014) A comparison of variable angle versus fixed angledistal femoral resection in primary total knee arthroplasty. J Arthroplasty 29(6):1133–1137. https://doi.org/10.1016/j.arth.2013.11.009 Epub 2013 Nov 22. PMID: 24355255
24. Christensen JC, Blackburn BE, Anderson LA et al (2023) Recovery curve for patient reported outcomes and Objective Physical Activity after primary total knee Arthroplasty-A Multicenter Study using Wearable Technology. J Arthroplasty 38(6S):S94–S102. https://doi.org/10.1016/j.arth.2023.03.060
25. Sodhi N, Jacofsky DJ, Chee A, Mont MA (2021) Benefits of CT scanning for the management of knee arthritis and arthroplasty. J Knee Surg 34(12):1296–1303. https://doi.org/10.1055/s-0040-1708041 Epub 2020 Apr 8. PMID: 32268407
26. Minoda Y, Yoshida T, Sugimoto K, Baba S, Ikebuchi M, Nakamura H (2014) Detection of small periprosthetic bone defects after total knee arthroplasty. J Arthroplasty 29(12):2280–2284. https://doi.org/10.1016/j.arth.2014.05.013 Epub 2014 May 24. PMID: 24961891

27. Berger RA, Rubash HE, Seel MJ, et al. Determining the rotational alignment of the femoral component in total knee arthroplasty using the epicondylar axis. Clin Orthop Relat Res. 1993;286:40–7.
28. Churchill DL, Incavo SJ, Johnson CC, et al. The transepicondylar axis approximates the optimal flexion axis of the knee. Clin Orthop Relat Res. 1998;356:111–8. https://doi.org/10.1097/00003086-199811000-00016.
29. Griffin FM, Insall JN, Scuderi GR. The posterior condylar angle in osteoarthritic knees. J Arthroplast. 1998;13(7):812–5. https://doi.org/10.1016/s0883-5403(98)90036-5.
30. Miller MC, Berger RA, Petrella AJ, Karmas A, Rubash HE. Optimizing femoral component rotation in total knee arthroplasty. Clin Orthop Relat Res. 2001;392:38–45.
31. Anouchi YS, Whiteside LA, Kaiser AD, et al. The effects of axial rotational alignment of the femoral component on knee stability and patellar tracking in total knee arthroplasty demonstrated on autopsy specimens. Clin Orthop Relat Res. 1993;287:170–7.
32. Victor J (2009) Rotational alignment of the distal femur: a literature review. Orthop Traumatol Surg Res 95:365–372
33. Lei K, Liu LM, Xiang Y, et al. Clinical value of ct-based patient-specific 3d preoperative design combined with conventional instruments in primary total knee arthroplasty: a propensity score-matched analysis. J Orthop Surg Res. 2020;15(1):591. https://doi.org/10.1186/s13018-020-02123-5.
34. Koo, T. K., and Li, M. Y. (2016). A guideline of selecting and reporting intraclass correlation coefficients for reliability research. *Journal of Chiropractic Medicine, 15*(2), 155–163. https://doi.org/10.1016/j.jcm.2016.02.012
35. Agarwal N, To K, Mcdonnell S, et al. Clinical and radiological outcomes in robotic-assisted total knee arthroplasty: a systematic review and meta-analysis. J Arthroplast. 2020;35(11):3393–3409.e3392. https://doi.org/10.1016/j.arth.2020.03.005.
36. Jones CW, Jerabek SA. Current Role of Computer Navigation in Total Knee Arthroplasty. J Arthroplasty. 2018;33:1989–93.
37. Lin, Y., et al. (2020). Patient-specific or conventional instrumentations: A meta-analysis of randomized controlled trials. *BioMed Research International.* https://doi.org/10.1155/2020/2164371
38. Jenny JY, Boeri C. Low reproducibility of the intra-operative measurement of the transepicondylar axis during total knee replacement. Acta Orthop Scand. 2004;75(1):74–7. https://doi.org/10.1080/00016470410001708150.
39. Jerosch J, Peuker E, Philipps B, et al. Interindividual reproducibility in perioperative rotational alignment of femoral components in knee prosthetic surgery using the transepicondylar axis. Knee Surg Sports Traumatol Arthrosc. 2002;10(3):194–7. https://doi.org/10.1007/s00167-001-0271-x.
40. Kinzel V, Ledger M, Shakespeare D. Can the epicondylar axis be defined accurately in total knee arthroplasty? Knee. 2005;12(4):293–6. https://doi.org/10.1016/j.knee.2004.09.003.

41. Siston RA, Patel JJ, Goodman SB, et al. The variability of femoral rotational alignment in total knee arthroplasty. J Bone Joint Surg Am. 2005;87(10):2276–80. https://doi.org/10.2106/jbjs.D.02945.
42. Stoeckl B, Nogler M, Krismer M, Beimel C, Moctezuma de la Barrera J-L, Kessler O (2006) Reliability of the transepicondylar axis as an anatomical landmark in total knee arthroplasty. J Arthroplasty 21:878–882
43. Yan CH, Yau WP, Ng TP, et al. Inter- and intra-observer errors in identifying the transepicondylar axis and whiteside's line. J Orthop Surg (Hong Kong). 2008;16(3):316–20. https://doi.org/10.1177/230949900801600310.
44. Dennis DA: Evaluation of painful total knee arthroplasty. J Arthroplasty. 2004, 19 (4 Suppl 1): 35-40. 10.1016/j.arth.2004.03.003.
45. Sharkey PF, Hozack WJ, Rothman RH, Shastri S, Jacoby SM: Insall Award paper. Why are total knee arthroplasties failing today?. Clin Orthop Relat Res. 2002, 7-13. 10.1097/00003086-200211000-00003. 404
46. Toms AD, Mandalia V, Haigh R, Hopwood B. The management of patients with painful total knee replacement. J Bone Joint Surg (Br). 2009;91(2):143–50.
47. Hirschmann MT, Iranpour F, Davda K, Rasch H, Hugli R, Friederich NF. Combined single-photon emission computerized tomography and conventional computerized tomography (SPECT/CT): clinical value for the knee surgeons? Knee Surg Sports Traumatol Arthrosc. 2010;18(3):341–5.
48. Gratz S, Hoffken H, Kaiser JW, Behr TM, Strosche H, Reize P: [Nuclear medical imaging in case of painful knee arthroplasty]. Radiologe. 2009, 49 (1): 59-67. 10.1007/s00117-008-1703-0.
49. Kantor SG, Schneider R, Insall JN, Becker MW: Radionuclide imaging of asymptomatic versus symptomatic total knee arthroplasties. Clin Orthop Relat Res. 1990, 118-123. 260
50. Awengen R, Rasch H, Amsler F, Hirschmann MT. Symptomatic versus asymptomatic knees after bilateral total knee arthroplasty: what is the difference in SPECT/CT? Eur J Nucl Med Mol Imaging. 2016;43(4):762–72.
51. van der Bruggen V, Hirschmann MT, Strobel K, Kampen WU, Kuwert T, Gnanasegaran G et al (2018) SPECT/CT in the postoperative painful knee. Semin Nucl Med 48(5):439–453
52. Van den Wyngaert T, Strobel K, Kampen WU, Kuwert T, van der Bruggen W, Mohan HK, et al. The EANM practice guidelines for bone scintigraphy. Eur J Nucl Med Mol Imaging. 2016;43(9):1723–38.
53. Hsu, A. R., Kim, J. D., Bhatia, S., and Levine, B. R. (2012). Effect of training level on accuracy of digital templating in primary total hip and knee arthroplasty. *Orthopedics, 35*, e179-183. https://doi.org/10.3928/01477447-20120123-15
54. Laskin, R. S. (2001). Intramedullary instrumentation: Safer and more accurate than extramedullary instrumentation. *Orthopedics, 24*, 739. https://doi.org/10.3928/0147-7447-20010801-14
55. Trickett R, Hodgson P, Forster M, Robertson A (2009) The reliability and accuracy of digital templating in total knee replacement. J Bone Joint Surg Br 91(8):903–906

56. Marchand, R. C., Sodhi, N., Bhowmik-Stoker, M., Scholl, L., Condrey, C., et al. (2019). Does the robotic arm and preoperative CT planning help with 3D intraoperative total knee arthroplasty planning? *The Journal of Knee Surgery, 32*, 742–749. https://doi.org/10.1055/s-0038-1668122
57. Pietrzak, J. R. T., Rowan, F. E., Kayani, B., Donaldson, M. J., Huq, S. S., and Haddad, F. S. (2019). Preoperative CT-based three-dimensional templating in robot-assisted total knee arthroplasty more accurately predicts implant sizes than two-dimensional templating. *The Journal of Knee Surgery, 32*, 642–648. https://doi.org/10.1055/s-0038-1666829
58. Wan, X., Qiang, Su., Wang, D., Yuan, M., Yahao, L., Xu, H., and Zhou, Z. (2021). Robotic arm-assisted total knee arthroplasty improves preoperative planning and intraoperative decision-making. *Journal Orthopaedic Surgery and Research*. https://doi.org/10.1186/s13018-021-02815-6
59. Koch PP, Müller D, Pisan M, Fucentese SF. Radiographic accuracy in TKA with a CT-based patient-specific cutting block technique. Knee Surg Sport Traumatol Arthrosc. 2013;21:2200–5.
60. Kotela, A., Lorkowski, J., Kucharzewski, M., Wilk-Frańczuk, M., Śliwiński, Z., Frańczuk, B., Łęgosz, P., et al. (2015). Patient-specific CT-based instrumentation versus conventional instrumentation in total knee arthroplasty: A prospective randomized controlled study on clinical outcomes and in-hospital data. *BioMed Research International, 2015*, 165908. https://doi.org/10.1155/2015/165908
61. Vaishya, R., Vijay, V., Krishnan, M., and Agarwal, A. K. (2018). Fallacies of CT based component size prediction in total knee arthroplasty-are patient specific instruments the answer? *Journal of Clinical Orthopaedics Trauma, 9*, 34–39. https://doi.org/10.1016/j.jcot.2017.11.001
62. Schotanus, M. G. M., Schoenmakers, D. A. L., Sollie, R., and Kort, N. P. (2017). Patient-specific instruments for total knee arthroplasty can accurately predict the component size as used peroperative. *Knee Surgery, Sports Traumatology, Arthroscopy, 25*, 3844–3848. https://doi.org/10.1007/s00167-016-4345-1
63. Cucchi, D., Menon, A., Compagnoni, R., Ferrua, P., Fossati, C., and Randelli, P. (2018). Significant differences between manufacturer and surgeon in the accuracy of final component size prediction with CT-based patient-specific instrumentation for total knee arthroplasty. *Knee Surgery, Sports Traumatology, Arthroscopy, 26*, 3317–3324. https://doi.org/10.1007/s00167-018-4876-8
64. Biant, L. C., Yeoh, K., Walker, P. M., Bruce, W. J., and Walsh, W. R. (2008). The accuracy of bone resections made during computer navigated total knee replacement. Do we resect what the computer plans we resect? *The Knee, 15*, 238–241. https://doi.org/10.1016/j.knee.2008.01.012
65. Hafez MA (2012) The use of computer-assisted orthopaedic surgery in complex cases of hip and knee arthroplasty: experience from a developing country. Biomed Tech 57(4):301–306
66. Rubin LE, Murgo KT (2013) Brief report: total knee arthroplasty performed with patient-specific, pre-operative CT-guided navigation. R I Med J 96(3):34–37

67. White D, Chelule KL, Seedhom BB. Accuracy of MRI vs CT imaging with particular reference to patient specific templates for total knee replacement surgery. Int J Med Robot. 2008;4(3):224–31.
68. Boonen B, Schotanus MG, Kerens B et al (2013) Intra-operative results and radiological outcome of conventional and patient-specific surgery in total knee arthroplasty: a multicentre, randomised controlled trial. Knee Surg Traumatol Arthrosc
69. Bouché P-A, Corsia S, Dechartres A, Resche-Rigon M, Nizard R. Are there differences in accuracy or outcomes scores among navigated, robotic, patient-specific instruments or standard cutting guides in TKA? A network meta-analysis. Clinical Orthopaedics and Related Research. 2020;478:2105–16. https://doi.org/10.1097/corr.0000000000001324.
70. Li JT, Gao X, Li X. Comparison of iASSIST navigation system with conventional techniques in total knee arthroplasty: a systematic review and meta-analysis of radiographic and clinical outcomes. Orthop Surg. 2019;11:985–93. https://doi.org/10.1111/os.12550.
71. Lonner JH, Fillingham YA. Pros and cons: a balanced view of robotics in knee arthroplasty. J Arthroplasty. 2018;33:2007–13. https://doi.org/10.1016/j.arth.2018.03.056.
72. Liow MHL, Goh GS, Wong MK, Chin PL, Tay DK, Yeo SJ. Robotic-assisted total knee arthroplasty may lead to improvement in quality-of-life measures: a 2-year follow-up of a prospective randomized trial. Knee Surg Sports Traumatol Arthrosc. 2017;25:2942–51. https://doi.org/10.1007/s00167-016-4076-3.
73. Swank ML, Alkire M, Conditt M, Lonner JH. Technology and cost-effectiveness in knee arthroplasty: computer navigation and robotics. Am J Orthop (Belle Mead NJ). 2009;38:32–6.
74. Park SE, Lee CT. Comparison of robotic-assisted and conventional manual implantation of a primary total knee arthroplasty. J Arthroplasty. 2007;22:1054–9. https://doi.org/10.1016/j.arth.2007.05.036.
75. Parratte S, Blanc G, Boussemart T, et al. Rotation in total knee arthroplasty: no difference between patient-specific and conventional instrumentation. Knee Surg Sports Traumatol Arthrosc. 2013;21(10):2213–9. https://doi.org/10.1007/s00167-013-2623-8.
76. Yan CH, Chiu KY, Ng FY, Chan PK, Fang CX. Comparison between patient-specific instruments and conventional instruments and computer navigation in total knee arthroplasty: a randomized controlled trial. Knee Surg Sports Traumatol Arthrosc. 2015;23:3637–45. https://doi.org/10.1007/s00167-014-3264-2.
77. Victor J, Dujardin J, Vandenneucker H, Arnout N, Bellemans J. Patient-specific guides do not improve accuracy in total knee arthroplasty: a prospective randomized controlled trial. Clin Orthop Relat Res. 2014;472(1):263–71.
78. Woolson ST, Harris AH, Wagner DW, Giori NJ. Component alignment during total knee arthroplasty with use of standard or custom instrumentation: a randomized clinical trial using computed tomography for postoperative alignment

measurement. J Bone Joint Surg Am. 2014;96:366–72. https://doi.org/10.2106/JBJS.L.01722.
79. Stronach BM, Pelt CE, Erickson JA, Peters CL. Patient-specific instrumentation in total knee arthroplasty provides no improvement in component alignment. J Arthroplasty. 2014;29:1705–8. https://doi.org/10.1016/j.arth.2014.04.025.
80. Hofmann S, Seitlinger G, Djahani O, Pietsch M. The painful knee after TKA: a diagnostic algorithm for failure analysis. Knee Surg Sports Traumatol Arthrosc. 2011;19(9):1442–52.
81. Mandalia V, Eyres K, Schranz P, Toms AD. Evaluation of patients with a painful total knee replacement. J Bone Joint Surg (Br). 2008;90(3):265–71.
82. Berger RA, Rubash HE (2001) Rotational instability and malrotation after total knee arthroplasty. Orthop Clin North Am 32:639–647
83. Bedard M, Vince KG, Redfern J, Collen SR. Internal rotation of the tibial component is frequent in stiff total knee arthroplasty. *Clin Orthop Relat Res.* 2011;8:2346–2355.
84. Konigsberg B, Hess R, Hartman C, Smith L, Garvin KL (2014) Inter- and intraobserver reliability of two-dimensional CT scan for total knee arthroplasty component malrotation. Clin Orthop Relat Res 472(1):212–217. https://doi.org/10.1007/s11999-013-3111-7
85. Watanabe, Shotaro; Akagi, Ryuichiro; Shiko, Yuki; Ono, Yoshimasa; Kawasaki, Yohei; Ohdera, Toshihiro; Ohtori, Seiji; Sasho, Takahisa Intra- and inter-observer reliability of implant positioning evaluation on a CT-based three-dimensional postoperative matching system for total knee arthroplasty. BMC Musculoskeletal Disorders (2021). https://doi.org/10.1186/s12891-021-04228-2
86. Awengen, R.; Rasch, H.; Amsler, F.; Hirschmann, M. T. Symptomatic versus asymptomatic knees after bilateral total knee arthroplasty: what is the difference in SPECT/CT?. European Journal of Nuclear Medicine and Molecular Imaging (2015). https://doi.org/10.1007/s00259-015-3278-0
87. Reilly, Keryn; Munro, Jacob; Pandit, Salil; Kress, Alexander; Walker, Cameron; Pitto, Rocco Paolo Inter-observer validation study of quantitative CT-osteodensitometry in total knee arthroplasty. Archives of Orthopaedic and Trauma Surgery (2007). https://doi.org/10.1007/s00402-007-0351-6
88. Rasch, Helmut; Falkowski, Anna L.; Forrer, Flavio; Henckel, Johann; Hirschmann, Michael T. 4D-SPECT/CT in orthopaedics: a new method of combined quantitative volumetric 3D analysis of SPECT/CT tracer uptake and component position measurements in patients after total knee arthroplasty. Skeletal Radiology (2013). https://doi.org/10.1007/s00256-013-1643-2
89. Konigsberg, Beau; Hess, Ryan; Hartman, Curtis; Smith, Lynette; Garvin, Kevin L. Inter- and Intraobserver Reliability of Two-dimensional CT Scan for Total Knee Arthroplasty Component Malrotation. Clinical Orthopaedics and Related Research® (2013). https://doi.org/10.1007/s11999-013-3111-7
90. Hirschmann, Michael T.; Amsler, Felix; Rasch, Helmut Clinical value of SPECT/CT in the painful total knee arthroplasty (TKA): a prospective study in

a consecutive series of 100 TKA. European Journal of Nuclear Medicine and Molecular Imaging (2015). https://doi.org/10.1007/s00259-015-3095-5
91. Mhaskar, Vikram Arun; Saggar, Rachit; Karan, Satyabrat; Maheshwari, Jitendra Comparing supine CT scanogram and standing long-leg radiograph for postoperative alignment in total knee arthroplasty: a prospective study. Archives of Orthopaedic and Trauma Surgery (2024). https://doi.org/10.1007/s00402-024-05743-2
92. Lei, Kai; Liu, Li Ming; Luo, Jiang Ming; Ma, Chao; Feng, Qing; Yang, Liu; Guo, Lin Could surgical transepicondylar axis be identified accurately in preoperative 3D planning for total knee arthroplasty? A reproducibility study based on 3D-CT. Arthroplasty (2022). https://doi.org/10.1186/s42836-022-00147-2
93. Hirschmann, Michael T; Konala, Praveen; Iranpour, Farhad; Kerner, Anna; Rasch, Helmut; Friederich, Niklaus F Clinical value of SPECT/CT for evaluation of patients with painful knees after total knee arthroplasty- a new dimension of diagnostics?. BMC Musculoskeletal Disorders (2011). https://doi.org/10.1186/1471-2474-12-36
94. Verschueren, Jolien; Albert, Adrien; Carp, Laurens; Ceyssens, Sarah; Huyghe, Ivan; Stroobants, Sigrid; Paycha, Frédéric; Gnanasegaran, Gopinath; Van den Wyngaert, Tim Bloodpool SPECT as part of bone SPECT/CT in painful total knee arthroplasty (TKA): validation and potential biomarker of prosthesis biomechanics. European Journal of Nuclear Medicine and Molecular Imaging (2019). https://doi.org/10.1007/s00259-018-4244-4
95. Adkar, Neeraj; Patil, Mangesh; Vaidya, Swapnil; Kumbar, Rajendra; Kerhalkar, Ravi; Mote, Girish; Thareja, Satwik; Sadalagi, Prajwal; Bajwa, Supreet The Accuracy of CT-Based Three-Dimensional Templating in Predicting Implant Sizes in Patients Undergoing Robot-Assisted Total Knee Arthroplasty. Indian Journal of Orthopaedics (2024). https://doi.org/10.1007/s43465-024-01244-x
96. Schotanus, M. G. M.; van Haaren, E. H.; Hendrickx, R. P. M.; Jansen, E. J. P.; Kort, N. P. Accuracy of CT-based patient-specific guides for total knee arthroplasty in patients with post-traumatic osteoarthritis. European Journal of Orthopaedic Surgery & Traumatology (2015). https://doi.org/10.1007/s00590-015-1677-3
97. Lei, Kai; Liu, Li Ming; Xiang, Yi; Chen, Xin; Fan, Hua Quan; Peng, Yang; Luo, Jiang Ming; Guo, Lin Clinical value of CT-based patient-specific 3D preoperative design combined with conventional instruments in primary total knee arthroplasty: a propensity score-matched analysis. Journal of Orthopaedic Surgery and Research (2020). https://doi.org/10.1186/s13018-020-02123-5
98. Sharma, D.; Shukla, A.; Kumar, K. Role of preoperative calculation of condylar twist angle (CTA) by CT scan in optimizing femoral component rotation during TKA. MUSCULOSKELETAL SURGERY (2017). https://doi.org/10.1007/s12306-017-0466-z
99. Figueroa, José; Guarachi, Juan Pablo; Matas, José; Arnander, Magnus; Orrego, Mario Is computed tomography an accurate and reliable method for measuring total knee arthroplasty component rotation?. International Orthopaedics (2015). https://doi.org/10.1007/s00264-015-2917-1

3.4 Fluoroscopy

Machine Generated Summaries

Disclaimer: The summaries in this chapter were generated from Springer Nature publications using abstractive AI auto-summarization: An abstraction-based summarizer creates new text based on deep learning. New phrases are created to summarize the content. As the constituted sentences are machine selected, they may not fully reflect the body of the work, so we strongly advise that the original content is read and cited. The auto-generated summaries were curated by the editor to meet Springer Nature publication standards.

3.4.1 3D Kinematics of Mobile-Bearing Total Knee Arthroplasty Using X-Ray Fluoroscopy [11]

This is a machine-generated summary of:

Yamazaki, Takaharu; Futai, Kazuma; Tomita, Tetsuya; Sato, Yoshinobu; Yoshikawa, Hideki; Tamura, Shinichi; Sugamoto, Kazuomi 3D kinematics of mobile-bearing total knee arthroplasty using X-ray fluoroscopy [11].

Published in: International Journal of Computer Assisted Radiology and Surgery (2014).

Link to original: https://doi.org/10.1007/s11548-014-1093-x

If you want to cite the papers, please refer to the original.

For technical reasons we could not place the page where the original quote is coming from.

3.4.1.1 Research Highlights

In the field of orthopedics, total knee arthroplasty (TKA) is a widely used treatment for patients with functional disabilities and arthritic knees, where the articular cartilage is damaged. TKA implants typically consist of metallic femoral and tibial components with a polyethylene-bearing insert in between, which replaces the damaged cartilage and provides a low-friction surface. The success of TKA depends on the design of the joint surface and surgical technique, as improper movement can lead to implant wear and postoperative pain. Accurate assessment of TKA kinematics is crucial for evaluating surgical outcomes and improving implant designs. However, current imaging techniques like CT and MRI face limitations in capturing dynamic knee motion due to metal artifacts and environmental restrictions. The study by

Yamazaki et al. proposes a novel technique using X-ray fluoroscopy to analyze the kinematics of mobile-bearing inserts in TKA, addressing these challenges.

The study utilized X-ray fluoroscopy combined with computer-aided design (CAD) models to estimate the three-dimensional pose of knee implants. The researchers inserted tantalum beads into the polyethylene insert during surgery to track its movement, as these beads are visible in X-ray images unlike the radiolucent insert itself. A contour-based registration technique was employed to estimate the pose of femoral and tibial components by matching their silhouettes in X-ray images with CAD models. For the mobile-bearing insert, a feature-based registration technique was used to determine its pose based on the positions of the tantalum beads. The accuracy of this method was validated through experiments involving synthetic images and clinical application on nine TKA patients during dynamic motion.

The study demonstrated that this new technique allows for accurate kinematic analysis of mobile-bearing inserts in TKA, even when only three bead projections are visible in fluoroscopic images. This advancement provides valuable insights into implant performance during activities such as deep knee bending. Future study could focus on integrating preoperative and intraoperative data with postoperative kinematic analysis to further enhance implant design and surgical techniques. Additionally, automating certain manual processes involved in image analysis could improve efficiency and reduce labor-intensive tasks. This research contributes significantly to understanding TKA kinematics and optimizing patient outcomes through improved implant designs.

3.4.2 A 3D Kinematic Estimation of Knee Prosthesis Using X-Ray Projection Images: Clinical Assessment of the Improved Algorithm for Fluoroscopy Images [12]

This is a machine-generated summary of:

Hirokawa, Shunji; Abrar Hossain, M.; Kihara, Yuichi; Ariyoshi, Shogo A 3D kinematic estimation of knee prosthesis using X-ray projection images: clinical assessment of the improved algorithm for fluoroscopy images [12].

Published in: Medical & Biological Engineering & Computing (2008).

Link to original: https://doi.org/10.1007/s11517-008-0398-8

If you want to cite the papers, please refer to the original.

For technical reasons we could not place the page where the original quote is coming from.

3.4.2.1 Research Highlights

The demand for total knee arthroplasty (TKA) has increased, necessitating improvements in the durability and design of TKA prostheses. In vivo measurement of prosthetic kinematics is crucial for enhancing these designs, yet direct measurement methods are impractical, leading to reliance on indirect techniques such as X-ray image-based registration. Existing methods, including those by Zuffi et al. and Mahfouz et al., have limitations in accuracy and require manual processing. Now, a new study by Shunji Hirokawa and colleagues proposes a two-step estimation algorithm that enhances the accuracy of prosthetic position/orientation estimation while maintaining simplicity and reducing computation time.

The study introduces a two-step estimation algorithm that builds upon Banks and Hodge's pattern matching method. The first step involves using a library of pre-computed images to estimate the initial position/orientation of the prosthesis. The second step refines this estimate by generating a localized image library around the initial estimate, reducing inaccuracies caused by weak perspective projection assumptions. Additionally, the researchers incorporate a geometric articulation model to improve depth translation accuracy, particularly for z-translation, which has been challenging with single-plane images. The algorithm was tested through simulations and experiments using an industrial robot to position prosthetic components in swine knees for X-ray photography, as well as clinical assessments with fluoroscopy images from a TKA patient.

The study advances TKA kinematic assessment by significantly improving estimation accuracy, especially for z-translations, through the incorporation of an articulation model. This improvement allows for more accurate introduction of contact point trajectories between prosthetic components. Future study could focus on further refining the algorithm's application in clinical settings and exploring its use across different knee motions and patient conditions. The researchers plan to continue experiments with various subjects to validate the algorithm's effectiveness in diverse scenarios, potentially enhancing its utility in clinical practice for assessing knee kinematics post-TKA.

Bibliography

1. Banks SA, Hodge WA (1996) Accurate measurement of three-dimensional knee replacement kinematics using single-plane fluoroscopy. IEEE Trans Biomed Eng 43:638–649
2. Hirokawa S, Abrar Hossain M (2008) A 3D kinematic estimation of knee prosthesis using X-ray projection images: clinical assessment of the improved algorithm for fluoroscopy images. Med Biol Eng Comput 46:1253–1262
3. Fantozzi S, Leardini A, Banks SA, Marcacci M, Giannini S, Cantani F (2004) Dynamic in-vivo tibio-femoral and bearing motions in mobile bearing knee arthroplasty. Knee Surg Sports Traumatol Arthrosc 12:144–151
4. Wolterbeek N, Garling EH, Mertens B, Valstar ER, Nelissen RGHH (2009) Mobile bearing knee kinematics change over time. A fluoroscopic study in rheumatoid arthritis patients. Clin Biomech 24:441–445

5. Canny J (1986) A computational approach to edge detection. IEEE Trans Pattern Anal Mach Intell 8:679–698
6. Grood ES, Suntay WJ (1983) A joint coordinate system for the clinical description of three-dimensional motions: application to the knee. J Biomech Eng 105:136–144
7. Mahfouz MR, Hoff WA, Komistek RD et al (2005) Effect of segmentation errors on 3D-to-2D registration of implant models in X-ray images. J Biomech 38:229–239. https://doi.org/10.1016/j.jbiomech.2004.02.025
8. Banks SA (1992) Model based 3D kinematic estimation from 2D perspective silhouettes: application with total knee prostheses. Doctorial thesis of Massachusetts Institute of Technology, Cambridge, 5
9. Banks SA, Hodge WA (1996) Accurate measurement of three-dimensional knee replacement kinematics using single-plane fluoroscopy. IEEE Trans Biomed Eng 43:638–649. https://doi.org/10.1109/10.495283
10. Zuffi S, Leardini A, Catani F, Fantozzi S, Cappello A (1999) A model-based method for the reconstruction of total knee replacement kinematics. IEEE Trans Med Imaging 18:981–991
11. Yamazaki, Takaharu; Futai, Kazuma; Tomita, Tetsuya; Sato, Yoshinobu; Yoshikawa, Hideki; Tamura, Shinichi; Sugamoto, Kazuomi 3D kinematics of mobile-bearing total knee arthroplasty using X-ray fluoroscopy. International Journal of Computer Assisted Radiology and Surgery (2014). https://doi.org/10.1007/s11548-014-1093-x
12. Hirokawa, Shunji; Abrar Hossain, M.; Kihara, Yuichi; Ariyoshi, Shogo A 3D kinematic estimation of knee prosthesis using X-ray projection images: clinical assessment of the improved algorithm for fluoroscopy images. Medical & Biological Engineering & Computing (2008). https://doi.org/10.1007/s11517-008-0398-8

3.5 Scans

Machine Generated Summaries

Disclaimer: The summaries in this chapter were generated from Springer Nature publications using abstractive AI auto-summarization: An abstraction-based summarizer creates new text based on deep learning. New phrases are created to summarize the content. As the constituted sentences are machine selected, they may not fully reflect the body of the work, so we strongly advise that the original content is read and cited. The auto-generated summaries were curated by the editor to meet Springer Nature publication standards.

3.5.1 Three-Phase Technetium-99 M Bone Scanning in Patients with Pain in the Knee Region After Cemented Total Knee Arthroplasty [8]

This is a machine-generated summary of:

Hill, Daniel S.; Kinsella, Denis; Toms, Andrew D. Three-phase Technetium-99 m bone scanning in patients with pain in the knee region after cemented total knee arthroplasty [8].

Published in: European Journal of Orthopaedic Surgery & Traumatology (2019).

Link to original: https://doi.org/10.1007/s00590-019-02407-5

If you want to cite the papers, please refer to the original.

For technical reasons we could not place the page where the original quote is coming from.

3.5.1.1 Research Highlights

Total knee replacement (TKR) surgery is a common procedure, but persistent pain in the knee region post-surgery can be challenging to diagnose, particularly when differentiating between prosthetic joint infection and component loosening. A three-phase bone scan (TPBS) is often used due to its high sensitivity in detecting bone turnover, but it suffers from poor specificity, as increased radionuclide uptake can occur in various conditions. The study by Hill et al. questions the diagnostic value of TPBS in evaluating knee pain after TKR, suggesting that abnormal TPBS results have a poor association with infection or loosening and do not provide additional diagnostic information beyond standard investigations.

The study conducted by Hill et al. was a retrospective analysis of patients who underwent TPBS for unexplained knee pain following primary cemented TKR at their institution over a 12-month period. The researchers utilized a standardized quadruple assessment approach, including clinical evaluation, serological investigation, diagnostic imaging, and microbiological analysis. TPBS was performed when other evaluations failed to clarify the cause of pain. The scans were interpreted independently by experienced radiologists, and clinical outcomes were assessed through medical records and follow-up data. The study found that while TPBS had high sensitivity, its specificity was low, leading to numerous false positives for infection or loosening.

The findings of this study highlight the limited diagnostic role of TPBS in assessing post-TKR knee pain. Hill et al. emphasize that an abnormal TPBS does not reliably indicate the need for revision surgery and often fails to provide additional insights beyond existing diagnostic methods. The authors suggest that better, more cost-effective alternatives exist for diagnosing peri-prosthetic infections and recommend that TPBS should only be considered after thorough evaluation by a specialist revision knee arthroplasty surgeon. Future study could explore more accurate imaging techniques or biomarkers to improve the diagnosis of complications following TKR surgery.

Bibliography

1. Toms AD, Mandalia V, Haigh R, Hopwood B (2009) The management of patients with painful total knee replacement. J Bone Joint Surg Br 91(2):143–150
2. Greidanus NV, Masri BA, Garbuz DS, Wilson SD, McAlinden MG, Xu M et al (2007) Use of erythrocyte sedimentation rate and C-reactive protein level to diagnose infection before revision total knee arthroplasty. A prospective evaluation. J Bone Joint Surg Am 89(7):1409–1416
3. Mandalia V, Eyres K, Schranz P, Toms AD (2008) Evaluation of patient with a painful total knee replacement. J Bone Joint Surg (British) 90-B(3):265–271
4. Henderson JJ, Bamford DJ, Noble J, Brown JD (1996) The value of skeletal scintigraphy in predicting the need for revision surgery in total knee replacement. Orthopedics 19(4):295–299
5. Smith SL, Wastie ML, Forster I (2001) Radionuclide bone scintigraphy in the detection of significant complications after total knee joint replacement. Clin Radiol 56(3):221–224
6. Rubello D, Caricasulo D, Borsato N, Chierichetti F, Zanco P, Ferlin G (1996) Three-phase bone scan pattern in asymptomatic uncemented total knee arthroplasty. Eur J Nucl Med 23(10):1400–1403
7. Verlooy H, Victor J, Renson L, Vandecruys A, Drent P, Mortelmans L et al (1993) Limitations of quantitative radionuclide bone scanning in the evaluation of total knee replacement. Clin Nucl Med 18(8):671–674
8. Hill, Daniel S.; Kinsella, Denis; Toms, Andrew D. Three-phase Technetium-99m bone scanning in patients with pain in the knee region after cemented total knee arthroplasty. European Journal of Orthopaedic Surgery & Traumatology (2019). https://doi.org/10.1007/s00590-019-02407-5

3.6 Arthrogram

Machine Generated Summaries

Disclaimer: The summaries in this chapter were generated from Springer Nature publications using abstractive AI auto-summarization: An abstraction-based summarizer creates new text based on deep learning. New phrases are created to summarize the content. As the constituted sentences are machine selected, they may not fully reflect the body of the work, so we strongly advise that the original content is read and cited. The auto-generated summaries were curated by the editor to meet Springer Nature publication standards.

3.6.1 *Detection of Aseptic Loosening in Total Knee Replacements: A Systematic Review and Meta-analysis [15]*

This is a machine-generated summary of:

Barnslcy, Lara; Barnsley, Les Detection of aseptic loosening in total knee replacements: a systematic review and meta-analysis [15].

Published in: Skeletal Radiology (2019).

Link to original: https://doi.org/10.1007/s00256-019-03215-y

If you want to cite the papers, please refer to the original.

For technical reasons we could not place the page where the original quote is coming from.

3.6.1.1 Research Highlights

Total knee arthroplasty (TKA) is a widely performed surgical procedure for managing osteoarthritis, with over 50,000 operations conducted annually in Australia. Aseptic loosening, characterized by the failure of the prosthesis-bone integration without infection, is the leading cause of revision surgeries for TKA. The challenge lies in the insidious progression of tissue damage around the implant due to particulate deposition, which often remains undetected until advanced stages. The study by Barnsley et al. aims to address this issue by evaluating the diagnostic accuracy of various nuclear medical imaging modalities for detecting aseptic loosening in knee prostheses.

The study conducted a systematic review and meta-analysis following PRISMA (Preferred Reporting Items for Systematic Reviews and Meta-Analyses) guidelines, searching databases such as MEDLINE, EMBASE, and the Cochrane Database. The researchers included studies that compared nuclear imaging modalities like bone scintigraphy, Single Photon Emission Computed Tomography/CT (SPECT/CT) arthrography, radionuclide arthrography, and FDG-PET against a criterion standard for diagnosing aseptic loosening. Data extraction was performed independently by two authors using a standardized tool, and risk of bias was assessed using the QUADAS-2 tool. The study did not calculate pooled estimates but used summary receiver operating characteristic (SROC) curves to compare diagnostic accuracy. Among the modalities assessed, SPECT/CT arthrography emerged as the most accurate technique for identifying aseptic loosening.

The study highlights that while SPECT/CT arthrography shows promise as a diagnostic tool for aseptic loosening in TKA, the findings are limited by the small sample sizes and high risk of bias in included studies. Future studies should focus on larger sample sizes and incorporate CT and MRI assessments with contemporary metal artifact reduction techniques to enhance diagnostic accuracy. Additionally, reporting detailed data on diagnosis combinations and time intervals between procedures could improve future research outcomes. These steps are crucial given the significant clinical implications of misdiagnosis in TKA patients.

3.6.2 Diagnostic Accuracy of SPECT/CT Arthrography in Patients with Suspected Aseptic Joint Prostheses Loosening [16]

This is a machine-generated summary of:

Bao, Bo; Liu, Crystal S.; Masson, Edward C. O.; Abele, Jonathan T. Diagnostic accuracy of SPECT/CT arthrography in patients with suspected aseptic joint prostheses loosening [16].

Published in: European Journal of Hybrid Imaging (2021).

Link to original: https://doi.org/10.1186/s41824-021-00098-y

If you want to cite the papers, please refer to the original.

For technical reasons we could not place the page where the original quote is coming from.

3.6.2.1 Research Highlights

Hip and knee arthroplasties are widely performed procedures to manage osteoarthritis, with millions of individuals in the USA having undergone these surgeries. Despite their general success, a significant number of patients experience persistent pain post-surgery, often due to aseptic loosening—a complication that necessitates major revision surgery. Accurate detection of aseptic loosening is crucial for guiding management decisions in these cases. The study by et al. investigates the diagnostic accuracy of Single Photon Emission Computed Tomogaphy/CT (SPECT/CT) arthrography in detecting aseptic loosening in patients with persistent pain following hip or knee arthroplasty.

The study conducted a retrospective analysis of SPECT/CT arthrograms performed at their center between February 2015 and July 2020. Patients included in the study had undergone initial standard radiograph exams followed by SPECT/CT arthrograms as part of their diagnostic pathway. The researchers analyzed demographic information, radiographic diagnoses, clinical findings, and surgical reports. They excluded cases with failed tracer injections or without a reference standard for diagnosis. The imaging procedure involved injecting a tracer into the joint space under fluoroscopic guidance, followed by SPECT/CT imaging to detect tracer activity along the bone-prosthetic interface. The study found that SPECT/CT arthrography demonstrated high sensitivity and specificity for detecting aseptic loosening, with true-positive results confirmed during revision surgeries.

The findings suggest that SPECT/CT arthrography is a highly accurate diagnostic tool for identifying aseptic loosening in patients experiencing persistent pain after hip or knee arthroplasty. This technique could serve as an important adjunct to conventional imaging methods, particularly in complex cases where clinical uncertainty exists. Future study could explore optimizing the timing between tracer injection and imaging to potentially improve diagnostic accuracy further. Additionally, comparing SPECT/CT arthrography with other imaging modalities like bone scintigraphy may provide insights into enhancing diagnostic protocols for aseptic loosening detection.

Bibliography

1. Sneag DB, Bogner EA, Potter HG. Magnetic resonance imaging evaluation of the painful total knee arthroplasty. Semin Musculoskelet Radiol. 2015;19:40–8.
2. Jones CM, Athanasiou T. Summary receiver operating characteristic curve analysis techniques in the evaluation of diagnostic tests. Ann Thorac Surg. 2005;79:16–20.
3. Macaskill P, Gatsonis C, Deeks J, Harbord R, Takwoingi Y. Chapter 10: analysing and presenting results. In: Deeks J, Bossuyt P, Gatsonis C, eds. Cochrane handbook for systematic reviews of diagnostic test accuracy version 10: The Cochrane Collaboration; 2010.
4. Whiting P, Rutjes A, Westwood M, Mallett S, Deeks J, Reitsma J, et al. QUADAS-2: a revised tool for the quality assessment of diagnostic accuracy studies. Ann Intern Med. 2011;155(8):529–36.
5. Zweig M, Campbell G. Receiver-operating characteristic (ROC) plots: a fundamental evaluation tool in clinical medicine. Clin Chem. 1993;39(4):561–77.
6. Mandegaran R, Agrawal K, Vijayanathan S, Gnanasegaran G. The value of 99mTc-MDP bone SPECT/CT in evaluation of patients with painful knee prosthesis. Nucl Med Commun. 2018;39(5):397–404.

7. Chew CG, Lewis P, Middleton F, Wijngaard R, Deshaies A. Radionuclide arthrogram with SPECT/CT for the evaluation of mechanical loosening of hip and knee prostheses. Ann Nucl Med. 2010;24:735–43.
8. Marx A, Saxler G, Landgraeber S, Löer F, Holland-Letz T, Mv K. Comparison of subtraction arthrography, radionuclide arthrography and conventional plain radiography to assess loosening of total knee arthroplasty. Biomed Tech. 2005;50:143–7.
9. Wylde V, Hewlett S, Learmonth ID, Dieppe P (2011) Persistent pain after joint replacement: prevalence, sensory qualities, and postoperative determinants. Pain 152(3):566–572
10. Piscitelli P, Iolascon G, Innocenti M, Civinini R, Rubinacci A, Muratore M et al (2013) Painful prosthesis: approaching the patient with persistent pain following total hip and knee arthroplasty. Clin Cases Miner Bone Metab 10(2):97–110
11. Becker R, Bonnin M, Hofmann S. The painful knee after total knee arthroplasty. Knee Surg Sports Traumatol Arthrosc. 2011;19(9):1409–10.
12. Sharkey PF, Lichstein PM, Shen C, Tokarski AT, Parvizi J (2014) Why are total knee arthroplasties failing today—has anything changed after 10 years? J Arthroplasty 29:1774–1778
13. Lohmann CH, Rampal S, Lohrengel M, Singh G (2017) Imaging in periprosthetic assessment: an orthopaedic perspective. EFORT Open Rev 2(5):117–125
14. Abele JT, Swami VG, Russell G, Masson ECO, Flemming JP. The accuracy of single photon emission computed tomography/computed tomography arthrography in evaluating aseptic loosening of hip and knee prostheses. J Arthroplast. 2015;30:1647–51.
15. Barnsley, Lara; Barnsley, Les Detection of aseptic loosening in total knee replacements: a systematic review and meta-analysis. Skeletal Radiology (2019). https://doi.org/10.1007/s00256-019-03215-y
16. Bao, Bo; Liu, Crystal S.; Masson, Edward C. O.; Abele, Jonathan T. Diagnostic accuracy of SPECT/CT arthrography in patients with suspected aseptic joint prostheses loosening. European Journal of Hybrid Imaging (2021). https://doi.org/10.1186/s41824-021-00098-y

3.7 Advanced Techniques

Machine Generated Summaries

Disclaimer: The summaries in this chapter were generated from Springer Nature publications using abstractive AI auto-summarization: An abstraction-based summarizer creates new text based on deep learning. New phrases are created to summarize the content. As the constituted sentences are machine selected, they may not fully reflect the body of the work, so we strongly advise that the original content is read and cited. The auto-generated summaries were curated by the editor to meet Springer Nature publication standards.

3.7.1 Do Size, Shape, and Alignment Parameters of the Femoral Condyle Affect the Trochlear Groove Tracking? A Morphometric Study Based on 3D-Computed Tomography Models in Chinese People [5]

This is a machine-generated summary of:

Du, Zhe; Chen, Shichang; Yan, Mengning; Yue, Bing; Zeng, Yiming; Wang, You Do size, shape, and alignment parameters of the femoral condyle affect the trochlear groove tracking? A morphometric study based on 3D- computed tomography models in Chinese people [5].

Published in: BMC Musculoskeletal Disorders (2017).

Link to original: https://doi.org/10.1186/s12891-016-1374-3

If you want to cite the papers, please refer to the original.

For technical reasons we could not place the page where the original quote is coming from.

3.7.1.1 Research Highlights

Evaluating the morphology of the trochlear groove is crucial for understanding differences between natural and prosthetic knees, as well as between healthy and pathological knees. Previous studies have classified the trochlear groove into four main types based on the position of the groove turning point relative to the femoral mechanical axis, providing a foundation for anatomical category definitions in groove tracking. However, it remains unclear which specific geometrical features of the trochlear groove influence its morphology, especially beyond factors like sex, morphotype, and race. The study by Du et al. investigates whether certain morphological parameters of the femoral condyle affect the shape of the trochlear groove in Chinese individuals.

The study utilized computerized tomography (CT) images from a previous cohort to analyze three-dimensional knee models of healthy individuals. The researchers established three-dimensional planes based on anatomical landmarks and classified the trochlear groove into four types using coaxial cutting planes along the trochlear groove axis. They measured various size, shape, and alignment parameters of the femoral condyle to determine their influence on trochlear groove morphology. Statistical analyses were conducted to assess differences among groups classified by trochlear groove type. The study found that size-related parameters did not significantly influence trochlear groove morphology. However, shape- and alignment-related parameters showed partial influence, particularly affecting types 0° and 90°.

The findings suggest that shape- and alignment-related parameters are key factors influencing trochlear groove morphology. Specifically, type 0° grooves are associated with relatively flat femoral condyles, while type 90° grooves are linked to valgus knee alignment. These insights could inform individualized prosthesis design for Chinese populations by considering these morphological characteristics. Future study could explore these relationships in arthritic knees to enhance prosthetic implant design further. The study's limitations include reliance on CT data that excludes cartilage layer considerations and its focus on healthy adults, indicating areas for future research expansion.

3.7.2 Validation of a Measuring Technique with Computed Tomography for Cement Penetration into Trabecular Bone underneath the Tibial Tray in Total Knee Arthroplasty on a Cadaver Model [6]

This is a machine-generated summary of:

Verburg, Hennie; van de Ridder, Laurens C; Verhoeven, Vincent WJ; Pilot, Peter Validation of a measuring technique with computed tomography for cement penetration into trabecular bone underneath the tibial tray in total knee arthroplasty on a cadaver model [6].

Published in: BMC Medical Imaging (2014).

Link to original: https://doi.org/10.1186/1471-2342-14-29

If you want to cite the papers, please refer to the original.

For technical reasons we could not place the page where the original quote is coming from.

3.7.2.1 Research Highlights

In total knee arthroplasty (TKA), cement is commonly used to fixate the tibial component, yet loosening due to micro motion at the cement-bone interface remains a significant cause of late failure. Optimal cement penetration into the trabecular bone is crucial for preventing this micro motion, but current in vivo measurement techniques, such as conventional radiographs, are limited by their two-dimensional nature and difficulty in achieving precise alignment. The study by Verburg et al. addresses this challenge by developing and validating a novel in vivo technique using computerized tomography (CT) imaging to measure cement penetration beneath tibial prostheses.

The study utilized femoral heads from total hip arthroplasty patients to simulate the tibial environment. Researchers defined radiodensity ranges for trabecular bone, polymethylmethacrylate (PMMA) cement, and cement-penetrated bone using CT scans. They then assessed cement penetration by applying PMMA cement to tibial prostheses implanted in femoral heads and conducted spiral CT scans to analyze the distribution and depth of cement penetration. The influence of metal prostheses on CT image quality was also evaluated by comparing scans with and without the prosthesis in place. The results showed that modern CT imaging could accurately differentiate between trabecular bone and cement-penetrated bone without significant interference from metal artifacts.

The study's findings suggest that CT imaging can reliably measure the three-dimensional extent of cement penetration in TKA, providing a valuable tool for clinical assessment and comparison of different cementing techniques. Future study could explore the optimal percentage of cement penetration required at various depths to prevent prosthesis loosening. This advancement holds promise for improving TKA outcomes by enabling more precise evaluation of cement fixation quality in vivo, potentially guiding surgical practices toward enhanced long-term stability of knee implants.

3.7.3 Computed Tomography Radiomics in Predicting Patient Satisfaction after Robotic-Assisted Total Knee Arthroplasty [7]

This is a machine-generated summary of:

Tian, Run; Duan, Xudong; Xing, Fangze; Zhao, Yiwei; Liu, ChengYan; Li, Heng; Kong, Ning; Cao, Ruomu; Guan, Huanshuai; Li, Yiyang; Li, Xinghua; Zhang, Jiewen; Wang, Kunzheng; Yang, Pei; Wang, Chunsheng Computed tomography radiomics in predicting patient satisfaction after robotic-assisted total knee arthroplasty [7].

Published in: International Journal of Computer Assisted Radiology and Surgery (2024).

If you want to cite the papers, please refer to the original.

For technical reasons we could not place the page where the original quote is coming from.

3.7.3.1 Research Highlights

Total knee arthroplasty (TKA) is a widely accepted surgical intervention for end-stage knee joint pathologies, offering significant pain relief and improved joint function. Despite advancements in conventional TKA, challenges such as suboptimal prosthetic alignment and soft tissue balance persist, affecting patient satisfaction. Robot-assisted TKA systems have been introduced to address these issues, yet some patients still experience dissatisfaction post-surgery. Identifying risk factors for postoperative dissatisfaction remains a challenge, with limited research available. The study by Tian et al. explores the use of radiomics combined with clinical data to develop a predictive model for patient satisfaction following robot-assisted TKA.

The study involved patients who underwent primary unilateral TKA at a hospital between July and October. Patients were selected based on specific inclusion criteria, such as age range and follow-up duration, while those with complications or low-quality imaging data were excluded. The researchers utilized computerized tomography (CT) scans to extract radiomic features from preoperative images using Slicer software and Pyradiomics(van Griethuysen, et al., Cancer Research, 77(21), e104–e107). A total of 1000 radiomic features were initially extracted, with 10 selected for further analysis based on statistical significance and reliability. The study employed logistic regression to develop a clinical model using factors like postoperative hip-knee-ankle (HKA) angle and visual analog scale (VAS) score. By combining these clinical factors with radiomic features, the researchers constructed a Radiomics-Clinical nomogram model to predict patient satisfaction 6 months post-surgery.

The combined clinical-radiomic model demonstrated superior predictive performance compared to models using only clinical or radiomic data. Calibration curves indicated good agreement between predicted and actual outcomes, while decision curve analysis showed the nomogram's potential clinical utility. Future study could focus on addressing limitations such as manual segmentation bias and short-term follow-up by incorporating artificial intelligence techniques and conducting multicenter prospective studies with larger sample sizes. This research highlights the potential of integrating radiomics into predictive models to enhance personalized medicine approaches in TKA procedures.

Bibliography

1. Lutz MJ, Pincus PF, Whitehouse SL, Halliday BR: The effect of cement gun and cement syringe use on the tibial cement mantle in total knee arthroplasty. J Arthroplast. 2009, 24 (3): 461–467. https://doi.org/10.1016/j.arth.2007.10.028.
2. Lee GC (2016) Patient-specific cutting blocks: of unproven value. Bone Jt J 98-b:78–80. https://doi.org/10.1302/0301-620x.98b1.36370
3. Verbeek JFM, Hannink G, Defoort KC, Wymenga AB, Heesterbeek PJC (2019) Age, gender, functional KSS, reason for revision and type of bone defect predict functional outcome 5 years after revision total knee arthroplasty: a multivariable prediction model. Knee Surg Sports Traumatol Arthrosc 27:2289–2296. https://doi.org/10.1007/s00167-019-05365-x
4. Muertizha M, Cai X, Ji B, Aimaiti A, Cao L (2022) Factors contributing to 1-year dissatisfaction after total knee arthroplasty: a nomogram prediction model. J Orthop Surg Res 17:367. https://doi.org/10.1186/s13018-022-03205-2
5. Du, Zhe; Chen, Shichang; Yan, Mengning; Yue, Bing; Zeng, Yiming; Wang, You Do size, shape, and alignment parameters of the femoral condyle affect the trochlear groove tracking? A morphometric study based on 3D- computed tomography models in Chinese people. BMC Musculoskeletal Disorders (2017). https://doi.org/10.1186/s12891-016-1374-3
6. Verburg, Hennie; van de Ridder, Laurens C; Verhoeven, Vincent WJ; Pilot, Peter Validation of a measuring technique with computed tomography for cement penetration into trabecular bone underneath the tibial tray in total knee arthroplasty on a cadaver model. BMC Medical Imaging (2014). https://doi.org/10.1186/1471-2342-14-29
7. Tian, Run; Duan, Xudong; Xing, Fangze; Zhao, Yiwei; Liu, ChengYan; Li, Heng; Kong, Ning; Cao, Ruomu; Guan, Huanshuai; Li, Yiyang; Li, Xinghua; Zhang, Jiewen; Wang, Kunzheng; Yang, Pei; Wang, Chunsheng Computed tomography radiomics in predicting patient satisfaction after robotic-assisted total knee arthroplasty. International Journal of Computer Assisted Radiology and Surgery (2024). https://doi.org/10.1007/s11548-024-03192-1

Chapter 4
Prosthetic Designs for Primary Total Knee Arthroplasty

Alfred J. Tria Jr. and Giles R. Scuderi

Introduction by the Editors

The current prostheses for primary total knee arthroplasty (TKA) have all come from three main designs: PCL sparing, posterior stabilized, and mobile bearing. Since the very first TKA by Insall, Ranawat, and Walker, the issue of the cruciate ligaments and their importance in knee range of motion (ROM), balance, and proprioception has been ever present. The original total condylar knee sacrificed both cruciates and relied upon the surface anatomy for stability. The polycentric knee attempted to retain both cruciates and was fraught with loosening. Then, designers decided to sacrifice the anterior cruciate ligament and rely upon the posterior cruciate ligament (PCL) for stability or resect both cruciates and substitute for the PCL. The mobile bearing design looked toward addressing wear with mobile surfaces and initially sacrificed the cruciate ligaments. The 15 percent dissatisfaction rate continues to trouble designers and the final solution is yet to come. This chapter addresses the present-day prostheses including PCL sparing, medial pivot, PCL substituting, bicruciate retaining, partial knee replacements, and constrained knees.

Using our editorial prerogative, we reviewed each of the referenced articles and summarized our own conclusions, as detailed below. As you read each of the computer-generated summaries that follow in this chapter you can draw your own conclusions.

With regard to PCL sparing designs, Razak et al. looked at the joint line changes in the posterior cruciate sparing (CR) versus the posterior stabilized (PS) knees. The CR knees showed less joint line changes, but the differences were not significant. This information is not new. Several of the authors looked at PCL preservation

A. J. Tria Jr. (✉)
Department of Orthopedics, Rutgers-Robert Wood Johnson Medical School, New Brunswick, NJ, USA

G. R. Scuderi
Department of Orthopedic Surgery, Northwell Health, Garden City, NY, USA

A. J. Tria Jr., G. R. Scuderi (eds.), *Total Knee Arthroplasty*,
https://doi.org/10.1007/978-3-032-00175-7_4

during the CR surgery. Cinotti et al. reviews the surgical technique for tibial resection in a CR knee. Th data showed that the two-cut technique preserved the PCL better. However, the en-block resection was not protected with retractors as was the double cut. Xin et al. showed that the presence of a discoid lateral meniscus made PCL preservation more difficult. Yue et al. showed that the retained PCL elongates much more in flexion than in the osteoarthritic knee restricting motion. When it comes to coronal deformity, McAuley et al. reviewed the valgus knee with PCL preservation and concluded that preservation of the lateral collateral ligament and the popliteus insertion was associated with a better clinical result. This is not new information but affirms previous publications. Savov et al. favored the PS over the CR knee in the valgus deformity but admitted that the CR knee probably needed a more constrained insert. When the deformity is greater than 10 degrees, more release are usually required demanding more constraint in the associated tibial insert.

Jawhar et al. suggested using the fibular head for PCL location and this is another surgical landmark that is helpful.

Chen et al. looked at stability with PCL retention versus resection with a highly congruent tibial insert. The results were judged with respect to post operative complications but without any objective kinematic information. Fiedler et al. looked at pain with the PCL retention and found no difference from the PS design. Ersin et al. looked at the tibial slope and showed its relationship to anterior translation. While it appeared to have minimal clinical affect, the angle does affect translation. Zhao et al. measured compartment pressures at different angles and concluded that the data supported use of a CR prosthesis even when the PCL is resected. This conclusion is not well supported by this data and further study is warranted. Fujimoto et al. used an offset tensor to evaluate the surgical gaps and the conclusions affirm previous knowledge that the gaps do affect rollback. Matsumoto et al. looked at CR and PS knees with two techniques: measured resection and gap balancing. The gap balancing was favored slightly.

Tsuji et al. looked at rollback and mobile bearing modifications. The modified implant did have greater flexion; however, the numbers were not that large. Seon et al. studied kinematics to affirm our knowledge that the final ROM after surgery correlates well with the preop. Peters et al. compared a highly congruent anterior stabilized knee to a CR design. While the anterior stabilized had fewer revisions, this may have been biased by the surgical choice in the operating room. Elorza et al. showed that increased medal conformity in the PCL retaining knee increased internal rotation and stability. This is information that is already documented in the literature.

Lee et al. evaluated outcome scores and compared the PS knee to the medal congruent CR knee with no long-term clinical difference and some slight faster early recovery with the PS, which is not significant. Obada et al. also compared the PS and medial pivot favoring the medial pivot but in a study with no randomization and no indication how the surgeons chose the prostheses. Therefore, the findings are not strong enough to support a particular implant design. Nakamura et al. compared a flat tibial surface design to a medial pivot both PCL sparing and favored the medial pivot. However, this was a retrospective study without any information on indications and patient selection.. I search of an implant that best replicates normal knee kinematics, numerous comparative studies have been performed. Groot et al. compared three designs: PS, rotating platform, ad medial pivot. The medial pivot had more AP stability, but clinical results were the same. Xu et al. in a comparison of PS and medial pivot showed the only difference was less patellar cluck in the medial pivot. This is not a new finding. Shi et al. compared medial pivot and PS with no clinical differences. Iwakiri et al. compared the medial pivot and the PS in the valgus knee setting and found not significant differences. Iwakiri et al. performed a comparison with a valgus deformity, but there were only 15 valgus knees, and the degree of deformity was not reported. Risitano et al. compared the medial pivot and PS designs with respect to gait analysis and showed that the two have significant kinematic differences.

Ueyama et al. reported on 10-year clinical results of a alumina ceramic medial pivot design with 97% without ceramic complications. This group also reported on a comparison of 2 medial pivot designs with kinematic improvements with the modified knee that had and enlarged single radius and asymmetric tibial trays. While the results were statistically significant the ROM only improved by 9 degrees and the Forgotten Joint Score score by 7 points.

Implant selection will always be surgeon choice based upon experience and their patient outcomes. Wittig et al. reported that the fixed bearing and PS implants are favored over the mobile and medial pivot in the countries included in their study. However, this data does not conform to the present-day experience in the United States. Chinzei et al. offered a study of the Advance TKA. The real value of the paper is the ability compare a simple post-operative x-ray to a preoperative CT scan. In reviewing implant kinematics, Nakajima et al. noted that there can be a lateral shift of the femoral component in the medial pivot design. This is design specific and cannot be applied to all such designs. In contrast, Putame et al. observed that increased constraint in the medial pivot design allows for less internal tibial rotation.

Longevity and durability are very desirable. The study by Xiang et al. included 1128 medial pivot knees with 95.6% survival at an average of 5 years. Simmarily, Cacciola et al. looked at 297 medial pivot knees with a 97.5% survival at 5 years.

The PS has been a popular design since it reproducible kinematics even with complex deformities. Kim et al., Ishii et al., Gotz et al., Ritter et al., and Ozturk et al. all compared various aspects of the PS and the PCL sparing knees with minimal differences. Mne et al. report on a single PS knee design showing good stability but variant kinematics versus the normal knee. These findings are not surprising as the degree of deformity will impact kinematics. In that regard surgical technique and implant placement is important. Chiang et al. discuss their observations with femoral posterior condylar offset choosing either posterior referencing or anterior referencing for placement and sizing of the femoral component, It was interesting that they reported no difference, as one would have suspected that posterior referencing provided a more predictable posterior condylar offset.

Realizing the importance of both the ACL and PCL in knee kinematics, designs have attempted to replicate this with the bicruciate substituting knee design. Chisten et al. reported on 226 knees with a complication rate of 10.3% thought to be due to a steep learning curve. In contrast attempts to design bicruciate retaining implants have been entertained. While Kono et al. report on the altered kinematics of the design, Zhao et al. showed that the bicruciate retaining design had promising kinematics. This has been a challenging design as Christensen et al. report poor results with the implant due either to the design itself or difficulty with the surgical technique. Furtherance to these observations, Inui et al. reported short term results comparing the the bicruciate retaining design to unicompartmental knee arthroplasty with similar findings. They did indicate that the management of the soft tissues was critical to success. Bauman et al. reported that the the bicruciate retaining design had reduced joint awareness perhaps related to improved proprioception. Pritchett's study has the longest follow up with the the bicruciate retaining design and showed satisfactory survivorship of 94%. These results are certainly related both to the design and the surgical technique. Singh et al. showed good results at 2 years but admitted that the limitations of the study included the short term and the retrospective review. Not without complications, Biazzo et al. did a comparison of the the bicruciate retaining design to the posterior cruciate retaining design and reported more complications with the the bicruciate retaining design.

Unicompartmental knee arthroplasty (UKA) has gained some popularity. The Oxford implant has been reviewed in this chapter by Bray et al. Walker et al. and Hiranaka et al. They discuss some short-term results and accuracy studies with all agreeing that there is a learning curve to the surgery. Xie et al., Smith et al. look at TKA versus UKA from the aspect of cost and from identifying patient's needs. The results were mixed in both studies. Slamin et al. discuss evolution and is a good review of the approach to customization without addressing the costs involved. Mertens et al. look at the functional outcome of bicompartmental replacements, The modular implants are more effective, but the measuring was difficult and there is no long-term follow-up. Mobile bearing and fixed bearing UKAs are reviewed by Kulshrestha et al. and D'Ambrosi et el. with similar results but they do involve a learning curve. Yeung et al. discuss robotic assisted UKA ad show similar results to other reports with greater accuracy but no clinical differences. Lee et al. favor UKA over HTO for survival. However, the study went out 12 years and this may not be long enough for a thorough comparison. Van Langeveld e al. conclude that the valgus stress x-ray for a medial UKA is not that helpful. This is not supported in the literature.

Elbardesy et al. compared the results of treatment of patellofemoral arthritis with either a TKA or a patellofemoral arthroplasty (PFA). They favor the PFA with 5 years of follow-up. The review has two flaws: short term follow up and no inclusion of surgical complications or difficulties. Woon et al. attempted to address these two factors and did show a higher rate of return to the operating room with the PFA.

With numerous designs available, it is surgeon preference what they choose for each of their patients. Some surgeons take an individualized approach and select a specific implant for a specific patient deformity. While others choose one implant and use it for all patients. What is apparent is that each implant design has a specific nuance to the surgical technique that impact the clinical outcome. Hopefully this chapter gives you further insights into some of the designs.

4.1 PCL Sparing

Machine Generated Summaries
Disclaimer: The summaries in this chapter were generated from Springer Nature publications using abstractive AI auto-summarization: An abstraction-based summarizer creates new text based on deep learning. New phrases are created to summarize the content. As the constituted sentences are machine selected, they may not fully reflect the body of the work, so we strongly advise that the original content is read and cited. The auto-generated summaries were curated by the editor to meet Springer Nature publication standards.

4.1.1 Joint Line Changes in Cruciate-Retaining Versus Posterior-Stabilized Computer-Navigated Total Knee Arthroplasty [106]

This is a machine-generated summary of:

Bin Abd Razak, Hamid Rahmatullah; Pang, Hee Nee; Yeo, Seng Jin; Tan, Mann Hong; Lo, Ngai Nung; Chong, Hwei Chi Joint line changes in cruciate-retaining versus posterior-stabilized computer-navigated total knee arthroplasty [106].

Published in: Archives of Orthopaedic and Trauma Surgery (2013).

Link to original: https://doi.org/10.1007/s00402-013-1738-1

If you want to cite the papers, please refer to the original.

For technical reasons we could not place the page where the original quote is coming from.

4.1.1.1 Research Highlights

Restoration of the native joint line is a critical objective in total knee arthroplasty (TKA), with computer-navigated TKA gaining popularity for its precision in implant positioning and improved functional outcomes. Despite this, the impact of computer navigation on joint line restoration, particularly between cruciate-retaining (CR) and posterior-stabilized (PS) prostheses, remains underexplored. Razak et al. compared the joint line changes in computer-navigated CR and PS TKAs and evaluating their impact on clinical outcomes.

The study utilized a retrospective design, analyzing data from patients who underwent primary computer-navigated TKA for severe osteoarthritis. Patients were categorized into CR or PS groups based on the condition of their posterior cruciate ligament and other surgical considerations. The researchers employed

BrainLab (Depuy, Warswa, IN) Mi TKR software for precise anatomical mapping and surgical planning. Key measurements included joint line changes, mechanical axis alignment, and range of motion, assessed through standardized radiographs and goniometry. Statistical analyses revealed that while CR TKAs exhibited significantly lesser joint line changes compared to PS TKAs, the absolute difference was minimal. Both groups achieved similar mechanical axis alignment and functional outcomes over a follow-up period extending to several years.

This study concluded that although there is a statistically significant difference in joint line changes between CR and PS TKAs, the clinical relevance of this difference is negligible. The findings suggest that the choice between CR and PS designs should be guided by individual patient factors rather than concerns over joint line restoration alone. Future study could focus on prospective trials to further validate these findings and explore mid-flexion stability issues not addressed in this research. The results underscore the importance of personalized surgical planning in achieving optimal outcomes in TKA procedures.

4.1.2 *Higher Rates of Fully Preserved Posterior Cruciate Ligament in Total Knee Arthroplasty Using a Double Tibial Cut: A Prospective Randomized Controlled Trial [107]*

This is a machine-generated summary of:

Cinotti, Gianluca; Ripani, Francesca Romana; Perciballi, Beatrice; La Torre, Giuseppe; Giannicola, Giuseppe Higher rates of fully preserved posterior cruciate ligament in total knee arthroplasty using a double tibial cut: a prospective randomized controlled trial [107].

Published in: Knee Surgery & Related Research (2024).

Link to original: https://doi.org/10.1186/s43019-023-00208-z

If you want to cite the papers, please refer to the original.

For technical reasons we could not place the page where the original quote is coming from.

4.1.2.1 Research Highlights

Clinical and experimental studies have established the critical role of the posterior cruciate ligament (PCL) in maintaining normal knee biomechanics, particularly as a primary constraint against posterior tibial translation and a secondary stabilizer under rotatory loading. In total knee arthroplasty (TKA), designs that either retain or sacrifice the PCL have been developed, with each approach presenting unique challenges and outcomes. Despite satisfactory results with cruciate retaining (CR) implants, issues such as paradoxical femoral rollback and decreased tibial rotation persist, potentially leading to patient dissatisfaction. A study by Cinotti et al. investigates the effectiveness of a novel double tibial cutting technique aimed at preserving the PCL during TKA, compared to traditional methods.

The study was conducted as a prospective randomized controlled trial involving patients scheduled for primary TKA due to knee osteoarthritis. Participants were randomly assigned to one of three groups: the novel double tibial cut technique, bone island preservation, or en bloc resection. The double cut technique involved an initial tibial cut followed by a second cut to achieve the necessary thickness for implant placement while protecting the PCL fibers with a retractor. The effectiveness of each technique was assessed through intraoperative visualization of PCL integrity and postoperative evaluations including femoral rollback using fluoroscopy, range of motion (ROM), and clinical scores such as the Oxford Knee Score (OKS) and Western Ontario and McMaster Universities Osteoarthritis Index (WOMAC).

The study found that the double tibial cut technique resulted in significantly higher rates of complete PCL preservation compared to the other methods. This approach also led to improved femoral rollback and ROM without compromising clinical outcomes. While all groups showed significant improvements in clinical scores postoperatively, no significant differences were observed between them. Future study could explore larger sample sizes or different implant designs to further validate these findings. The research highlights the potential for improved surgical techniques in TKA to enhance ligament preservation and patient satisfaction.

4.1.3 The Effect of Sacrificing the Posterior Cruciate Ligament on Total Knee Arthroplasty with Cruciate Retaining Highly Congruent Rotating Platform Prosthesis [108]

This is a machine-generated summary of:

Chen, Long; Xu, Jie; Lin, Yuan; Luo, Fen Qi; Yu, Yu Guo The effect of sacrificing the posterior cruciate ligament on total knee arthroplasty with cruciate retaining highly congruent rotating platform prosthesis [108].

Published in: Journal of Orthopaedic Surgery and Research (2021).

Link to original: https://doi.org/10.1186/s13018-021-02433-2

If you want to cite the papers, please refer to the original.

For technical reasons we could not place the page where the original quote is coming from.

4.1.3.1 Research Highlights

Total knee arthroplasty (TKA) is a common treatment for end-stage knee osteoarthritis, with the posterior cruciate ligament (PCL) playing a crucial role in prosthesis stability. Previous studies have shown no significant difference in clinical outcomes when comparing PCL retention and sacrifice in various TKA designs. However, in cruciate retaining (CR) highly congruent rotating platform TKA, excessive PCL tension can lead to complications such as bearing dislocation, necessitating PCL release. Although it is known that sacrificing the PCL does not affect the stability of CR highly congruent fixed platform prostheses, its impact on CR highly congruent rotating platform prostheses remains unexplored. The study by Chen et al. investigates the effects of PCL sacrifice on knee function following TKA with CR highly congruent rotating platform prostheses.

The study retrospectively analyzed cases of TKA performed between May and September 2018–19, focusing on patients who received CR highly congruent rotating platform prostheses. Patients were divided into two groups based on PCL continuity and tension: a sacrifice group and a retention group. All surgeries were conducted by the same senior orthopedic surgeon using standardized procedures, including general anesthesia and specific osteotomy techniques to balance extension and flexion gaps. Postoperative management involved early mobilization and regular follow-ups to assess range of motion (ROM) and Hospital for Special Surgery (HSS) scores. Statistical analyses revealed significant improvements in postoperative ROM and HSS scores in both groups, with no significant differences. Additionally, no postoperative complications such as joint instability or prosthesis loosening were observed.

The study's findings suggest that sacrificing the PCL in CR highly congruent rotating platform TKA does not compromise joint stability or function, aligning with previous research on fixed platform prostheses. The deep disk design of the highly congruent gasket enhances prosthesis stability by increasing contact area and limiting excessive femoral movement during flexion. Future study could focus on larger sample sizes and longer follow-up periods to better understand the long-term effects of PCL sacrifice on prosthesis survival. Additionally, developing precise objective indicators for assessing PCL tension could improve surgical decision-making and outcomes.

4.1.4 Posterior Cruciate Ligament Tibial Attachment Sacrifice Percentage Is Higher in Cruciate-Retaining Total Knee Arthroplasty in Patients with Discoid Lateral Meniscus [109]

This is a machine-generated summary of:

Xin, Weiwei; Gao, Yingjian; Zheng, Liangjun; Qu, Xinhua; Yue, Bing Posterior cruciate ligament tibial attachment sacrifice percentage is higher in cruciate-retaining total knee arthroplasty in patients with discoid lateral meniscus [109].

Published in: Arthroplasty (2024).

Link to original: https://doi.org/10.1186/s42836-024-00238-2

If you want to cite the papers, please refer to the original.

For technical reasons we could not place the page where the original quote is coming from.

4.1.4.1 Research Highlights

Cruciate-retaining total knee arthroplasty (CR-TKA) is a common surgical procedure where the posterior cruciate ligament (PCL) is preserved to maintain knee stability. However, preserving the PCL can be challenging due to the fragility of the bony island that supports it, leading many surgeons to opt for complete resection of the proximal tibia, which can damage the PCL attachment. The impact of this resection on PCL preservation varies among patients due to differences in knee morphology. The study by Xin et al. investigates how the presence of a discoid lateral meniscus (DLM), a common anatomical variant, affects PCL attachment preservation in CR-TKA.

The study involved a retrospective analysis of MRI scans from patients with and without DLM who underwent CR-TKA. Using a detailed imaging protocol, the researchers simulated tibial osteotomies at various slopes and measured the percentage of PCL attachment sacrificed. The study included matched groups based on age, sex, and body size to minimize bias. The MRI scans were reviewed by experienced orthopedic surgeons using a standardized method to ensure accuracy. Statistical analyses were conducted to compare the extent of PCL sacrifice between DLM and non-DLM groups and to explore correlations with morphological parameters such as meniscus width and tibial slope.

The findings revealed that patients with DLM experienced significantly greater PCL attachment sacrifice compared to those without DLM, particularly at steeper osteotomy slopes. This suggests that DLM is an independent risk factor for increased PCL damage during CR-TKA. The study highlights the need for alternative surgical techniques or prostheses for patients with DLM to preserve knee function postoperatively. Future studies could explore three-dimensional modelling based on MRI data to provide more detailed insights into PCL preservation strategies in CR-TKA, especially for patients with anatomical variations like DLM.

4.1.5 In Vivo Function of Posterior Cruciate Ligament Before and After Posterior Cruciate Ligament-Retaining Total Knee Arthroplasty [110]

This is a machine-generated summary of:

Yue, Bing; Varadarajan, Kartik M.; Rubash, Harry E.; Li, Guoan In vivo function of posterior cruciate ligament before and after posterior cruciate ligament-retaining total knee arthroplasty [110].

Published in: International Orthopaedics (2012).

Link to original: https://doi.org/10.1007/s00264-011-1481-6

If you want to cite the papers, please refer to the original.

For technical reasons we could not place the page where the original quote is coming from.

4.1.5.1 Research Highlights

The posterior cruciate ligament (PCL) is often retained during total knee arthroplasty (TKA) with the assumption that it aids in femoral rollback and enhances knee range of motion (ROM). However, previous studies have shown that knee kinematics and ROM after PCL-retaining TKA differ significantly from those of a native knee. Despite this, clinical outcomes such as stability, loosening rate, and patient satisfaction appear similar whether the PCL is retained or not. The role of the PCL in TKA remains a critical area of research, as in vitro studies suggest that normal PCL force is not restored post-surgery. The study by Yue et al. investigates the in vivo function of the PCL in patients before and after undergoing PCL-retaining TKA.

In this study, eleven patients with advanced medial-compartment knee osteoarthritis (OA) were recruited to assess the function of the PCL before and after TKA. Preoperative magnetic resonance imaging (MRI) was used to model the knee anatomy, focusing on the attachment sites of the PCL bundles. Patients performed weight-bearing single-leg lunges while dual fluoroscopic imaging captured knee positions at various flexion angles. Post-surgery, patients underwent high-flexion PCL-retaining TKA performed by a single surgeon. The same imaging technique was used postoperatively to evaluate changes in PCL kinematics. The study found that elongation of both anterolateral (AL) and posteromedial (PM) bundles increased with flexion across all groups. However, elongation was significantly greater in TKA knees during late flexion compared to OA and normal knees.

The findings suggest that current PCL-retaining TKA systems may not fully restore normal biomechanics of the PCL bundles. The study highlights that over-stretching of the PCL could limit further knee flexion or lead to ligament failure due to reduced posterior femoral translation. Future study could explore other TKA designs and evaluate knee function during dynamic activities like gait to better understand these biomechanical changes. Additionally, examining knees with different OA patterns could provide further insights into optimizing surgical techniques for improved patient outcomes.

4.1.6 Posterior Cruciate-Retaining Total Knee Arthroplasty for Valgus Osteoarthritis [111]

This is a machine-generated summary of:

McAuley, James P.; Collier, Matthew B.; Hamilton, W. G.; Tabaraee, Ehsan; Engh, G. A. Posterior Cruciate-retaining Total Knee Arthroplasty for Valgus Osteoarthritis [111].

Published in: Clinical Orthopaedics and Related Research® (2008).

Link to original: https://doi.org/10.1007/s11999-008-0436-8

If you want to cite the papers, please refer to the original.

For technical reasons we could not place the page where the original quote is coming from.

4.1.6.1 Research Highlights

Performing total knee arthroplasty (TKA) in patients with valgus osteoarthritis presents significant challenges due to the unique anatomical and biomechanical characteristics of the condition. The typical dysplastic lateral femoral condyle and contracted lateral soft tissues complicate the restoration of mechanical alignment and soft tissue balancing. Traditionally, posterior cruciate ligament (PCL)-substituting implants have been recommended to address these issues, but there is a lack of prospective studies comparing clinical outcomes between PCL-retaining and PCL-substituting designs in valgus knees. The study by McAuley et al. investigates the impact of surgical techniques, implant characteristics, and patient factors on implant survival and clinical outcomes in TKA for valgus osteoarthritis.

The study retrospectively reviewed data from patients who underwent primary PCL-retaining TKA for valgus osteoarthritis. The researchers analysed various factors, including surgical techniques for lateral soft tissue release, implant characteristics such as polyethylene shelf age, and patient demographics. The surgeries were performed using either an "outside-in" or "inside-out" approach for lateral soft tissue release. Clinical outcomes were assessed using Knee Society scores, and implant survival was evaluated through Kaplan-Meier analysis. The study found that preserving the lateral collateral ligament (LCL) and popliteus tendon was associated with better implant survival and higher clinical outcome scores. Conversely, releasing both structures increased the likelihood of revision due to wear, osteolysis, or instability.

The findings suggest that preserving lateral stabilizing structures during TKA can improve both survivorship and clinical outcomes in patients with valgus osteoarthritis. The study highlights the importance of surgical technique in achieving optimal results and suggests that using polyethylene with a shorter shelf life may further enhance implant survival. Future study could explore refining surgical techniques to maximize preservation of stabilizing structures while considering individual patient anatomy and biomechanics. Additionally, further research could investigate long-term outcomes across diverse patient populations to validate these findings more broadly.

4.1.7 Fibula Head Is a Useful Landmark to Predict the Location of Posterior Cruciate Ligament Footprint Prior to Total Knee Arthroplasty [112]

This is a machine-generated summary of:

Jawhar, Ahmed; Wasnik, Sandeep; Scharf, Hanns-Peter; Roehl, Henning Fibula head is a useful landmark to predict the location of posterior cruciate ligament footprint prior to total knee arthroplasty [112].

Published in: International Orthopaedics (2013).

Link to original: https://doi.org/10.1007/s00264-013-2100-5

If you want to cite the papers, please refer to the original.

For technical reasons we could not place the page where the original quote is coming from.

4.1.7.1 Research Highlights

The role of the posterior cruciate ligament (PCL) in primary total knee arthroplasty (TKA) has been a subject of debate, with no significant outcome differences reported between cruciate retaining and cruciate substituting techniques. While the cruciate retaining approach may offer advantages such as proprioceptive function and stabilization, flexion instability due to insufficient PCL can lead to pain and poor outcomes. A critical challenge is predicting PCL damage during surgery, as its exposure is difficult with routine TKA approaches. The study by Jawhar et al. addresses this issue by quantifying the relationship between tibial cutting planes and the fibula head to predict PCL damage risk.

The study involved a large patient cohort undergoing primary cruciate retaining TKA for osteoarthritis. Researchers measured vertical distances between the tibial cutting plane and fibula head using calibrated radiographs and MRI scans. The study aimed to determine the probability of partial or total PCL footprint removal with routine tibial cuts. Measurements were conducted using Syngo fast view software (Siemens, Munich, Germany) for radiographs and OSIRIX software (Pixmeo SARL, Geneva, Switzerland) for MRI images, ensuring high intra- and interobserver reliability. The vertical distance between the tibial cut and the most proximal point of the fibula head averaged 6.1 mm ±4.8 mm. The mean vertical distance from fibula head to the proximal and distal PCL footprint revealed to be 11.4 mm ±3.7 mm and 5.4 mm ±2.9 mm, respectively. The location of the insertion was not significantly different between subgroups such as age (<50 or > 50 years), sex and laterality. Based on these results 11 (7%) knees were considered at high risk of an entire PCL removal after implantation of a cruciate retaining TKA design.

This research provides valuable insights into preoperative planning for TKA by identifying reliable anatomical landmarks that predict PCL damage risk. The study suggests that using the fibula head as a landmark can help surgeons estimate potential PCL disruption during surgery, potentially improving surgical outcomes. Future study could explore alternative surgical techniques or implant designs that minimize PCL damage while maintaining joint stability. Additionally, further investigation into the impact of severe osteoarthritic deformities on these measurements could refine surgical strategies for complex cases.

4.1.8 Intra-operative Gaps Affect Outcome and Postoperative Kinematics In Vivo Following Cruciate-Retaining Total Knee Arthroplasty [113]

This is a machine-generated summary of:

Fujimoto, Eisaku; Sasashige, Yoshiaki; Tomita, Tetsuya; Sasaki, Hirofumi; Touten, Yoriko; Fujiwara, Yuusuke; Ochi, Mitsuo Intra-operative gaps affect outcome and postoperative kinematics in vivo following cruciate-retaining total knee arthroplasty [113].

Published in: International Orthopaedics (2015).

Link to original: https://doi.org/10.1007/s00264-015-2847-y

If you want to cite the papers, please refer to the original.

For technical reasons we could not place the page where the original quote is coming from.

4.1.8.1 Research Highlights

Total knee arthroplasty (TKA) aims to relieve pain and restore knee function, requiring a stable range of motion and proper soft-tissue balance. Achieving accurate intra-operative gap and soft-tissue balance is challenging, prompting the development of an offset-type tensor for TKA procedures. This device allows for gap and soft tissue balance assessments under physiological conditions. While cruciate retaining (CR) TKA designs control both posterior cruciate and collateral ligaments, the influence of posterior cruciate ligament (PCL) tension on postoperative kinematics remains unclear. The study by Fujimoto et al. investigates how intra-operative component gaps affect in vivo kinematics and outcomes in CR TKA.

The study utilized a two-dimensional/three-dimensional registration technique to analyse anterior-posterior translation and axial rotation kinematics between narrow and wide component gaps in CR TKA under weight-bearing and non-weight-bearing conditions. Thirty patients with primary varus osteoarthritis underwent implantation of a NRG CR cementless TKA. The surgeries employed a modified gap-balance technique with the Stryker Joint Dependent Kinematics system to ensure ligament balance and satisfactory alignment. The offset tensor device measured ligament balance and joint gaps by applying a constant distraction force. Patients performed deep knee bends under fluoroscopic monitoring to assess kinematic differences between narrow and wide gap groups. Significant differences were observed in medial condyle positions during non-weight-bearing conditions, while no significant differences were found under weight-bearing conditions.

The study advances understanding of how intra-operative joint gaps influence postoperative kinematics in CR TKA. It suggests that a wide flexion gap may lead to late rollback under non-weight-bearing conditions, while a tight flexion gap could hinder daily activities. The findings indicate that 1–2 mm laxity at 0°–90° component gaps may be necessary for comfortable daily activities. Future study could explore increasing the sample size to include patients with poor clinical outcomes, providing further insights into in vivo kinematics after TKA. Additionally, evaluating other daily motions such as gait or stair navigation could offer a more comprehensive understanding of functional outcomes post-TKA.

4.1.9 Can Pain Be Improved with Retention of the Posterior Cruciate Ligament During Total Knee Arthroplasty? [114]

This is a machine-generated summary of:

Fiedler, Benjamin; Bieganowski, Thomas; Anil, Utkarsh; Lin, Charles C.; Habibi, Akram A.; Schwarzkopf, Ran Can pain be improved with retention of the posterior cruciate ligament during total knee arthroplasty? [114].

Published in: European Journal of Orthopaedic Surgery & Traumatology (2023).

Link to original: https://doi.org/10.1007/s00590-023-03562-6

If you want to cite the papers, please refer to the original.

For technical reasons we could not place the page where the original quote is coming from.

4.1.9.1 Research Highlights

Total knee arthroplasty (TKA) is a common surgical intervention for patients with degenerative knee arthritis who do not respond to non-surgical treatments. The choice of implant in TKA involves complex decisions influenced by factors such as fixation method, material, and degrees of constraint. While constrained implants are typically reserved for severe cases, unconstrained designs like cruciate-retaining (CR) and posterior-stabilized (PS) are more commonly used. Despite ongoing debates about the superiority of PS versus CR TKA, few studies have focused on immediate post-operative outcomes. The study by Fiedler et al. examines the effects of these implant types on early post-operative pain and opioid use.

The study conducted a retrospective review at an urban academic institution, analyzing patients who underwent primary TKA for knee arthritis. Participants were stratified into groups based on whether they received CR or PS implants, with further sub-analysis comparing constrained and non-constrained PS designs. Propensity score matching was used to ensure comparable groups based on demographics and clinical characteristics. The researchers collected data on visual analog scale (VAS) pain scores and opioid consumption within 48 hours post-operatively, converting opioid usage into morphine milligram equivalents for comparison. Statistical analyses were performed to identify any significant differences in pain levels, opioid use, and 30-day readmission rates between the different implant groups.

The study found no significant differences in immediate post-operative pain scores or opioid consumption between CR and PS TKA patients. Similarly, there were no differences in 30-day pain-related readmissions or length of stay between the groups. These findings suggest that both CR and PS implants provide comparable outcomes in terms of early post-operative pain management. Future study could explore longer-term outcomes and assess the impact of patient-specific factors on implant choice to further refine surgical decision-making in TKA. The results indicate that surgeons can select implants based on individual patient needs without compromising immediate post-operative recovery.

4.1.10 Higher Revision Rate for Posterior Cruciate-Retaining Than Posterior-Stabilized Total Knee Arthroplasty for the Treatment of Valgus Osteoarthritis [115]

This is a machine-generated summary of:

Savov, Peter; Mielke, Evelyn; Windhagen, Henning; Calliess, Tilman; Richter, Alena; Ettinger, Max Higher revision rate for posterior cruciate-retaining than posterior-stabilized total knee arthroplasty for the treatment of valgus osteoarthritis [115].

Published in: Archives of Orthopaedic and Trauma Surgery (2020).

Link to original: https://doi.org/10.1007/s00402-020-03618-w

If you want to cite the papers, please refer to the original.

For technical reasons we could not place the page where the original quote is coming from.

4.1.10.1 Research Highlights

The debate surrounding cruciate-retaining (CR) and posterior-stabilized (PS) designs in total knee arthroplasty (TKA) continues, particularly regarding their effectiveness in stabilizing the knee joint post-surgery. In CR TKA, the posterior cruciate ligament (PCL) is preserved, potentially enhancing proprioception and balance, while PS designs are thought to offer greater flexion and femoral rollback. However, a recent meta-analysis found no significant differences in knee scores or complication rates between these designs. The study by Savov et al. investigates the mid-term outcomes of CR versus PS TKA specifically for treating valgus osteoarthritis, a condition that presents unique surgical challenges due to limb alignment issues.

The study was a retrospective analysis approved by the local ethical board, focusing on patients with preoperative valgus deformity greater than 10 degrees who underwent TKA using either CR or PS implants. The choice of prosthesis was made intraoperatively based on the condition of the PCL and other soft tissues. The primary endpoint was the Knee injury and Osteoarthritis Outcome Score (KOOS), with additional assessments of implant survival and revision rates. Patients were categorized by the severity of their valgus deformity and body mass index (BMI). Statistical analyses included Mann–Whitney U tests for KOOS comparisons and Chi-square tests for evaluating the impact of deformity severity and BMI on outcomes.

The study found no significant difference in clinical outcomes between CR and PS TKA groups in terms of KOOS subscores or overall limb alignment post-surgery. However, CR TKA showed a higher failure rate due to instability, which may be attributed to the low-conforming design used in this cohort. Despite similar mid-term clinical outcomes, the high revision rate for instability in CR TKAs suggests that PS designs might be more suitable for patients with severe valgus deformities. Future study could focus on prospective randomized trials to validate these findings further and explore alternative prosthetic designs that mitigate instability risks while preserving knee function.

4.1.11 The Effect of Posterior Tibial Slope on Anteroposterior Stability in Posterior Cruciate Retaining Total Knee Arthroplasty [116]

This is a machine-generated summary of:

Ersin, Mehmet; Demirel, Mehmet; Civan, Melih; Ekinci, Mehmet; Akgül, Turgut; Şen, Cengiz The effect of posterior tibial slope on anteroposterior stability in posterior cruciate retaining total knee arthroplasty [116].

Published in: BMC Musculoskeletal Disorders (2023).

Link to original: https://doi.org/10.1186/s12891-023-06507-6

If you want to cite the papers, please refer to the original.

For technical reasons we could not place the page where the original quote is coming from.

4.1.11.1 Research Highlights

Total knee arthroplasty (TKA) aims to improve the functional range of motion while maintaining joint stability, with anteroposterior stability being crucial for clinical success. The posterior cruciate ligament (PCL) is believed to play a significant role in this stability by limiting posterior translation, and the posterior tibial slope (PTS) is thought to influence PCL function and knee biomechanics. Despite extensive research on PCL's role in TKA, the relationship between PTS and anteroposterior stability remains unclear. The study by Ersin et al. investigates the effects of PTS on anteroposterior stability in PCL-retaining TKA.

The study retrospectively reviewed patients who underwent TKA for osteoarthritis, focusing on the association between PTS and anteroposterior laxity. Using AUTOCAD software (Autodesk, San Francisco, California, USA), postoperative PTS was measured from lateral radiographs, while anteroposterior displacement was assessed using KT-1000 arthrometer measurements and sagittal drawer radiographic images. Clinical outcomes were evaluated through knee flexion range of motion, WOMAC scores, and VAS pain scores. Statistical analyses were conducted to determine correlations between PTS and these measures. The study found no significant correlation between tibial slope and clinical outcome scores or maximal knee flexion. However, subgroup analyses suggested that a tibial slope of $\geq 3°$ to $<6°$ might reduce anterior translation at certain flexion angles.

The study highlights that while increasing PTS may slightly reduce anterior-posterior translation at specific flexion angles, the correlation is weak, indicating limited clinical significance. Future study could explore other factors influencing PCL tension and TKA stability, such as flexion gap adjustments or implant positioning. Despite its limitations, this research provides valuable insights into the nuanced role of PTS in TKA outcomes and suggests that achieving optimal anteroposterior stability may require considering multiple biomechanical factors beyond just tibial slope adjustments.

4.1.12 Effect of Posterior Design Changes on Postoperative Flexion Angle in Cruciate Retaining Mobile-Bearing Total Knee Arthroplasty [117]

This is a machine-generated summary of:

Tsuji, Shigeyoshi; Tomita, Tetsuya; Hashimoto, Hideo; Fujii, Masakazu; Yoshikawa, Hideki; Sugamoto, Kazuomi Effect of posterior design changes on postoperative flexion angle in cruciate retaining mobile-bearing total knee arthroplasty [117].

Published in: International Orthopaedics (2010).

Link to original: https://doi.org/10.1007/s00264-010-1060-2

Copyright of the summarized publication:

4.1.12.1 Research Highlights

Total knee arthroplasty (TKA) is widely recognized for its effectiveness in alleviating pain and restoring gait, yet there is a growing demand for TKA designs that allow for deeper knee flexion, such as sitting or kneeling. While preoperative range of motion is generally considered the most critical factor influencing postoperative outcomes, the impact of posterior design changes in cruciate-retaining (CR) mobile-bearing TKA on range of motion remains uncertain. The study by Tsuji et al. investigates the effects of specific design modifications on postoperative flexion angles in TKA patients.

The study involved the development of a fully congruent mobile-bearing knee replacement in collaboration with Finsbury UK, featuring a reduced curvature radius of the posterior condyle and a posteriorly shifted base of the insert dish. The research included patients with preoperative flexion angles over 90 degrees who underwent either Hi-Flex or Standard-design Dual Bearing Knee (DBK) TKA (MMT Co. Ltd. (Kneeopus System), Osaka, Japan). The surgical team employed a medial parapatellar approach with cement fixation, conserving the posterior cruciate ligament. Postoperative outcomes were assessed using various parameters, including Knee Society Scores and range of motion measurements taken by physical therapists. Statistical analyses revealed that while both groups showed improvements in extension angles, the high flexion group demonstrated significantly greater postoperative flexion angles and range of motion compared to the Standard group.

The study's findings suggest that specific design changes—namely, decreasing the curvature radius of the posterior condyle and shifting the insert dish base posteriorly—can enhance postoperative flexion angles in CR mobile-bearing TKA. These modifications appear to facilitate an improved rollback mechanism and reduce posterior impingement. Future study could explore further refinements to prosthesis design or investigate long-term outcomes associated with these changes. Additionally, understanding patient-specific factors that influence postoperative improvements could guide personalized approaches to TKA.

4.1.13 Correlation Between Preoperative and Postoperative Knee Kinematics in Total Knee Arthroplasty Using Cruciate Retaining Designs [119]

This is a machine-generated summary of:

Seon, Jong Keun; Park, Ju Kwon; Jeong, Mun Su; Jung, Woo Bin; Park, Kyung Soon; Yoon, Taek Rim; Song, Eun Kyoo Correlation between preoperative and postoperative knee kinematics in total knee arthroplasty using cruciate retaining designs [119].

Published in: International Orthopaedics (2010).

Link to original: https://doi.org/10.1007/s00264-010-1029-1

If you want to cite the papers, please refer to the original.

For technical reasons we could not place the page where the original quote is coming from.

4.1.13.1 Research Highlights

Total knee arthroplasty (TKA) is a common surgical procedure aimed at improving knee function and patient satisfaction. However, some patients report unsatisfactory outcomes, potentially due to abnormal knee kinematics post-surgery. While factors such as preoperative knee conditions, prosthesis design, and surgical technique are believed to influence postoperative kinematics, most studies have focused on the latter. There is a lack of research exploring the relationship between preoperative and postoperative knee kinematics. The study by Seon et al. investigates this relationship by evaluating anterior-posterior translation and internal-external rotation kinematics before and after TKA.

The study involved 56 patients with varus osteoarthritis scheduled for cruciate-retaining TKA using a navigation system. Exclusions were made for patients with prior knee surgeries or severe deformities. The researchers used a standard medial parapatellar approach to perform the surgeries, employing navigation systems to measure passive knee kinematics at various flexion angles both preoperatively and postoperatively. Anterior-posterior translation and internal-external rotation were assessed using coordinate systems established through anatomical landmarks on the femur and tibia. The study found significant correlations between preoperative and postoperative kinematic variables, particularly in posterior femoral roll back and external femoral rotation.

The findings suggest that knees after TKA exhibit similar posterior femoral roll back but reduced external femoral rotation compared to preoperative osteoarthritic knees during passive flexion. Importantly, the study highlights that postoperative passive knee kinematics are significantly correlated with preoperative conditions, which may explain why preoperative range of motion is a strong predictor of postoperative outcomes. Future study could explore the relationship between intraoperative passive knee kinematics and postoperative active knee kinematics under weight-bearing conditions to further understand these dynamics. This research provides valuable insights into the role of preoperative conditions in determining postoperative success in TKA.

4.1.14 Soft-Tissue Balancing in Total Knee Arthroplasty: Cruciate-Retaining Versus Posterior-Stabilised, and Measured-Resection Versus Gap Technique [120]

This is a machine-generated summary of:

Matsumoto, Tomoyuki; Muratsu, Hirotsugu; Kawakami, Yohei; Takayama, Koji; Ishida, Kazunari; Matsushita, Takehiko; Akisue, Toshihiro; Nishida, Kotaro; Kuroda, Ryosuke; Kurosaka, Masahiro Soft-tissue balancing in total knee arthroplasty: cruciate-retaining versus posterior-stabilised, and measured-resection versus gap technique [120].

Published in: International Orthopaedics (2013).

Link to original: https://doi.org/10.1007/s00264-013-2133-9

If you want to cite the papers, please refer to the original.

For technical reasons we could not place the page where the original quote is coming from.

4.1.14.1 Research Highlights

Total knee arthroplasty (TKA) requires precise soft tissue balancing and accurate bony alignment to ensure optimal outcomes. Despite advancements in surgical instruments, achieving accurate intra-operative soft tissue balance remains challenging, particularly for less experienced surgeons. Traditional methods rely on the surgeon's subjective assessment, but new tools like the offset-type tensor have been developed to objectively assess soft-tissue balance throughout the range of motion. However, the best method for achieving appropriate soft-tissue balance and rotational alignment of the femur is still debated, with measured-resection and gap techniques being the primary contenders. The study by Matsumoto et al. explores the efficacy of using a gap technique with a navigation system for soft tissue balancing in knees undergoing cruciate retaining (CR) or posterior-stabilized (PS) TKA.

The study involved patients with osteoarthritis who underwent TKA using either the gap technique or the measured resection technique. The researchers used an offset-type tensor to assist in achieving soft tissue balance during surgery. The tensor allowed for intra-operative measurement of joint center gaps and varus ligament balance under a constant distraction force. The surgeries were performed by experienced surgeons using a navigation system to ensure accurate bone cuts and range of motion measurements. The study compared outcomes between CR and PS knees, as well as between the gap and measured-resection techniques, focusing on achieving an equalised rectangular gap at extension and flexion.

The study found that while the gap technique showed a trend towards superior soft tissue balancing compared to the measured-resection technique, this did not translate into significant differences in clinical outcomes at a minimum 2-year follow-up. Future study could explore combining elements of both techniques to enhance clinical outcomes further. Additionally, prospective randomized trials using consistent implant types could provide more definitive comparisons between these surgical approaches. Expanding research to include different types of osteoarthritis, such as valgus deformities, may also offer insights into optimizing TKA procedures across diverse patient populations.

4.1.15 Comparison of Total Knee Arthroplasty with Highly Congruent Anterior-Stabilized Bearings Versus a Cruciate-Retaining Design [121]

This is a machine-generated summary of:

Peters, Christopher L.; Mulkey, Patrick; Erickson, Jill; Anderson, Michael B.; Pelt, Christopher E. Comparison of Total Knee Arthroplasty With Highly Congruent Anterior-stabilized Bearings versus a Cruciate-retaining Design [121].

Published in: Clinical Orthopaedics and Related Research® (2013).

Link to original: https://doi.org/10.1007/s11999-013-3068-6

If you want to cite the papers, please refer to the original.

For technical reasons we could not place the page where the original quote is coming from.

4.1.15.1 Research Highlights

Total knee arthroplasty (TKA) is a well-established procedure for alleviating pain and enhancing function in patients with knee issues. Despite the variety of surgical techniques and implant options available, the management of the posterior cruciate ligament (PCL) remains a topic of debate. The PCL is crucial for stabilizing the knee by preventing posterior translation of the tibia. Strategies for managing the

PCL during TKA include retaining it or substituting it with different implant designs, yet there is little consensus on which approach yields the best outcomes. The study by Peters et al. investigates the clinical performance of anterior-stabilized bearings compared to cruciate-retaining (CR) bearings in TKA.

The study involved a retrospective review of patients who underwent primary TKA with either an anterior-stabilized or CR bearing. The researchers analysed data from patients with a minimum follow-up period of several years(From 2003 to 2008, minimum follow up of 2 years), focusing on Knee Society scores, radiographic results, complication rates, revision rates, and overall survival. All surgeries were performed using a medial parapatellar approach with a single FDA-approved implant type. The decision to use an anterior-stabilized or CR bearing was made intraoperatively based on the competence and balance of the PCL. Statistical analyses, including mixed effects modelling and Kaplan-Meier survival analysis, were employed to compare outcomes between the two groups.

The study found that while knee scores and radiographic results were comparable between anterior-stabilized and CR TKAs, there was better survival in the anterior-stabilized group due to fewer revisions related to instability. This suggests that anterior-stabilized bearings may offer adequate clinical stability when the PCL is deficient or absent. However, limitations such as selection bias and non-randomization should be considered when interpreting these findings. Future study could explore long-term outcomes like polyethylene wear and detailed kinematic analyses to further evaluate the benefits of anterior-stabilized bearings in TKA.

4.1.16 Effect of Posterior Cruciate Ligament on Knee Pressure and Gap Measured by an Electronic Sensor During Total Knee Arthroplasty [122]

This is a machine-generated summary of:

Zhao, Ran; Liu, Yanqing; Tian, Hua Effect of posterior cruciate ligament on knee pressure and gap measured by an electronic sensor during total knee arthroplasty [122].

Published in: Journal of Orthopaedic Surgery and Research (2023).

Link to original: https://doi.org/10.1186/s13018-023-03643-6

If you want to cite the papers, please refer to the original.

For technical reasons we could not place the page where the original quote is coming from.

4.1.16.1 Research Highlights

Total knee arthroplasty (TKA) is a widely used treatment for end-stage knee osteoarthritis, with two primary types of prostheses: cruciate retaining (CR) and cruciate sacrificing (CS). Both types have a high survival rate, but the CR prosthesis offers advantages in maintaining knee biomechanics and proprioception. However, issues such as tightness or excessive relaxation of the posterior cruciate ligament (PCL) can lead to complications like increased polyethylene wear or knee instability, affecting prosthesis longevity and patient satisfaction. The study by Zhao et al. investigates the effects of PCL retention, recession, and resection on joint pressure during TKA using an electronic sensor.

The study involved patients undergoing TKA who met specific inclusion criteria, such as genu varum and limited flexion contracture. Exclusions included conditions like rheumatoid arthritis or severe deformities requiring metal gaskets. The researchers used a wireless electronic pressure sensor to measure medial and lateral compartment pressures at various knee flexion angles. The study compared three groups: PCL retention, tibial recession, and complete resection. Data were collected prospectively with ethical approval, and statistical analysis was performed using non-parametric tests due to non-normal data distribution. The results showed that total joint pressure decreased with increased flexion angle across all groups, with the highest pressure observed in the retention group during extension.

The findings suggest that even after tibial recession or resection of the PCL, some tension remains, indicating partial functionality. This supports the use of CR prostheses without routinely converting to PS designs after PCL release. The study highlights that PCL resection affects both flexion and extension gaps but may not be effective for adjusting flexion gap tension alone. Future study could explore larger sample sizes or different prosthesis designs to further understand intra-articular pressure changes post-PCL resection. These insights contribute to optimizing surgical techniques and improving outcomes in TKA procedures.

4.1.17 Faster Improvement in Outcome Scores in Posterior Stabilised Total Knee Arthroplasty Compared to Medial Congruent System with Posterior Cruciate Ligament Retained [124]

This is a machine-generated summary of:

Lee, W. C.; Foong, C. M. B.; Khoo, K. M. S.; Kwan, Y. H.; Kunnasegaran, R. Faster improvement in outcome scores in posterior stabilised total knee arthroplasty compared to medial congruent system with posterior cruciate ligament retained [124].

Published in: MUSCULOSKELETAL SURGERY (2023).

Link to original: https://doi.org/10.1007/s12306-023-00797-8

If you want to cite the papers, please refer to the original.

For technical reasons we could not place the page where the original quote is coming from.

4.1.17.1 Research Highlights

End-stage knee osteoarthritis is frequently treated with total knee arthroplasty (TKA), which generally has a good survival rate. However, only a small percentage of patients report satisfaction with the outcomes, potentially due to the inability of current designs to replicate normal knee kinematics. The posterior-stabilized (PS) design is commonly used in primary TKA, but it may contribute to dissatisfaction by failing to restore the medial pivot mechanism of a normal knee. The medial congruent (MC) TKA design aims to address this by providing more congruence in the medial compartment while allowing for natural femoral rollback. The study by Lee et al. investigates the outcomes of MC TKA with posterior cruciate ligament retention (MC-PCLR) compared to PS TKA, hypothesizing that MC-PCLR may offer improved outcomes.

The study retrospectively analyzed data from an institutional registry, focusing on primary TKAs performed for osteoarthritis between October 2018 and July 2021. Exclusions were made for cases involving inflammatory diseases, avascular necrosis, or complications. Surgeries were conducted using either PS or MC-PCLR implants, with the latter retaining the PCL and avoiding femoral box cuts. Both groups followed an Enhanced Recovery After Surgery protocol with standardized postoperative care. Outcomes measured included range of motion (ROM), Knee Society Score (KSS), and Oxford Knee Score (OKS), assessed preoperatively and at several postoperative intervals. Statistical analyses were performed to compare these outcomes between the two groups.

The study found that both PS and MC-PCLR TKAs achieved similar 1-year postoperative outcomes in terms of ROM, OKS, and KSS. However, the PS group showed faster improvement in these metrics within the first 3 months post-surgery. The MC-PCLR group demonstrated significant improvement from 6 months to 1-year post-operation, particularly in functional scores exceeding the minimum clinically important difference (MCID). Despite these findings, no significant differences were observed in pain levels or walking distance on postoperative day one between the groups. Future studies could explore comparisons between different TKA designs or investigate long-term outcomes to further elucidate these findings.

4.1.18 Ball-in-Socket Medial Conformity with Posterior Cruciate Ligament Retention Neither Limits Internal Tibial Rotation and Knee Flexion nor Lowers Clinical Outcome Scores After Unrestricted Kinematically Aligned Total Knee Arthroplasty [125]

This is a machine-generated summary of:

Elorza, Saúl Pacheco; O'Donnell, Ed; Nedopil, Alexander; Howell, Stephen M.; Hull, Maury L. Ball-in-socket medial conformity with posterior cruciate ligament retention neither limits internal tibial rotation and knee flexion nor lowers clinical outcome scores after unrestricted kinematically aligned total knee arthroplasty [125].

Published in: International Orthopaedics (2023).

Link to original: https://doi.org/10.1007/s00264-023-05834-6

4.1.18.1 Research Highlights

Total knee arthroplasty (TKA) has traditionally involved designs such as cruciate retaining and posterior stabilized knees, where the cruciate ligaments are either retained or resected to provide stability. Recently, interest has shifted towards the medial stabilized design, which aims to guide femoral-tibial motion differently from conventional designs. This design is typically implemented with mechanical alignment and posterior cruciate ligament (PCL) resection to avoid over-constraining the knee. However, when surgeons prefer to retain the PCL, as in kinematic alignment, it becomes crucial to determine the appropriate level of medial constraint needed to restore native knee kinematics without compromising function and patient satisfaction. The study by Elorza et al. evaluates whether a new tibial insert design with a ball-in-socket medial compartment can be used in kinematic alignment with PCL retention without compromising knee flexion and clinical outcomes.

The study involved 25 patients who underwent bilateral unrestricted caliper-verified kinematically aligned TKA with PCL retention. Each patient received a ball-in-socket medial compartment (B-in-S MC + PCL) insert in one knee and an intermediate medial conformity (I MC + PCL) insert in the other. The researchers used fluoroscopic imaging during weight-bearing exercises such as deep knee bends, step-ups, and chair rises to assess internal tibial rotation and flexion. The study also evaluated patient-reported outcomes using scores like the Forgotten Joint Score and Western Ontario and McMaster Universities Arthritis Index. Statistical analyses were conducted to compare internal tibial rotation, flexion angles, and clinical outcome scores between the two insert designs.

The findings revealed that the B-in-S MC + PCL insert allowed greater internal tibial rotation during deep knee bends compared to the I MC + PCL insert but did not significantly differ in other exercises or affect flexion or patient-reported outcomes negatively. This suggests that the new insert design provides high anteroposterior stability without compromising function, making it potentially beneficial for patients interested in high-level activities post-TKA. Future study could explore the long-term effects of this design on implant survivorship, considering potential risks like polyethylene bearing failure or baseplate subsidence due to increased internal rotation. The ongoing research by the senior author aims to address these aspects further.

Bibliography

1. Selvarajah E, Hooper G (2009) Restoration of the joint line in total knee. Arthroplast J Arthroplast 24:1099–1103
2. Maruyama S, Yoshiya S, Matsui N et al (2004) Functional comparison of posterior cruciate-retaining versus posterior stabilized total knee arthroplasty. J Arthroplast 19:349–353
3. Snider MG, MacDonald SJ (2009) The influence of the posterior cruciate ligament and component design on joint line position after primary total knee arthroplasty. J Arthroplast 24:1093–1098

4. Cinotti G, Sessa P, Amato M, Ripani FR, Giannicola G (2017) Preserving the PCL during the tibial cut in total knee arthroplasty. Knee Surg Sport Traumatol Artrosc 25(8):2594–2601
5. Meneghini RM, Mont MA, Backstein DB, Bourne RB, Dennis DA, Scuderi GR (2015) Development of a modern knee society radiographic evaluation system and methodology for total knee arthroplasty. J Arthroplasty 30:2311–2314
6. Dion C-AB, Howard JL, Lanting BA, McAuley JP (2019) Does recession of the posterior cruciate ligament influence outcome in total knee arthroplasty? J Arthroplasty 34:2383–2397
7. Rosemberg AG, Knaple DM (2006) Posterior cruciate-retaining total knee arthroplasty. In: Scott NW (ed) Insall and Scott, surgery of the knee, 4th edn. Churcill Livingstone Elsevier, Philadelphia, p 1522
8. Jiang C, Liu Z, Wang Y, Bian Y, Feng B, Weng X. Posterior cruciate ligament retention versus posterior stabilization for total knee arthroplasty: a meta-analysis. PLoS One. 2016;11(1):e0147865. https://doi.org/10.1371/journal.pone.0147865.
9. Stronach BM, Adams JC, Jones LC, Farrell SM, Hydrick JM. The effect of sacrificing the posterior c ligament in total knee arthroplasties that use a highly congruent polyethylene component. J Arthroplasty. 2019;34(2):286–9. https://doi.org/10.1016/j.arth.2018.10.006.
10. Lynch JT, Scarvell JM, Galvin CR, et al. Influence of component design on in vivo tibiofemoral contact patterns during kneeling after total knee arthroplasty: a systematic review and meta-analysis. Knee Surg Sports Traumatol Arthrosc. 2020;29:446-66. https://doi.org/10.1007/s00167-020-05949-y.
11. Daniilidis K, Skwara A, Vieth V, Fuchs-Winkelmann S, Heindel W, Stuckmann V, et al. Highly conforming polyethylene inlays reduce the in vivo variability of knee joint kinematics after total knee arthroplasty. Knee. 2012;19(4):260–5. https://doi.org/10.1016/j.knee.2011.04.001.
12. Aoki M, Shishido T, Takahashi Y, Katori Y, Kubo K, Takamatsu T, et al. Functional evaluation in cruciate-retaining-type TKA: anatomical relationship between tibial osteotomy level and PCL attachment. Eur J Orthop Surg Traumatol. 2014;24:1531–7. https://doi.org/10.1007/s00590-014-1414-3.
13. Inou Y, Tomita T, Kiyotomo D, Yoshikawa H, Sugamoto K. What kinds of posterior cruciate ligament bundles are preserved in cruciate-retaining total knee arthroplasty? a three-dimensional morphology study. J Knee Surg. 2019;32:989–4. https://doi.org/10.1055/s-0038-1675184.
14. Shannon FJ, Cronin JJ, Cleary MS, Eustace SJ, O'Byrne JM (2007) The posterior cruciate ligament-preserving total knee replacement: do we 'preserve' it? A radiological study. J Bone Joint Surg Br 89:766–771
15. Goyal T, Singla M, Paul S. Anatomy of posterior cruciate ligament retained in a posterior cruciate ligament retaining total knee replacement: a cadaveric study. SICOT J. 2018;4:40. https://doi.org/10.1051/sicotj/2018013.
16. Totlis T, Iosifidis M, Melas I, KonstantinosApostolidis K, Agapidis A, Eftychiakos N, DimitriosAlvanos D, Kyriakidis A (2017) Cruciate-retaining

total knee arthroplasty: how much of the PCL is really retained. Knee Surg Sport Traumatol Arthrosc. 25:3556
17. Onishi Y, Hino K, Watanabe S, Watamori K, Kutsuna T, Miura H. The influence of tibial resection on the PCL in PCL-retaining total knee arthroplasty: a clinical and cadaveric study. J Orthop Sci. 2016;21:798–803. https://doi.org/10.1016/j.jos.2016.07.008.
18. Sessa P, Fioravanti G, Giannicola G, Cinotti G (2015) The risk of sacrificing the PCL in cruciate retaining total knee arthroplasty and the relationship to the sagittal inclination of the tibial plateau. Knee 22:51–55
19. Liabaud B, Patrick DA Jr, Geller JA (2013) Is the posterior cruciate ligament destabilized after the tibial cut in a cruciate retaining total knee replacement? Knee 20:412–415
20. Matziolis G, Mehlhorn S, Schattat N, Diederichs G, Hube R, Perka C et al (2012) How much of the PCL is really preserved during the tibial cut? Knee Surg Sports Traumatol Arthrosc 20:1083–1086
21. Feyen H, Van Opstal N, Bellemans J (2013) Partial resection of the PCL insertion site during tibial preparation in cruciate-retain- ing TKA. Knee Surg Sports Traumatol Arthrosc 21:2674–2726
22. Song GY, Liu X, Zhang H, Wang QQ, Zhang J, Li Y, et al. Increased medial meniscal slope is associated with greater risk of ramp lesion in noncontact anterior cruciate ligament injury. Am J Sports Med. 2016;44:2039–46. https://doi.org/10.1177/0363546516640516.
23. Kim SJ, Moon SH, Shin SJ. Radiographic knee dimensions in discoid lateral meniscus: comparison with normal control. Arthroscopy. 2000;16:511–6. https://doi.org/10.1053/jars.2000.4380.
24. Lu X, Qian J, Yang B, Li Z, Fan Y, Jiang B. A new radiographic finding of adult symptomatic discoid lateral meniscus. Medicine (Baltimore). 2020;99:e19646. https://doi.org/10.1097/MD.0000000000019646.
25. Rand JA, Trousdale RT, Ilstrup DM et al (2003) Factors affecting the durability of primary total knee prostheses. J Bone Joint Surg Am 85-A:259–265
26. Scott RD (2001) Would that it were so: save the PCL! Orthopedics 24:888–889
27. Tsuji S, Tomita T, Hashimoto H et al (2011) Effect of posterior design changes on postoperative flexion angle in cruciate retaining mobile-bearing total knee arthroplasty. Int Orthop 35:689–695
28. Fantozzi S, Catani F, Ensini A et al (2006) Femoral rollback of cruciate-retaining and posterior-stabilized total knee replacements: in vivo fluoroscopic analysis during activities of daily living. J Orthop Res 24:2222–2229
29. Seon JK, Park JK, Jeong MS et al (2011) Correlation between preoperative and postoperative knee kinematics in total knee arthroplasty using cruciate retaining designs. Int Orthop 35:515–520
30. Siston RA, Giori NJ, Goodman SB et al (2006) Intraoperative passive kinematics of osteoarthritic knees before and after total knee arthroplasty. J Orthop Res 24:1607–1614

31. Li G, Zayontz S, Most E et al (2004) In situ forces of the anterior and posterior cruciate ligaments in high knee flexion: an in vitro investigation. J Orthop Res 22:293–297
32. Most E, Li G, Sultan PG et al (2005) Kinematic analysis of conventional and high-flexion cruciate-retaining total knee arthroplasties: an in vitro investigation. J Arthroplasty 20:529–535
33. Yue B, Varadarajan KM, Moynihan AL et al (2011) Kinematics of medial osteoarthritic knees before and after posterior cruciate ligament retaining total knee arthroplasty. J Orthop Res 29:40–46
34. Defrate LE, Gill TJ, Li G (2004) In vivo function of the posterior cruciate ligament during weightbearing knee flexion. Am J Sports Med 32:1923–1928
35. Papannagari R, DeFrate LE, Nha KW, Moses JM, Moussa M, Gill TJ et al (2007) Function of posterior cruciate ligament bundles during in vivo knee flexion. Am J Sports Med 35:1507–1512
36. Li G, Defrate LE, Sun H et al (2004) In vivo elongation of the anterior cruciate ligament and posterior cruciate ligament during knee flexion. Am J Sports Med 32:1415–1420
37. Mahoney OM, Noble PC, Rhoads DD et al (1994) Posterior cruciate function following total knee arthroplasty. A biomechanical study. J Arthroplasty 9:569–578
38. Engh GA. The difficult knee severe varus and valgus. *Clin Orthop Relat Res.* 2003;416:588–563.
39. Politi J, Scott R. Balancing severe valgus deformity in total knee arthroplasty using a lateral cruciform retinacular release. *J Arthroplasty.* 2004;19:553–557.
40. Easely ME, Insall JN, Scuderi GR, Bullek DD. Primary constrained condylar knee arthroplasty for the arthritic valgus knee. *Clin Orthop Relat Res.* 2000;380:58–64.
41. Krackow KA, Jones MM, Teeny SM, Hungerford DS. Primary total knee arthroplasty in patients with fixed valgus deformity. *Clin Orthop Relat Res.* 1991;273:9–18.
42. Pagnano MW, Hanssen AD, Lewallen DG, Stuart MJ (1998) Flexion instability after primary posterior cruciate retaining total knee arthroplasty. Clin Orthop Relat Res 356:39–46
43. Waslewski GL, Marson BM, Benjamin JB (1998) Early, incapacitating instability of posterior cruciate ligament-retaining total knee arthroplasty. J Arthroplasty 13(7):763–767
44. Feyen H, Van Opstal N, Bellemans J (2012) Partial resection of the PCL insertion site during tibial preparation in cruciate-retaining TKA. Knee Surg Sports Traumatol Arthrosc. April 22 [Epub ahead of print]
45. Komistek RD, Mahfouz MR, Bertin KC, Rosenberg A, Kennedy W (2008) In vivo determination of total knee arthroplasty kinematics: a multicenter analysis of an asymmetrical posterior cruciate retaining total knee arthroplasty. J Arthroplasty 23(1):41–50

46. Bravi M, Santacaterina F, Bressi F et al (2021) Does posterior cruciate ligament retention or sacrifice in total knee replacement affect proprioception? A systematic review. J Clin Med 10:3470. https://doi.org/10.3390/jcm10163470
47. Orozco F, Ong A (2012) Posterior stabilized total knee arthroplasty. In: Fokter S (ed) Recent advances in hip and knee arthroplasty. InTech, London. https://doi.org/10.5772/25802
48. Keblish PA (1991) The lateral approach to the valgus knee. Surgical technique and analysis of 53 cases with over two-year follow-up evaluation. ClinOrthopRelat Res 271:52–62
49. Nabeyama R, Matsuda S, Miura H, Kawano T, Nagamine R, Mawatari T, Tanaka K, Iwamoto Y. Changes in anteroposterior stability following total knee arthroplasty. J Orthop Sci. 2003;8(4):526.
50. Yoshiya S, Matsui N, Komistek RD, Dennis DA, Mahfouz M, Kurosaka M (2005) In vivo kinematic comparison of posterior cruciate-retaining and posterior stabilized total knee arthroplasties under passive and weight-bearing conditions. J Arthroplasty 20(6):777–783
51. Oka S, Matsumoto T, Muratsu H, Kubo S, Matsushita T, Ishida K, Kuroda R, Kurosaka M. The influence of the tibial slope on intra-operative soft tissue balance in cruciate-retaining and posterior-stabilized total knee arthroplasty. Knee Surgery, Sports Traumatology, Arthroscopy 22: 1812, 2014.
52. Jones DPG, Locke C, Pennington J, Theis J-C. The Effect of Sagittal laxity on function after posterior cruciate–retaining total knee replacement. J Arthroplast. 2006;21(5):719.
53. Wolfe F, Kong SX. Rasch analysis of the western Ontario MacMaster questionnaire (WOMAC) in 2205 patients with osteoarthritis, rheumatoid arthritis, and fibromyalgia. Ann Rheum Dis. 1999;58(9):563.
54. Mizu-Uchi H, Matsuda S, Miura H, Nabeyama R, Okazaki K, Iwamoto Y. Anteroposterior Stability in posterior cruciate ligament–retaining total knee arthroplasty. J Arthroplast. 2006;21(4):592.
55. Ishii Y, Noguchi H, Sato J, Sakurai T, Toyabe S-i. Anteroposterior translation and range of motion after total knee arthroplasty using posterior cruciate ligament-retaining versus posterior cruciate ligament-substituting prostheses. Knee Surg Sports Traumatol Arthrosc. 2017;25(11):3536.
56. Ishii Y, Matsuda Y, Ishii R, Sakata S, Omori G. Sagittal laxity in vivo after total knee arthroplasty. Arch Orthop Trauma Surg. 2005;125(4):249.
57. Ritter MA, Harty LD, Davis KE, Meding JB, Berend ME (2003) Predicting range of motion after total knee arthroplasty. Clustering, log-linear regression, and regression tree analysis. J Bone Jt Surg Am 85–A:1278–1285
58. Anouchi YS, McShane M, Kelly F Jr., Elting J, Stiehl J (1996) Range of motion in total knee replacement. Clin Orthop Relat Res 87–92
59. Jacobs WC, Clement DJ, Wymenga AB: Retention versus removal of the posterior cruciate ligament in total knee replacement. Act Orth. 2005, 76 (6): 757-768. https://doi.org/10.1080/17453670510045345.
60. Cates HE, Komistek RD, Mahfouz MR, Schmidt MA, Anderle M (2008) In vivo comparison of knee kinematics for subjects having either a posterior

stabilized or cruciate retaining high-flexion total knee arthroplasty. J Arthroplasty 23:1057–1067
61. Dennis DA, Komistek RD, Mahfouz MR, Haas BD, Stiehl JB (2003) Multicenter determination of in vivo kinematics after total knee arthroplasty. Clin Orthop Relat Res 37–57
62. Hamai S, Miura H, Higaki H et al (2008) Kinematic analysis of kneeling in cruciate-retaining and posterior-stabilized total knee arthroplasties. J Orthop Res 26:435–442
63. Sharma A, Komistek RD, Scuderi GR, Cates HE Jr (2007) High-flexion TKA designs: what are their in vivo contact mechanics? Clin Orthop Relat Res 464:117–126
64. Suggs JF, Kwon YM, Durbhakula SM, Hanson GR, Li G (2009) In vivo flexion and kinematics of the knee after TKA: comparison of a conventional and a high flexion cruciate-retaining TKA design. Knee Surg Sports Traumatol Arthrosc 17:150–156
65. Wasielewski RC, Komistek RD, Zingde SM, Sheridan KC, Mahfouz MR (2008) Lack of axial rotation in mobile-bearing knee designs. Clin Orthop Relat Res 466:2662–2668
66. Casino D, Martelli S, Zaffagnini S et al (2009) Knee stability before and after total and unicondylar knee replacement: in vivo kinematic evaluation utilizing navigation. J Orthop Res 27:202–207
67. Casino D, Zaffagnini S, Martelli S et al (2009) Intraoperative evaluation of total knee replacement: kinematic assessment with a navigation system. Knee Surg Sports Traumatol Arthrosc 17:369–373
68. Mihalko WM, Ali M, Phillips MJ, Bayers-Thering M, Krackow KA (2008) Passive knee kinematics before and after total knee arthroplasty: are we correcting pathologic motion? J Arthroplasty 23:57–60
69. Saari T, Carlsson L, Karlsson J, Karrholm J (2005) Knee kinematics in medial arthrosis. Dynamic radiostereometry during active extension and weight-bearing. J Biomech 38:285–292
70. Lizaur A, Marco L, Cebrian R (1997) Preoperative factors influencing the range of movement after total knee arthroplasty for severe osteoarthritis. J Bone Joint Surg Br 79:626–629
71. Schurman DJ, Matityahu A, Goodman SB, et al (1998) Prediction of postoperative knee flexion in Insall-Burstein II total knee arthroplasty. Clin Orthop Relat Res 353:175–184
72. Berger RA, Rubash HE, Seel MJ, Thompson WH, Crossett LS (1993) Determining the rotational alignment of the femoral component in total knee arthroplasty using the epicondylar axis. Clin Orthop Relat Res (286):40–47
73. Griffin FM, Math K, Scuderi GR, Insall JN, Poilvache PL (2000) Anatomy of the epicondyles of the distal femur: MRI analysis of normal knees. J Arthroplasty 15(3):354–359
74. Matsumoto T, Kuroda R, Kubo S, Muratsu H, Mizuno K, Kurosaka M (2009) The intra-operative joint gap in cruciate-retaining compared with posterior-stabilised total knee replacement. J Bone Joint Surg (Br) 91(4):475–480

75. Matsumoto T, Muratsu H, Kubo S, Matsushita T, Kurosaka M, Kuroda R (2011) Soft tissue tension in cruciate-retaining and posterior-stabilized total knee arthroplasty. J Arthroplasty 26(5):788–795. https://doi.org/10.1016/j.arth.2010.06.006
76. Lee DH, Padhy D, Park JH, Jeong WK, Park JH, Han SB (2011) The impact of a rectangular or trapezoidal flexion gap on the femoral component rotation in TKA. Knee Surg Sports Traumatol Arthrosc 19(7):1141–1147. https://doi.org/10.1007/s00167-011-1422-3
77. Seon JK, Song EK, Park SJ, Lee DS (2011) The use of navigation to obtain rectangular flexion and extension gaps during primary total knee arthroplasty and midterm clinical results. J Arthroplasty 26(4):582–590. https://doi.org/10.1016/j.arth.2010.04.030
78. Aigner C, Windhager R, Pechmann M, Rehak P, Engeleke K. The influence of an anterior-posterior gliding mobile bearing on range of motion after total knee arthroplasty. A prospective, randomized, double-blinded study. *J Bone Joint Surg Am.* 2004;86:2257–2262.
79. Hofmann AA, Tkach TK, Evanich CJ, Camargo MP. Posterior stabilization in total knee arthroplasty with use of an ultracongruent polyethylene insert. *J Arthroplasty.* 2000;15:576–583.
80. Laskin RS, Maruyama Y, Villaneuva M, Bourne R. Deep-dish congruent tibial component use in total knee arthroplasty: a randomized prospective study. *Clin Orthop Relat Res.* 2000;380:36–44.
81. Sathappan SS, Wasserman B, Jaffe WL, Bong M, Walsh M, Di Cesare PE (2006) Midterm results of primary total knee arthroplasty using a dished polyethylene insert with a recessed or resected posterior cruciate ligament. J Arthroplasty 21:1012–1016
82. Scott RD, Thornhill TS. Posterior cruciate supplementing total knee replacement using conforming inserts and cruciate recession: effect on range of motion and radiolucent lines. *Clin Orthop Relat Res.* 1994;309:146.
83. Scott RD, Thornhill TS. Posterior cruciate supplementing total knee replacement using conforming inserts and cruciate recession. Effect on range of motion and radiolucent lines. Clin Orthop Relat Res. 1994;309:146–9.
84. Iwaki H, Pinskerova V, Freeman MA. Tibiofemoral movement 1: the shapes and relative movements of the femur and tibia in the unloaded cadaver knee. J Bone Jt Surg Br. 2000;82:1189–95. https://doi.org/10.1302/0301-620x.82b8.10717.
85. Schnaser E, Lee YY, Boettner F, Gonzalez Della Valle A. The position of the patella and extensor mechanism affects intraoperative compartmental loads during total knee arthroplasty: a pilot study using intraoperative sensing to guide soft tissue balance. J Arthroplast. 2015;30:1348-1353.e1343. https://doi.org/10.1016/j.arth.2015.03.004.
86. Baldini A, Anderson JA, Zampetti P, Pavlov H, Sculco TP: A new patellofemoral scoring system for total knee arthroplasty. Clin Orthop. 2006, 452: 150-154.

87. Burnett RS, Haydon CM, Rorabeck CH, Bourne RB: Patella resurfacing versus nonresurfacing in total knee arthroplasty - Results of a randomized controlled clinical trial at a minimum of 10 years' followup. Clin Orthop. 2004, 428: 12-25.
88. Smith AJ, Wood DJ, Li MG: Total knee replacement with and without patellar resurfacing - A prospective, randomised trial using the profix total knee system. J Bone Joint Surg Br. 2008, 90B (1): 43-49.
89. Pakos EE, Ntzani EE, Trikalinos TA: Patellar resurfacing in total knee arthroplasty - A meta-analysis. J Bone Joint Surg Am. 2005, 87A (7): 1438-1445.
90. Waters TS, Bentley G: Patellar resurfacing in total knee arthroplasty - A prospective, randomized study. J Bone Joint Surg Am. 2003, 85A (2): 212-217.
91. Wood DJ, Smith AJ, Collopy D, White B, Brankov B, Bulsara MK: Patellar resurfacing in total knee arthroplasty - A prospective, randomized trial. J Bone Joint Surg Am. 2002, 84A (2): 187-193.
92. Barrack RL, Bertot AJ, Wolfe MW, Waldman DA, Milicic M, Myers L: Patellar resurfacing in total knee arthroplasty - A prospective, randomized, double-blind study with five to seven years of follow-up. J Bone Joint Surg Am. 2001, 83A (9): 1376-1381.
93. Breeman S, Campbell M, Dakin H, Fiddian N, Fitzpatrick R, Grant A, Gray A, Johnston L, Maclennan G, Morris R, Murray D, KAT Trial Group: Patellar resurfacing in total knee replacement: five-year clinical and economic results of a large randomized controlled trial. J Bone Joint Surg Am. 2011, 93 (16): 1473-1481. https://doi.org/10.2106/JBJS.J.00725.
94. Feller JA, Bartlett RJ, Lang DM: Patellar resurfacing versus retention in total knee arthroplasty. J Bone Joint Surg Br. 1996, 78B: 226-228.
95. Insall JN, Dorr LD, Scott RD, Scott WN: Rationale of the knee-society clinical rating system. Clin Orthop. 1989, 248: 13-14.
96. Roos EM, Roos HP, Lohmander LS, Ekdahl C, Beynnon BD: Knee Injury and Osteoarthritis Outcome Score (KOOS)–development of a self-administered outcome measure. J Orthop Sports Phys Ther. 1998, 28 (2): 88-96. https://doi.org/10.2519/jospt.1998.28.2.88.
97. Baldini A, Anderson JA, Cerulli-Mariani P, Kalyvas J, Pavlov H, Sculco TP: Patellofemoral evaluation after total knee arthroplasty - Validation of a new weight-bearing axial radiographic view. J Bone Joint Surg Am. 2007, 89A (8): 1810-1817.
98. Elbardesy H, Salamah HM, McLeod A, Thada PK, Mohammed ER, Hanifa FA et al (2021) Medial pivot versus (cam post) posterior stabilised total knee arthroplasty, systematic review and meta-analysis of 3837 knees. Acta Orthop Belg 87(4):665–680
99. Clement ND, MacDonald D, Simpson AH (2014) The minimal clinically important difference in the Oxford knee score and Short Form 12 score after total knee arthroplasty. Knee Surg Sports Traumatol Arthrosc 22(08):1933–1939
100. Xie F, Li SC, Lo NN, Yeo SJ, Yang KY, Yeo W et al (2007) Cross-cultural adaptation and validation of Singapore English and Chinese Versions of the

Oxford Knee Score (OKS) in knee osteoarthritis patients undergoing total knee replacement. Osteoarthritis Cartilage 15(9):1019–1024
101. Insall JN, Dorr LD, Scott RD, Scott WN (1989) Rationale of the Knee Society clinical rating system. Clin Orthop Relat Res 248:13–14
102. Indelli PF, Risitano S, Halll KE, Leonardi E, Migliore E (2019) Effect of polyethylene conformity on total knee arthroplasty early clinical outcomes. Knee Surg Sports Traumatol Arthrosc 27(4):1028–1034
103. Moonot P, Mu S, Railton GT, Field RE, Banks SA (2009) Tibiofemoral kinematic analysis of knee flexion for a medial pivot knee. Knee Surg Sports Traumatol Arthrosc 17:927–934. https://doi.org/10.1007/s00167-009-0777-1
104. Moonot P, Shang M, Railton GT, Field RE, Banks SA (2010) In vivo weight-bearing kinematics with medial rotation knee arthroplasty. Knee 17:33–37. https://doi.org/10.1016/j.knee.2009.06.009
105. Shimmin A, Martinez-Martos S, Owens J, Iorgulescu AD, Banks S (2015) Fluoroscopic motion study confirming the stability of a medial pivot design total knee arthroplasty. Knee 22:522–526. https://doi.org/10.1016/j.knee.2014.11.011
106. Bin Abd Razak, Hamid Rahmatullah; Pang, Hee Nee; Yeo, Seng Jin; Tan, Mann Hong; Lo, Ngai Nung; Chong, Hwei Chi Joint line changes in cruciate-retaining versus posterior-stabilized computer-navigated total knee arthroplasty. Archives of Orthopaedic and Trauma Surgery (2013). https://doi.org/10.1007/s00402-013-1738-1
107. Cinotti, Gianluca; Ripani, Francesca Romana; Perciballi, Beatrice; La Torre, Giuseppe; Giannicola, Giuseppe Higher rates of fully preserved posterior cruciate ligament in total knee arthroplasty using a double tibial cut: a prospective randomized controlled trial. Knee Surgery & Related Research (2024). https://doi.org/10.1186/s43019-023-00208-z
108. Chen, Long; Xu, Jie; Lin, Yuan; Luo, Fen Qi; Yu, Yu Guo The effect of sacrificing the posterior cruciate ligament on total knee arthroplasty with cruciate retaining highly congruent rotating platform prosthesis. Journal of Orthopaedic Surgery and Research (2021). https://doi.org/10.1186/s13018-021-02433-2
109. Xin, Weiwei; Gao, Yingjian; Zheng, Liangjun; Qu, Xinhua; Yue, Bing Posterior cruciate ligament tibial attachment sacrifice percentage is higher in cruciate-retaining total knee arthroplasty in patients with discoid lateral meniscus. Arthroplasty (2024). https://doi.org/10.1186/s42836-024-00238-2
110. Yue, Bing; Varadarajan, Kartik M.; Rubash, Harry E.; Li, Guoan In vivo function of posterior cruciate ligament before and after posterior cruciate ligament-retaining total knee arthroplasty. International Orthopaedics (2012). https://doi.org/10.1007/s00264-011-1481-6
111. McAuley, James P.; Collier, Matthew B.; Hamilton, W. G.; Tabaraee, Ehsan; Engh, G. A. Posterior Cruciate-retaining Total Knee Arthroplasty for Valgus Osteoarthritis. Clinical Orthopaedics and Related Research® (2008). https://doi.org/10.1007/s11999-008-0436-8
112. Jawhar, Ahmed; Wasnik, Sandeep; Scharf, Hanns-Peter; Roehl, Henning Fibula head is a useful landmark to predict the location of posterior cruciate

ligament footprint prior to total knee arthroplasty. International Orthopaedics (2013). https://doi.org/10.1007/s00264-013-2100-5
113. Fujimoto, Eisaku; Sasashige, Yoshiaki; Tomita, Tetsuya; Sasaki, Hirofumi; Touten, Yoriko; Fujiwara, Yuusuke; Ochi, Mitsuo Intra-operative gaps affect outcome and postoperative kinematics in vivo following cruciate-retaining total knee arthroplasty. International Orthopaedics (2015). https://doi.org/10.1007/s00264-015-2847-y
114. Fiedler, Benjamin; Bieganowski, Thomas; Anil, Utkarsh; Lin, Charles C.; Habibi, Akram A.; Schwarzkopf, Ran Can pain be improved with retention of the posterior cruciate ligament during total knee arthroplasty?. European Journal of Orthopaedic Surgery & Traumatology (2023). https://doi.org/10.1007/s00590-023-03562-6
115. Savov, Peter; Mielke, Evelyn; Windhagen, Henning; Calliess, Tilman; Richter, Alena; Ettinger, Max Higher revision rate for posterior cruciate-retaining than posterior-stabilized total knee arthroplasty for the treatment of valgus osteoarthritis. Archives of Orthopaedic and Trauma Surgery (2020). https://doi.org/10.1007/s00402-020-03618-w
116. Ersin, Mehmet; Demirel, Mehmet; Civan, Melih; Ekinci, Mehmet; Akgül, Turgut; Şen, Cengiz The effect of posterior tibial slope on anteroposterior stability in posterior cruciate retaining total knee arthroplasty. BMC Musculoskeletal Disorders (2023). https://doi.org/10.1186/s12891-023-06507-6
117. Tsuji, Shigeyoshi; Tomita, Tetsuya; Hashimoto, Hideo; Fujii, Masakazu; Yoshikawa, Hideki; Sugamoto, Kazuomi Effect of posterior design changes on postoperative flexion angle in cruciate retaining mobile-bearing total knee arthroplasty. International Orthopaedics (2010). https://doi.org/10.1007/s00264-010-1060-2
118. Seon, Jong Keun; Park, Ju Kwon; Jeong, Mun Su; Jung, Woo Bin; Park, Kyung Soon; Yoon, Taek Rim; Song, Eun Kyoo Correlation between preoperative and postoperative knee kinematics in total knee arthroplasty using cruciate retaining designs. International Orthopaedics (2010). https://doi.org/10.1007/s00264-010-1029-1
119. Matsumoto, Tomoyuki; Muratsu, Hirotsugu; Kawakami, Yohei; Takayama, Koji; Ishida, Kazunari; Matsushita, Takehiko; Akisue, Toshihiro; Nishida, Kotaro; Kuroda, Ryosuke; Kurosaka, Masahiro Soft-tissue balancing in total knee arthroplasty: cruciate-retaining versus posterior-stabilised, and measured-resection versus gap technique. International Orthopaedics (2013). https://doi.org/10.1007/s00264-013-2133-9
120. Peters, Christopher L.; Mulkey, Patrick; Erickson, Jill; Anderson, Michael B.; Pelt, Christopher E. Comparison of Total Knee Arthroplasty With Highly Congruent Anterior-stabilized Bearings versus a Cruciate-retaining Design. Clinical Orthopaedics and Related Research® (2013). https://doi.org/10.1007/s11999-013-3068-6
121. Zhao, Ran; Liu, Yanqing; Tian, Hua Effect of posterior cruciate ligament on knee pressure and gap measured by an electronic sensor during total knee

arthroplasty. Journal of Orthopaedic Surgery and Research (2023). https://doi.org/10.1186/s13018-023-03643-6
122. Lee, W. C.; Foong, C. M. B.; Khoo, K. M. S.; Kwan, Y. H.; Kunnasegaran, R. Faster improvement in outcome scores in posterior stabilised total knee arthroplasty compared to medial congruent system with posterior cruciate ligament retained. MUSCULOSKELETAL SURGERY (2023). https://doi.org/10.1007/s12306-023-00797-8
123. Elorza, Saúl Pacheco; O'Donnell, Ed; Nedopil, Alexander; Howell, Stephen M.; Hull, Maury L. Ball-in-socket medial conformity with posterior cruciate ligament retention neither limits internal tibial rotation and knee flexion nor lowers clinical outcome scores after unrestricted kinematically aligned total knee arthroplasty. International Orthopaedics (2023). https://doi.org/10.1007/s00264-023-05834-6

4.2 Medial Pivot

Machine Generated Summaries
Disclaimer: The summaries in this chapter were generated from Springer Nature publications using abstractive AI auto-summarization: An abstraction-based summarizer creates new text based on deep learning. New phrases are created to summarize the content. As the constituted sentences are machine selected, they may not fully reflect the body of the work, so we strongly advise that the original content is read and cited. The auto-generated summaries were curated by the editor to meet Springer Nature publication standards.

4.2.1 Higher Use of Fixed-Bearing Over Mobile-Bearing and Posterior-Stabilized Over Medial Pivot Designs in Total Knee Arthroplasty (TKA): A Systematic Comparative Analysis Using Worldwide Arthroplasty Registers from England and Wales, Australia, Norway, New Zealand, Germany and Switzerland [146]

This is a machine-generated summary of:

Wittig, Ulrike; Moshammer, Maximilian; Vielgut, Ines; Hauer, Georg; Reinbacher, Patrick; Leithner, Andreas; Sadoghi, Patrick Higher use of fixed-bearing over mobile-bearing and posterior-stabilized over medial pivot designs in total knee arthroplasty (TKA): a systematic comparative analysis using worldwide arthroplasty registers from England and Wales, Australia, Norway, New Zealand, Germany and Switzerland [146].

Published in: Archives of Orthopaedic and Trauma Surgery (2022).
Link to original: https://doi.org/10.1007/s00402-022-04410-8

If you want to cite the papers, please refer to the original.
For technical reasons we could not place the page where the original quote is coming from.

4.2.1.1 Research Highlights

The establishment of arthroplasty registers has been pivotal in documenting the outcomes of total joint arthroplasty, evolving into regional or national registries to assess implant-related factors, surgical techniques, and patient-related outcomes. These registers aim to evaluate the efficacy of joint arthroplasties and identify potential failures. However, systematic comparisons of different design concepts in total knee arthroplasty (TKA) have been lacking, particularly concerning mobile- or fixed-bearing, posterior-stabilized, or medial pivot designs. The study by Wittig et al. addresses this gap by comparing the use of these TKA design concepts across various national arthroplasty registers.

The study utilized data from six national arthroplasty registers—England and Wales, Australia, Norway, New Zealand, Germany, and Switzerland—that met specific inclusion criteria such as language and data consistency. The researchers extracted data on the number of TKA procedures performed and the distribution of mobile- or fixed-bearing designs as well as posterior-stabilized or medial pivot designs. Descriptive statistics were employed to analyse these parameters across different countries. The findings revealed that fixed-bearing TKA was predominantly used across all registers, with its frequency slightly decreasing over time except in England and Wales. Mobile-bearing designs showed significant variation in usage among countries. Posterior-stabilized TKA usage also varied widely, with Switzerland reporting the highest frequency.

The study highlights significant differences in TKA design preferences across countries while underscoring the widespread use of fixed-bearing inserts due to their reduced risk of dislocation when properly inserted. Future study directions could focus on long-term outcomes associated with newer designs like medial pivot TKA, which aims to replicate natural knee kinematics but remains less commonly used due to its recent introduction. The authors suggest that an individualized approach considering implant design, patient selection, and surgical technique is crucial for optimizing prosthesis survival and functionality. Limitations include potential discrepancies in registry data quality and incomplete differentiation between design types in some registers.

4.2.2 Evaluation of Patellofemoral Joint in ADVANCE® Medial-Pivot Total Knee Arthroplasty [147]

This is a machine-generated summary of:

Chinzei, Nobuaki; Ishida, Kazunari; Matsumoto, Tomoyuki; Kuroda, Yuichi; Kitagawa, Atsushi; Kuroda, Ryosuke; Akisue, Toshihiro; Nishida, Kotaro; Kurosaka, Masahiro; Tsumura, Nobuhiro Evaluation of patellofemoral joint in ADVANCE® Medial-pivot total knee arthroplasty [147].

Published in: International Orthopaedics (2013).

Link to original: https://doi.org/10.1007/s00264-013-2043-x

If you want to cite the papers, please refer to the original.

For technical reasons we could not place the page where the original quote is coming from.

4.2.2.1 Research Highlights

Total knee arthroplasty (TKA) is a widely performed procedure for severe osteoarthritis and other cartilage degeneration conditions. Despite its success, complications related to the patellofemoral (PF) joint, such as pain and maltracking, remain a concern. The ADVANCE Medial-pivot prosthesis(Microport, Shanghai, China), known for its unique design aiming to replicate normal knee kinematics, has shown promising results in tibiofemoral joint studies. However, the PF joint's performance with this prosthesis is not well understood. The study by Chinzei et al. investigates the radiographic PF joint conditions in ADVANCE TKA using innovative three-dimensional digital templating software, "ATHENA KNEE,(Soft Cube, Osaka, Japan)" to assess postoperative changes.

The study involved ten patients with varus deformity undergoing ADVANCE MP TKA. Excluding those with valgus deformity or severe bony defects, the research focused on comparing pre- and postoperative PF joint conditions using ATHENA KNEE software. This tool allowed for precise visualization of the implanted knee's status by matching preoperative CT data with postoperative X-ray images. The study measured patella tilt and shift at various knee flexion angles and assessed the rotational profile of the femoral prosthesis. Statistical analysis revealed significant improvements in patella shift post-surgery but an increase in patella tilt at 0° flexion. The findings highlighted a positive correlation between postoperative condylar twist angle (CTA) and patella shift.

The study advances understanding of PF joint kinematics in ADVANCE MP TKA, emphasizing the influence of prosthesis design on joint motion rather than femoral rotation alone. The use of ATHENA KNEE software demonstrated its potential as a practical tool for postoperative assessment without requiring additional CT scans, thus reducing patient exposure to radiation. Future study could explore long-term outcomes and further refine surgical techniques to enhance PF joint congruity post-TKA. These insights contribute to improving surgical practices and patient outcomes in knee arthroplasty.

4.2.3 Lateral Shift of the Femoral Condyle After Total Knee Arthroplasty: Simulation Using 2D-Templates of the Medial Pivot Design on Knee Radiographs of Young Japanese Patients [148]

This is a machine-generated summary of:

Nakajima, Arata; Sonobe, Masato; Akatsu, Yorikazu; Yamada, Manabu; Yamamoto, Keiichiro; Saito, Junya; Norimoto, Masaki; Koyama, Keita; Taniguchi, Shinji; Takahashi, Hiroshi; Aoki, Yasuchika; Suguro, Toru; Nakagawa, Koichi Lateral shift of the femoral condyle after total knee arthroplasty: simulation using 2D-templates of the medial pivot design on knee radiographs of young Japanese patients [148].

Published in: Journal of Orthopaedic Surgery and Research (2022).

Link to original: https://doi.org/10.1186/s13018-022-03342-8

If you want to cite the papers, please refer to the original.

For technical reasons we could not place the page where the original quote is coming from.

4.2.3.1 Research Highlights

Total knee arthroplasty (TKA) generally yields satisfactory outcomes, yet a notable percentage of patients report dissatisfaction post-surgery. This dissatisfaction may stem from changes in the coronal positional relationship between the femur and tibia, particularly when using a medial pivot design that restricts femoral component positioning to the tibial inserts. Such alterations can impact the balance of major knee ligaments, including the medial and lateral collateral ligaments. The study by Nakajima et al. investigates these positional changes using radiographic simulations of TKA on young Japanese patients without osteoarthritic changes.

The study involved simulating TKA on knee radiographs from patients aged 20 to 40 who had undergone arthroscopic surgeries for various knee conditions. Using templates of the FINE total knee system (Teijin Nakashima Medical Co., Ltd. in Okayama, Japan), which features an oblique femorotibial joint line and a medial convex curve on the polyethylene insert, researchers assessed the lateral shift of the femoral condyle post-simulation. The femoral component was aligned with the medial concave of the tibial insert to estimate postoperative alignment. Measurements were conducted by three independent observers using SYNAPSE-PACS software (Fuji Film, Tokyo, Japan) ensuring reliability through inter- and intra-class correlation coefficients. Statistical analyses revealed that males exhibited a greater lateral shift than females, with significant correlations found between this shift and radiographic parameters like the medial proximal tibial angle (MPTA).

The findings suggest that TKA using a medial pivot design results in a lateral shift of the femoral condyle, potentially affecting ligament balance and leading to suboptimal clinical outcomes. The study highlights racial and gender differences in knee alignment, emphasizing the need for individualized approaches in TKA planning. Future studies could explore computational simulations or cadaver specimens to further evaluate ligament balance and knee kinematics post-TKA. Understanding these dynamics is crucial for improving surgical techniques and patient satisfaction in TKA procedures.

4.2.4 *Kinematics and Kinetics Comparison of Ultra-Congruent Versus Medial-Pivot Designs for Total Knee Arthroplasty by Multibody Analysis [149]*

This is a machine-generated summary of:

Putame, Giovanni; Terzini, Mara; Rivera, Fabrizio; Kebbach, Maeruan; Bader, Rainer; Bignardi, Cristina Kinematics and kinetics comparison of ultra-congruent versus medial-pivot designs for total knee arthroplasty by multibody analysis [149].

Published in: Scientific Reports (2022).

Link to original: https://doi.org/10.1038/s41598-022-06909-x

4.2.4.1 Research Highlights

Since the early development of total knee endoprostheses, collaboration between surgeons and bioengineers has led to increasingly sophisticated designs. Key considerations in implant design include range of motion, modularity, insert fixation type, and geometrical congruence between articulating surfaces. Despite advancements in materials and design concepts, complications such as joint instability and insert wear remain common causes of revision surgery. The study by Putame et al. investigates the biomechanical behaviour of two different insert designs—medial-pivot (MP) and ultra-congruent (UC)—using a multibody model to simulate knee kinematics during a weight-bearing deep squat.

The study employed a multibody dynamic analysis program to create a model of a right lower limb with standardized bone geometries fitted to patient-specific data. The model included two alternative insert designs: MP and UC. The researchers simulated a weight-bearing deep squat motion to evaluate the kinematics and kinetics of the artificial knee joint, focusing on contact force and pressure distributions on the inserts. Ligament structures were modelled as tension-only spring elements, while muscle forces were controlled using a proportional-integral-derivative controller. Contact forces were computed using an interpenetration formulation derived from Hertz's contact theory, with friction forces accounted for using Coulomb's model. The study found that while both designs showed similar ranges of internal tibial rotation, the MP design allowed for more physiological tibial rotation during early flexion and exhibited lower tibiofemoral contact pressures compared to the UC design.

The findings suggest that the MP design may offer improved post-operative outcomes by promoting more physiological knee kinematics and reducing contact pressures that could lead to wear. This could potentially enhance implant longevity by minimizing pressure peaks that contribute to insert deterioration. Future study could focus on integrating additional muscles into the model or incorporating motion capture data for more accurate simulations of in vivo movements. While direct experimental validation was not performed, comparisons with existing literature showed good agreement, indicating that these findings could inform future total knee implant development and optimization efforts.

4.2.5 Comparative Study of Outcomes with Total Knee Arthroplasty: Medial Pivot Prosthesis vs Posterior Stabilized Implant. Prospective Randomized Control [150]

This is a machine-generated summary of:

Obada, Bogdan; Iliescu, Madalina Gabriela; Costea, Dan Ovidiu; Petcu, Lucian; Popescu, Andrei Ion Comparative study of outcomes with total knee arthroplasty: medial pivot prosthesis vs posterior stabilized implant. Prospective randomized control [150].

Published in: International Orthopaedics (2025).

Link to original: https://doi.org/10.1007/s00264-025-06420-8

If you want to cite the papers, please refer to the original.

For technical reasons we could not place the page where the original quote is coming from.

4.2.5.1 Research Highlights

Total knee arthroplasty (TKA) is a widely used procedure to alleviate pain and restore function in patients with end-stage knee arthritis. Despite its effectiveness, patient satisfaction rates vary, often due to issues such as residual pain and abnormal gait, which may be linked to the kinematic limitations of conventional implant designs. To address these concerns, the medial stabilized prosthesis was developed to better mimic natural knee kinematics by allowing unrestricted posterolateral rollback of the lateral femoral condyle. The study by Obada et al. investigates whether the medial pivot (MP) knee system offers superior postoperative range of motion (ROM) and clinical outcomes compared to the posterior-stabilized (PS) knee system.

The study was conducted at the Emergency Clinical County Hospital "St Apostle Andrei" in Constanta, Romania, involving patients who underwent TKA between January and December 2017. Participants were divided into two groups based on the type of prosthesis received: MP or PS. The surgical technique involved a midline incision and medial parapatellar approach, with all components cemented in place. Patients were evaluated preoperatively and postoperatively at 1 and 2 years using various outcome measures, including ROM and patient-reported scores such as the Western Ontario McMaster Osteoarthritis Index (WOMAC) and Oxford Knee Score (OKS). The study employed statistical analyses to compare outcomes between the two groups while ensuring blinding for clinical assessments.

The findings suggest that patients with MP-TKA experienced better outcomes in terms of ROM and patient satisfaction compared to those with PS-TKA. The MP design's ability to replicate natural knee kinematics may contribute to these improved results. However, both designs showed comparable safety profiles with no significant differences in infection rates or component loosening. Future study could explore the interplay between implant design and other factors influencing patient satisfaction, as well as longer-term outcomes beyond the 2-year follow-up period. These insights could guide surgeons in selecting appropriate prosthesis designs tailored to individual patient needs.

4.2.6 A Comparative Study of Flat Surface Design and Medial Pivot Design in Posterior Cruciate-Retaining Total Knee Arthroplasty: A Matched Pair Cohort Study of Two Years [151]

This is a machine-generated summary of:

Nakamura, Junichi; Inoue, Takaki; Suguro, Toru; Suzuki, Masahiko; Sasho, Takahisa; Hagiwara, Shigeo; Akagi, Ryuichiro; Orita, Sumihisa; Inage, Kazuhide; Akazawa, Tsutomu; Ohtori, Seiji A comparative study of flat surface design and medial pivot design in posterior cruciate-retaining total knee arthroplasty: a matched pair cohort study of 2 years [151].

Published in: BMC Musculoskeletal Disorders (2018).

Link to original: https://doi.org/10.1186/s12891-018-2138-z

If you want to cite the papers, please refer to the original.

For technical reasons we could not place the page where the original quote is coming from.

4.2.6.1 Research Highlights

Total knee arthroplasty (TKA) is a common procedure aimed at alleviating pain and improving daily function in patients with knee issues. Surgeons often decide whether to retain or replace the posterior cruciate ligament and whether to use cement for prosthesis fixation based on individual cases. Previous studies have shown promising survival rates for cruciate-retaining TKA without cement in patients with rheumatoid arthritis. The study by Nakamura et al. compares the short-term clinical outcomes of two different TKA implants: the Hi-Tech Knee II and the FINE Knee (Teijin Nakashima Medical Co., Ltd. in Okayama, Japan), focusing on their design differences and impact on patient outcomes.

The study was a retrospective, case-control, observational cohort study conducted from January 2010 to December 2012. It involved a matched-pair analysis of patients undergoing TKA with either the Hi-Tech Knee II or the FINE Knee implants. The Hi-Tech Knee II used a cementless fixation method, while the FINE

Knee employed cemented fixation. The researchers collected data on various preoperative and perioperative factors, including age, body mass index, range of motion (ROM), and surgical time. Postoperative outcomes were assessed using metrics such as knee scores, ROM, and X-ray measurements over a 2-year follow-up period. Statistical analyses were performed to compare the two groups, revealing that the FINE Knee group had significantly better postoperative ROM, less pain, shorter surgical time, and lower estimated blood loss compared to the Hi-Tech Knee II group.

The study highlights that the medial pivot design of the FINE Knee offers advantages over the flat surface design of the Hi-Tech Knee II in terms of postoperative flexion angle and patient comfort. The findings suggest that implant design plays a crucial role in achieving better clinical outcomes following TKA. Future study could focus on long-term outcomes to further validate these findings and explore potential improvements in implant designs to enhance patient satisfaction and prosthesis longevity. Additionally, addressing limitations such as sample size and measurement errors could strengthen future research in this area.

4.2.7 Performance of Medial Pivot, Posterior Stabilized and Rotating Platform Total Knee Arthroplasty Based on Anteroposterior Stability and Patient-Reported Outcome Measures; A Multicentre Double-Blinded Randomized Controlled Trial of 210 Knees [152]

This is a machine-generated summary of:

De Groot, J. D.; Brokelman, R. B.G.; Lammers, P. G.; Van Stralen, G. M.J.; Kooijman, C. M.; Hokwerda, S. T. Performance of medial pivot, posterior stabilized and rotating platform total knee arthroplasty based on anteroposterior stability and patient-reported outcome measures; a multicentre double-blinded randomized controlled trial of 210 knees [152].

Published in: Archives of Orthopaedic and Trauma Surgery (2024).

Link to original: https://doi.org/10.1007/s00402-024-05340-3

If you want to cite the papers, please refer to the original.

For technical reasons we could not place the page where the original quote is coming from.

4.2.7.1 Research Highlights

Total Knee Arthroplasty (TKA) is widely recognized as the definitive treatment for advanced osteoarthritis when conservative measures fail. Despite significant advancements in surgical techniques, endoprosthetic materials, and designs, a notable percentage of patients remain dissatisfied post-surgery, often due to factors like postoperative pain and decreased knee biomechanics. A key area of debate is the performance differences among TKA designs, particularly concerning stability, which is crucial as instability can lead to early revision surgeries. The study by Groot et al. investigates the anteroposterior (AP) stability and patient-reported outcomes (PROMs) of medial pivot (MP), posterior-stabilized (PS), and rotating-platform (RP) TKA designs.

The study was conducted as a multicenter randomized controlled trial across three Dutch hospitals, involving patients with end-stage osteoarthritis eligible for TKA. Participants were randomly assigned to receive MP, PS, or RP implants. The surgical procedures were standardized across all groups, with similar perioperative care provided. AP stability was measured 1-year post-surgery using a KT-1000 arthrometer at various degrees of knee flexion. PROMs were assessed preoperatively and 1 year postoperatively using several validated scales. The study found that MP-TKA demonstrated significantly less AP translation at certain flexion angles compared to PS-TKA, indicating superior stability. However, while all PROMs improved post-surgery across all groups, only quality of life measures showed significant differences favouring MP-TKA.

The findings suggest that MP-TKA offers better AP stability at early and mid-flexion compared to non-MP designs, although this did not translate into broader improvements in PROMs beyond quality-of-life aspects. The study highlights the need for further research into non-implant-related factors that may influence TKA outcomes, as these could play a more significant role than previously thought. Future studies should focus on larger sample sizes and weight-bearing conditions to validate these findings and explore the impact of implant design on daily activities more comprehensively.

4.2.8 Medial Pivot Versus Posterior-Stabilized Prosthesis Design in Primary Total Knee Arthroplasty: A Systematic Review and Meta-analysis [153]

This is a machine-generated summary of:

Xu, Zihang; Tian, Shengyuan; Zhou, Xiang; Wei, Ya; Wu, Changbing; Jia, Xianghua; Wang, Hong Medial Pivot Versus Posterior-Stabilized Prosthesis Design in Primary Total Knee Arthroplasty: A Systematic Review and Meta-Analysis [153].

Published in: Indian Journal of Orthopaedics (2022).

Link to original: https://doi.org/10.1007/s43465-022-00678-5

If you want to cite the papers, please refer to the original.

For technical reasons we could not place the page where the original quote is coming from.

4.2.8.1 Research Highlights

Total knee arthroplasty (TKA) is a widely accepted treatment for end-stage knee osteoarthritis, known for its high survival rate and effectiveness in restoring knee function. However, dissatisfaction among patients persists, potentially due to the abnormal kinematics of conventional prosthetic designs like the posterior-stabilized (PS) prosthesis. The PS design, while providing stability and improved motion through a cam-and-post mechanism, may lead to complications such as paradoxical anterior movement and patellofemoral joint issues. To address these concerns, the medial pivot (MP) prosthesis was developed to mimic natural knee kinematics by adopting a ball-and-socket concept. The study by Xu et al. undertakes a meta-analysis to compare the clinical outcomes of MP and PS prostheses in TKA.

The study systematically reviewed literature from databases including PubMed, Embase, and Cochrane Library up to April 2023. The authors included randomized controlled trials and cohort studies that compared MP and PS prostheses in primary TKA, focusing on outcomes such as range of motion (ROM), patient-reported outcome measures (PROMs), complications, revision rates, and radiographic results. Data extraction and quality assessment were conducted independently by two researchers using standardized methods. The meta-analysis utilized RevMan software (Cochrane, Alberta Canada) for statistical analysis, employing fixed or random effect models based on heterogeneity assessments. The study found no significant differences between MP and PS prostheses in terms of ROM, PROMs, overall complication rates, or radiographic outcomes. However, the MP prosthesis showed a lower rate of patellar clunk or crepitus compared to the PS design.

The findings suggest that while the MP prosthesis may reduce certain patella-related complications like patellar clunk or crepitus, it does not demonstrate superiority over the PS prosthesis in other clinical outcomes or patient satisfaction measures. The study highlights the need for further high-quality randomized controlled trials to explore whether theoretical advantages of the MP design can translate into tangible benefits in clinical practice. Future studies should focus on long-term outcomes and patient satisfaction to better understand the potential advantages of different TKA prosthetic designs.

4.2.9 Comparative Study On Mid- and Long-Term Clinical Effects of Medial Pivot Prosthesis and Posterior-Stabilized Prosthesis After Total Knee Arthroplasty [154]

This is a machine-generated summary of:

Shi, Weipeng; Jiang, Yaping; Wang, Changyao; Zhang, Haining; Wang, Yingzhen; Li, Tao Comparative study on mid- and long-term clinical effects of medial pivot prosthesis and posterior-stabilized prosthesis after total knee arthroplasty [154].

Published in: Journal of Orthopaedic Surgery and Research (2020).

Link to original: https://doi.org/10.1186/s13018-020-01951-9

4.2.9.1 Research Highlights

Knee joint degenerative disease is increasingly prevalent among the aging population, with total knee arthroplasty (TKA) being the primary treatment for end-stage osteoarthrosis. The evolution of knee prostheses, from the first-generation designs by Gonston et al. to modern iterations, has significantly improved the restoration of natural knee kinematics and prosthesis survival rates. Posterior-stabilized (PS) prostheses are widely used due to their advantages in motion range and stability, but they pose challenges such as patella slip syndrome and complex revision surgeries. Medial pivot (MP) prostheses, designed with a "ball-and-socket" concept, aim to enhance joint stability and reduce wear. However, there is limited data on their efficacy in Chinese patients. The study by Shi et al. investigates the mid- and long-term clinical outcomes of TKA using MP and PS prostheses in Chinese patients.

The study conducted a retrospective analysis of patients who underwent TKA at the Affiliated Hospital of Qingdao University between June 2010–December 2013. Patients were selected based on specific criteria, excluding those with certain comorbidities or previous knee surgeries. The surgical procedure involved standard techniques for both MP and PS prostheses, with postoperative assessments including range of motion (ROM), Knee Society Score (KSS), Western Ontario and McMaster Universities Osteoarthritis Index (WOMAC), and Forgotten Joint Score (FJS). Data analysis was performed using SPSS software (SPSS Software, Chicago, USA) to compare outcomes between the two groups. Results showed no significant differences in postoperative ROM or KSS scores between MP and PS groups, although both groups exhibited significant improvements from preoperative levels. Complications were minimal, with some cases of infection and anterior knee pain reported.

The study concludes that both MP and PS prostheses offer similar clinical outcomes for Chinese patients undergoing TKA, with high patient satisfaction observed at mid- to long-term follow-up. Despite a high loss to follow-up rate, the findings suggest that both types of prostheses are safe and reliable options for this population. Future study could focus on addressing anatomical differences between populations to further optimize prosthesis design and improve patient outcomes. Additionally, exploring strategies to minimize complications such as anterior knee pain could enhance postoperative recovery experiences for patients undergoing TKA.

4.2.10 Long-Term Clinical Results of Alumina Ceramic Medial Pivot Total Knee Arthroplasty: A 10-Year Follow-Up Study [155]

This is a machine-generated summary of:

Ueyama, Hideki; Nakagawa, Shigeru; Kishimura, Yuichi; Minoda, Yukihide; Nakamura, Suguru; Koyanagi, Junichiro; Yamamura, Mitsuyoshi; Kadoya, Yoshinori Long-term clinical results of alumina ceramic medial pivot total knee arthroplasty: a 10-year follow-up study [155].

Published in: Arthroplasty (2023).

Link to original: https://doi.org/10.1186/s42836-023-00180-9

If you want to cite the papers, please refer to the original.

For technical reasons we could not place the page where the original quote is coming from.

4.2.10.1 Research Highlights

Total knee arthroplasty (TKA) is a widely successful surgical intervention for degenerative knee diseases, typically utilizing metal prostheses such as cobalt-chrome. However, alumina ceramic prostheses have also shown promising longevity and reduced intra-articular polyethylene wear particles, potentially decreasing the risk of aseptic loosening over time. Despite these benefits, ceramics are prone to fracture under mechanical stress, necessitating careful evaluation of their long-term survivorship. The study by Ueyama et al. investigates the clinical outcomes of a current model of alumina medial pivot TKA over a minimum follow-up period, hypothesizing favorable results in terms of clinical performance and survivorship.

The study employed a retrospective cohort design, including patients who underwent TKA using the Physio-knee system® (Kyocera, Kyoto, Japan) for osteoarthritis at a single institution. Exclusion criteria were applied to ensure a focus on osteoarthritis cases alone. All surgeries were performed by an experienced team using a standardized technique involving medial parapatellar approach and bone cement fixation. Clinical outcomes were assessed using the Knee Society Score (KSS) and radiological evaluations preoperatively and at final follow-up. Statistical analyses included Kaplan-Meier survival estimates and multivariate logistic regression to identify risk factors for revision or reoperation. The study reported significant improvements in KSS scores and knee alignment postoperatively, with survival rates of 97% for reoperation and 98% for revision at 5 years.

The study's findings suggest that the current alumina medial pivot TKA model offers good clinical results and survivorship comparable to metal counterparts, with no serious complications observed over the follow-up period. The design improvements tailored to East Asian anatomical features may enhance compatibility and ease of use. Future study could explore longer-term outcomes beyond 5 years and include control groups for more comprehensive comparisons. Additionally, alumina implants may be advantageous for patients with metal allergies due to their nickel-free composition. Despite inherent risks of ceramic fracture, no such incidents occurred in this study, indicating that alumina TKA can be safely implemented in clinical practice.

4.2.11 Comparison of Postoperative Knee Flexion and Patient Satisfaction Between Newly and Conventionally Designed Medial Pivot Total Knee Arthroplasty: A 5-Year Follow-Up Matched Cohort Study [156]

This is a machine-generated summary of:

Ueyama, Hideki; Kanemoto, Narihiro; Minoda, Yukihide; Yamamoto, Nobuo; Taniguchi, Yoshiki; Nakamura, Hiroaki Comparison of postoperative knee flexion and patient satisfaction between newly and conventionally designed medial pivot total knee arthroplasty: a 5-year follow-up matched cohort study [156].

Published in: Archives of Orthopaedic and Trauma Surgery (2021).

Link to original: https://doi.org/10.1007/s00402-021-04121-6

If you want to cite the papers, please refer to the original.

For technical reasons we could not place the page where the original quote is coming from.

4.2.11.1 Research Highlights

Total knee arthroplasty (TKA) is a common surgical procedure for treating degenerative knee disease, aiming to improve joint function and patient quality of life. Despite advancements in TKA designs, patient satisfaction remains suboptimal, partly due to unnatural knee kinematics post-surgery. The medial pivot TKA was developed to better mimic natural knee movement, yet earlier designs like the ADVANCE Medial Pivot (Microport Orthopaedics, Shanghai, China) have shown limitations in postoperative knee flexion. The study by Ueyama et al. investigates the performance of the next-generation EVOLUTION Medial Pivot Knee System (Microport Orthopaedics, Shanghai, China), designed to address these flexion limitations.

The study conducted a retrospective cohort analysis comparing the ADVANCE and EVOLUTION medial pivot prostheses. Patients who underwent TKA with either prosthesis at a single institution were included, with exclusions for specific conditions like rheumatoid arthritis or valgus deformity. The surgeries were performed by one expert surgeon using consistent techniques, and outcomes were assessed by an independent observer. Key metrics such as knee range of motion (ROM), Knee Society Score (KSS), and Forgotten Joint Score (FJS-12) were evaluated preoperatively and at multiple postoperative intervals. Statistical analyses, including multivariate regression, were used to identify factors influencing outcomes.

The findings suggest that the EVOLUTION prosthesis significantly improves postoperative knee flexion and patient satisfaction compared to its predecessor. The design changes—such as an enlarged single radius curvature and asymmetrical tibial tray—appear to enhance knee kinematics and reduce joint tension during flexion. While no critical failures were observed over the follow-up period, further studies are needed to explore long-term outcomes and clinical significance fully. Future study could focus on longitudinal changes in FJS-12 scores and determining minimal clinically important differences for enhanced patient-centered evaluations.

4.2.12 Comparative Analysis of Medial Pivot vs. Posterior Stabilized Total Knee Arthroplasty in Patients with Valgus Deformed Osteoarthritic Knees: A Retrospective Cohort Study [157]

This is a machine-generated summary of:

Iwakiri, Kentaro; Ohta, Yoichi; Minoda, Yukihide; Ueno, Shuhei; Kobayashi, Akio; Nakamura, Hiroaki Comparative analysis of medial pivot vs. posterior stabilized total knee arthroplasty in patients with valgus deformed osteoarthritic knees: a retrospective cohort study [157].

Published in: International Orthopaedics (2024).

Link to original: https://doi.org/10.1007/s00264-024-06337-8

4.2.12.1 Research Highlights

Total knee arthroplasty (TKA) is a highly effective surgical intervention for managing end-stage knee osteoarthritis, providing significant pain relief and improved function. While TKA is commonly performed for varus deformities, valgus deformities are less frequent but still present a clinical challenge. The Medial Pivot (MP)

TKA model, designed to mimic the natural pivot motion of the knee, has shown promising results in varus knees, but its efficacy in valgus knees remains uncertain. The study by Iwakiri et al. explores the comparative outcomes of MP-TKA versus posterior stabilized (PS) TKA in patients with valgus knee deformities.

The study was conducted as a retrospective, single-center cohort analysis involving patients with end-stage knee osteoarthritis and valgus deformity who underwent either MP-TKA or PS-TKA. The surgeries were performed by two experienced surgeons using a standardized medial parapatellar approach and modified gap technique. The primary outcome measured was the range of motion (ROM) of the knee joint, while secondary outcomes included clinical scores, operative time, blood loss, and postoperative complications. Both groups showed significant improvements in ROM and clinical scores postoperatively, with no significant differences between them. However, the PS group experienced longer operative times and greater blood loss compared to the MP group.

The study highlights that MP-TKA provides comparable mid-term clinical outcomes to PS-TKA for valgus deformed knees, suggesting it as a viable option for such cases. Despite concerns about its suitability due to potential joint instability in valgus knees, MP-TKA demonstrated favorable results similar to those seen in varus deformities. Future study could focus on larger patient populations and different implant models to enhance generalizability. Additionally, exploring the long-term outcomes beyond 2 years could provide further insights into the durability and effectiveness of MP-TKA in valgus knee deformities.

4.2.13 Is Medial Pivot Total Knee Arthroplasty Suitable for Patients with Valgus Knee Osteoarthritis? [158]

This is a machine-generated summary of:

Iwakiri, Kentaro; Ohta, Yoichi; Ohyama, Yohei; Minoda, Yukihide; Kobayashi, Akio; Nakamura, Hiroaki Is medial pivot total knee arthroplasty suitable for patients with valgus knee osteoarthritis? [158].

Published in: European Journal of Orthopaedic Surgery & Traumatology (2021).

Link to original: https://doi.org/10.1007/s00590-021-03007-y

If you want to cite the papers, please refer to the original.

For technical reasons we could not place the page where the original quote is coming from.

4.2.13.1 Research Highlights

Total knee arthroplasty (TKA) is a highly effective treatment for end-stage knee osteoarthritis, providing pain relief and improved function. While most TKA procedures address varus deformities, valgus deformities are less common and present unique challenges due to their distinct tibiofemoral articulation characteristics. The medial pivot-type TKA (MP-TKA) design, known for its stability and wear resistance, has shown promising long-term outcomes in varus knees. However, its efficacy in valgus knees remains unclear. The study by Iwakiri et al. investigates the mid-short-term postoperative outcomes of MP-TKA in patients with valgus knee osteoarthritis compared to those with varus deformities.

The study was a retrospective, single-center cohort analysis involving patients who underwent MP-TKA with a ceramic femoral component. Participants were selected based on specific criteria, including the ability to follow up for at least 2 years post-surgery. The surgical approach involved a standard medial parapatellar technique with modifications for gap balancing, including the pie crust technique for lateral soft tissue release in valgus knees. Outcomes were assessed through radiographic measurements, range of motion (ROM), and clinical scores such as the Western Ontario and McMaster Universities Arthritis Index (WOMAC). Statistical analyses compared results between the varus and valgus groups, focusing on ROM improvements and clinical outcomes.

The study found that MP-TKA provided equally favorable outcomes in both valgus and varus knee patients over the mid-term follow-up period. Despite initial concerns about medial conformity issues in valgus knees, the use of additional techniques like pie crusting allowed for effective alignment correction without extending surgical duration or increasing complications. Future study directions could explore larger sample sizes or different implant models to further validate these findings. The research suggests that MP-TKA is a viable option for patients with valgus knee deformity, expanding its applicability beyond traditional varus cases.

4.2.14 Mid-Term Clinical Outcomes and Survivorship of Medial-Pivot Total Knee Arthroplasty—A Mean Five Year Follow-Up Based on One Thousand, One Hundred and Twenty Eight Cases [159]

This is a machine-generated summary of:

Xiang, Shuai; Wang, Yingzhen; Lv, Chengyu; Wang, Changyao; Zhang, Haining Mid-term clinical outcomes and survivorship of medial-pivot total knee arthroplasty—a mean 5 year follow-up based on one thousand, one hundred and twenty eight cases [159].

Published in: International Orthopaedics (2021).
Link to original: https://doi.org/10.1007/s00264-021-05017-1

If you want to cite the papers, please refer to the original.
For technical reasons we could not place the page where the original quote is coming from.

4.2.14.1 Research Highlights

Total knee arthroplasty (TKA) is a widely used surgical procedure for treating advanced knee osteoarthritis, aiming to alleviate pain and restore normal knee function. Despite advancements in prosthetic designs and surgical techniques, many posterior-stabilized (PS) designs fail to replicate the natural kinematics of the knee, leading to complications such as patellar clunk syndrome and paradoxical anterior sliding of the femur. The study by Xiang et al. explores the clinical outcomes and survivorship of a medial pivotal (MP) design in TKA, specifically using the ADVANCE® prosthesis (Microport, Shanghai, China), in a large cohort of Chinese patients.

The study involved 1000 knees from patients diagnosed with end-stage osteoarthritis or rheumatoid arthritis who underwent TKA using the ADVANCE® MP design. The procedures were performed by six senior surgeons employing standard techniques, including medial parapatellar approach for knee exposure and specific resection methods for femur and tibia. Post-operative care included antibiotics and anticoagulants to prevent complications. Clinical outcomes were assessed pre- and post-operatively using various scoring systems such as the Knee Society Score (KSS) and Western Ontario and McMaster Universities Arthritis Index (WOMAC). The study reported significant improvements in range of motion (ROM), KSS, and WOMAC scores over an average follow-up period of 5 years. Complications were documented, including systemic issues like deep infections and patellofemoral joint problems.

The study demonstrated a mid-term cumulative survival rate of 95.6% when considering revisions for any reason as an endpoint. Despite these promising results, challenges remain, particularly regarding patellofemoral complications that may arise from altered joint kinematics. Future study could focus on addressing these issues through techniques like patellar resurfacing or further refining implant designs. Additionally, while this study provides valuable insights into MP systems' performance in a large cohort, longer-term follow-ups and larger sample sizes are necessary to fully understand the advantages and limitations of MP implants in diverse patient populations.

4.2.15 Clinical Radiographic Outcomes and Survivorship of Medial Pivot Design Total Knee Arthroplasty: A Systematic Review of the Literature [160]

This is a machine-generated summary of:

Alessio-Mazzola, Mattia; Clemente, Antonio; Russo, Antonio; Mertens, Peter; Burastero, Giorgio; Formica, Matteo; Felli, Lamberto Clinical radiographic outcomes and survivorship of medial pivot design total knee arthroplasty: a systematic review of the literature [160].

Published in: Archives of Orthopaedic and Trauma Surgery (2021).

Link to original: https://doi.org/10.1007/s00402-021-04210-6

If you want to cite the papers, please refer to the original.

For technical reasons we could not place the page where the original quote is coming from.

4.2.15.1 Research Highlights

Total knee arthroplasty (TKA) is a widely performed surgical procedure aimed at alleviating pain and improving function in patients with end-stage osteoarthritis. Despite advancements in prosthetic designs, a significant percentage of patients still report unsatisfactory outcomes post-surgery. The medial pivot design, which mimics the natural kinematics of the knee, has shown promising mid-term results, but its long-term effectiveness remains underexplored. The study by Alessio-Mazzola et al. systematically reviews the survivorship and clinical outcomes of medial pivot TKA to address this gap.

The study conducted a comprehensive systematic review following established guidelines, including the Cochrane Handbook and PRISMA. Researchers searched multiple databases for studies published between January 2000 and October 2023, focusing on clinical outcomes of medial pivot TKA. Eligible studies included those reporting objective and patient-reported outcomes without quality restrictions. Two independent reviewers screened titles and abstracts, resolving disagreements through discussion with a third reviewer. The primary endpoints were survivorship and revision rates, while secondary endpoints included radiological alignment and complications. The quality of evidence was assessed using the GRADE system, revealing that most included studies were of very low quality with high risk of bias.

The review found that medial pivot TKA demonstrated excellent overall survivorship with a revision rate of 0.5% after 5 years. Objective and patient-reported outcomes were generally good to excellent, although some studies reported higher complication rates compared to other designs. The study highlighted the need for further high-quality research due to limitations such as low evidence levels and potential conflicts of interest in several studies. Future study could focus on long-term outcomes and direct comparisons with other TKA designs to better understand the role of medial pivot implants in improving patient satisfaction and functional results.

4.2.16 Comparison Between Gaits After a Medial Pivot and Posterior Stabilized Primary Total Knee Arthroplasty: A Systematic Review of the Literature [161]

This is a machine-generated summary of:

Risitano, Salvatore; Cacciola, Giorgio; Capella, Marcello; Bosco, Francesco; Giustra, Fortunato; Fusini, Federico; Indelli, Pier Francesco; Massé, Alessandro; Sabatini, Luigi Comparison between gaits after a medial pivot and posterior stabilized primary total knee arthroplasty: a systematic review of the literature [161].

Published in: Arthroplasty (2023).

Link to original: https://doi.org/10.1186/s42836-023-00165-8

If you want to cite the papers, please refer to the original.

For technical reasons we could not place the page where the original quote is coming from.

4.2.16.1 Research Highlights

Total knee arthroplasty (TKA) is a widely used and cost-effective surgical intervention for end-stage knee osteoarthritis, with over 600,000 procedures performed annually in the United States. Despite the procedure's success in terms of implant longevity, with a revision rate of 6% after 10 years, approximately 20% of patients remain dissatisfied post-surgery. This dissatisfaction is often attributed to the failure of current prosthetic designs to replicate natural knee kinematics. The study by Risitano et al. systematically reviews comparative gait analysis studies to explore the kinematic and kinetic differences between medial pivot (MP) and posterior stabilized (PS) TKA designs.

The study conducted a systematic review following PRISMA guidelines (Preferred Reporting Items for Systematic Reviews and Meta-Analyses), analysing nine studies that compared gait analysis outcomes between MP and PS TKA designs. The researchers searched databases such as PubMed, Embase, Scopus, and Cochrane using specific MeSH (Medical Subject headings) terms related to TKA designs and gait analysis. The inclusion criteria focused on studies reporting knee kinematic data in frontal or sagittal planes or relative tibiofemoral movement. Data extraction involved demographic information, surgical details, gait analysis protocols, and clinical scores. Statistical analyses were performed using R software to evaluate differences in kinematic and kinetic parameters between the two prosthetic designs.

The review identified significant kinematic and kinetic differences between MP and PS TKA designs. MP TKA showed greater tibial external rotation but was associated with a "stiff-knee pattern" during gait. In contrast, PS TKA demonstrated increased anterior femoral roll and translation during knee flexion but failed to replicate the screw-home mechanism observed in healthy knees. Both designs exhibited paradoxical anterior femoral motion; however, this was less pronounced in MP TKA. Future study could focus on refining prosthetic designs to better mimic natural knee mechanics and improve patient satisfaction post-TKA. The study highlights the need for more standardized protocols in gait analysis to enhance data validity across different prosthetic models.

4.2.17 Does the Medial Pivot Knee Improve the Clinical and Radiographic Outcome of Total Knee Arthroplasty? A Single Centre Study on Two Hundred and Ninety Seven Patients [162]

This is a machine-generated summary of:

Cacciola, Giorgio; De Martino, Ivan; De Meo, Federico Does the medial pivot knee improve the clinical and radiographic outcome of total knee arthroplasty? A single centre study on two hundred and ninety seven patients [162].

Published in: International Orthopaedics (2019).
Link to original: https://doi.org/10.1007/s00264-019-04462-3

If you want to cite the papers, please refer to the original.
For technical reasons we could not place the page where the original quote is coming from.

4.2.17.1 Research Highlights

Total knee arthroplasty (TKA) is a common orthopedic procedure performed to alleviate pain and restore function in patients with severe knee osteoarthritis. Despite advancements in surgical techniques and prosthetic designs, patient satisfaction post-surgery varies, with dissatisfaction often linked to factors such as prosthesis design and post-operative pain. A key challenge is replicating natural knee kinematics, which many prosthetic designs fail to achieve. The study by Cacciola et al. investigates the medium-term clinical and radiological outcomes of the K-Mod dynamic congruence (DC) medial pivot (MP) TKA system, designed to mimic natural knee motion and improve patient satisfaction.

The study retrospectively analysed data from patients who underwent primary TKA using the K-Mod DC system at a single institution between January 2014 and August 2015. All surgeries were performed by the same experienced surgeon using a standardized surgical approach. The K-Mod DC system features a unique design intended to restore normal joint kinematics by allowing the medial femoral condyle to act as a pivot while permitting anteroposterior movement of the lateral femoral condyle. Patients were evaluated clinically and radiographically pre-operatively and at regular intervals up to a minimum follow-up of 5 years. Outcomes were assessed using various scoring systems, including the Knee Society score and the Forgotten Joint Score (FJS), with statistical analyses conducted to compare pre- and post-operative results.

The study found that the K-Mod DC TKA system achieved excellent clinical, radiographic, and patient-reported outcomes over 5 years, with a cumulative implant survivorship of 97.5%. No revisions were required due to implant-related failures such as aseptic loosening or instability. The results suggest that this MP design may help bridge the gap between clinical outcomes and patient-reported measures by restoring natural knee kinematics. Future study could focus on longer-term outcomes and comparisons with other prosthetic designs to further validate these findings.

4.2.18 A Mid-Term Comparison of the Functional Outcomes of Medial Pivot and Rotating Platform Mobile-Bearing Total Knee Arthroplasty in the Indian Population [163]

This is a machine-generated summary of:

Shakya, Akash; Singh, Vijay; Agrawal, Romit A.; Sharma, Ayush; Mangale, Nilesh; Wadgave, Venkatramana; Jaiswal, Ajay A Mid-term Comparison of the Functional Outcomes of Medial Pivot and Rotating Platform Mobile-Bearing Total Knee Arthroplasty in the Indian Population [163].

Published in: Indian Journal of Orthopaedics (2021).

Link to original: https://doi.org/10.1007/s43465-021-00472-9

If you want to cite the papers, please refer to the original.

For technical reasons we could not place the page where the original quote is coming from.

4.2.18.1 Research Highlights

Total knee arthroplasty (TKA) is a widely used surgical intervention for alleviating pain and restoring function in patients with knee osteoarthritis. The design of TKA implants is crucial for improving patient outcomes, knee function, and implant longevity. Among the various designs, the medial pivot (MP) and rotating platform (RP) designs have been developed to mimic natural knee kinematics and reduce wear. However, there is limited data comparing these designs in the Indian population, particularly in mid- or long-term studies. The study by Shakya et al. addresses this gap by comparing the clinical and functional outcomes of MP-TKA and RP-TKA in an Indian cohort at mid-term follow-up.

The study was conducted as a retrospective, comparative analysis at a tertiary care hospital in Western India. It included patients who underwent primary TKA with either MP or RP designs between January 2015 and May 2018. The decision to use either design was based on implant availability, and all surgeries were performed by a single surgeon using standardized techniques. Patients were assessed preoperatively and postoperatively using various clinical scores such as WOMAC, Knee Society Score, and Forgotten Joint Score (FJS). Radiological assessments were also performed to evaluate component positioning and alignment. Statistical analyses were conducted to compare outcomes between the two groups.

The study found that both MP-TKA and RP-TKA significantly improved range of motion postoperatively, with no significant difference between the two groups. However, patients with MP-TKA showed better functional outcomes as indicated by higher Functional Knee Society Scores and FJS compared to those with RP-TKA. The MP design's inherent stability may contribute to these superior subjective outcomes. Despite these differences, other clinical and radiological outcomes were comparable between the groups. The authors suggest that future studies could focus on long-term outcomes with larger sample sizes to further validate these findings.

Bibliography

1. Blaha JD (2002) A medial pivot geometry. Orthopaedics 25:963
2. Li N, Tan Y, Deng Y, Chen L (2014) Posterior cruciate-retaining versus posterior stabilized total knee arthroplasty: a meta-analysis of randomized controlled trials. Knee Surg Sports Traumatol Arthrosc 22:556–564
3. Baldini A, Anderson JA, Cerulli-Mariani P, Kalyvas J, Pavlov H, Sculco TP: Patellofemoral evaluation after total knee arthroplasty - Validation of a new weight-bearing axial radiographic view. J Bone Joint Surg Am. 2007, 89A (8): 1810-1817.
4. Kanekasu K, Kondo M, Kadoya Y (2005) Axial radiography of the distal femur to assess rotational alignment in total knee arthroplasty. Clin Orthop Relat Res 434:193–197
5. Chia SL, Merican AM, Devadasan B, Strachan RK, Amis AA (2009) Radiographic features predictive of patellar maltracking during total knee arthroplasty. Knee Surg Sports Traumatol Arthrosc 17:1217–1224
6. Heegaard J, Leyvraz PF, Van Kampen A, Rakotomanana L, Rubin PJ, Blankevoort L (1994) Influence of soft structures on patellar three-dimensional tracking. Clin Orthop Relat Res 299:235–243
7. Kessler O, Patil S, Colwell CW Jr, D'Lima DD (2008) The effect of femoral component malrotation on patellar biomechanics. J Biomech 41:3332–3339
8. Konig C, Sharenkov A, Matziolis G, Taylor WR, Perka C, Duda GN et al (2010) Joint line elevation in revision TKA leads to increased patellofemoral contact forces. J Orthop Res 28:1–5
9. Miller MC, Berger RA, Petrella AJ, Karmas A, Rubash HE (2001) Optimizing femoral component rotation in total knee arthroplasty. Clin Orthop Relat Res 392:38–45
10. Moreland JR, Bassett LW, Hanker GJ. Radiographic analysis of the axial alignment of the lower extremity. J Bone Joint Surg Am. 1987;69(5):745–9.
11. Hsu RW, Himeno S, Coventry MB, Chao EY. Normal axial alignment of the lower extremity and load-bearing distribution at the knee. Clin Orthop Relat Res. 1990;225:215–27.
12. Baker PN, van der Meulen JH, Lewsey J, Gregg PJ. National Joint Registry for England and Wales. The role of pain and function in determining patient satisfaction after total knee replacement. Data from the National Joint Registry for England and Wales. J Bone Joint Surg Br. 2007;89(7):893–900.
13. Hirschmann MT, Behrend H. Functional knee phenotypes: a call for a more personalized and individualized approach to total knee arthroplasty? Knee Surg Sports Traumatol Arthrosc. 2018;26(10):2873–4.
14. Hirschmann MT, Amsler PK, Iranpour F, Friederich NF, Cobb JP. The position and orientation of total knee replacement components: a comparison of

conventional radiographs, transverse 2D-CT slices and 3D-CT reconstruction. J Bone Joint Surg Br. 2011;93(5):629–33.
15. Jabalameli M, Moghimi J, Yeganeh A, Nojomi M. Parameters of lower extremities alignment view in Iranian adult populations. Acta Med Iran. 2015;53(5):293–6.
16. Kawakami H, Sugano N, Yonenobu K, Yoshikawa H, Ochi T, Hattori A, Suzuki N. Effects of rotation on measurement of lower limb alignment for knee osteotomy. J Orthop Res. 2004;22(6):1248–53.
17. Lampart M, Behrend H, Moser L, Hirschmann MT. Due to great variability fixed HKS angle for alignment of the distal cut leads to a significant error in coronal TKA orientation. Knee Surg Sports Traumatol Arthrosc. 2019;27(5):1434–41.
18. Mullaji AB, Marawar SV, Mittal V. A comparison of coronal plane axial femoral relationships in Asian patients with varus osteoarthritic knees and healthy knees. J Arthroplasty. 2009;24(6):861–7.
19. Cooke D, Scudamore A, Li J, Wyss U, Bryant T, Costigan P. Axial lower-limb alignment: comparison of knee geometry in normal volunteers and osteoarthritic patients. Osteoarthritis Cartilage. 1997;5(1):39–47.
20. Hovinga KR, Lerner AL. Anatomical variations between Japanese and Caucasian populations in the healthy young adult knee joint. J Orthop Res. 2009;27(9):1191–6.
21. Nayak M, Kumar V, Yadav R, Maredupaka S, Srivastava DN, Malhotra R, Pandit H. Coronal alignment of the lower extremity: a gender-based ratiographic analysis in Indian patients. Indian J Orthop. 2020;54(4):504–12.
22. Tang WM, Zhu YH, Chiu KY. Axial alignment of the lower extremity in Chinese adults. J Bone Joint Surg Am. 2000;82(11):1603–8.
23. Toguchi K, Nakajima A, Akatsu Y, Sonobe M, Yamada M, Takahashi H, Saito J, Aoki Y, Suguro T, Nakagawa K. Predicting clinical outcomes after total knee arthroplasty from preoperative radiographic factors of the knee osteoarthritis. BMC Musculoskelet Disord. 2020;21(1):9.
24. Zhang, Q. *et al.* Insert conformity variation affects kinematics and wear performance of total knee replacements. *Clin. Biomech. 65*, 19–25 (2019).
25. Koh, Y., Jung, K., Hong, H., Kim, K. and Kang, K.-T. Optimal design of patient-specific total knee arthroplasty for improvement in wear performance. *J. Clin. Med. 8*(11), 2023 (2019).
26. Ardestani, M. M., Moazen, M. and Jin, Z. Contribution of geometric design parameters to knee implant performance: Conflicting impact of conformity on kinematics and contact mechanics. *Knee 22*(3), 217–224 (2015).
27. Shu, L., Yamamoto, K., Kai, S., Inagaki, J. and Sugita, N. Symmetrical cruciate-retaining versus medial pivot prostheses: The effect of intercondylar sagittal conformity on knee kinematics and contact mechanics. *Comput. Biol. Med. 108*, 101–110 (2019).
28. Vaishya R, Scarlat MM, Bhadani J et al (2024) Ethics in orthopaedic surgery practice: balancing patient care and technological advances. Int Orthopaedics (SICOT) 48:2769–2774. https://doi.org/10.1007/s00264-024-06335-w

29. Lee QJ, Wai Yee EC, Wong YC (2020) No difference in patient preference for medial pivot versus posterior-stabilized design in staged bilateral total knee arthroplasty: a prospective study. Knee Surg Sports Traumatol Arthrosc 28:3805–3809. https://doi.org/10.1007/s00167-020-05867-z
30. Nisar S, Ahmad K, Palan J et al (2002) Medial stabilised total knee arthroplasty achieves comparable clinical outcomes when compared to other TKA designs: a systematic review and meta-analysis of the current literature. Knee Surg Sports Traumatol Arthrosc 30:638–665. https://doi.org/10.1007/s00167-020-06358-x
31. Dennis DA, Komistek RD, Mahfouz MR, Haas BD, Stiehl JB (2003) Multicenter determination of in vivo kinematics after total knee arthroplasty. Clin Orthop Relat Res 416:37
32. Kaneyama R, Suzuki M, Moriya H, Banks SA, Hodge WA. Fluoroscopic analysis of knee kinematics after total knee arthroplasty in osteoarthritis and rheumatoid arthritis. Chiba Med J. 2002;78:193–201.
33. Watanabe E, Suzuki M, Nagata K, Kaneeda T, Harada Y, Utsumi M, Mori A, Moriya H. Oxidation-induced dynamic changes in morphology reflected on freeze-fractured surface of gamma-irradiated ultra-high molecular weight polyethylene components. J Biomed Mater Res. 2002;62:540–9.
34. Insall JN, Dorr LD, Scott RD, Scott WN. Rationale of the knee society clinical rating system. Clin Orthop Relat Res. 1989;248:13–4.
35. Ewald FC. The knee society total knee arthroplasty roentgenographic evaluation and scoring system. Clin Orthop Relat Res. 1989;248:9–12.
36. Tamai H, Suzuki M, Tsuneizumi Y, Tsukeoka T, Banks SA, Moriya H, Takahashi K. Knee kinematics do not influence the long-term results in posterior cruciate-retaining total knee arthroplasties. Chiba Med J. 2008;84:269–76.
37. Miyazaki Y, Nakamura T, Kogame K, Saito M, Yamamoto K, Suguro T (2011) Analysis of the kinematics of total knee prostheses with a medial pivot design. J Arthroplasty 26:1038–1044
38. Elbardesy H, Salamah HM, McLeod A, Thada PK, Mohammed ER, Hanifa FA et al (2021) Medial pivot versus (cam post) posterior stabilised total knee arthroplasty, systematic review and meta-analysis of 3837 knees. Acta Orthop Belg 87(4):665–680
39. Shi W, Jiang Y, Wang Y, Zhao X, Yu T, Li T (2022) Medial pivot prosthesis has a better functional score and lower complication rate than posterior-stabilized prosthesis: a systematic review and meta-analysis. J Orthop Surg Res 17(1):395. https://doi.org/10.1186/s13018-022-03285-0
40. Kakoulidis P, Panagiotidou S, Profitiliotis G, Papavasiliou K, Tsiridis E, Topalis C (2022) Medial pivot design does not yield superior results compared to posterior-stabilised total knee arthroplasty: a systematic review and meta-analysis of randomised control trials. Knee Surg Sports Traumatol Arthrosc. https://doi.org/10.1007/s00167-022-07238-2. Epub
41. Hoskins W, Smith G, Spelman T, Vince KG (2022) Medial pivot designs Versus Conventional bearing types in primary total knee arthroplasty: a systematic review and Meta-analysis of Randomized controlled trials. J Am Acad

Orthop Surg Glob Res Rev 6(12):e22. https://doi.org/10.5435/JAAOSGlobal-D-22-00170
42. Xu Z, Tian S, Zhou X, Wei Y, Wu C, Jia X, Wang H (2022) Medial pivot versus posterior-stabilized Prosthesis Design in primary total knee arthroplasty: a systematic review and Meta-analysis. Indian J Orthop 56(9):1506–1524. https://doi.org/10.1007/s43465-022-00678-5
43. Sabatini L, Risitano S, Parisi G, Tosto F, Indelli PF, Atzori F, Masse A (2018) Medial pivot in total knee arthroplasty: literature review and our first experience. Clin Med Insights Arthritis Musculoskelet Disord 11:1–4. https://doi.org/10.1177/1179544117751431
44. Tsubosaka M, Ishida K, Kodato K, Shibanuma N, Hayashi S, Kurosaka M, Kuroda R, Matsumoto T (2021) Mid-flexion stability in the anteroposterior plane is achieved with a medial congruent insert in cruciate-retaining total knee arthroplasty for varus osteoarthritis. Knee Surg Sports Traumatol Arthrosc 29(2):467–473. https://doi.org/10.1007/s00167-020-05927-4
45. Moonot P, Shang M, Railton GT, Field RE, Banks SA (2010) In vivo weight-bearing kinematics with medial rotation knee arthroplasty. Knee 17:33–37. https://doi.org/10.1016/j.knee.2009.06.009
46. Wautier D, Thienpont E (2017) Changes in anteroposterior stability and proprioception after different types of knee arthroplasty. Knee Surg Sports Traumatol Arthrosc 25(6):1792–1800. https://doi.org/10.1007/s00167-016-4038-9
47. Edelstein AI, Bhatt S, Wright-Chisem J, Sullivan R, Beal M, Manning DW (2020) The Effect of Implant Design on Sagittal Plane Stability: a randomized trial of medial- versus posterior-stabilized total knee arthroplasty. J Knee Surg 33(5):452–458. https://doi.org/10.1055/s-0039-1678524
48. Jones CW, Jacobs H, Shumborski S, Talbot S, Redgment A, Brighton R, Walter WL. Sagittal stability and implant design affect patient reported outcomes after total knee arthroplasty. J Arthroplast. 2020;35(3):747.
49. Kato M, Warashina H, Mitamura S, Kataoka A (2022) Medial pivot-based total knee arthroplasty achieves better clinical outcomes than posterior-stabilized total knee arthroplasty. Knee Surg Sports Traumatol Arthrosc 1–13. https://doi.org/10.1007/s00167-022-07149-2
50. Scott DF, Hellie AA, Mid-Flexion (2023) Anteroposterior Stability of Total Knee Replacement Implanted with Kinematic Alignment: a Randomized, quantitative Radiographic Laxity Study with posterior-stabilized and medial-stabilized implants. J Bone Joint Surg Am 105(1):9–19. https://doi.org/10.2106/JBJS.22.00549
51. Konno, T., Onodera, T., Nishio, Y., et al. (2014). Correlation between knee kinematics and patellofemoral contact pressure in total knee arthroplasty. *Journal of Arthroplasty, 29*(12), 2305–2308.
52. Dorr, L. D., Ochsner, J. L., Gronley, J., et al. (1988). Functional comparison of posterior cruciate-retained versus cruciate-sacrificed total knee arthroplasty. *Clinical Orthopaedics and Related Research, 236*, 36–43.

53. Dennis DA, Komistek RD, Mahfouz MR (2003) In vivo fluoroscopic analysis of fixed-bearing total knee replacements. Clin Orthop Relat Res 410:114–130
54. Walker PS, Yildirim G, Sussman-Fort J, Roth J, White B, Klein GR (2007) Factors affecting the impingement angle of fixed- and mobile-bearing total knee replacements: a laboratory study. J Arthroplasty 22:745–752
55. Gill, U. N., Shiraz, H. M., Rehman, M. K. U., et al. (2019). Comparison of functional outcome of medial pivot total knee arthroplasty with posterior stabilizing (PS) total knee arthroplasty - A randomized trial. *Pakistan Journal of Medical and Health Sciences, 13*(2), 385–388.
56. Blaha, J. D., Mancinelli, C. A., Simons, W. H., et al. (2003). Kinematics of the human knee using an open chain cadaver model. *Clinical Orthopaedics and Related Research, 410*, 25–34.
57. Bae, D. K., Cho, S. D., Im, S. K., et al. (2016). Comparison of midterm clinical and radiographic results between total knee arthroplasties using medial pivot and posterior-stabilized prosthesis-a matched pair analysis. *Journal of Arthroplasty, 31*(2), 419–424.
58. Choi NY, In Y, Bae JH, Do JH, Chung SJ, Koh IJ (2017) Are Midterm patient-reported outcome measures between rotating-platform Mobile-Bearing prosthesis and medial-pivot prosthesis different? A Minimum of 5-Year Follow-Up study. J Arthroplasty 32(3):824–829. https://doi.org/10.1016/j.arth.2016.08.028
59. Papagiannis GI, Roumpelakis IM, Triantafyllou AI, Makris IN, Babis GC (2016) No differences identified in transverse plane biomechanics between medial pivot and rotating platform total knee implant designs. J Arthroplasty 31(8):1814–1820
60. Zhang, Z. A., Feng, H., Yan, W. N., et al. (2020). Comparison of postoperative effects between medial pivot prosthesis and posterior stabilized prosthesis. *Orthopaedic Surgery, 12*(6), 1843–1853.
61. Chang, J. S., Kayani, B., Moriarty, P. D., et al. (2021). A prospective randomized controlled trial comparing medial-pivot versus posterior-stabilized total knee arthroplasty. *Journal of Arthroplasty, 36*(5), 1584-1589.e1.
62. Hossain F, Patel S, Rhee SJ, Haddad FS (2011) Knee arthroplasty with a medially conforming ball-and-socket tibiofemoral articulation provides better function. Clin Orthop Relat Res 469:55–63
63. Kim YH, Yoon SH, Kim JS (2009) Early outcome of TKA with a medial pivot fixed bearing prosthesis is worse than with a PFC mobile-bearing prosthesis. Clin Orthop Relat Res 467:493–503
64. Wang, Z., Zhang, Y. Q., Ding, C. R., et al. (2021). Early patellofemoral function of medial pivot prostheses compared with posterior-stabilized prostheses for unilateral total knee arthroplasty. *Orthopaedic Surgery, 13*(2), 417–425.
65. Anderson, M. J., Becker, D. L., and Kieckbusch, T. (2002). Patellofemoral complications after posterior-stabilized total knee arthroplasty: A comparison of 2 different implant designs. *Journal of Arthroplasty, 17*(4), 422–426.
66. Lin Y, Chen X, Li L, Li Z, Zhang Y, Fan P (2020) Comparison of patient satisfaction between medial pivot prostheses and posterior-stabilized prostheses

in total knee arthroplasty. Orthop Surg 12(3):836–842. https://doi.org/10.1111/os.12687
67. Shi W, Jiang Y, Wang C, Zhang H, Wang Y, Li T (2020) Comparative study on mid- and long-term clinical effects of medial pivot prosthesis and posterior-stabilized prosthesis after total knee arthroplasty. J Orthop Surg Res 15(1):421. https://doi.org/10.1186/s13018-020-01951-9
68. Samy DA, Wolfstadt JI, Vaidee I, Backstein DJ (2018) A retrospective comparison of a medial pivot and posterior-stabilized total knee arthroplasty with respect to patient-reported and radiographic outcomes. J Arthroplasty 33(5):1379–1383. https://doi.org/10.1016/j.arth.2017.11.049
69. Batra S, Malhotra R, Kumar V, Srivastava DN, Backstein D, Pandit H (2021) Superior patient satisfaction in medial pivot as compared to posterior stabilized total knee arthroplasty: a prospective randomized study. Knee Surg Sports Traumatol Arthrosc 29(11):3633–3640
70. Indelli PF, Risitano S, Halll KE, Leonardi E, Migliore E (2019) Effect of polyethylene conformity on total knee arthroplasty early clinical outcomes. Knee Surg Sports Traumatol Arthrosc 27(4):1028–1034
71. Kulshrestha V, Sood M, Kanade S, Kumar S, Datta B, Mittal G (2020) Early outcomes of medial pivot total knee arthroplasty compared to posterior-stabilized design: a randomized controlled trial. Clin Orthop Surg 12(2):178–186. https://doi.org/10.4055/cios19141
72. Jacobs WC, Clement DJ, Wymenga AB: Retention versus removal of the posterior cruciate ligament in total knee replacement. Act Orth. 2005, 76 (6): 757-768. 10.1080/17453670510045345.
73. Fitch, D. A., Sedacki, K., and Yang, Y. (2014). Mid- to long-term outcomes of a medial-pivot system for primary total knee replacement: A systematic review and meta-analysis. *Bone Joint Research, 3*(10), 297–304.
74. Causero A, Di Benedetto P, Beltrame A, Gisonni R, Cainero V, Pagano M. Design evolution in total knee replacement: which is the future? Acta Biomed. 2014;85(Suppl 2):5–19 Published 2014 Sep 24.
75. Warth LC, Ishmael MK, Deckard ER, Ziemba-Davis M, Meneghini RM (2017) Do medial pivot kinematics correlate with patient-reported outcomes after total knee arthroplasty? J Arthroplasty 32:2411–2416. https://doi.org/10.1016/j.arth.2017.03.019
76. Carvalho Júnior LH, Teixeira BP, Bernardes CO, Soares LF, Gonçalves MB, Temponi EF. Range of motion predictability after total knee arthroplasty with medial pivot prosthesis. Rev Bras Ortop. 2017;52(2):197–202Published 2017 Mar 9. https://doi.org/10.1016/j.rboe.2017.03.001.
77. Macheras George A, Galanakos Spyridon P, Panagiotis L, Anastasopoulos Panagiotis P, Papadakis SA. A long term clinical outcome of the medial pivot knee arthroplasty system. Knee. 2017;24(2):447–53. https://doi.org/10.1016/j.knee.2017.01.008.
78. Evans JPTP, Walker RW, Evans JPTP, Blom AW, Sayers A, Whitehouse MR. How long does a knee replacement last? A systematic review and meta-

analysis of case series and national registry reports with more than 15 years of follow-up. Lancet. 2019;393:655–63.
79. Nakamura S, Minoda Y, Nakagawa S, Kadoya Y, Takemura S, Kobayashi A, et al. Clinical results of alumina medial pivot total knee arthroplasty at a minimum follow-up of 10 years. Knee. 2017;24:434–8.
80. Insall JN, Dorr LD, Scott RD, Scott WN (1989) Rationale of the Knee Society clinical rating system. Clin Orthop Relat Res 248:13–14
81. Karachalios T, Komnos G, Amprazis V, Antoniou I, Athanaselis S. A 9-year outcome study comparing cancellous titanium-coated cementless to cemented tibial components of a single knee arthroplasty design. J Arthroplasty. 2018;33:3672–7.
82. Minoda Y, Kobayashi A, Iwaki H, Iwakiri K, Inori F, Sugama R, et al. In vivo analysis of polyethylene wear particles after total knee arthroplasty: the influence of improved materials and designs. J Bone Joint Surg Am. 2009;91:67–73.
83. Minoda Y, Kobayashi A, Iwaki H, Miyaguchi M, Kadoya Y, Ohashi H, et al. Polyethylene wear particle generation in vivo in an alumina medial pivot total knee prosthesis. Biomaterials. 2005;26:6034–40.
84. Dalury DF, Barrett WP, Mason JB et al (2008) Midterm survival of a contemporary modular total knee replacement: a multicentre study of 1970 knees. J Bone Jt Surg Br 90:1594–1596. https://doi.org/10.1302/0301-620X.90B12.21064
85. Karachalios T, Varitimidis S, Bargiotas K, Hantes M, Roidis N, Malizos KN. An 11- to 15-year clinical outcome study of the Advance Medial Pivot total knee arthroplasty. Bone Joint J. 2016;98-B:1050–5.
86. Ha CW, Park YB, Song YS, Kim JH, Park YG (2016) Increased range of motion is important for functional outcome and satisfaction after total knee arthroplasty in Asian Patients. J Arthroplasty 31(6):1199–1203
87. Ewald FC (1989) The knee society total knee arthroplasty roentgenographic evaluation and scoring system. Clin Orthop Relat Res 248:9–12
88. Bauer GC, Insall J, Koshino T (1969) Tibial osteotomy in gonarthrosis (osteoarthritis of the knee). J Bone Jt Surg Am 51:1545–1563. https://doi.org/10.5035/nishiseisai.21.87
89. Ritter MA, Harty LD, Davis KE et al (2003) Predicting range of motion after total knee arthroplasty. Clustering, log-linear regression, and regression tree analysis. J Bone Jt Surg Am 85:1278–1285. https://doi.org/10.2106/00004623-200307000-00014
90. Iwakiri K, Ohta Y, Ohyama Y, Minoda Y, Kobayashi A, Nakamura H (2022) Is medial pivot total knee arthroplasty suitable for patients with valgus knee osteoarthritis? Eur J Orthop Surg Traumatol 32(3):p551–557
91. Okuda M, Omokawa S, Tanaka Y, Okahashi K, Akahane M (2012) Validity and reliability of the Japanese orthopaedic association score for osteoarthritic knees. J Orthop Sci 17(6):p750–756
92. Nadler SB, Hidalgo JH, Bloch T (1962) Prediction of blood volume in normal human adults. Surgery 51(2):p224-232

93. Indelli PF, Spinello P, Zepeda K, Campi S, Rossi SMP, Engl M, Papalia R, Benazzo F (2023) Medially congruent total knee arthroplasty in valgus knee deformities yields satisfactory outcomes: a multicenter, international study. Knee Surg Sports Traumatol Arthrosc 31(2):p407-412
94. Ando G, Tsukimoto T (2002) Osteoarthritis of knee joint–standard concept and diagnosis. Clin Calcium 12(1):47–52
95. Krackow KA, Jones MM, Teeny SM, Hungerford DS (1991) Primary total knee arthroplasty in patients with fixed valgus deformity. Clin Orthop Relat Res 273:p9–18
96. Pritchett JW (2011) Patients prefer a bicruciate-retaining or the medial pivot total knee prosthesis. J Arthroplasty 26:224–228. https://doi.org/10.1016/j.arth.2010.02.012
97. Moro-oka TA, Shiraishi H, Iwamoto Y, Banks SA (2010) Modified gap-balancing technique in total knee arthroplasty: evaluation of the post-operative coronal laxity. Knee Surg Sports Traumatol Arthrosc 18(3):p375–380
98. Shu L, Yamamoto K, Kai S, Inagaki J, Sugita N (2019) Symmetrical cruciate-retaining versus medial pivot prostheses: the effect of intercondylar sagittal conformity on knee kinematics and contact mechanics. Comput Biol Med 108:101–110. https://doi.org/10.1016/j.compbiomed.2019.03.005
99. Minoda Y, Kobayashi A, Iwaki H, et al. Polyethylene wear particles in synovial fluid after total knee arthroplasty. Clin Orthop Relat Res. 2003;410:165–72. https://doi.org/10.1097/01.blo.0000063122.39522.c2.
100. Castellarin G, Pianigiani S, Innocenti B (2019) Asymmetric polyethylene inserts promote favorable kinematics and better clinical outcome compared to symmetric inserts in a mobile bearing total knee arthroplasty. Knee Surg Sports Traumatol Arthrosc 27(4):1096–1105. https://doi.org/10.1007/s00167-018-5207-9
101. Cheng-Yu F, Tzung-Shian HJ, Ming-Shium H, Ying-Chieh S, Lee C-H. Primitive results after medial-pivot knee arthroplasties: a minimum 5-year follow-up study. J Arthroplast. 2010;25(3):492–6. https://doi.org/10.1016/j.arth.2009.05.008.
102. Chinzei N, Ishida K, Tsumura N, Matsumoto T, Kitagawa A, Iguchi T et al (2014) Satisfactory results at 8 years mean follow-up after ADVANCE® medial-pivot total knee arthroplasty. Knee 21:387–390
103. Karachalios T, Roidis N, Giotikas D, Bargiotas K, Varitimidis S, Malizos KN (2009) A mid-term clinical outcome study of the Advance Medial Pivot knee arthroplasty. Knee 16(6):484–488. https://doi.org/10.1016/j.knee.2009.03.002
104. Youm YS, Cho SD, Lee SH, Cho HY (2014) Total knee arthroplasty using a posterior cruciate ligament sacrificing medial pivot knee: minimum 5-year follow-up results. Knee Surg Relat Res 26(3):135–140. https://doi.org/10.5792/ksrr.2014.26.3.135
105. Ishida K, Matsumoto T, Tsumura N, Iwakura T, Kubo S, Iguchi T, Akisue T, Nishida K, Kurosaka M, Kuroda R (2014) No difference between double-high insert and medial-pivot insert in TKA. Knee Surg Sports Traumatol Arthrosc 22(3):576–580. https://doi.org/10.1007/s00167-012-2314-x

106. Vecchini E, Christodoulidis A, Magnan B, Ricci M, Regis D, Bartolozzi P (2012) Clinical and radiologic outcomes of total knee arthroplasty using the Advance Medial Pivot prosthesis. A mean 7 years follow-up. Knee 19(6):851–855. https://doi.org/10.1016/j.knee.2012.04.002
107. Kitagawa A, Ishida K, Chin T, Tsumura N, Iguchi T (2014) Partial restoration of knee kinematics in severe valgus deformity using the medial-pivot total knee arthroplasty. Knee Surg Sports Traumatol Arthrosc 22(7):1599–1606. https://doi.org/10.1007/s00167-012-2315-9
108. Mugnai R, Digennaro V, Ensini A et al (2014) Can TKA design affect the clinical outcome? Comparison between two guided-motion systems. Knee Surg Sport Traumatol Arthrosc. https://doi.org/10.1007/s00167-013-2509-9
109. Freeman MA, Pinskerova V (2005) The movement of the normal tibio-femoral joint. J Biomech 38(2):197–208
110. Robert S, Steven O, David BJ, Angelia A, Fitch David A, Lowry BC. Midterm clinical and radiographic results of the medial pivot total knee system. Int Orthop. 2014;38(12):2495–8. https://doi.org/10.1007/s00264-014-2444-5.
111. Guyatt GH, Oxman AD, Vist GE et al (2008) GRADE: an emerging consensus on rating quality of evidence and strength of recommendations. BMJ. https://doi.org/10.1136/bmj.39489.470347.ad
112. Kim YH, Park JW, Kim JS (2017) Clinical outcome of medial pivot compared with press-fit condylar sigma cruciate-retaining mobile-bearing total knee arthroplasty. J Arthroplast 32(10):3016–3023. https://doi.org/10.1016/j.arth.2017.05.022
113. Nakamura J, Inoue T, Suguro T, Suzuki M, Sasho T, Hagiwara S, Akagi R, Orita S, Inage K, Akazawa T, Ohtori S. A comparative study of flat surface design and medial pivot design in posterior cruciate-retaining total knee arthroplasty: a matched pair cohort study of two years. BMC Musculoskelet Disord. 2018;19(1):234.
114. Jeremić DV, Massouh WM, Sivaloganathan S et al (2020) Short-term follow-up of kinematically vs mechanically aligned total knee arthroplasty with medial pivot components: a case-control study. Orthop Traumatol Surg Res. https://doi.org/10.1016/j.otsr.2020.04.005
115. Nishitani K, Furu M, Nakamura S et al (2018) No differences in patient-reported outcomes between medial pivot insert and symmetrical insert in total knee arthroplasty: a randomized analysis. Knee 25:1254–1261. https://doi.org/10.1016/j.knee.2018.08.005
116. Cacciola G, De Martino I, De Meo F (2020) Does the medial pivot knee improve the clinical and radiographic outcome of total knee arthroplasty? A single centre study on two hundred and ninety seven patients. Int Orthop 44:291–299. https://doi.org/10.1007/s00264-019-04462-3
117. Mannan K, Scott G (2009) The Medial Rotation total knee replacement: a clinical and radiological review at a mean followup of six years. J Bone Jt Surg Ser B 91:750–756. https://doi.org/10.1302/0301-620X.91B6.22124
118. Dehl M, Bulaïd Y, Chelli M, Belhaouane R, Gabrion A, Havet E, et al. Total knee arthroplasty with the medial-pivot knee system: clinical and radiological

outcomes at 9.5 years' mean follow-up. Orthop Traumatol Surg Res. 2018;104(2):185–91. https://doi.org/10.1016/j.otsr.2017.10.016.
119. Gill UN, Shiraz HM, Rehman MKU et al (2019) Comparison of functional outcome of medial pivot total knee arthroplasty with posterior stabilizing (PS) total knee arthroplasty—a randomized trial. Pak J Med Health Sci 13:385–388
120. French SR, Munir S, Brighton R (2020) A single surgeon series comparing the outcomes of a cruciate retaining and medially stabilized total knee arthroplasty using kinematic alignment principles. J Arthroplast 35:422–428. https://doi.org/10.1016/j.arth.2019.09.021
121. Mancino F, Di Matteo V, Mocini F, Cacciola G, Malerba G, Perisano C, et al. Survivorship and clinical outcomes of proximal femoral replacement in non-neoplastic primary and revision total hip arthroplasty: a systematic review. BMC Musculoskelet Disord. 2021;22(Suppl 2):933. https://doi.org/10.1186/s12891-021-04711-w.
122. Liberati A, Altman DG, Tetzlaff J, Mulrow C, Gøtzsche PC, Ioannidis JP, et al. The PRISMA statement for reporting systematic reviews and meta-analyses of studies that evaluate health care interventions: explanation and elaboration. PLoS Med. 2009;6(7):e1000100. https://doi.org/10.1371/journal.pmed.1000100.
123. Artiaco S, Bosco F, Lusso A, Cioffi LL, Battiston B, Massè A. Flexor tendon pulley injuries: a systematic review of the literature and current treatment options. J Hand Microsurg. 2022. https://doi.org/10.1055/s-0042-1749420.
124. Via RG, F. Bosco, F. Giustra et al. Acute Rockwood type III ACJ dislocation: Conservative vs surgical approach. A systematic review and meta-analysis of current concepts in literature, Injury, 2022. https://doi.org/10.1016/j.injury.2022.07.050.
125. Sideri S, Papageorgiou SN, Eliades T. Registration in the international prospective register of systematic reviews (PROSPERO) of systematic review protocols was associated with increased review quality. J Clin Epidemiol. 2018;100:103–10. https://doi.org/10.1016/j.jclinepi.2018.01.003.
126. Ranawat CS. History of total knee replacement. J South Orthop Assoc. 2002;11(4):218–26 PMID: 12597066.
127. Insall JN, Lachiewicz PF, Burstein AH. The posterior stabilized condylar prosthesis: a modification of the total condylar design Two to four-year clinical experience. J Bone Joint Surg Am. 1982;64(9):1317–23 PMID: 7142239.
128. Stolarczyk A, Maciąg BM, Mostowy M, Maciąg GJ, Stępiński P, Szymczak J, et al. Comparison of biomechanical gait parameters and patient-reported outcome in patients after total knee arthroplasty with the use of fixed-bearing medial pivot and multi-radius design implants-retrospective matched-cohort study. Arthroplast Today. 2022;14:29–35. https://doi.org/10.1016/j.artd.2021.10.002.
129. Ghirardelli S, Asay JL, Leonardi EA, Amoroso T, Andriacchi TP, Indelli PF. Kinematic comparison between medially congruent and posterior-stabilized third-generation TKA designs. J Funct Morphol Kinesiol. 2021;6(1):27. https://doi.org/10.3390/jfmk6010027.

130. Tan J, Zou D, Zhang X, Zheng N, Pan Y, Ling Z, et al. Loss of knee flexion and femoral rollback of the medial-pivot and posterior-stabilized total knee arthroplasty during early-stance of walking in chinese patients. Front Bioeng Biotechnol. 2021;9:675093. https://doi.org/10.3389/fbioe.2021.675093.
131. Bianchi N, Facchini A, Mondanelli N, Sacchetti F, Ghezzi R, Gesi M, et al. Medial pivot vs posterior stabilized total knee arthroplasty designs: a gait analysis study. Med Glas (Zenica). 2021;18(1):252–9. https://doi.org/10.17392/1312-21.
132. Miura K, Ohkoshi Y, Ino T, Ukishiro K, Kawakami K, Suzuki S, et al. Kinematics and center of axial rotation during walking after medial pivot type total knee arthroplasty. J Exp Orthop. 2020;7(1):72. https://doi.org/10.1186/s40634-020-00286-y.
133. Esposito F, Freddolini M, Marcucci M, Latella L, Corvi A (2020) Biomechanical analysis on total knee replacement patients during gait: Medial pivot or posterior stabilized design? Clin Biomech 78:105068. https://doi.org/10.1016/j.clinbiomech.2020.105068
134. Gray HA, Guan S, Young TJ, Dowsey MM, Choong PF, Pandy MG (2020) Comparison of posterior-stabilized, cruciate-retaining, and medial-stabilized knee implant motion during gait. J Orthop Res 38:1753–1768. https://doi.org/10.1002/jor.24613
135. Benjamin B, Pietrzak JRT, Tahmassebi J, Haddad FS (2018) A functional comparison of medial pivot and condylar knee designs based on patient outcomes and parameters of gait. Bone Jt J 100B:76–82. https://doi.org/10.1302/0301-620X.100B1.BJJ-2017-0605.R1
136. Burns PB, Rohrich RJ, Chung KC. The levels of evidence and their role in evidence-based medicine. Plast Reconstr Surg. 2011;128(1):305–10. https://doi.org/10.1097/PRS.0b013e318219c171.
137. Kurtz S, Ong K, Lau E et al (2007) Projections of primary and revision hip and knee arthroplasty in the United States from 2005 to 2030. J Bone Jt Surg Ser A. https://doi.org/10.2106/JBJS.F.00222
138. Insall JN, Dorr LD, Scott RD, Scott WN (1989) Rationale of the knee society clinical rating system. Clin Orthop Relat Res 248:13–14
139. Roos EM, Roos HP, Lohmander LS, Ekdahl C, Beynnon BD: Knee Injury and Osteoarthritis Outcome Score (KOOS)–development of a self-administered outcome measure. J Orthop Sports Phys Ther. 1998, 28 (2): 88-96. https://doi.org/10.2519/jospt.1998.28.2.88.
140. Behrend H, Giesinger K, Giesinger JM, Kuster MS (2012) The "forgotten joint" as the ultimate goal in joint arthroplasty: validation of a new patient-reported outcome measure. J Arthroplasty 27:430-436 e1
141. Ware J Jr, Kosinski M, Keller SD (1996) A 12-item short-form health survey: construction of scales and preliminary tests of reliability and validity. MedCare. 34(3):220–233
142. Arauz P, Peng Y, Kwon YM (2018) Knee motion symmetry was not restored in patients with unilateral bi-cruciate retaining total knee arthroplasty-in vivo

three-dimensional kinematic analysis. Int Orthop 42(12):2817–2823. https://doi.org/10.1007/s00264-018-3986-8
143. Murray DW, Carr AJ, Bulstrode C (1993) Survival analysis of joint replacements. J Bone Joint Surg Br 75(5):697–704
144. Katchky AM, Jones CW, Walter WL, Shimmin AJ (2019) Medial ball and socket total knee arthroplasty. Bone Joint J 101-B(1_Supple_A):59–65. https://doi.org/10.1302/0301620X.101B1.BJJ-2018-0434.R1
145. Schmidt R, Komistek RD, Blaha JD, Penenberg BL, Maloney WJ (2003) Fluoroscopic analyses of cruciate-retaining and medial pivot knee implants. Clin Orthop Relat Res 410:139–147. https://doi.org/10.1097/01.blo.0000063565.90853.a4
146. Wittig, Ulrike; Moshammer, Maximilian; Vielgut, Ines; Hauer, Georg; Reinbacher, Patrick; Leithner, Andreas; Sadoghi, Patrick Higher use of fixed-bearing over mobile-bearing and posterior-stabilized over medial pivot designs in total knee arthroplasty (TKA): a systematic comparative analysis using worldwide arthroplasty registers from England and Wales, Australia, Norway, New Zealand, Germany and Switzerland. Archives of Orthopaedic and Trauma Surgery (2022). https://doi.org/10.1007/s00402-022-04410-8
147. Chinzei, Nobuaki; Ishida, Kazunari; Matsumoto, Tomoyuki; Kuroda, Yuichi; Kitagawa, Atsushi; Kuroda, Ryosuke; Akisue, Toshihiro; Nishida, Kotaro; Kurosaka, Masahiro; Tsumura, Nobuhiro Evaluation of patellofemoral joint in ADVANCE® Medial-pivot total knee arthroplasty. International Orthopaedics (2013). https://doi.org/10.1007/s00264-013-2043-x
148. Nakajima, Arata; Sonobe, Masato; Akatsu, Yorikazu; Yamada, Manabu; Yamamoto, Keiichiro; Saito, Junya; Norimoto, Masaki; Koyama, Keita; Taniguchi, Shinji; Takahashi, Hiroshi; Aoki, Yasuchika; Suguro, Toru; Nakagawa, Koichi Lateral shift of the femoral condyle after total knee arthroplasty: simulation using 2D-templates of the medial pivot design on knee radiographs of young Japanese patients. Journal of Orthopaedic Surgery and Research (2022). https://doi.org/10.1186/s13018-022-03342-8
149. Putame, Giovanni; Terzini, Mara; Rivera, Fabrizio; Kebbach, Maeruan; Bader, Rainer; Bignardi, Cristina Kinematics and kinetics comparison of ultra-congruent versus medial-pivot designs for total knee arthroplasty by multi-body analysis. Scientific Reports (2022). https://doi.org/10.1038/s41598-022-06909-x
150. Obada, Bogdan; Iliescu, Madalina Gabriela; Costea, Dan Ovidiu; Petcu, Lucian; Popescu, Andrei Ion Comparative study of outcomes with total knee arthroplasty: medial pivot prosthesis vs posterior stabilized implant. Prospective randomized control. International Orthopaedics (2025). https://doi.org/10.1007/s00264-025-06420-8
151. Nakamura, Junichi; Inoue, Takaki; Suguro, Toru; Suzuki, Masahiko; Sasho, Takahisa; Hagiwara, Shigeo; Akagi, Ryuichiro; Orita, Sumihisa; Inage, Kazuhide; Akazawa, Tsutomu; Ohtori, Seiji A comparative study of flat surface design and medial pivot design in posterior cruciate-retaining total knee

arthroplasty: a matched pair cohort study of two years. BMC Musculoskeletal Disorders (2018). https://doi.org/10.1186/s12891-018-2138-z
152. De Groot, J. D.; Brokelman, R. B.G.; Lammers, P. G.; Van Stralen, G. M.J.; Kooijman, C. M.; Hokwerda, S. T. Performance of medial pivot, posterior stabilized and rotating platform total knee arthroplasty based on anteroposterior stability and patient-reported outcome measures; a multicentre double-blinded randomized controlled trial of 210 knees. Archives of Orthopaedic and Trauma Surgery (2024). https://doi.org/10.1007/s00402-024-05340-3
153. Xu, Zihang; Tian, Shengyuan; Zhou, Xiang; Wei, Ya; Wu, Changbing; Jia, Xianghua; Wang, Hong Medial Pivot Versus Posterior-Stabilized Prosthesis Design in Primary Total Knee Arthroplasty: A Systematic Review and Meta-Analysis. Indian Journal of Orthopaedics (2022). https://doi.org/10.1007/s43465-022-00678-5
154. Shi, Weipeng; Jiang, Yaping; Wang, Changyao; Zhang, Haining; Wang, Yingzhen; Li, Tao Comparative study on mid- and long-term clinical effects of medial pivot prosthesis and posterior-stabilized prosthesis after total knee arthroplasty. Journal of Orthopaedic Surgery and Research (2020). https://doi.org/10.1186/s13018-020-01951-9
155. Ueyama, Hideki; Nakagawa, Shigeru; Kishimura, Yuichi; Minoda, Yukihide; Nakamura, Suguru; Koyanagi, Junichiro; Yamamura, Mitsuyoshi; Kadoya, Yoshinori Long-term clinical results of alumina ceramic medial pivot total knee arthroplasty: a 10-year follow-up study. Arthroplasty (2023). https://doi.org/10.1186/s42836-023-00180-9
156. Ueyama, Hideki; Kanemoto, Narihiro; Minoda, Yukihide; Yamamoto, Nobuo; Taniguchi, Yoshiki; Nakamura, Hiroaki Comparison of postoperative knee flexion and patient satisfaction between newly and conventionally designed medial pivot total knee arthroplasty: a 5-year follow-up matched cohort study. Archives of Orthopaedic and Trauma Surgery (2021). https://doi.org/10.1007/s00402-021-04121-6
157. Iwakiri, Kentaro; Ohta, Yoichi; Minoda, Yukihide; Ueno, Shuhei; Kobayashi, Akio; Nakamura, Hiroaki Comparative analysis of medial pivot vs. posterior stabilized total knee arthroplasty in patients with valgus deformed osteoarthritic knees: a retrospective cohort study. International Orthopaedics (2024). https://doi.org/10.1007/s00264-024-06337-8
158. Iwakiri, Kentaro; Ohta, Yoichi; Ohyama, Yohei; Minoda, Yukihide; Kobayashi, Akio; Nakamura, Hiroaki Is medial pivot total knee arthroplasty suitable for patients with valgus knee osteoarthritis?. European Journal of Orthopaedic Surgery & Traumatology (2021). https://doi.org/10.1007/s00590-021-03007-y
159. Xiang, Shuai; Wang, Yingzhen; Lv, Chengyu; Wang, Changyao; Zhang, Haining Mid-term clinical outcomes and survivorship of medial-pivot total knee arthroplasty—a mean five year follow-up based on one thousand, one hundred and twenty eight cases. International Orthopaedics (2021). https://doi.org/10.1007/s00264-021-05017-1
160. Alessio-Mazzola, Mattia; Clemente, Antonio; Russo, Antonio; Mertens, Peter; Burastero, Giorgio; Formica, Matteo; Felli, Lamberto Clinical radio-

graphic outcomes and survivorship of medial pivot design total knee arthroplasty: a systematic review of the literature. Archives of Orthopaedic and Trauma Surgery (2021). https://doi.org/10.1007/s00402-021-04210-6
161. Risitano, Salvatore; Cacciola, Giorgio; Capella, Marcello; Bosco, Francesco; Giustra, Fortunato; Fusini, Federico; Indelli, Pier Francesco; Massé, Alessandro; Sabatini, Luigi Comparison between gaits after a medial pivot and posterior stabilized primary total knee arthroplasty: a systematic review of the literature. Arthroplasty (2023). https://doi.org/10.1186/s42836-023-00165-8
162. Cacciola, Giorgio; De Martino, Ivan; De Meo, Federico Does the medial pivot knee improve the clinical and radiographic outcome of total knee arthroplasty? A single centre study on two hundred and ninety seven patients. International Orthopaedics (2019). https://doi.org/10.1007/s00264-019-04462-3
163. Shakya, Akash; Singh, Vijay; Agrawal, Romit A.; Sharma, Ayush; Mangale, Nilesh; Wadgave, Venkatramana; Jaiswal, Ajay A Mid-term Comparison of the Functional Outcomes of Medial Pivot and Rotating Platform Mobile-Bearing Total Knee Arthroplasty in the Indian Population. Indian Journal of Orthopaedics (2021). https://doi.org/10.1007/s43465-021-00472-9

4.3 PCL Substituting

Machine Generated Summaries

Disclaimer: The summaries in this chapter were generated from Springer Nature publications using abstractive AI auto-summarization: An abstraction-based summarizer creates new text based on deep learning. New phrases are created to summarize the content. As the constituted sentences are machine selected, they may not fully reflect the body of the work, so we strongly advise that the original content is read and cited. The auto-generated summaries were curated by the editor to meet Springer Nature publication standards.

4.3.1 No Difference of Survival Between Cruciate Retaining and Substitution Designs in High Flexion Total Knee Arthroplasty [38]

This is a machine-generated summary of:

Kim, Gun-Woo; Jin, Quan He; Lim, Jun-Hyuk; Song, Eun-Kyoo; Seon, Jong-Keun No difference of survival between cruciate retaining and substitution designs in high flexion total knee arthroplasty [38].

Published in: Scientific Reports (2021).

Link to original: https://doi.org/10.1038/s41598-021-85892-1

4.3.1.1 Research Highlights

Total knee arthroplasty (TKA) aims to provide pain relief and ensure long-term implant survival. With increasing patient expectations, achieving higher flexion post operatively has become a priority, leading to the development of high-flexion prosthesis designs. These designs incorporate subtle geometric changes to enhance contact areas at high-flexion angles, potentially improving posterior femoral translation compared to conventional designs. However, the clinical benefits of these high-flexion prostheses remain undocumented, and questions persist regarding their motion patterns and stress impacts. The study by Kim et al. investigates the long-term outcomes of high-flexion cruciate-retaining (CR) and posterior-stabilized (PS) prostheses in TKA.

The study conducted a retrospective analysis of prospectively collected data from primary knee arthroplasties performed at Chonnam National University Hwasun Hospital. Patients were divided into CR and PS groups, with exclusions for prior knee surgeries or severe deformities. The surgical procedures were standardized across both groups, differing only in the retention or sacrifice of the posterior cruciate ligament. Clinical outcomes were assessed using various scoring systems, while radiographic evaluations focused on hip-knee-ankle angles and radiolucent lines. Statistical analyses compared functional outcomes, range of motion (ROM), and survival rates between the two groups over a minimum follow-up period of several years.

The study found no significant differences in ROM, clinical scores, or survival rates between the CR and PS groups after long-term follow-up. Both prosthesis designs showed similar improvements in clinical outcomes post-TKA. Despite concerns about aseptic loosening associated with high-flexion designs, no significant differences in radiolucent lines or loosening rates were observed between the two groups. Future study could explore broader patient populations or different implant systems to validate these findings further. The results suggest that both high-flexion CR and PS knee designs offer comparable long-term benefits in terms of ROM and clinical outcomes for patients undergoing TKA.

4.3.2 Kinematic Analysis of Posterior-Stabilized Total Knee Arthroplasty During Standing Up from and Sitting Down on a Chair [39]

This is a machine-generated summary of:

Mine, Takatomo; Hoshi, Kenji; Gamada, Kazuyoshi; Ihara, Koichiro; Kawamura, Hiroyuki; Kuriyama, Ryutaro; Date, Ryo Kinematic analysis of posterior-stabilized total knee arthroplasty during standing up from and sitting down on a chair [39].

Published in: Journal of Orthopaedic Surgery and Research (2016).

Link to original: https://doi.org/10.1186/s13018-016-0482-y

4.3.2.1 Research Highlights

Kinetic and gait analyses are crucial for understanding the effects of total knee arthroplasty (TKA), with in vivo kinematic studies using fluoroscopy providing insights into postoperative outcomes. Knee implants, such as the Bi-Surface PS (Kyocera Corp kyoto, Japan), are designed to mimic the natural constraints of the knee joint, featuring a ball and socket joint structure and an asymmetric tibial plate. Despite advancements in implant design, there remains a need to better understand how these designs influence functional knee motion during daily activities like standing up from and sitting down on a chair. The study by Mine et al. investigates the in vivo kinematics of the Bi-Surface PS knee system during these activities.

The study involved 15 patients who had undergone successful TKA with the Bi-Surface PS prosthesis. Using a two-dimensional to three-dimensional registration technique, researchers analysed knee motion while participants stood up from and sat down on a chair under fluoroscopic surveillance. The study measured various parameters, including flexion angle, axial rotation angle, anteroposterior translation, and post-cam engagement. The results showed distinct kinematic patterns: slight anterior femoral translation from minimum to 30° flexion, a medial pivot pattern from 30° to 90° flexion, and bicondylar rollback beyond 90° flexion. These patterns differ from normal knee kinematics and are attributed to the unique design of the Bi-Surface PS implant.

The findings suggest that while the Bi-Surface PS implant provides stability during shallow knee flexion, its kinematic patterns differ from those of a natural knee due to its design features like post-cam engagement. Future study should explore how these kinematic differences impact long-term outcomes of TKA and consider factors such as muscular strength and ligament balance. Although limited by sample size and lack of a control group, this research contributes valuable insights into improving knee prosthesis design for better functional outcomes.

4.3.3 Rotational Alignment of Tibial Components in Mobile-Bearing TKA: Posterior Substituted vs. PCL Retaining [40]

This is a machine-generated summary of:

Ishii, Yoshinori; Noguchi, Hideo; Sato, Junko; Todoroki, Koji; Toyabe, Shin-Ichi Rotational alignment of tibial components in mobile-bearing TKA: posterior substituted vs. PCL retaining [40].

Published in: Archives of Orthopaedic and Trauma Surgery (2015).

Link to original: https://doi.org/10.1007/s00402-015-2275-x

If you want to cite the papers, please refer to the original.

For technical reasons we could not place the page where the original quote is coming from.

4.3.3.1 Research Highlights

Total knee arthroplasty (TKA) often encounters challenges in achieving proper rotational alignment of the tibial component, which is crucial for optimal knee function. Traditional methods using fixed anatomical landmarks can lead to malalignment due to anatomical variations and deformities. The study by Ishii et al. explores the use of the medial border of the tibial tubercle (MBTT) as an initial reference point for tibial rotation in mobile-bearing TKA, examining its reliability and the impact of posterior cruciate ligament (PCL) retention on rotational alignment.

The study involved 222 TKA procedures performed on patients with primary osteoarthritis or rheumatoid arthritis, using a quasi-randomized approach to allocate patients to either PCL-retaining or PCL-substituting prostheses. The surgeries were conducted by a single surgeon using standardized techniques, with the MBTT cleared of soft tissues and marked as the anterior reference point. A quantitative three-dimensional imaging technique was employed to assess postoperative alignment relative to both the MBTT and the transepicondylar axis (TEA) of the femur. The results showed no significant difference in rotational alignment between PCL-retaining and PCL-substituting designs, with all knees achieving alignment within ±3° of both reference axes.

The study advances our understanding of tibial component rotation in TKA by demonstrating that using the MBTT as an initial landmark, followed by adjustments during knee flexion-extension exercises, provides reliable rotational placement. This approach compensates for anatomical variability and supports the use of mobile-bearing designs that allow self-alignment. Future study could explore this method's applicability to fixed-bearing designs and its clinical significance compared to other anatomical landmarks. The findings suggest that combining anatomical landmarks with mobile-bearing technology may enhance surgical outcomes in TKA.

4.3.4 Posterior Condylar Offset Changes and Its Effect on Clinical Outcomes After Posterior-Substituting, Fixed-Bearing Total Knee Arthroplasty: Anterior Versus Posterior Referencing [41]

This is a machine-generated summary of:

Chang, Moon Jong; Kang, Seung-Baik; Chang, Chong Bum; Han, Do Hwan; Park, Hyung Jun; Hwang, Keummin; Park, Jisu; Hwang, Il-Ung; Lee, Seung Ah.; Oh, Sohee Posterior condylar offset changes and its effect on clinical outcomes after posterior-substituting, fixed-bearing total knee arthroplasty: anterior versus posterior referencing [41].

Published in: Knee Surgery & Related Research (2020).

Link to original: https://doi.org/10.1186/s43019-019-0022-2

If you want to cite the papers, please refer to the original.

For technical reasons we could not place the page where the original quote is coming from.

4.3.4.1 Research Highlights

Proper implant positioning and sizing are critical for successful total knee arthroplasty (TKA), with anterior referencing (AR) and posterior referencing (PR) systems being the primary methods used. Each system has its own advantages and disadvantages, such as the risk of femoral notching in AR and less predictable anterior femoral cutting in PR. However, recent advancements in surgical techniques and implant designs may mitigate these drawbacks. The study by Chang et al. investigates whether there are differences in posterior condylar offset (PCO) and posterior condylar offset ratio (PCOR) after TKA between AR and PR systems, and how these factors relate to range of motion (ROM) and clinical outcomes.

The study was a retrospective analysis involving patients who underwent primary TKA using the same prosthesis for end-stage osteoarthritis. Patients were divided into AR and PR groups, with surgeries performed by a single senior surgeon using consistent techniques except for the referencing system. Radiographic evaluations were conducted to measure PCO and PCOR pre- and postoperatively, while clinical outcomes were assessed using ROM measurements and Western Ontario and McMaster University Osteoarthritis Index (WOMAC) scores. Statistical analyses compared demographic data, PCO/PCOR changes, ROM, and WOMAC scores between the two groups. The results showed that while PCO was more consistently preserved in the PR group, there was no significant difference in PCOR or postoperative ROM between the groups. The preoperative ROM was found to be the only factor significantly related to postoperative ROM.

The study concludes that both AR and PR systems can achieve satisfactory clinical outcomes in TKA using contemporary surgical techniques and implants. Although PCO preservation was more consistent in the PR group, it did not translate into differences in postoperative ROM or WOMAC score improvements between the groups. Future study could explore longer follow-up periods or different implant designs to further understand their impact on TKA outcomes. The findings suggest that both referencing systems are viable options for achieving successful TKA results with a PCL-substituting fixed-bearing implant.

4.3.5 Retrospective Comparative Study Shows No Significant Difference in Postural Stability Between Cruciate-Retaining (CR) and Cruciate-Substituting (PS) Total Knee Implant Systems [42]

This is a machine-generated summary of:

Götz, Juergen; Beckmann, Johannes; Sperrer, Ingo; Baier, Clemens; Dullien, Silvia; Grifka, Joachim; Koeck, Franz Retrospective comparative study shows no significant difference in postural stability between cruciate-retaining (CR) and cruciate-substituting (PS) total knee implant systems [42].

Published in: International Orthopaedics (2015).

Link to original: https://doi.org/10.1007/s00264-015-3067-1

If you want to cite the papers, please refer to the original.

For technical reasons we could not place the page where the original quote is coming from.

4.3.5.1 Research Highlights

Total knee arthroplasty (TKA) is a prevalent procedure in orthopedic surgery, primarily aimed at alleviating pain and restoring knee function when conservative treatments fail. With the increasing demand for TKA in Western countries, various implant designs have emerged, with choices often influenced by surgeon preference and hospital contracts. A critical decision in TKA is whether to retain or substitute the posterior cruciate ligament (PCL), as this can impact knee kinematics and postural stability. The study by Götz et al. investigates whether PCL-retaining implants offer superior postural stability and clinical outcomes compared to PCL-substituting designs.

The study was conducted prospectively on patients with primary osteoarthritis undergoing TKA, using either cruciate-retaining (CR) or posterior-stabilized (PS) implants based on stability needs. Exclusion criteria included metabolic diseases, previous surgeries, and unwillingness to participate. Postoperative assessments included the Western Ontario and McMaster Universities Arthritis Index (WOMAC), Knee Society Score (KSS), and postural stability measured using the Biodex Balance System (Biodexrehab, New York, USA). The study found no significant differences in postural stability between CR and PS groups during one-leg stance tests. However, the PS group showed better WOMAC scores, indicating superior clinical outcomes compared to the CR group.

The findings suggest that PCL substitution does not negatively impact postural stability or functional outcomes in TKA patients. The study highlights that factors such as pain relief and restoration of soft tissue tension may play more significant roles in postoperative proprioception than PCL retention. Future study directions could explore the long-term effects of implant design on knee function and consider biomechanical factors like shear forces on tibial interfaces. While both implant types are equivalent regarding postural stability, the PS design's better WOMAC scores suggest it may offer advantages in clinical outcomes. The study's limitations include its retrospective nature and early follow-up period, which should be considered when interpreting results.

4.3.6 The Surgeon's Role in Relative Success of PCL-Retaining and PCL-Substituting Total Knee Arthroplasty [43]

This is a machine-generated summary of:

Ritter, Merrill A.; Davis, Kenneth E.; Farris, Alex; Keating, E. Michael; Faris, Philip M. The Surgeon's Role in Relative Success of PCL-Retaining and PCL-Substituting Total Knee Arthroplasty [43].

Published in: HSS Journal ® (2014).

Link to original: https://doi.org/10.1007/s11420-014-9389-5

If you want to cite the papers, please refer to the original.

For technical reasons we could not place the page where the original quote is coming from.

4.3.6.1 Research Highlights

Total knee arthroplasty (TKA) often involves a critical decision regarding the retention or substitution of the posterior cruciate ligament (PCL). The two prevailing approaches—PCL retention and PCL substitution—are based on differing philosophies, with each method offering distinct advantages such as joint structure preservation and increased range of motion, respectively. Despite extensive research, the literature has not consistently demonstrated significant differences in clinical outcomes between these methods, except for increased flexion associated with PCL substitution. The study by Ritter et al. at The Center for Hip and Knee Surgery, St. Francis Hospital, Mooresville, IN, explores these differences further by examining the impact of individual prosthesis designs and other variables such as surgeon experience on TKA outcomes.

The study involved a retrospective analysis of 3000 total knee arthroplasties performed between January 2000 and April 2010. The authors focused on four predominant prosthesis designs used at their center: AGC PCL-retaining, Legacy PCL-substituting, Vanguard PCL-retaining, and Vanguard PCL-substituting (Zimmer-Biiomet, Warsaw, Indiana, USA). Patients were followed up at regular intervals post-surgery to assess Knee Society scores, flexion measurements, and other clinical outcomes. Statistical analyses using ANOVA and multiple linear regression were employed to evaluate the influence of various factors including prosthesis type, surgeon experience, and patient demographics on TKA results. The study found significant differences in flexion favoring PCL substitution but noted that function scores often favored retention. Importantly, the analysis revealed that surgeon-specific factors significantly influenced outcomes across different prosthesis designs.

The findings suggest that while prosthesis design plays a role in TKA outcomes, the operating surgeon's experience and technique may be equally or more influential. This underscores the need for future studies to consider nested models that account for both surgeon and implant variables to better understand their interaction in determining TKA success. Such research could help surgeons identify which prosthesis design aligns best with their surgical approach to achieve optimal patient outcomes. The study highlights the complexity of TKA decision-making and suggests that personalized approaches considering both surgical expertise and implant characteristics may be necessary for improving long-term results.

4.3.7 Posterior Cruciate-Substituting Total Knee Replacement Recovers the Flexion ARC Faster in the Early Postoperative Period In Knees with High Varus Deformity: A Prospective Randomized Study [44]

This is a machine-generated summary of:

Öztürk, Alpaslan; Akalın, Yavuz; Çevik, Nazan; Otuzbir, Ali; Özkan, Yüksel; Dostabakan, Yasin Posterior cruciate-substituting total knee replacement recovers the flexion arc faster in the early postoperative period in knees with high varus deformity: a prospective randomized study [44].

Published in: Archives of Orthopaedic and Trauma Surgery (2016).

Link to original: https://doi.org/10.1007/s00402-016-2482-0

If you want to cite the papers, please refer to the original.

For technical reasons we could not place the page where the original quote is coming from.

4.3.7.1 Research Highlights

Total knee replacement (TKR) surgery often involves a decision between preserving or sacrificing the posterior cruciate ligament (PCL). While some surgeons opt to retain the PCL for its potential benefits, such as more natural knee kinematics and reduced blood loss, others prefer to substitute it for advantages like increased range of motion and easier surgical procedures. Despite these considerations, the superiority of one design over the other remains unclear, with conflicting results from gait analysis studies and long-term survivorship reports. The study by Öztürk et al. investigates the early postoperative outcomes of PCL-retaining (CR) versus PCL-substituting (PS) TKR designs in patients with significant preoperative deformity.

The study was conducted as a prospective randomized controlled trial in the Netherlands, involving patients with knee osteoarthritis and deformities greater than 10 degrees. Participants were randomly assigned to receive either CR or PS TKR, with surgeries performed by a single surgeon using DePuy prostheses. The researchers measured various outcomes, including range of motion (ROM), pain levels, walking ability, stair climbing, and quadriceps function at multiple postoperative intervals. Statistical analyses were performed using the Mann–Whitney U test due to non-normal distribution of variables. The study found that PS knees achieved larger flexion arcs and faster recovery of function compared to CR knees in the early postoperative period.

The findings suggest that PS TKR may offer advantages in terms of faster recovery of ROM and function without compromising pain levels or long-term outcomes. However, CR knees showed better performance in unaided walking and straight leg raising. Future study could explore these differences further to optimize surgical decisions based on patient-specific factors. The study's strengths include its randomized design and consistent surgical technique, though its sample size may limit broader applicability. Overall, both CR and PS designs provide satisfactory functional outcomes in osteoarthritic knees with high varus deformity.

Bibliography

1. Han, H. S., Kang, S. B. and Yoon, K. S. High incidence of loosening of the femoral component in legacy posterior stabilised-flex total knee replacement. *J. Bone Joint Surg. Br. 89*, 1457–1461 (2007).
2. Zelle, J., Janssen, D., Van Eijden, J., DeWaalMalefijt, M. and Verdonschot, N. Does high-flexion total knee arthroplasty promote early loosening of the femoral component?. *J. Orthop. Res. 29*, 976–983 (2011).
3. Sharma, A., Komistek, R. D., Scuderi, G. R. and Cates, H. E. Jr. High-flexion TKA designs: what are their in vivo contact mechanics?. *Clin. Orthop. Relat. Res. 464*, 117–126 (2007).
4. Seon JK, Park JK, Shin YJ, Seo HY, Lee KB, Song EK (2011) Comparisons of kinematics and range of motion in high-flexion total knee arthroplasty: cruciate retaining vs. substituting designs. Knee Surg Sports Traumatol Arthrosc 19(12):2016–2022. https://doi.org/10.1007/s00167-011-1434-z

5. Yagishita, K. *et al.* High-flex posterior cruciate-retaining vs posterior cruciate-substituting designs in simultaneous bilateral total knee arthroplasty: a prospective, randomized study. *J. Arthroplasty 27*, 368–374 (2012).
6. Harato, K. *et al.* Midterm comparison of posterior cruciate-retaining versus-substituting total knee arthroplasty using the Genesis II prosthesis: a multicenter prospective randomized clinical trial. *Knee 15*, 217–221 (2008).
7. Wang, C. J., Wang, J. W. and Chen, H. S. Comparing cruciate-retaining total knee arthroplasty and cruciate-substituting total knee arthroplasty: a prospective clinical study. *Chang Gung Med. J. 27*, 578–585 (2004).
8. Han, C. W., Yang, I. H., Lee, W. S., Park, K. K. and Han, C. D. Evaluation of postoperative range of motion and functional outcomes after cruciate-retaining and posterior-stabilized high-flexion total knee arthroplasty. *Yonsei Med. J. 53*, 794–800 (2012).
9. Merkow RL, Soundry M, Insall JN (1985) Patellar dislocation following total knee arthroplasty. J Bone Joint Surg Am 67:1321–1327
10. Insall JN, Easley ME (2001) Surgical techniques and instrumentation in total knee arthroplasty. In: Insall JN, Scott WN (eds) Surgery of the knee, 3rd edn. Churchill-Livingstone, New York, pp 1553–1620
11. Dalury DF, Jiranek W, Pierson J, Pearson SE (2003) The long-term outcome of total knee patients with moderate loss of motion. J Knee Surg 16:215–220
12. Uehara K, Kadoya Y, Kobayashi A, Ohashi H, Yamano Y (2002) Bone anatomy and rotational alignment in total knee arthroplasty. Clin Orthop Relat Res 402:196–201
13. Aglietti P, Sensi L, Cuomo P, Ciardullo A (2008) Rotational position of femoral and tibial components in TKA using the femoral transepicondylar axis. Clin Orthop Relat Res 466:2751–2755
14. Kawahara S, Matsuda S, Okazaki K, Tashiro Y, Mitsuyasu H, Nakahara H, Iwamoto Y (2012) Relationship between the tibial anteroposterior axis and the surgical epicondylar axis in varus and valgus knees. Knee Surg Sports Traumatol Arthrosc 20:2077–2081
15. Moreland JR (1988) Mechanism of failure in total knee arthroplasty. Clin Orthop Relat Res 226:49–64
16. Eckhoff DG, Metzger RJ, Stamm ER, Kilcoyne RE, Wiedel JD (1994) Version of osteoarthritic knee. J Arthroplasty 9:73–79
17. Yoshioka Y, Siu DW, Scudamore RA, Cooke TD (1989) Tibial anatomy and functional axes. J Orthop Res 7:132–137
18. Sahin N, Atıcı T, Kurtoğlu Ü, Turgut A, Ozkaya G, Ozkan Y (2013) Centre of the posterior cruciate ligament and the sulcus between tubercle spines are reliable landmarks for tibial component placement. Knee Surg Sports Traumatol Arthrosc 21:2384–2391
19. Ishii Y, Terajima K, Koga Y, Bechtold JE (1999) Screw home motion after total knee replacement. Clin Orthop Relat Res 358:181–187
20. Sato T, Koga Y, Omori G (2004) Three-dimensional lower extremity alignment assessment system: application to evaluation of component positioning after total knee arthroplasty. J Arthroplasty 19:620–628

21. Sato T, Koga Y, Sobue T, Omori G, Tanabe Y, Sakamoto M (2007) Quantitative 3-dimensional analysis of preoperative and postoperative joint lines in total knee arthroplasty: a new concept for evaluation of component alignment. J Arthroplasty 22:560–568
22. Bellemans J, Banks S, Victor J, Vandenneucker H, Moemans A (2002) Fluoroscopic analysis of the kinematics of deep flexion in total knee arthroplasty: influence of posterior condylar offset. J Bone Joint Surg 84(1):50–53
23. Hanratty B, Thompson N, Wilson R, Beverland D (2007) The influence of posterior condylar offset on knee flexion after total knee replacement using a cruciate-sacrificing mobile-bearing implant. J Bone Joint Surg 89(7):915–918
24. Ishii Y, Noguchi H, Takeda M, Sato J, Toyabe S-i (2013) Posterior condylar offset does not correlate with knee flexion after TKA. Clin Orthop Relat Res 471(9):2995–3001
25. Malviya A, Lingard E, Weir D, Deehan D (2009) Predicting range of movement after knee replacement: the importance of posterior condylar offset and tibial slope. Knee Surg Sports Traumatol Arthrosc 17(5):491–498
26. Kansara D, Markel DC (2006) The effect of posterior tibial slope on range of motion after total knee arthroplasty. J Arthroplasty 21(6):809–813
27. Kurosaka M, Yoshiya S, Mizuno K, Yamamoto T (2002) Maximizing flexion after total knee arthroplasty: the need and the pitfalls. J Arthroplasty 17(4):59–62
28. Freeman MA, Pinskerova V (2005) The movement of the normal tibio-femoral joint. J Biomech 38(2):197–208
29. Kapandji I (2006) Funktionelle Anatomie der Gelenke, vol 2, 4th edn. Thieme, Stuttgart, p 84
30. Bachmann M, Bolliger L, Ilchmann T, Clauss M (2014) Long-term survival and radiological results of the Duracon™ total knee arthroplasty. Int Orthop 38(4):747–752. https://doi.org/10.1007/s00264-013-2154-4
31. Becher C, Heyse TJ, Kron N, Ostermeier S, Hurschler C, Schofer MD et al (2009) Posterior stabilized TKA reduce patellofemoral contact pressure compared with cruciate retaining TKA in vitro. Knee Surg Sports Traumatol Arthrosc 17:1159–1165
32. Wang CJ, Wang JW, Chen HS (2004) Comparing cruciate-retaining total knee arthroplasty and cruciate-substituting total knee arthroplasty: a prospective clinical study. Chang Gung Med J 27(8):578–585
33. van den Boom LG, Brouwer RW, van den Akker-Scheek I, Bulstra SK, van Raaij JJ (2009) Retention of the posterior cruciate ligament versus the posterior stabilized design in total knee arthroplasty: a prospective randomized controlled clinical trial. BMC Musculoskelet Disord 10:119
34. McCormack HM, Horne DJ, Sheather S (1988) Clinical applications of visual analogue scales: a critical review. Psychol Med 18(4):1007–1019
35. Kolisek FR, McGrath MS, Marker DR, Jessup N, Seyler TM, Mont MA, Lowry Barnes C (2009) Posterior-stabilized versus posterior cruciate ligament-retaining total knee arthroplasty. Iowa Orthop J 29:23–27

36. Chaudhary R, Beaupre LA, Johnston DW (2008) Knee range of motion during the first two years after use of posterior cruciate-stabilizing or posterior cruciate-retaining total knee prostheses. A randomized clinical trial. J Bone Joint Surg Am 90(12):2579–2586
37. Clark CR, Rorabeck CH, MacDonald S, MacDonald D, Swafford J, Cleland D (2001) Posterior-stabilized and cruciate-retaining total knee replacement: A randomized study. Clin Orthop Relat Res 392:208–212
38. Kim, Gun-Woo; Jin, Quan He; Lim, Jun-Hyuk; Song, Eun-Kyoo; Seon, Jong-Keun No difference of survival between cruciate retaining and substitution designs in high flexion total knee arthroplasty. Scientific Reports (2021). https://doi.org/10.1038/s41598-021-85892-1
39. Mine, Takatomo; Hoshi, Kenji; Gamada, Kazuyoshi; Ihara, Koichiro; Kawamura, Hiroyuki; Kuriyama, Ryutaro; Date, Ryo Kinematic analysis of posterior-stabilized total knee arthroplasty during standing up from and sitting down on a chair. Journal of Orthopaedic Surgery and Research (2016). https://doi.org/10.1186/s13018-016-0482-y
40. Ishii, Yoshinori; Noguchi, Hideo; Sato, Junko; Todoroki, Koji; Toyabe, Shin-Ichi Rotational alignment of tibial components in mobile-bearing TKA: posterior substituted vs. PCL retaining. Archives of Orthopaedic and Trauma Surgery (2015). https://doi.org/10.1007/s00402-015-2275-x
41. Chang, Moon Jong; Kang, Seung-Baik; Chang, Chong Bum; Han, Do Hwan; Park, Hyung Jun; Hwang, Keummin; Park, Jisu; Hwang, Il-Ung; Lee, Seung Ah.; Oh, Sohee Posterior condylar offset changes and its effect on clinical outcomes after posterior-substituting, fixed-bearing total knee arthroplasty: anterior versus posterior referencing. Knee Surgery & Related Research (2020). https://doi.org/10.1186/s43019-019-0022-2
42. Götz, Juergen; Beckmann, Johannes; Sperrer, Ingo; Baier, Clemens; Dullien, Silvia; Grifka, Joachim; Koeck, Franz Retrospective comparative study shows no significant difference in postural stability between cruciate-retaining (CR) and cruciate-substituting (PS) total knee implant systems. International Orthopaedics (2015). https://doi.org/10.1007/s00264-015-3067-1
43. Ritter, Merrill A.; Davis, Kenneth E.; Farris, Alex; Keating, E. Michael; Faris, Philip M. The Surgeon's Role in Relative Success of PCL-Retaining and PCL-Substituting Total Knee Arthroplasty. HSS Journal ® (2014). https://doi.org/10.1007/s11420-014-9389-5
44. Öztürk, Alpaslan; Akalın, Yavuz; Çevik, Nazan; Otuzbir, Ali; Özkan, Yüksel; Dostabakan, Yasin Posterior cruciate-substituting total knee replacement recovers the flexion arc faster in the early postoperative period in knees with high varus deformity: a prospective randomized study. Archives of Orthopaedic and Trauma Surgery (2016). https://doi.org/10.1007/s00402-016-2482-0

4.4 Bicruciate Substituting

Machine Generated Summaries
Disclaimer: The summaries in this chapter were generated from Springer Nature publications using abstractive AI auto-summarization: An abstraction-based summarizer creates new text based on deep learning. New phrases are created to summarize the content. As the constituted sentences are machine selected, they may not fully reflect the body of the work, so we strongly advise that the original content is read and cited. The auto-generated summaries were curated by the editor to meet Springer Nature publication standards.

4.4.1 Consecutive Series of 226 Journey Bicruciate Substituting Total Knee Replacements: Early Complication and Revision Rates [5]

This is a machine-generated summary of:

Christen, Bernhard; Neukamp, Michal; Aghayev, Emin Consecutive series of 226 journey bicruciate substituting total knee replacements: early complication and revision rates [5].

Published in: BMC Musculoskeletal Disorders (2014).

Link to original: https://doi.org/10.1186/1471-2474-15-395

If you want to cite the papers, please refer to the original.

For technical reasons we could not place the page where the original quote is coming from.

4.4.1.1 Research Highlights

Total knee replacement (TKR) is a common procedure aimed at alleviating pain and improving function in patients with severe knee arthritis. However, a significant number of patients remain dissatisfied due to persistent pain, functional deficits, and unmet expectations. Traditional TKR designs often fail to restore normal knee kinematics, particularly due to challenges in replicating the functions of the anterior and posterior cruciate ligaments. The study by Christen et al. investigates the safety and early complication rates of the Journey bicruciate substituting (BCS) knee system, which aims to improve knee kinematics by more closely mimicking a natural knee.

The study conducted a retrospective analysis of consecutive patients who underwent TKR with the Journey BCS prosthesis (Smith and Nephew, Memphis, Tenn., USA). Excluding those with significant ligament instability, the analysis included 113 knees operated on by a single surgeon. The surgical approach varied between mini-midvastus and lateral approaches depending on deformity type, with techniques evolving from conventional instrumentation to CT-less navigation for improved precision. Follow-ups were conducted at regular intervals up to several years postoperatively, assessing complications and revision rates. Statistical analyses were performed to identify predictors of complications and revisions, considering factors such as patient demographics and surgical techniques.

The findings revealed an overall joint-based complication rate of 10.3%, with midflexion instability being the most common issue leading to revisions. The study noted a learning curve effect, with higher complication rates in the initial treatment year that decreased over time. Despite using advanced navigation techniques, no significant reduction in complication rates was observed compared to conventional methods. The study highlights that while the Journey BCS system aims for improved kinematics, it presents higher complication and revision rates than established systems. Future study could focus on refining surgical techniques or exploring alternative designs to enhance outcomes for patients undergoing TKR with this system.

Bibliography

1. Ward TR, Burns AW, Gillespie MJ, Scarvell JM, Smith PN: Bicruciate-stabilised total knee replacements produce more normal sagittal plane kinematics than posterior-stabilised designs. J Bone Joint Surg Br. 2011, 93: 907-913.
2. Luyckx L, Luyckx T, Bellemans J, Victor J: Iliotibial band traction syndrome in guided motion TKA. A new clinical entity after TKA. Acta Orthop Belg. 2010, 76: 507-512.
3. van Duren BH, Pandit H, Price M, Tilley S, Gill HS, Murray DW, Thomas NP: Bicruciate substituting total knee replacement: how effective are the added kinematic constraints in vivo?. Knee Surg Sports Traumatol Arthrosc. 2012, 20 (10): 2002-2010. https://doi.org/10.1007/s00167-011-1796-2.
4. Catani F, Ensini A, Belvedere C, Feliciangeli A, Benedetti MG, Leardini A, Giannini S: In vivo kinematics and kinetics of a bi-cruciate substituting total knee arthroplasty: a combined fluoroscopic and gait analysis study. J Orthop Res. 2009, 27: 1569-1575. 10.1002/jor.20941.
5. Christen, Bernhard; Neukamp, Michal; Aghayev, Emin Consecutive series of 226 journey bicruciate substituting total knee replacements: early complication and revision rates. BMC Musculoskeletal Disorders (2014). https://doi.org/10.1186/1471-2474-15-395

4.5 Bicruciate Retaining

Machine Generated Summaries

Disclaimer: The summaries in this chapter were generated from Springer Nature publications using abstractive AI auto-summarization: An abstraction-based summarizer creates new text based on deep learning. New phrases are created to summarize the content. As the constituted sentences are machine selected, they may not fully reflect the body of the work, so we strongly advise that the original content is read and cited. The auto-generated summaries were curated by the editor to meet Springer Nature publication standards.

4.5.1 In Vivo Kinematics and Cruciate Ligament Forces in Bicruciate-Retaining Total Knee Arthroplasty [64]

This is a machine-generated summary of:

Kono, Kenichi; Inui, Hiroshi; Tomita, Tetsuya; Yamazaki, Takaharu; Konda, Shoji; Taketomi, Shuji; Tanaka, Sakae; D'Lima, Darryl D. In vivo kinematics and cruciate ligament forces in bicruciate-retaining total knee arthroplasty [64].

Published in: Scientific Reports (2021).

Link to original: https://doi.org/10.1038/s41598-021-84942-y

If you want to cite the papers, please refer to the original.

For technical reasons we could not place the page where the original quote is coming from.

4.5.1.1 Research Highlights

Osteoarthritis (OA) of the knee significantly alters knee kinematics, and while total knee arthroplasty (TKA) can alleviate pain, it often fails to restore normal knee movement. Traditional TKA designs, which sacrifice the anterior cruciate ligament (ACL), do not fully replicate natural knee kinematics. Bicruciate-retaining total knee arthroplasty (BCR-TKA) aims to address this by preserving both cruciate ligaments, potentially improving stability and function. However, the impact of BCR-TKA on knee kinematics and cruciate ligament forces during high-flexion activities remains unclear. The study by Kono et al. investigates these effects, focusing on the relationship between knee kinematics and cruciate ligament forces during specific high-flexion activities.

The study involved patients undergoing BCR-TKA for bicompartmental or tricompartmental OA with an intact ACL. Researchers used fluoroscopic imaging to record knee kinematics during closed-kinetic chain deep knee bends and open-kinetic chain high-flexion activities both pre- and postoperatively. The analysis included measuring femoral rotation, varus-valgus angulation, and anteroposterior translation of the femoral condyles relative to the tibia. Cruciate ligament forces were calculated using a nonlinear force-strain model based on the relative movement of bony attachment points during flexion. The study found that BCR-TKA altered femoral external rotation and anteroposterior translation patterns during flexion, with significant changes in varus-valgus angulation observed during squatting.

The findings suggest that BCR-TKA can modify knee kinematics in ways that correlate with changes in cruciate ligament forces, potentially improving clinical outcomes. The study highlights that different high-flexion activities affect ACL forces differently, with squatting inducing greater femoral external rotation compared to cross-legged sitting. Future study could explore long-term effects of BCR-TKA on kinematics and ligament forces beyond the short follow-up period of this research. These insights are valuable for refining BCR-TKA designs and developing strategies for optimal ligament balancing in surgical practice.

4.5.2 CORR Insights®: Higher Frequency of Reoperation with a New Bicruciate-Retaining Total Knee Arthroplasty [65]

This is a machine-generated summary of:

Colwell, Clifford W. CORR Insights®: Higher Frequency of Reoperation With a New Bicruciate-retaining Total Knee Arthroplasty [65].

Published in: Clinical Orthopaedics and Related Research® (2016).

Link to original: https://doi.org/10.1007/s11999-016-4872-6

If you want to cite the papers, please refer to the original.
For technical reasons we could not place the page where the original quote is coming from.

4.5.2.1 Research Highlights

Total knee replacement (TKR) surgeries are common, yet many patients report dissatisfaction due to unnatural knee kinematics resulting from standard prostheses. Traditional cruciate-retaining or cruciate-substituting implants may not mimic natural knee movement, prompting researchers to explore alternative designs. Now, a new study by Clifford W. Colwell and colleagues investigates the efficacy of a bicruciate-retaining prosthesis compared to a standard posterior cruciate-retaining implant. The study found that patients with the new implant had a higher likelihood of reoperation and longer surgery times, without significant improvements in clinical outcomes or range of motion.

The study conducted by Christensen and colleagues involved a large comparative analysis between the new bicruciate-retaining prosthesis and the standard posterior cruciate-retaining device. Despite the innovative approach, the results indicated that the new implant did not enhance patient outcomes as anticipated. The research faced limitations such as non-randomized patient selection, which could have influenced the results. Additionally, it remains unclear whether the increased reoperation risk and extended surgery duration were due to a surgical learning curve or an inherent flaw in the prosthesis design. The authors commendably reported these findings, emphasizing that the new prosthesis should not replace standard options at this time.

Future study directions include conducting randomized clinical trials to better assess the potential benefits of bicruciate-retaining prostheses. Such trials should involve surgeons experienced with the new device to mitigate learning curve effects and focus on evaluating patient-reported outcomes over various timeframes. Additionally, initial cadaveric studies under dynamic load conditions could provide insights into kinematic improvements before proceeding to human trials. These efforts aim to determine whether bicruciate-retaining designs can match or surpass the long-term success rates of existing TKR implants, ultimately improving patient satisfaction and outcomes in knee replacement surgeries.

4.5.3 Short-Term Clinical Results of Bicruciate-Retaining Total Knee Arthroplasty Using Personalized Alignment [66]

This is a machine-generated summary of:

Inui, Hiroshi; Yamagami, Ryota; Kono, Kenichi; Kawaguchi, Kohei; Kage, Tomofumi; Murakami, Ryo; Nakamura, Haruhiko; Saita, Kazuo; Taketomi, Shuji; Tanaka, Sakae Short-term clinical results of bicruciate-retaining total knee arthroplasty using personalized alignment [66].

Published in: BMC Musculoskeletal Disorders (2023).

Link to original: https://doi.org/10.1186/s12891-023-07083-5

If you want to cite the papers, please refer to the original.

For technical reasons we could not place the page where the original quote is coming from.

4.5.3.1 Research Highlights

Total knee arthroplasty (TKA) is the standard treatment for late-stage osteoarthritis, yet a significant percentage of patients remain dissatisfied with their surgically restored knees. Recent efforts have focused on improving knee prosthesis designs to enhance clinical outcomes and patient satisfaction, with bicruciate-retaining (BCR) prostheses being introduced to preserve both the anterior and posterior cruciate ligaments. While some studies suggest BCR TKAs may offer advantages over traditional ACL-sacrificing TKAs, the evidence remains mixed, with reports of similar clinical outcomes and higher complication rates. The study by Inui et al. explores the use of personalized alignment in BCR TKA to improve outcomes by comparing it with unicompartmental knee arthroplasty (UKA).

The study conducted by Inui et al. was a retrospective case-control analysis involving patients who underwent either PA-BCR TKA or UKA using an image-free navigation system. The surgical indications for each procedure were carefully defined, and all patients had a minimum follow-up period of 1 year. The research team meticulously recorded preoperative demographics and clinical scores using standardized scoring systems. Surgical procedures were performed by experienced surgeons employing a consistent technique, focusing on precise bone resection and soft tissue balance. Postoperative evaluations included radiographic assessments and clinical outcome measures such as range of motion and Knee Society Scores. Statistical analyses were performed to compare joint laxity and clinical outcomes between the two groups.

The study found that PA-BCR TKA achieved comparable or slightly superior short-term clinical outcomes compared to UKA, with significant improvements in patient expectation scores and maximum extension angles. The use of personalized alignment may contribute to these positive results by ensuring appropriate soft tissue balance, particularly moderate lateral joint laxity, which is crucial for successful BCR TKA outcomes. Future study could focus on long-term evaluations to confirm these findings and further refine surgical techniques to optimize patient satisfaction and functional results. Additionally, exploring larger patient cohorts could provide more robust data to support the widespread adoption of PA-BCR TKA in clinical practice.

4.5.4 Does Contemporary Bicruciate Retaining Total Knee Arthroplasty Restore the Native Knee Kinematics? A Descriptive Literature Review [67]

This is a machine-generated summary of:

Zhou, Chaochao; Peng, Yun; An, Shuai; Bedair, Hany; Li, Guoan Does contemporary bicruciate retaining total knee arthroplasty restore the native knee kinematics? A descriptive literature review [67].

Published in: Archives of Orthopaedic and Trauma Surgery (2021).

Link to original: https://doi.org/10.1007/s00402-021-04116-3

If you want to cite the papers, please refer to the original.

For technical reasons we could not place the page where the original quote is coming from.

4.5.4.1 Research Highlights

Total knee arthroplasty (TKA) is a widely performed procedure for patients with severe knee arthritis, yet approximately 20% of patients remain dissatisfied post-surgery. This dissatisfaction has spurred the development of new TKA designs aimed at restoring native knee kinematics. The anterior cruciate ligament (ACL) plays a crucial role in knee kinematics, and most TKAs involve sacrificing or substituting the ACL and posterior cruciate ligament (PCL). The bicruciate retaining (BCR) TKA, which retains both ligaments, offers a promising alternative to achieve native knee kinematics and potentially improve patient satisfaction. However, despite its potential benefits, BCR TKA has not gained widespread acceptance due to mixed evidence regarding its outcomes. The study by Zhou et al. provides an updated review of the kinematics of modern BCR TKA systems.

The study conducted a comprehensive literature search using databases such as PubMed and Web of Science to gather data on BCR TKA systems from 2010 onwards. The inclusion criteria focused on studies reporting at least one kinematic parameter during knee flexion for BCR systems. After screening, five in vitro cadaveric studies and six in vivo clinical studies were included for analysis. The review identified two main BCR TKA systems: the Vanguard XP and Journey II XR (Vanguard XP is Zimmer-Biomet, Warsaw, Indiana, USA, the Journey XR is Smith and Nephew, Memphis, Tenn., USA). In vitro studies showed that BCR TKAs exhibited low internal rotation throughout flexion compared to native knees, with significant differences during early and late flexion phases. In vivo studies revealed that native knee kinematics were not fully restored after BCR TKA during various activities, with asymmetric kinematics observed during gait cycles.

The findings suggest that while BCR TKA systems show promise in mimicking native knee kinematics, they do not fully restore them. Future study could focus on more challenging activities beyond level walking to better capture differences between BCR TKAs and normal knees. Additionally, the tibial component's influence on kinematics highlights the importance of implant design choices. The role of the ACL in maintaining joint stability is confirmed, suggesting that preserving its function is crucial in BCR TKA procedures. Further research is needed to explore these aspects and refine BCR TKA designs to enhance their ability to replicate natural knee movement fully.

4.5.5 Reduced Joint-Awareness in Bicruciate-Retaining Total Knee Arthroplasty Compared to Cruciate-Sacrificing Total Knee Arthroplasty [68]

This is a machine-generated summary of:

Baumann, Florian; Krutsch, Werner; Worlicek, Michael; Kerschbaum, Maximilian; Zellner, Johannes; Schmitz, Paul; Nerlich, Michael; Tibesku, Carsten

Reduced joint-awareness in bicruciate-retaining total knee arthroplasty compared to cruciate-sacrificing total knee arthroplasty [68].

Published in: Archives of Orthopaedic and Trauma Surgery (2017).

Link to original: https://doi.org/10.1007/s00402-017-2839-z

If you want to cite the papers, please refer to the original.

For technical reasons we could not place the page where the original quote is coming from.

4.5.5.1 Research Highlights

In recent years, patient-reported outcome measurements (PROMs) have gained prominence in evaluating the quality of life following joint arthroplasty, particularly in knee surgeries. Traditional questionnaires often emphasize functional aspects such as range of motion and ligament stability. However, the "Forgotten Joint Score" (FJS) has emerged as a revolutionary tool, focusing on the patient's ability to forget the presence of an artificial joint, which is considered the pinnacle of patient satisfaction. Despite its proven validity and reliability post-total knee arthroplasty (TKA), there remains a gap in understanding how bicruciate-retaining total knee arthroplasty (BCR-TKA) affects PROMs compared to other surgical options. The study by Baumann et al. addresses this gap by comparing PROMs in patients undergoing BCR-TKA with those receiving medial unicompartmental knee arthroplasty (UKA) and standard TKA that sacrifices both cruciate ligaments.

The study was conducted as a prospective, controlled trial involving patients who underwent knee arthroplasty for advanced osteoarthritis. Participants were divided into three groups: those receiving BCR-TKA, medial UKA, and posterior-stabilized TKA. Preoperative assessments included medical history, clinical examination, and radiographic analysis. The BCR implant used was designed to retain both cruciate ligaments with specific structural features to enhance strength and stability. Postoperative care was standardized across all groups, including analgesia, physiotherapy, and routine follow-ups. The primary outcome measure was the FJS at 12 months postoperatively. Statistical analyses were performed using SPSS software to compare mean FJS values among the groups.

The study found that patients with BCR-TKA reported significantly reduced joint awareness compared to those with standard TKA, aligning their scores more closely with those of the UKA group. This suggests that preserving both cruciate ligaments may enhance proprioception and patient satisfaction. While these findings are promising, the authors note that further research is needed to explore long-term outcomes and survivorship of BCR implants. Future study could focus on randomized trials comparing BCR-TKA with standard implants to better understand the impact of ligament preservation on joint perception and overall patient satisfaction in knee osteoarthritis treatment.

4.5.6 Bicruciate-Retaining Total Knee Replacement Provides Satisfactory Function and Implant Survivorship at 23 Years [69]

This is a machine-generated summary of:

Pritchett, James W. Bicruciate-retaining Total Knee Replacement Provides Satisfactory Function and Implant Survivorship at 23 Years [69].

Published in: Clinical Orthopaedics and Related Research® (2015).

Link to original: https://doi.org/10.1007/s11999-015-4219-8

If you want to cite the papers, please refer to the original.

For technical reasons we could not place the page where the original quote is coming from.

4.5.6.1 Research Highlights

Normal knee function relies on smooth, uninterrupted motion, which is facilitated by stable, well-lubricated, low-friction articular surfaces. Traditional knee replacement surgeries often involve the removal of one or both cruciate ligaments, which can compromise the natural movement of the knee. To address this issue, a bicruciate-retaining knee prosthesis was developed to preserve these ligaments, minimize bone resection, and limit constraint, thereby allowing more natural knee movement. Despite the potential benefits of bicruciate-retaining total knee arthroplasty (TKA), few studies have evaluated its long-term performance and durability. The study by Pritchett et al. investigates the functional results and reasons for revision of bicruciate-retaining knee arthroplasty over a 10-year period.

The study involved 216 patients who underwent TKA with a bicruciate-retaining prosthesis between January 2003 and September 2010. Patients were selected based on having an intact anterior cruciate ligament (ACL) and acceptable deformity. The surgical technique emphasized ligamentous balancing without recessing the ACL or posterior cruciate ligament (PCL). The tibial component was placed with slight external rotation to align with ACL fibers, and patellar resurfacing was performed for all patients. The study assessed range of motion (ROM), laxity, and American Knee Society scores at regular follow-ups over a minimum of 10 years. Radiographs were used to monitor implant failure signs such as wear and loosening. The Kaplan-Meier survivorship analysis showed an implant survival rate of 88% at a mean follow-up of 10 years. Improvements were noted in postoperative flexion and Knee Society scores compared to preoperative values.

The study found that the bicruciate-retaining prosthesis provided satisfactory long-term survivorship and function, with a low rate of complications such as polyethylene wear being the most common reason for revision. While preserving both cruciate ligaments may offer more natural kinematics compared to other prostheses, the procedure is technically demanding and requires meticulous surgical technique to avoid complications like intraoperative ACL rupture or tibial eminence fracture. Future studies using validated patient-reported outcomes are recommended to further assess the appropriateness of retaining both cruciates during TKA in selected patients. This research contributes valuable insights into the potential benefits and challenges associated with bicruciate-retaining knee arthroplasty.

4.5.7 Early Outcomes of a Novel Bicruciate-Retaining Knee System: a 2-Year Minimum Retrospective Cohort Study [70]

This is a machine-generated summary of:

Singh, Vivek; Yeroushalmi, David; Christensen, Thomas H.; Bieganowski, Thomas; Tang, Alex; Schwarzkopf, Ran Early outcomes of a novel bicruciate-retaining knee system: a 2-year minimum retrospective cohort study [70].

Published in: Archives of Orthopaedic and Trauma Surgery (2022).

Link to original: https://doi.org/10.1007/s00402-022-04351-2

If you want to cite the papers, please refer to the original.

For technical reasons we could not place the page where the original quote is coming from.

4.5.7.1 Research Highlights

Total knee arthroplasty (TKA) is a widely successful procedure, yet a significant percentage of patients remain dissatisfied with their knee replacements. To address this issue, bicruciate-retaining (BCR) TKA designs have been developed to better mimic natural knee kinematics by retaining both the anterior and posterior cruciate ligaments. Previous studies suggest that BCR TKA may offer advantages over traditional TKA systems but concerns about implant survivorship and technical challenges have persisted. The study by Singh et al. evaluates the short-term functional outcomes and implant survivorship of a novel BCR design aimed at overcoming these limitations.

The study was conducted as a multi-institutional, retrospective analysis involving patients who underwent primary TKA using the novel BCR implant across ten institutions. This implant combines a kinematic femoral design with a unique tibial component that retains both cruciate ligaments, featuring an asymmetric notch and independently designed medial and lateral inserts for improved fixation and strength. The study included patients with at least 2 years of follow-up data, excluding those with severe deformities or inadequate follow-up. Data on patient demographics, surgical details, and outcomes were collected from electronic medical records. Outcomes assessed included operative time, length of stay, complications, readmissions, reoperations, and patient-reported outcome measures such as the Knee Injury and Osteoarthritis Outcome Score (KOOS).

The novel BCR design demonstrated promising short-term results with a high survival rate for aseptic implant revision and mechanical failure at 2 years postoperatively. The study reported no cases of aseptic loosening or polyethylene wear, addressing previous concerns about tibial component fixation. While these early results are encouraging, the authors acknowledge limitations such as the retrospective design and limited follow-up duration. Future studies should focus on long-term outcomes to fully assess the durability of this BCR system. Additionally, further research could explore outcomes in patients with specific preoperative conditions to refine patient selection criteria for this implant.

4.5.8 *Early Results with a Bicruciate-Retaining Total Knee Arthroplasty: A Match-Paired Study [71]*

This is a machine-generated summary of:

Biazzo, Alessio; D'Ambrosi, Riccardo; Staals, Eric; Masia, Francesco; Izzo, Vincenzo; Verde, Francesco Early results with a bicruciate-retaining total knee arthroplasty: a match-paired study [71].

Published in: European Journal of Orthopaedic Surgery & Traumatology (2020).

Link to original: https://doi.org/10.1007/s00590-020-02834-9

If you want to cite the papers, please refer to the original.

For technical reasons we could not place the page where the original quote is coming from.

4.5.8.1 Research Highlights

Reproducing the anatomy and kinematics of the knee is a critical goal in total knee arthroplasty (TKA) to enhance patient satisfaction and improve long-term outcomes. Previous studies have shown that preserving the anterior cruciate ligament (ACL) during TKA can restore normal knee function, as the ACL contains proprioceptive nerve cells crucial for proprioception. Despite promising results from early adopters like Cloutier and Prichett, the technical challenges of bicruciate-retaining

(BCR) TKA have limited its widespread adoption. The study by Biazzo et al. compares BCR-TKA with conventional cruciate-retaining (CR) TKA to evaluate short-term functional outcomes.

The study involved a retrospective review of patients who underwent TKA between February and December, with some receiving BCR implants and others CR implants. The inclusion criteria for BCR included intact ACLs and no history of ACL injury, while CR criteria allowed for partial or total ACL degeneration. The researchers used clinical evaluations such as the visual analogue score (VAS) and the Western Ontario and McMaster Universities Osteoarthritis Index (WOMAC), along with radiological assessments, to compare outcomes between the two groups. Surgical techniques varied slightly between BCR and CR procedures, particularly in how the tibial component was handled to preserve or sacrifice the ACL.

The study found no statistically significant differences in functional or radiological outcomes between BCR and CR groups, although BCR procedures had longer operative times. Complications were more frequent in the BCR group, primarily due to aseptic loosening of the tibial component. These findings suggest that while BCR-TKA can achieve similar short-term outcomes to CR-TKA, it presents challenges such as increased surgical complexity and higher complication rates. Future studies could focus on refining surgical techniques and improving implant designs to address these issues, potentially enhancing the viability of BCR-TKA as a standard practice in knee arthroplasty.

Bibliography

1. Okada, Y. *et al.* ACL function in bicruciate-retaining total knee arthroplasty. *J. Bone Jt. Surg. Am. 100*, e114. https://doi.org/10.2106/jbjs.18.00099 (2018).
2. Tsai, T. Y. *et al.* Bi-cruciate retaining total knee arthroplasty does not restore native tibiofemoral articular contact kinematics during gait. *J. Orthop. Res. Off. Publ. Orthop. Res. Soc. 37*, 1929–1937. https://doi.org/10.1002/jor.24333 (2019).
3. Kono, K. *et al.* In vivo kinematics of bicruciate-retaining total knee arthroplasty with anatomical articular surface under high-flexion conditions. *J. Knee Surg.* https://doi.org/10.1055/s-0039-1696959 (2019).
4. Kono, K. *et al.* Bicruciate-retaining total knee arthroplasty reproduces in vivo kinematics of normal knees to a lower extent than unicompartmental knee arthroplasty. *Knee Surg. Sports Traumatol. Arthrosc. Off. J. ESSKA* https://doi.org/10.1007/s00167-019-05754-2 (2019).
5. Arauz, P., Klemt, C., Limmahakhun, S., An, S. and Kwon, Y. M. Stair climbing and high knee flexion activities in Bi-cruciate retaining total knee arthroplasty: in vivo kinematics and articular contact analysis. *J. Arthroplast. 34*, 570–576. https://doi.org/10.1016/j.arth.2018.11.013 (2018).
6. Kono K, Tomita T, Futai K, Yamazaki T, Tanaka S, Yoshikawa H, Sugamoto K (2018) In vivo three-dimensional kinematics of normal knees during different high-flexion activities. Bone Joint J 100-B(1):50–55. https://doi.org/10.1302/0301-620X.100B1.BJJ-2017-0553.R2

7. Patil S, Colwell CW Jr, Ezzet KA, D'Lima DD. Can normal knee kinematics be restored with unicompartmental knee replacement? *J Bone Joint Surg Am.* 2005;87:332–338.
8. Patil S, McCauley JC, Pulido P, Colwell CW Jr. How do knee implants perform past the second decade? Nineteen- to 25-year followup of the press-fit condylar design TKA. *Clin Orthop Rel Res.* 2015;473:135–140.
9. American Joint Replacement Registry. AJRR publishes annual report on data from its registry. Available at: http://www.ajrr.net/media-news/press--releases/239-ajrr-publishes-annual-report-on-data-from-its-registry. Accessed April 27, 2016.
10. Callaghan JJ, Martin CT, Gao Y, Pugely AJ, Liu SS, Goetz DD, Kelley SS, Johnston RC. What can be learned from minimum 20-year followup studies of knee arthroplasty? *Clin Orthop Relat Res.* 2015;473:94–100.
11. Christensen JC, Brothers J, Stoddard GJ, Anderson MB, Pelt CE, Gililland JM, Peters CL. Higher frequency of reoperation with a new bicruciate-retaining total knee arthroplasty. Clin Orthop Relat Res. 2017;475(1):62–9. https://doi.org/10.1007/s11999-016-4812-5.
12. Perreault C, Al-Shakfa F, Lavoie F. Complications of bicruciate-retaining total knee arthroplasty: the importance of alignment and balance. J Knee Surg. https://doi.org/10.1055/a-2037-6261. Online ahead of print.
13. Boese CK, Ebohon S, Ries C, De Faoite D. Bi-cruciate retaining total knee arthroplasty: a systematic literature review of clinical outcomes. Arch Orthop Trauma Surg. 2021;141(2):293–304. https://doi.org/10.1007/s00402-020-03622-0.
14. Lavoie F, Denis A, Chergui S, Al-Shakfa F, Sabouret P. Bicruciate-retaining total knee arthroplasty non-inferior to posterior-stabilized prostheses after 5 years: a randomized, controlled trial. Knee Surg Sports Traumatol Arthrosc. 2023;31(3):1034–42. https://doi.org/10.1007/s00167-022-07210-0.
15. Biazzo A, D'Ambrosi R, Staals E, Masia F, Izzo V, Verde F. Early results with a bicruciate-retaining total knee arthroplasty: a match-paired study. Eur J Orthop Surg Traumatol. 2021;31(4):785–90. https://doi.org/10.1007/s00590-020-02834-9.
16. Inui H, Yamagami R, Kono K, Kawaguchi K, Sameshima S, Kage T, Tanaka T, Taketomi S, Tanaka S. Comparison of the joint laxity of total knee arthroplasty evaluated by the distraction force and the varus-valgus force. Knee. 2022;34:98–107. https://doi.org/10.1016/j.knee.2021.10.019.
17. Lustig S, Sappey-Marinier E, Fary C, Servien E, Parratte S, Batailler C. Personalized alignment in total knee arthroplasty: current concepts. SICOT J. 2021;7:19. https://doi.org/10.1051/sicotj/2021021.
18. Baumann F, Bahadin Ö, Krutsch W, Zellner J, Nerlich M, Angele P, Tibesku CO. Proprioception after bicruciate-retaining total knee arthroplasty is comparable to unicompartmental knee arthroplasty. Knee Surg Sports Traumatol Arthrosc. 2017;25(6):1697–704. https://doi.org/10.1007/s00167-016-4121-2.

19. Okazaki K, Miura H, Matsuda S, Takeuchi N, Mawatari T, Hashizume M, Iwamoto Y. Asymmetry of mediolateral laxity of the normal knee. J Orthop Sci. 2006;11:264–6.
20. Kaneko T, Mochizuki Y, Hada M, Toyoda S, Takada K, Ikegami H, Musha Y. Greater postoperative relatively medial loose gap at 90 of flexion for varus knees improves patient-reported outcome measurements in anatomical bi-cruciate retaining total knee arthroplasty. Knee. 2020;27:1534–41. https://doi.org/10.1016/j.knee.2020.08.005.
21. Takasago T, Hamada D, Wada K, Nitta A, Tamaki Y, Goto T, Tsuruo Y, Sairyo K. Insufficient lateral joint laxity after bicruciate-retaining total knee arthroplasty potentially influences kinematics during flexion: A biomechanical cadaveric study. Knee. 2021;28:311–8. https://doi.org/10.1016/j.knee.2020.12.008.
22. Matsumoto T, Takayama K, Ishida K, Kuroda Y, Tsubosaka M, Muratsu H, Hayashi S, Hashimoto S, Matsushita T, Niikura T, Kuroda R. Intraoperative Soft Tissue Balance/Kinematics and Clinical Evaluation of Modified Kinematically versus Mechanically Aligned Total Knee Arthroplasty. J Knee Surg. 2020;33(8):777–84. https://doi.org/10.1055/s-0039-1688504.
23. Wada K, Hamada D, Takasago T, Nitta A, Goto T, Tonogai I, Tsuruo Y, Sairyo K (2019) The medial constrained insert restores native knee rotational kinematics after bicruciate-retaining total knee arthroplasty. Knee Surg Sports Traumatol Arthrosc 27(5):1621–1627. https://doi.org/10.1007/s00167-018-5249-z
24. Hamada, D. *et al.* Native rotational knee kinematics are lost in bicruciate-retaining total knee arthroplasty when the tibial component is replaced. *Knee Surg. Sports Traumatol. Arthrosc. Off. J. ESSKA 26*, 3249–3256. https://doi.org/10.1007/s00167-018-4842-5 (2018).
25. Arauz P, Peng Y, Kwon YM (2018) Knee motion symmetry was not restored in patients with unilateral bi-cruciate retaining total knee arthroplasty-in vivo three-dimensional kinematic analysis. Int Orthop 42(12):2817–2823. https://doi.org/10.1007/s00264-018-3986-8
26. Zumbrunn T, Varadarajan KM, Rubash HE, Malchau H, Li G, Muratoglu OK. Regaining native knee kinematics following joint arthroplasty: A novel biomimetic design with ACL and PCL preservation. J Arthroplasty. 2015;30(12):2143–8. https://doi.org/10.1016/j.arth.2015.06.017.
27. Baumann F, Ernstberger T, Loibl M, Zeman F, Nerlich M, Tibesku C (2016) Validation of the German Forgotten Joint Score (G-FJS) according to the COSMIN checklist: does a reduction in joint awareness indicate clinical improvement after arthroplasty of the knee? Arch Orthop Trauma Surg 136(2):257–264. https://doi.org/10.1007/s00402-015-2372-x
28. Behrend H, Giesinger K, Giesinger JM, Kuster MS (2012) The "forgotten joint" as the ultimate goal in joint arthroplasty: validation of a new patient-reported outcome measure. J Arthroplasty 27:430-436 e1
29. Cao S, Liu N, Han W, Zi Y, Peng F, Li L, Fu Q, Chen Y, Zheng W, Qian Q (2017) Simplified Chinese version of the Forgotten Joint Score (FJS) for patients who underwent joint arthroplasty: cross-cultural adaptation and validation. J Orthop Surg Res 12(1):6. https://doi.org/10.1186/s13018-016-0508-5

30. Shadid MB, Vinken NS, Marting LN, Wolterbeek N (2016) The Dutch version of the Forgotten Joint Score: test–retesting reliability and validation. Acta Orthop Belg 82(1):112–118
31. Thienpont E, Opsomer G, Koninckx A, Houssiau F (2014) Joint awareness in different types of knee arthroplasty evaluated with the Forgotten Joint Score. J Arthroplasty 29:48–51
32. Thomsen MG, Latifi R, Kallemose T, Husted H, Troelsen A (2016) Does knee awareness differ between different knee arthroplasty prostheses? A matched, case-control, cross-sectional study. BMC Musculoskelet Disord 17:141. https://doi.org/10.1186/s12891-016-1001-3
33. Fuchs S, Frisse D, Tibesku CO, Laass H, Rosenbaum D (2002) Proprioceptive function, clinical results, and quality of life after unicondylar sledge prostheses. Am J Phys Med Rehabil Assoc Acad Physiatr 81(7):478–482
34. Komistek RD, Allain J, Anderson DT, Dennis DA, Goutallier D (2002) In vivo kinematics for subjects with and without an anterior cruciate ligament. Clin Orthop Relat Res 404:315–325
35. Peersman G, Slane J, Dirckx M, Vandevyver A, Dworschak P, Heyse TJ, Scheys L (2017) The influence of polyethylene bearing thickness on the tibiofemoral kinematics of a bicruciate retaining total knee arthroplasty. Knee 24(4):751–760. https://doi.org/10.1016/j.knee.2017.03.010
36. Ward TR, Burns AW, Gillespie MJ, Scarvell JM, Smith PN: Bicruciate-stabilised total knee replacements produce more normal sagittal plane kinematics than posterior-stabilised designs. J Bone Joint Surg Br. 2011, 93: 907-913.
37. Cloutier JM (1983) Results of total knee arthroplasty with a non-constrained prosthesis. J Bone Joint Surg Am 65(7):906–919
38. Lombardi AV (2015) THE BI-CRUCIATE RETAINING TKA: "A THING OF BEAUTY IS A JOY FOREVER"—AFFIRMS. Bone Jt J Orthop Proc Suppl 97-B(SUPP 1):69
39. Moro-oka, T. A., Muenchinger, M., Canciani, J. P. and Banks, S. A. Comparing in vivo kinematics of anterior cruciate-retaining and posterior cruciate-retaining total knee arthroplasty. *Knee Surg. Sports Traumatol. Arthrosc. Off. J. ESSKA 15*, 93–99. https://doi.org/10.1007/s00167-006-0134-6 (2007).
40. Zuiderbaan HA, van der List JP, Khamaisy S, Nawabi DH, Thein R, Ishmael C, Paul S, Pearle AD (2017) Unicompartmental knee arthroplasty versus total knee arthroplasty: Which type of artificial joint do patients forget? Knee Surg Sports Traumatol Arthrosc 3:681–686. https://doi.org/10.1007/s00167-015-3868-1
41. Townley CO. Total knee arthroplasty: a personal retrospective and prospective review. *Clin Orthop Relat Res*. 1988;236:8–22.
42. Sabouret, P., Lavoie, F. and Cloutier, J. M. Total knee replacement with retention of both cruciate ligaments: a 22-year follow-up study. *Bone Jt. J. 95-b*, 917–922. https://doi.org/10.1302/0301-620x.95b7.30904 (2013).
43. Howell SM, Howell SJ, Kuznik KT, Cohen J, Hull ML. Does a kinematically aligned total knee athroplasty restore function without failure regardless of alignment category? *Clin Orthop Relat Res.* 2013;471:1000–1007.

44. Barrington JW, Sah A, Malchau H, Burke DW. Contemporary cruciate-retaining total knee arthroplasty with a pegged tibial baseplate: results at a minimum of ten years. *J Bone Joint Surg Am.* 2009;91:874–878.
45. Insall JN, Dorr LD, Scott RD, Scott WN. Rationale of the Knee Society clinical rating system. *Clin Orthop Relat Res.* 1989;248:13–14.
46. Pritchett JW (2011) Patients prefer a bicruciate-retaining or the medial pivot total kncc prosthesis. J Arthroplasty 26:224–228. https://doi.org/10.1016/j.arth.2010.02.012
47. Pritchett JW. J Bone Joint Surg Br. 2004;86(7):979–82. https://doi.org/10.1302/0301-620x.86b7.14991.
48. Barrett TJ, Shi L, Parsley BS (2017) Bicruciate-retaining total knee arthroplasty, a promising technology, that's not quite there. Ann Transl Med 5(Suppl 1):S17. https://doi.org/10.21037/atm.2017.03.77
49. Halewood, C., Traynor, A., Bellemans, J., Victor, J. and Amis, A. A. Anteroposterior laxity after bicruciate-retaining total knee arthroplasty is closer to the native knee than ACL-resecting TKA: a biomechanical cadaver study. *J. Arthroplast. 30*, 2315–2319. https://doi.org/10.1016/j.arth.2015.06.021 (2015).
50. Wodowski AJ, Swigler CW, Liu H, Nord KM, Toy PC, Mihalko WM (2016) Proprioception and knee arthroplasty: a literature review. Orthop Clin N Am 47(2):301–309. https://doi.org/10.1016/j.ocl.2015.09.005
51. Stiehl, J. B., Komistek, R. D., Cloutier, J. M. and Dennis, D. A. The cruciate ligaments in total knee arthroplasty: a kinematic analysis of 2 total knee arthroplasties. *J. Arthroplast. 15*, 545–550 (2000).
52. Pritchett, J. W. Bicruciate-retaining total knee replacement provides satisfactory function and implant survivorship at 23 years. *Clin. Orthop. Relat. Res. 473*, 2327–2333. https://doi.org/10.1007/s11999-015-4219-8 (2015).
53. Pelt CE, Sandifer PA, Gililland JM, Anderson MB, Peters CL (2019) Mean three-year survivorship of a new bicruciate-retaining total knee arthroplasty: are revisions still higher than expected? J Arthroplasty 34(9):1957–1962. https://doi.org/10.1016/j.arth.2019.04.030
54. Osmani FA, Thakkar SC, Collins K, Schwarzkopf R (2017) The utility of bicruciate-retaining total knee arthroplasty. Arthroplast Today 3(1):61–66. https://doi.org/10.1016/j.artd.2016.11.004
55. Cloutier JM, Sabouret P, Deghrar A (1999) Total knee arthroplasty with retention of both cruciate ligaments. A nine to eleven-year follow-up study. J Bone Jt Surg Am Vol 81(5):697–702
56. Haefeli M, Elfering A (2006) Pain assessment. Eur Spine J 15:S17-24. https://doi.org/10.1007/s00586-005-1044-x
57. Salaffi F, Leardini G, Canesi B, Mannoni A, Fioravanti A, Caporali R, Lapadula G, Punzi L; GOnorthrosis and Quality Of Life Assessment (GOQOLA) (2003) Reliability and validity of the Western Ontario and McMaster universities (WOMAC) osteoarthritis index in Italian patients with osteoarthritis of the knee. Osteoarthr Cartil 11:551–560. https://doi.org/10.1016/s1063-4584(03)00089-x

58. Klemt C, Drago J, Oganesyan R, Smith EJ, Yeo I, Kwon YM (2020) Gait and knee flexion in vivo kinematics of asymmetric tibial polyethylene geometry cruciate retaining total knee arthroplasty. J Knee Surg. https://doi.org/10.1055/s-0040-1718681
59. Koh IJ, Chalmers CE, Lin CC, Park SB, McGarry MH, Lee TQ (2020) Posterior stabilized total knee arthroplasty reproduces natural joint laxity compared to normal in kinematically aligned total knee arthroplasty: a matched pair cadaveric study. Arch Orthop Trauma Surg. https://doi.org/10.1007/s00402-020-03624-y
60. Zhang Q, Chen Z, Zhang Z, Jin Z, Muratoglu OK, Varadarajan KM (2020) Leveraging subject-specific musculoskeletal modeling to assess effect of anterior cruciate ligament retaining total knee arthroplasty during walking gait. Proc Inst Mech Eng H. https://doi.org/10.1177/0954411920947204
61. Parcells BW, Tria AJ Jr (2016) The cruciate ligaments in total knee arthroplasty. Am J Orthop (Belle Mead NJ) 45:E153–E160
62. Huang W, Zhang Y, Yao Z, Ma L (2016) Clinical examination of anterior cruciate ligament rupture: a systematic review and meta-analysis. Acta Orthop Traumatol Turc 50:22–31. https://doi.org/10.3944/AOTT.2016.14.0283
63. De FD, Ries C, Foster M et al (2020) Indications for bi-cruciate retaining total knee replacement: an international survey of 346 knee surgeons. PLoS ONE. https://doi.org/10.1371/journal.pone.0234616
64. Kono, Kenichi; Inui, Hiroshi; Tomita, Tetsuya; Yamazaki, Takaharu; Konda, Shoji; Taketomi, Shuji; Tanaka, Sakae; D'Lima, Darryl D. In vivo kinematics and cruciate ligament forces in bicruciate-retaining total knee arthroplasty. Scientific Reports (2021). https://doi.org/10.1038/s41598-021-84942-y
65. Colwell, Clifford W. CORR Insights®: Higher Frequency of Reoperation With a New Bicruciate-retaining Total Knee Arthroplasty. Clinical Orthopaedics and Related Research® (2016). https://doi.org/10.1007/s11999-016-4872-6
66. Inui, Hiroshi; Yamagami, Ryota; Kono, Kenichi; Kawaguchi, Kohei; Kage, Tomofumi; Murakami, Ryo; Nakamura, Haruhiko; Saita, Kazuo; Taketomi, Shuji; Tanaka, Sakae Short-term clinical results of bicruciate-retaining total knee arthroplasty using personalized alignment. BMC Musculoskeletal Disorders (2023). https://doi.org/10.1186/s12891-023-07083-5
67. Zhou, Chaochao; Peng, Yun; An, Shuai; Bedair, Hany; Li, Guoan Does contemporary bicruciate retaining total knee arthroplasty restore the native knee kinematics? A descriptive literature review. Archives of Orthopaedic and Trauma Surgery (2021). https://doi.org/10.1007/s00402-021-04116-3
68. Baumann, Florian; Krutsch, Werner; Worlicek, Michael; Kerschbaum, Maximilian; Zellner, Johannes; Schmitz, Paul; Nerlich, Michael; Tibesku, Carsten Reduced joint-awareness in bicruciate-retaining total knee arthroplasty compared to cruciate-sacrificing total knee arthroplasty. Archives of Orthopaedic and Trauma Surgery (2017). https://doi.org/10.1007/s00402-017-2839-z
69. Pritchett, James W. Bicruciate-retaining Total Knee Replacement Provides Satisfactory Function and Implant Survivorship at 23 Years. Clinical

Orthopaedics and Related Research® (2015). https://doi.org/10.1007/s11999-015-4219-8
70. Singh, Vivek; Yeroushalmi, David; Christensen, Thomas H.; Bieganowski, Thomas; Tang, Alex; Schwarzkopf, Ran Early outcomes of a novel bicruciate-retaining knee system: a 2-year minimum retrospective cohort study. Archives of Orthopaedic and Trauma Surgery (2022). https://doi.org/10.1007/s00402-022-04351-2
71. Biazzo, Alessio; D'Ambrosi, Riccardo; Staals, Eric; Masia, Francesco; Izzo, Vincenzo; Verde, Francesco Early results with a bicruciate-retaining total knee arthroplasty: a match-paired study. European Journal of Orthopaedic Surgery & Traumatology (2020). https://doi.org/10.1007/s00590-020-02834-9

4.6 Partial Knee Replacements

Machine Generated Summaries

Disclaimer: The summaries in this chapter were generated from Springer Nature publications using abstractive AI auto-summarization: An abstraction-based summarizer creates new text based on deep learning. New phrases are created to summarize the content. As the constituted sentences are machine selected, they may not fully reflect the body of the work, so we strongly advise that the original content is read and cited. The auto-generated summaries were curated by the editor to meet Springer Nature publication standards.

4.6.1 Medium Term Results of the Cementless Oxford Mobile Bearing Medial Unicompartmental Knee Replacement [122]

This is a machine-generated summary of:

Bray, R.; Macdonald-Taylor, K.; Miller, S.; Nugent, C. Medium term results of the cementless Oxford mobile bearing medial unicompartmental knee replacement [122].

Published in: European Journal of Orthopaedic Surgery & Traumatology (2022).

Link to original: https://doi.org/10.1007/s00590-022-03289-w

If you want to cite the papers, please refer to the original.

For technical reasons we could not place the page where the original quote is coming from.

4.6.1.1 Research Highlights

End-stage anteromedial arthritis of the medial compartment of the knee can be treated with either Unicompartmental Knee Replacement (UKR) or Total Knee Replacement (TKR), with UKR gaining popularity due to its improved functional outcomes and cost-effectiveness. Despite these advantages, UKR has a higher revision rate compared to TKR, particularly in low-volume centers and among low-volume surgeons, possibly due to incorrect patient selection or ease of revision. The study by Manara et al. investigates the initial experience with cementless Oxford mobile bearing UKR, hypothesizing that revision rates would align with national joint registry data and that Patient Reported Outcome Measures (PROMs) would be comparable to existing literature.

The study included all patients who underwent cementless Oxford UKR between April 2014 and December 2016, ensuring a minimum of 5 years follow-up. The primary outcome was implant survivorship, with re-operation as the endpoint, while secondary outcomes included PROMs such as the Oxford Knee Score and WOMAC index. Data were collected through postal questionnaires and follow-up calls, with survival analysis performed at monthly intervals. The study found an overall survivorship of 94.5% at 5 years, with most re-operations occurring within the first 18 months due to tibial component issues. PROMs showed significant improvements post-surgery, indicating sustained benefits over time.

The findings suggest that cementless Oxford UKR offers good medium-term survivorship and clinical outcomes, although a learning curve may exist for surgeons transitioning from cemented systems. The study highlights the importance of proper tibial component positioning to avoid early revisions. Future study could focus on standardizing patient selection criteria and further investigating the learning curve associated with cementless instrumentation to optimize surgical outcomes. Additionally, exploring radiographic analyses could provide insights into implant fixation and long-term performance.

4.6.2 Total or Partial Knee Replacement? Cost-Utility Analysis in Patients with Knee Osteoarthritis Based on a 2-Year Observational Study [123]

This is a machine-generated summary of:

Xie, Feng; Lo, Ngai-Nung; Tarride, Jean-Eric; O'Reilly, Daria; Goeree, Ron; Lee, Hin-Peng Total or partial knee replacement? Cost-utility analysis in patients with knee osteoarthritis based on a 2-year observational study [123].

Published in: The European Journal of Health Economics (2009).

Link to original: https://doi.org/10.1007/s10198-009-0154-5

If you want to cite the papers, please refer to the original.

For technical reasons we could not place the page where the original quote is coming from.

4.6.2.1 Research Highlights

Knee osteoarthritis (OA) in the medial compartment is a degenerative condition that significantly affects patients' physical and psychosocial well-being, while also imposing a substantial economic burden on society. Total knee replacement (TKR) and unicompartmental knee arthroplasty (UKA) are two surgical options for patients with severe medial compartmental knee OA who have not responded to conservative treatments. While TKR is known for its effectiveness in improving patient functioning and quality of life, UKA offers potential advantages such as less invasive surgery and quicker rehabilitation, albeit with a potentially higher revision rate. The choice between these surgical treatments has been controversial due to conflicting findings in the literature, often based on model simulations rather than empirical evidence from clinical practice. The study by Xie et al. aims to address this gap by evaluating the incremental cost-utility of TKR versus UKA in patients with knee OA of the medial compartment through a five-year observational study.

The study was conducted as a non-randomized prospective observational cohort study from a societal perspective at Singapore General Hospital. Patients diagnosed with medial compartment knee OA who underwent either TKR or UKA were included. Data collection involved interviews conducted 1 week before surgery, 6 months after, and 5 years post-surgery using standardized questionnaires like the Oxford Knee Score (OKS) and SF-6D for utility measurement. Costs were estimated using a unit costing method from hospital administrative data, focusing on direct costs such as health professional fees, prosthesis costs, and ward costs. The effectiveness was measured by changes in OKS scores and quality-adjusted life years (QALYs). The incremental cost-utility ratio (ICUR) was calculated using mean values of incremental costs and QALYs for TKR versus UKA, with bootstrapping methods employed to estimate confidence intervals.

The study found that TKR gained more QALYs at higher costs compared to UKA over the five-year period. However, due to significant individual variations, it was not possible to conclude with certainty whether TKR or UKA is more cost-effective. The ICUR was less favorable for TKR from societal and patient perspectives but more favorable from a governmental perspective due to differences in cost distribution. Future study could focus on long-term controlled trials to provide comprehensive profiles for these surgeries, considering factors like clinical manifestation and patient preferences. Additionally, reviewing reimbursement policies could help optimize healthcare resource allocation based on patient benefit levels.

4.6.3 Partial or Total Knee Replacement? Identifying Patients' Information Needs on Knee Replacement Surgery: A Qualitative Study to Inform a Decision Aid [124]

This is a machine-generated summary of:

Smith, Stephanie; Alvand, Abtin; Locock, Louise; Ryan, Sara; Smith, James; Bayliss, Lee; Wilson, Hannah; Price, Andrew Partial or total knee replacement? Identifying patients' information needs on knee replacement surgery: a qualitative study to inform a decision aid [124].

Published in: Quality of Life Research (2019).

Link to original: https://doi.org/10.1007/s11136-019-02381-9

If you want to cite the papers, please refer to the original.

For technical reasons we could not place the page where the original quote is coming from.

4.6.3.1 Research Highlights

Osteoarthritis is a prevalent form of knee arthritis, particularly affecting older adults, and can lead to significant pain, stiffness, and reduced function. In severe cases, knee replacement surgery is often recommended when non-surgical treatments fail to provide relief. Patients eligible for knee replacement may choose between partial or total knee replacement, with each option offering distinct benefits and risks. Despite the advantages of partial knee replacement, such as faster recovery and better functional outcomes, it has a higher revision rate compared to total knee replacement. The study by Smith et al. explores the decision-making process for patients considering knee replacement surgery and evaluates the potential of a decision aid to support shared decision-making.

The study employed qualitative research methods, including focus groups with patients who were either candidates for or had undergone knee replacement surgery.

Participants were recruited from outpatient clinics in Oxford, UK, using purposive sampling to ensure a diverse range of experiences. The focus groups aimed to gather insights into patients' experiences before surgery and their views on a decision aid based on the Option Grid format (Ebsco Health, Ipswich, Mass., USA). This format provides evidence-based summaries of treatment options in a table format with frequently asked questions. The study involved four focus groups facilitated by a qualitative researcher and two orthopaedic surgeons who provided expert input during discussions. Data from the focus groups were analysed using Framework Analysis to identify key themes related to patient information needs and preferences.

The findings underscore the importance of providing patients with clear, concise information about surgical options to facilitate informed decision-making. Participants expressed a need for detailed information on surgical outcomes, risks, recovery times, and cosmetic concerns such as scarring. The study highlights the potential of decision aids like Option Grids to enhance shared decision-making by presenting balanced information in an accessible format. Future study directions include user-testing the decision aid in clinical settings and incorporating patient narratives alongside factual information to address emotional and social aspects of decision-making. These efforts aim to improve patient satisfaction and outcomes by aligning treatment choices with individual preferences and expectations.

4.6.4 No Difference in Mobile and Fixed Bearing Partial Knee Arthroplasty in Octogenarians: A Clinical Trial [125]

This is a machine-generated summary of:

D'Ambrosi, Riccardo; Valli, Federico; Nuara, Alessandro; Mariani, Ilaria; Di Feo, Fabrizio; Ursino, Nicola; Formica, Matteo; Mangiavini, Laura; Hantes, Michael; Migliorini, Filippo No difference in mobile and fixed bearing partial knee arthroplasty in octogenarians: a clinical trial [125].

Published in: European Journal of Orthopaedic Surgery & Traumatology (2023).

Link to original: https://doi.org/10.1007/s00590-023-03537-7

If you want to cite the papers, please refer to the original.

For technical reasons we could not place the page where the original quote is coming from.

4.6.4.1 Research Highlights

The concept of an aging population is a relatively new issue, with the World Health Organization estimating that by 2050, 38% of the global population will be over 60 years old. Osteoarthritis of the knee is prevalent among the elderly, significantly affecting their quality of life. Total knee arthroplasty is often recommended for advanced cases, but partial knee arthroplasty (PKA) may be suitable when only the medial compartment is affected. Previous studies have shown that PKA can lead to better patient-reported outcomes and quicker recovery times compared to total knee arthroplasty. However, it remains unclear whether mobile bearing (MB) implants outperform fixed bearing (FB) implants in octogenarians undergoing PKA. The study by D'Ambrosi et al. investigates this question by comparing MB and FB implants in terms of patient-reported outcome measures (PROMs), range of motion (ROM), implant positioning, and survivorship in octogenarians.

The study was conducted as a clinical trial following ethical standards and involved patients with idiopathic or secondary osteoarthritis of the medial femoral compartment. Participants were divided into two groups: one receiving FB PKA and the other MB PKA. Surgeries were performed using minimally invasive techniques, with pre-operative MRI confirming ligament integrity. Post-operative rehabilitation included passive mobilization from day one and progressive weight-bearing exercises. The primary outcomes assessed were PROMs, ROM, implant positioning, and survivorship over a follow-up period. Statistical analyses were conducted to compare outcomes between the two groups, with no significant differences found in PROMs, ROM, or implant positioning. The study also evaluated implant survivorship using Kaplan-Meier curves.

The findings indicate that MB implants perform similarly to FB implants in octogenarians undergoing PKA, with no significant differences in PROMs, ROM, or implant positioning. The FB group demonstrated shorter surgical times; however, both groups showed comparable implant survivorship rates. The study highlights that while MB implants offer theoretical advantages in terms of biomechanics and stress distribution, these did not translate into clinically significant benefits over FB implants in this population. Future studies could explore larger sample sizes or randomized designs to further validate these findings and investigate potential long-term outcomes or complications associated with each implant type.

4.6.5 Evolution of Customization Design for Total Knee Arthroplasty [126]

This is a machine-generated summary of:

Slamin, John; Parsley, Brian Evolution of customization design for total knee arthroplasty [126].

Published in: Current Reviews in Musculoskeletal Medicine (2012).

Link to original: https://doi.org/10.1007/s12178-012-9141-z

If you want to cite the papers, please refer to the original.

For technical reasons we could not place the page where the original quote is coming from.

4.6.5.1 Research Highlights

Traditionally, custom implants have been utilized in orthopedic surgery for cases where standard implants do not suffice, such as in patients with juvenile rheumatoid arthritis or unusual bone geometry. These custom solutions have been particularly valuable in revision surgeries where bone erosion is present, requiring additional fixation features. However, the process of creating these implants has evolved significantly over the years. The study by Slamin et al. explores the advancements in patient-specific instrumentation and implants, highlighting the potential benefits of these innovations in improving surgical outcomes and patient satisfaction.

The study delves into the methods used to create patient-specific implants, which involve advanced imaging techniques like MRI and CT scans to capture detailed anatomical data. This data is then processed through segmentation to create a point cloud representing the joint's outer surface. The point cloud is imported into computer-assisted design (CAD) software to develop a solid model for designing customized implants. The research emphasizes the advantages of using MRI for soft tissue analysis and CT for hard tissue imaging, allowing for precise customization of implants that better fit individual patients' anatomy. The study also reviews various approaches by different manufacturers, including complete patient-specific systems that incorporate both custom instrumentation and implants.

The main advances highlighted by Slamin and colleagues include the potential for improved surgical precision and reduced operative time with patient-specific systems. These systems can lead to better postoperative alignment and potentially restore near-normal joint kinematics, addressing common issues like implant overhang that contribute to patient dissatisfaction. Future study directions could focus on further refining these technologies to enhance their cost-effectiveness and accessibility, ensuring broader adoption in clinical practice. By continuing to innovate in this field, there is potential to significantly improve outcomes for patients undergoing joint replacement surgeries.

4.6.6 Functional Outcome After Bicompartmental Knee Replacement for Medial and Patellofemoral Osteoarthritis [127]

This is a machine-generated summary of:

Mertens, Joren; Floor, Valerie; Stuyts, Bart Functional outcome after bicompartmental knee replacement for medial and patellofemoral osteoarthritis [127].

Published in: Archives of Orthopaedic and Trauma Surgery (2024).

Link to original: https://doi.org/10.1007/s00402-024-05543-8

If you want to cite the papers, please refer to the original.

For technical reasons we could not place the page where the original quote is coming from.

4.6.6.1 Research Highlights

Unicompartmental knee arthroplasty (UKA) is often preferred for isolated unicompartmental osteoarthritis due to its ability to preserve native knee kinematics and proprioception, while total knee arthroplasty (TKA) is typically used for tricompartmental osteoarthritis. However, when osteoarthritis affects two of the three knee compartments, the choice between UKA and TKA remains debated, particularly regarding the patellofemoral joint's role. The study by Mertens et al. explores the outcomes of medial and patellofemoral bicompartmental knee arthroplasty using modular implants, aiming to address this knowledge gap by evaluating clinical and functional outcomes over a minimum follow-up period of 2 years.

The study was conducted as a single-center descriptive cohort study with ethical approval. Patients with medial and patellofemoral osteoarthritis were retrospectively selected based on specific clinical and radiographic criteria. All surgeries were performed using a medial parapatellar approach, employing the Zimmer Biomet Oxford Partial Knee system for the medial compartment and the

Zimmer Biomet Gender Solution Patello-Femoral Joint System for the patello-femoral compartment. Postoperative care included standardized physiotherapy regimens. Data on demographics, adverse events, and patient-reported outcomes were collected through patient records and follow-up assessments. Statistical analyses were performed to compare pre- and postoperative outcomes, focusing on patient-reported outcome measures, range of motion, complication rates, and length of hospital stay.

The study found that bicompartmental knee replacement using modular implants offers promising results in terms of pain relief and functional improvement. The majority of patients reported good to excellent outcomes on standardized assessment tools like the Knee Society Score. However, challenges such as poor inter- and intrarater variability in measuring pre- and postoperative alignment were noted. Future studies could focus on long-term implant survival rates and compare bicompartmental knee arthroplasty with total knee replacement in larger randomized trials to better understand their relative advantages. The findings suggest that bicompartmental knee replacement could be a viable alternative for patients with specific patterns of osteoarthritis, though further research is needed to confirm these results over longer follow-up periods.

4.6.7 Early Outcomes of Modified Technique of Mobile Bearing Unicondylar Knee Replacement [128]

This is a machine-generated summary of:

Kulshrestha, Vikas; Sood, Munish; Kumar, Santhosh; Kharat, Kiran; Padhi, Prashanth P.; Kumar, Pardeep; Shrama, Saurabh; Stanley, Abin Early Outcomes of Modified Technique of Mobile Bearing Unicondylar Knee Replacement [128].

Published in: Indian Journal of Orthopaedics (2023).

Link to original: https://doi.org/10.1007/s43465-023-00907-5

If you want to cite the papers, please refer to the original.

For technical reasons we could not place the page where the original quote is coming from.

4.6.7.1 Research Highlights

Recent advancements in knee replacement surgery have led to a resurgence in the use of unicompartmental knee replacement (UKR) due to its benefits over total knee replacement (TKR), such as higher patient satisfaction and reduced perioperative morbidity. Despite registry data indicating higher revision rates for UKR, this may be attributed to the ease of revising UKR compared to TKR. With the increasing adoption of UKR, there is a focus on improving implant design and surgical techniques. The study by Kulshrestha et al. explores the outcomes of a modified surgical technique for Oxford mobile bearing UKR (Zimmer Biomet, Warsaw, IN) in an Asian patient population with smaller bone stock.

The study was conducted as a prospective cohort study at two state-sponsored tertiary care military hospitals, comparing two-year outcomes between patients undergoing Oxford UKR using a modified technique versus the standard technique. The modified technique involved minimizing tibial bone resection and adjusting femoral preparation to preserve tibial bone stock while maintaining knee balance. Patients with medial compartment osteoarthritis were enrolled after meeting specific inclusion criteria, and surgeries were performed by fellowship-trained surgeons using standardized protocols. The primary objective was to compare patient-reported outcomes using the New Knee Society Score and Forgotten Joint Score, while secondary objectives included assessing performance with the Delaware Osteoarthritis Profile score and monitoring complications.

The study found no significant differences in patient-reported outcomes or complication rates between the modified and standard technique groups at two-year follow-up. Both groups showed improved satisfaction and activity scores postoperatively. The modified technique effectively preserved tibial bone stock without affecting early function or patient satisfaction. However, the study's limitation lies in its short follow-up period, which does not allow for assessment of long-term survival benefits against aseptic loosening of the tibial component. Future study could focus on mid- to long-term follow-up to evaluate potential survival advantages of this novel modification in patients with varying bone quality.

4.6.8 Midterm Results of Modern Patellofemoral Arthroplasty Versus Total Knee Arthroplasty for Isolated Patellofemoral Arthritis: Systematic Review and Meta-analysis of Comparative Studies [129]

This is a machine-generated summary of:

Elbardesy, Hany; McLeod, André; Gul, Rehan; Harty, James Midterm results of modern patellofemoral arthroplasty versus total knee arthroplasty for isolated patellofemoral arthritis: systematic review and meta-analysis of comparative studies [129].

Published in: Archives of Orthopaedic and Trauma Surgery (2021).
Link to original: https://doi.org/10.1007/s00402-021-03882-4

If you want to cite the papers, please refer to the original.
For technical reasons we could not place the page where the original quote is coming from.

4.6.8.1 Research Highlights

The surgical treatment for end-stage patellofemoral osteoarthritis (PFOA) often involves either patellofemoral arthroplasty (PFA) or total knee arthroplasty (TKA). While PFA has been used for over 40 years, its early adoption was limited due to high failure rates, which were attributed to suboptimal implant design and poor patient selection. However, advancements in prosthetic design and refined patient selection have improved outcomes for PFA, making it a viable option alongside TKA, which is known for its predictable long-term results. Despite these advancements, there remains a lack of comprehensive reviews comparing the outcomes of PFA and TKA using randomized controlled trials (RCTs). The study by Elbardesy et al. addresses this gap by conducting a meta-analysis to evaluate the effectiveness of PFA versus TKA in treating isolated PFOA.

The study employed a systematic approach following the Preferred Reporting Items for Systematic Reviews and Meta-analyses (PRISMA) guidelines and the Cochrane Handbook. The researchers conducted an extensive literature search across multiple databases, including MEDLINE-OVID, Web of Science, PubMed, EMBASE-OVID, Google Scholar, and the Cochrane Library. They also explored grey literature sources to ensure comprehensive coverage. The inclusion criteria focused on full-text RCTs and high-quality observational cohort studies comparing complications and patient-reported outcome measures (PROMs) for both PFA and TKA. The meta-analysis assessed primary outcomes such as University of California Los Angeles (UCLA) activity scores, patient satisfaction scores, and Western Ontario and McMaster Universities Osteoarthritis Index (WOMAC) scores. Secondary outcomes included operative time and mean postoperative inpatient time. Statistical analysis was performed using Review Manager with a random-effects model to account for heterogeneity among studies.

The findings suggest that there is no significant difference between PFA and TKA regarding PROMs such as UCLA scores, patient satisfaction, and WOMAC scores after 5 years of follow-up. However, PFA demonstrated significantly shorter postoperative inpatient times compared to TKA. Additionally, PFA was associated with less postoperative blood loss and was found to be an economically beneficial joint-preserving procedure that could delay the need for TKA until implant failure or progression of tibiofemoral osteoarthritis occurs. Future study could focus on larger RCTs to further elucidate whether PFA offers better early functional outcomes compared to TKA. These findings provide valuable insights for patients and surgeons in selecting appropriate treatment options for isolated PFOA.

4.6.9 Return to the Operating Room After Patellofemoral Arthroplasty Versus Total Knee Arthroplasty for Isolated Patellofemoral Arthritis—A Systematic Review [130]

This is a machine-generated summary of:

Woon, Colin Y. L.; Christ, Alexander B.; Goto, Rie; Shanaghan, Kate; Shubin Stein, Beth E.; Gonzalez Della Valle, Alejandro Return to the operating room after patellofemoral arthroplasty versus total knee arthroplasty for isolated patellofemoral arthritis—a systematic review [130].

Published in: International Orthopaedics (2019).

Link to original: https://doi.org/10.1007/s00264-018-04280-z

If you want to cite the papers, please refer to the original.

For technical reasons we could not place the page where the original quote is coming from.

4.6.9.1 Research Highlights

End-stage, isolated patellofemoral arthritis (PFOA) can be surgically treated with patellofemoral arthroplasty (PFA), a procedure that has been in use for over four decades. Despite its potential benefits, such as reduced operative and recovery time and preservation of bone and soft tissue, PFA's widespread adoption has been limited due to high early failure rates, often attributed to implant design and patient selection. The evidence comparing PFA to total knee arthroplasty (TKA) for treating isolated PFOA is of relatively poor quality, with TKA showing predictable outcomes. The study by Woon et al. aims to address this knowledge gap by reporting the rate of return to the operating room for patients who underwent modern PFA and TKA for PFOA.

The study was conducted following Preferred Reporting Items for Systematic Reviews and Meta-analyses (PRISMA) guidelines, with comprehensive searches performed across multiple databases without year restrictions. Articles were screened and selected based on specific inclusion criteria, focusing on studies that reported reasons for re-operation in English. The analysis included data from various studies reporting on patients undergoing PFAs and TKAs, with data extraction focusing on patient demographics, type of prosthesis, follow-up duration, and subsequent surgeries. The researchers used statistical methods to calculate pooled proportions for conversion, revision, and other surgical outcomes. The study found that the weighted pooled proportion of conversion and revision to TKA was higher in the PFA group compared to the TKA group.

The findings suggest a higher likelihood of revision and conversion after modern PFA compared to TKA. However, the study acknowledges several limitations, including the younger average age of PFA patients and lower methodological quality scores for PFA studies. Future study could focus on larger prospective trials to better understand whether PFA offers improved early functional outcomes compared to TKA and if it allows patients to return to higher-level sporting activities. These insights can aid patients and surgeons in making informed decisions about the risks associated with PFA and TKA for isolated PFOA.

4.6.10 Robotic Arm-Assisted Unicondylar Knee Arthroplasty Resulted in Superior Radiological Accuracy: A Propensity Score-Matched Analysis [131]

This is a machine-generated summary of:

Yeung, Matthew H. Y.; Fu, Henry; Cheung, Amy; Kwan, Vincent Chan Wai; Cheung, Man Hong; Chan, Ping Keung; Chiu, Kwong Yuen; Yan, Chun Hoi Robotic arm-assisted unicondylar knee arthroplasty resulted in superior radiological accuracy: a propensity score-matched analysis [131].

Published in: Arthroplasty (2023).

Link to original: https://doi.org/10.1186/s42836-023-00210-6

If you want to cite the papers, please refer to the original.

For technical reasons we could not place the page where the original quote is coming from.

4.6.10.1 Research Highlights

Osteoarthritis prevalence has been increasing, leading to a projected rise in knee replacement surgeries. Unicompartmental knee arthroplasty (UKA) is a less invasive surgical option for medial knee osteoarthritis, offering quicker recovery but facing higher revision rates due to surgical technique challenges. Prior research has linked prosthesis malalignment to early UKA failure and highlighted racial differences in post-UKA fracture risks. The study by Yeung et al. investigates the early clinical and radiological outcomes of robotic arm-assisted UKA compared to conventional manual UKA, hypothesizing that robotic assistance would yield superior results.

The study employed a retrospective case-control design, analysing 74 knees that underwent robotic arm-assisted UKA at a single institution. Propensity score matching was used to compare these cases with manually instrumented UKAs performed during the same period, ensuring balanced covariates such as age and BMI. The Mako robotic arm system (MAKO, Stryker Orthopedics, Mahwah, new jersey) facilitated preoperative planning with 3D knee models and intraoperative alignment adjustments using optical motion capture technology. Manual instrumentation involved traditional jig-based techniques for component placement. Radiological outcomes focused on component alignment, while clinical outcomes included Knee Society scores and range of motion assessments at various postoperative intervals.

The study found that robotic arm-assisted UKA achieved more accurate component alignment than manual techniques, particularly in femoral and tibial coronal alignments. However, clinical outcomes such as Knee Society scores and range of motion showed no significant differences between the two groups over the follow-up period. The study suggests that while robotic assistance improves alignment precision, its impact on long-term implant survivorship remains uncertain. Future studies with larger sample sizes and extended follow-up periods are needed to validate these findings and assess whether improved alignment translates into better long-term outcomes for patients undergoing UKA.

4.6.11 Minimally Invasive Oxford Medial Unicompartmental Knee Replacement in Patients 50 Years of Age or Younger [132]

This is a machine-generated summary of:

Walker, Tilman; Stupp, Julius; Reiner, Tobias; Panzram, Benjamin; Nees, Timo A.; Innmann, Moritz M.; Gotterbarm, Tobias; Merle, Christian Minimally invasive Oxford medial unicompartmental knee replacement in patients 50 years of age or younger [132].

Published in: Archives of Orthopaedic and Trauma Surgery (2022).

Link to original: https://doi.org/10.1007/s00402-022-04539-6

If you want to cite the papers, please refer to the original.

For technical reasons we could not place the page where the original quote is coming from.

4.6.11.1 Research Highlights

Unicompartmental knee arthroplasty (UKA) is a well-established treatment for severe isolated medial arthritis of the knee joint, offering advantages over total knee arthroplasty such as bone preservation, faster recovery, and better range of motion. The Oxford mobile bearing prosthesis (Zimmer-Biomet, Warsaw, Indiana, USA) has shown excellent long-term results, prompting its use in younger, more active patients. However, concerns about higher revision rates in this demographic persist due to their high activity levels and longer life expectancy. The study by Walker et al. evaluates the clinical and radiological outcomes, as well as mid-term survivorship, of minimally invasive medial UKA in patients aged 50 years or younger using a mobile-bearing prosthesis.

The study is a single-centre retrospective cohort analysis conducted at the University Hospital of Heidelberg. It included 92 patients who underwent medial UKA for advanced osteoarthritis or avascular necrosis of the femoral condyle. The surgeries were performed using a minimally invasive technique with cemented fixation prior to 2014 and cementless fixation thereafter based on bone quality. Patients were followed up for a minimum of 24 months, with clinical data collected through regular check-ups and structured interviews. Survivorship analysis was conducted using the Kaplan–Meier estimator for endpoints such as revision surgery and dislocation of the bearing. The study found significant improvements in functional scores and pain levels postoperatively, with survival rates of 94.5% at 5 years and 91.2% at 10 years for device-related revisions.

The findings suggest that medial UKA offers high functional outcomes and good mid-term survivorship in young patients, comparable to results in older populations. Despite these promising results, the study acknowledges limitations such as its retrospective design and relatively short follow-up period. Future study should focus on long-term outcomes and factors influencing the progression of arthritis in this patient group. Nonetheless, this research supports the viability of OUKA as a treatment option for young patients with end-stage osteoarthritis of the medial compartment.

4.6.12 Agreement and Accuracy of Radiographic Assessment Using a Decision Aid for Medial Oxford Partial Knee Replacement: Multicentre Study [133]

This is a machine-generated summary of:

Hiranaka, Takafumi; Furuhashi, Ryosuke; Takashiba, Kenichiro; Kodama, Takao; Michishita, Kazuhiko; Inui, Hiroshi; Togashi, Eita Agreement and accuracy of radiographic assessment using a decision aid for medial Oxford partial knee replacement: multicentre study [133].

Published in: Knee Surgery & Related Research (2022).

Link to original: https://doi.org/10.1186/s43019-022-00140-8

If you want to cite the papers, please refer to the original.

For technical reasons we could not place the page where the original quote is coming from.

4.6.12.1 Research Highlights

Partial knee replacement (PKR) is gaining attention as an effective treatment for knee osteoarthritis, offering benefits such as faster recovery and superior patient satisfaction compared to total knee replacement (TKR). However, national registry data indicate a higher revision rate for PKR than TKR, highlighting the importance of patient selection for successful outcomes. The study by Hiranaka et al. investigates the inter-rater reproducibility and accuracy of a radiological decision aid designed to assist experienced surgeons in determining the suitability of patients for mobile-bearing PKR.

The study involved experienced surgeons evaluating pre-operative radiographs of patients who underwent single-sided total knee replacement. The decision aid included criteria based on anteroposterior, lateral, valgus, and varus stress radiographs to assess medial bone-on-bone contact, ACL functionality, lateral cartilage integrity, MCL condition, and patellofemoral joint status. Surgeons rated each section as "yes" or "no" to determine overall PKR suitability. The accuracy of these assessments was validated against intra-operative findings. Despite the expertise of the raters, the study found moderate agreement on PKR suitability, with significant variability in predictions of ACL status and lateral cartilage condition. The predictability did not correlate with the surgeons' experience or volume of surgeries performed.

The study highlights challenges in accurately diagnosing ACL deficiencies and partial-thickness lateral cartilage defects using radiographs alone. It suggests that MRI could enhance diagnostic accuracy by providing more detailed information on cartilage and meniscus conditions. Future study could focus on integrating MRI into the decision-making process to improve patient selection for PKR and reduce failure rates. Additionally, developing more quantitative criteria based on larger clinical datasets may enhance the reliability of radiographic assessments. Despite its limitations, this research offers valuable insights into improving PKR outcomes through better patient selection strategies.

4.6.13 Valgus Stress Radiographs Have a Minor Additional Value in Detecting Lateral Cartilage Wear When Selecting Patients for Medial Partial Knee Replacement [134]

This is a machine-generated summary of:

van Langeveld, Stephan J.; Janssen, Stein J.; Oost, Iris Koenraadt-van; Terra, Maaike P.; van Geenen, Rutger C. I. Valgus stress radiographs have a minor additional value in detecting lateral cartilage wear when selecting patients for medial partial knee replacement [134].

Published in: Archives of Orthopaedic and Trauma Surgery (2024).

4.6.13.1 Research Highlights

Medial partial knee replacement (PKR) is often preferred over total knee replacement (TKR) for isolated medial compartmental knee osteoarthritis due to better clinical outcomes. However, PKR is associated with higher revision rates, which has sparked debate regarding its efficacy. These higher revision rates may be attributed to factors such as lower surgical caseloads and inadequate patient selection. Traditional indications for PKR have evolved, and current criteria focus on specific cartilage wear patterns and ligament sufficiency. The study by Langeveld et al. investigates the potential added value of valgus stress radiographs in assessing lateral cartilage wear in patients with medial knee osteoarthritis.

The study was a retrospective cross-sectional analysis involving patients with medial knee osteoarthritis who underwent both Rosenberg and valgus stress radiographs at a single urban center. The researchers aimed to determine the clinical relevance of valgus stress radiographs by comparing joint space width (JSW) measurements between the two radiographic techniques. The study included patients who subsequently underwent knee replacement surgery, excluding those with inflammatory diseases or other forms of osteoarthritis. Radiographic measurements were performed using digital calipers, and interobserver reliability was assessed. The results showed that valgus stress radiographs measured a narrower lateral JSW compared to Rosenberg radiographs, but the additional value in detecting joint space narrowing was limited to a small percentage of patients.

The findings suggest that while valgus stress radiographs can measure narrower JSW, their additional clinical value in patient selection for PKR is limited. The study highlights that optimal radio-anatomic alignment of Rosenberg radiographs reduces the need for additional valgus stress imaging. Future study could explore specific patient or disease characteristics that might predict when valgus stress radiographs are beneficial. Despite its potential utility in certain cases, the routine use of valgus stress radiographs may not be justified given the increased radiation exposure and costs associated with this technique.

4.6.14 Risk of Revision and Adverse Outcomes Following Partial Knee Replacement and High Tibial Osteotomy for Unicompartmental Knee Osteoarthritis: A Nationwide Cohort Study [135]

This is a machine-generated summary of:

Lee, Sun-Ho; Kim, Hae-Rim; Song, Eun-Kyoo; Seon, Jong-Keun Risk of Revision and Adverse Outcomes Following Partial Knee Replacement and High Tibial Osteotomy for Unicompartmental Knee Osteoarthritis: A Nationwide Cohort Study [135].

Published in: Indian Journal of Orthopaedics (2021).

Link to original: https://doi.org/10.1007/s43465-021-00517-z

If you want to cite the papers, please refer to the original.

For technical reasons we could not place the page where the original quote is coming from.

4.6.14.1 Research Highlights

Osteoarthritis (OA) of the knee joint is a prevalent condition that significantly impacts quality of life worldwide. While total knee arthroplasty (TKA) is a common treatment for late-stage OA, it is not typically the first choice for OA confined to the medial compartment. Instead, high tibial osteotomy (HTO) and unicompartmental knee arthroplasty (UKA) are often considered. Despite extensive research, the optimal choice between UKA and HTO remains debated due to varying patient factors and surgical outcomes. The study by Lee et al. investigates trends in utilization, revision rates, and perioperative complications of these two surgical methods using data from South Korea's National Health Insurance Service.

The study conducted a nationwide cohort analysis using data from the Korean NHIS, which covers nearly the entire population of South Korea. Researchers extracted data on patients who underwent UKA or HTO for knee OA between January 2007 and May 2019. To ensure accurate comparisons, they employed propensity score matching (PSM) to balance baseline characteristics such as age, sex, comorbidities, and type of hospital. The study analysed conversion rates to TKA, adverse medical outcomes, and perioperative complications using statistical methods including Kaplan-Meier curves and Cox regression models. Subgroup analyses were performed based on age to further explore differences in outcomes between UKA and HTO.

The study found that while both UKA and HTO have increased in utilization over recent years, UKA demonstrated a higher survival rate compared to HTO over a 12-year follow-up period. However, UKA was associated with higher incidences of deep vein thrombosis (DVT) and surgical site infections compared to HTO. The findings suggest that while UKA may offer better long-term survival for medial compartment knee OA, it also carries specific risks that should be considered when selecting a surgical method. Future study could extend follow-up periods beyond 12 years and address limitations such as potential selection bias due to surgeons' preferences and lack of detailed clinical data in the NHIS database.

Bibliography

1. National Joint Registry Annual report 2020, www.njrcentre.org.uk. Accessed January 2021
2. Chawla H, van der List JP, Christ AB, Sobrero MR, Zuiderbaan HA, Pearle AD (2017) Annual revision rates of partial versus total knee arthroplasty: a comparative meta-analysis. Knee 24(2):179–190
3. Evans JPTP, Walker RW, Evans JPTP, Blom AW, Sayers A, Whitehouse MR. How long does a knee replacement last? A systematic review and meta-analysis of case series and national registry reports with more than 15 years of follow-up. Lancet. 2019;393:655–63.
4. Nakama GY, Peccin MS, Almeida GJM, de Lira Neto OA, Queiroz AAB, Navarro RD (2012) Cemented, cementless or hybrid fixation options in total knee arthroplasty for osteoarthritis and other non-traumatic diseases. Cochrane Database Syst Rev 10:CD006193
5. Buly, R.L., Sculco, T.P.: Recent advances in total knee replacement surgery. Curr. Opin. Rheumatol. *7*, 107–113 (1995). https://doi.org/10.1097/00002281-199503000-00007
6. Iorio, R., Healy, W.L.: Unicompartmental arthritis of the knee. J. Bone Joint Surg. Am. *85-A*, 1351–1364 (2003)
7. Gioe, T.J., Killeen, K.K., Hoeffel, D.P., Bert, J.M., Comfort, T.K., Scheltema, K., et al.: Analysis of unicompartmental knee arthroplasty in a community-based implant registry. Clin. Orthop. Relat. Res. 111–119 (2003). https://doi.org/10.1097/01.blo.0000093004.90435.d1
8. Knutson, K., Lewold, S., Robertsson, O., Lidgren, L.: The Swedish knee arthroplasty register. A nation-wide study of 30,003 knees 1976–1992. Acta Orthop. Scand. *65*, 375–386 (1994)
9. Robertsson, O.: Unicompartmental arthroplasty. Results in Sweden 1986–1995. Orthopade *29*(Suppl 1), S6–S8 (2000). https://doi.org/10.1007/PL00003689

10. Newman, J.H., Ackroyd, C.E., Shah, N.A.: Unicompartmental or total knee replacement? Five-year results of a prospective, randomised trial of 102 osteoarthritic knees with unicompartmental arthritis. J. Bone Joint Surg. Br. *80*, 862–865 (1998). https://doi.org/10.1302/0301-620X.80B5.8835
11. Laurencin, C.T., Zelicof, S.B., Scott, R.D., Ewald, F.C.: Unicompartmental versus total knee arthroplasty in the same patient. A comparative study. Clin. Orthop. Relat. Res. *15*, 1–156 (1991)
12. Scott, R.D., Santore, R.F.: Unicondylar unicompartmental replacement for osteoarthritis of the knee. J. Bone Joint Surg. Am. *63*, 536–544 (1981)
13. Robertsson, O., Borgquist, L., Knutson, K., Lewold, S., Lidgren, L.: Use of unicompartmental instead of tricompartmental prostheses for unicompartmental arthrosis in the knee is a cost-effective alternative. 15, 437 primary tricompartmental prostheses were compared with 10, 624 primary medial or lateral unicompartmental prostheses. Acta Orthop. Scand. *70*, 170–175 (1999)
14. Slover, J., Espehaug, B., Havelin, L.I., Engesaeter, L.B., Furnes, O., Tomek, I., et al.: Cost-effectiveness of unicompartmental and total knee arthroplasty in elderly low-demand patients. A Markov decision analysis. J. Bone Joint Surg. Am. *88*, 2348–2355 (2006). https://doi.org/10.2106/JBJS.E.01033
15. Soohoo, N.F., Sharifi, H., Kominski, G., Lieberman, J.R.: Cost-effectiveness analysis of unicompartmental knee arthroplasty as an alternative to total knee arthroplasty for unicompartmental osteoarthritis. J. Bone Joint Surg. Am. *88*, 1975–1982 (2006). https://doi.org/10.2106/JBJS.E.00597
16. Liddle AD, Pandit H, Judge A, Murray DW (2015) Patient-reported outcomes after total and unicompartmental knee arthroplasty: a study of 14,076 matched patients from the National Joint Registry for England and Wales. Bone Jt J 97-B(6):793–801
17. Burn, E., Sanchez-Santos, M., Pandit, H., Hamilton, T., Liddle, A., Murray, D., et al. (2016). Ten-year patient-reported outcomes following total and minimally invasive unicompartmental knee arthroplasty: A propensity score-matched cohort analysis. *Knee Surgery, Sports Traumatology, Arthroscopy,26*(5), 1455–1464.
18. Khatri, P. J., O'Connor, A. M., and Dervin, G. F. (2011). Decision Support Needs of Patients Choosing Between Unicompartmental and Total Knee Arthroplasty for Advanced Medial Compartment Osteoarthritis of the Knee. *Journal of Arthroplasty,26*(8), 1343–1349. https://doi.org/10.1016/j.arth.2010.12.016.
19. Suarez-Almazor, M. E., Richardson, M., Kroll, T. L., and Sharf, B. F. (2010). A qualitative analysis of decision-making for total knee replacement in patients with osteoarthritis. *Journal of Clinical Rheumatology: Practical Reports on Rheumatic* and *Musculoskeletal Diseases,16*(4), 158. https://doi.org/10.1097/RHU.0b013e3181df4de4.
20. Kinsey, K., Firth, J., Elwyn, G., Edwards, A., Brain, K., Marrin, K., et al. (2017). Patients' views on the use of an Option Grid for knee osteoarthritis in physiotherapy clinical encounters: An interview study. *Health Expectations,20*(6), 1302–1310. https://doi.org/10.1111/hex.12570.

21. Migliorini F, Maffulli N, Cuozzo F, Elsner K, Hildebrand F, Eschweiler J, Driessen A (2022) Mobile bearing versus fixed bearing for unicompartmental arthroplasty in monocompartmental osteoarthritis of the knee: a meta-analysis. J Clin Med 11:2837. https://doi.org/10.3390/jcm11102837
22. Johal S, Nakano N, Baxter M, Hujazi I, Pandit H, Khanduja V (2018) Unicompartmental knee arthroplasty: the past, current controversies, and future perspectives. J Knee Surg 31:992–998. https://doi.org/10.1055/s-0038-1625961
23. Migliorini F, Tingart M, Niewiera M, Rath B, Eschweiler J (2019) Unicompartmental versus total knee arthroplasty for knee osteoarthritis. Eur J Orthop Surg Traumatol. 29:947–955
24. Morales-Avalos R, Perelli S, Raygoza-Cortez K, Padilla-Medina JR, Peña-Martínez VM, Guzmán-López S, Zavala JMD, Barrera FJ, Vilchez-Cavazos F, Monllau JC (2022) Fixed-bearing unicompartmental knee arthroplasty provides a lower failure rate than mobile-bearing unicompartimental knee arthroplasty when used after a failed high tibial osteotomy: a systematic review and meta-analysis. Knee Surg Sport Traumatol Arthrosc 30:3228–3235. https://doi.org/10.1007/s00167-021-06707-4
25. Zhang W, Wang J, Li H, Wang W, George DM, Huang T (2020) Fixed- versus mobile-bearing unicompartmental knee arthroplasty: a meta-analysis. Sci Rep 10:19075. https://doi.org/10.1038/s41598-020-76124-z
26. Bruce DJ, Hassaballa M, Robinson JR, Porteous AJ, Murray JR, Newman JH (2020) Minimum 10-year outcomes of a fixed bearing all-polyethylene unicompartmental knee arthroplasty used to treat medial osteoarthritis. Knee 27:1018–1027. https://doi.org/10.1016/j.knee.2020.02.018
27. Ko YB, Gujarathi MR, Oh KJ (2015) Outcome of unicompartmental knee arthroplasty: a systematic review of comparative studies between fixed and mobile bearings focusing on complications. Knee Surg Relat Res 27:141–148. https://doi.org/10.5792/ksrr.2015.27.3.141
28. Goodfellow JW, Kershaw CJ, Benson MK, O'Connor JJ (1988) The Oxford knee for unicompartmental osteoarthritis. The first 103 cases. J Bone Jt Surg Br 70:692–701. https://doi.org/10.1302/0301-620X.70B5.3192563
29. Howell SM, Kuznik K, Hull ML, Siston RA. Results of an initial experience with custom-fit positioning total knee arthroplasty in a series of 48 patients. Orthopedics. 2008;31:857–63.
30. Parratte S, Ollivier M, Opsomer G, Lunebourg A, Argenson JN, Thienpont E (2015) Is knee function better with contemporary modular bicompartmental arthroplasty compared to total knee arthroplasty? Short-term outcomes of a prospective matched study including 68cases. Orthop Traumatol Surg Res 101(5):547–552. https://doi.org/10.1016/j.otsr.2015.03.019
31. Rolston L et al Bicompartmental knee arthroplasty: a Bone-sparing, Ligament-sparing, and minimally invasive alternative for active patients. [Online]. Available: https://www.ORTHOSuperSite.com
32. Kooner S, Johal H, Clark M (Dec. 2017) Bicompartmental knee arthroplasty vs total knee arthroplasty for the treatment of medial compartment and patel-

lofemoral osteoarthritis. Arthroplast Today 3(4):309–314. https://doi.org/10.1016/j.artd.2017.02.006
33. Beard DJ, Davies LJ, Cook JA, MacLennan G, Price A, Kent S et al (2019) The clinical and cost-effectiveness of total versus partial knee replacement in patients with medial compartment osteoarthritis (TOPKAT): 5-year outcomes of a randomised controlled trial. Lancet Lond Engl 394(10200):746–756
34. Keudell, A. V., Sodha, S., Collins, J., Minas, T., Fitz, W., and Gomoll, A. H. (2014). Patient satisfaction after primary total and Unicompartmental knee arthroplasty: An age-dependent analysis. *The Knee, 21*, 180–184. https://doi.org/10.1016/j.knee.2013.08.004
35. Jansen, K., Beckert, M., Deckard, E. R., Davis, M. Z., and Meneghini, M. (2020). Satisfaction and Functional Outcomes in Unicompartmental Compared with Total Knee Arthroplasty. *JBJS Open Access., 5*(3), 2000051. https://doi.org/10.2106/JBJS.OA.20.00051
36. Fredborg C, Odgaard A, Sørensen J (2020) Patellofemoral arthroplasty is cheaper and more effective in the short term than total knee arthroplasty for isolated patellofemoral osteoarthritis: Cost-effectiveness analysis based on a randomized trial. Bone Jt J 102:449–457. https://doi.org/10.1302/0301-620X.102B4.BJJ-2018-1580.R3
37. Joseph MN, Achten J, Parsons NR, Costa ML (2020) The PAT randomized clinical trial. Bone Jt J 102:310–318. https://doi.org/10.1302/0301-620X.102B3.BJJ-2019-0723.R1
38. Wada K, Price A, Gromov K et al (2020) Clinical outcome of bi-unicompartmental knee arthroplasty for both medial and lateral femorotibial arthritis: a systematic review—is there proof of concept? Arch Orthop Trauma Surg 140:1503–1513. https://doi.org/10.1007/s00402-020-03492-6
39. Feucht MJ, Lutz PM, Ketzer C et al (2020) Preoperative patellofemoral anatomy affects failure rate after isolated patellofemoral inlay arthroplasty. Arch Orthop Trauma Surg 140:2029–2039. https://doi.org/10.1007/s00402-020-03651-9
40. Julian P.T. Higgins JT, Jacqueline Chandler, Miranda Cumpston TL, Welch MJP and VA (2019) Cochrane Handbook for Systematic Reviews of Interventions
41. Dy CJ, Franco N, Ma Y et al (2012) Complications after patello-femoral versus total knee replacement in the treatment of isolated patello-femoral osteoarthritis. A meta-analysis. Knee Surg Sport Traumatol Arthrosc 20:2174–2190. https://doi.org/10.1007/s00167-011-1677-8
42. Leadbetter WB, Kolisek FR, Levitt RL et al (2009) Patellofemoral arthroplasty: a multi-centre study with minimum 2-year follow-up. Int Orthop 33:1597–1601. https://doi.org/10.1007/s00264-008-0692-y
43. Ackroyd CE, Newman JH, Evans R et al (2007) The Avon patellofemoral arthroplasty. J Bone Joint Surg Br 89:310–315. https://doi.org/10.1302/0301-620X.89B3.18062
44. Sisto DJ, Sarin VK. Custon patellofemoral arthroplasty of the knee. JBJS. 2006;88:1475–80.

45. Ackroyd CE, Chir B (2005) Development and early results of a new patellofemoral arthroplasty. Clin Orthop Relat Res 2:7–13. https://doi.org/10.1097/01.blo.0000171914.94503.d1
46. Butler JE, Shannon R (2009) Patellofemoral arthroplasty with a custom-fit femoral prosthesis. Orthopedics 32:81
47. Kazarian GS, Tarity TD, Hansen EN, Cai J, Lonner JH (2016) Significant functional improvement at 2 years after isolated patellofemoral arthroplasty with an onlay trochlear implant, but low mental health scores predispose to dissatisfaction. J Arthroplast 31:389–394. https://doi.org/10.1016/j.arth.2015.08.033
48. Akhbari P, Malak T, Dawson-Bowling S, East D, Miles K, Butler-Manuel PA (2015) The Avon patellofemoral joint replacement: mid-term prospective results from an independent centre. Clin Orthop Surg 7:171–176. https://doi.org/10.4055/cios.2015.7.2.171
49. Al-Hadithy N, Patel R, Navadgi B, Deo S, Hollinghurst D, Satish V (2014) Mid-term results of the FPV patellofemoral joint replacement. Knee 21:138–141. https://doi.org/10.1016/j.knee.2013.08.010
50. Benazzo F, Rossi SMP, Ghiara M (2014) Partial knee arthroplasty: patellofemoral arthroplasty and combined unicompartmental and patellofemoral arthroplasty implants - general considerations and indications, technique and clinical experience. Knee 21:S43–S46. https://doi.org/10.1016/S0968-0160(14)50009-9
51. Dahm DL, Al-Rayashi W, Dajani K, Shah JP, Levy BA, Stuart MJ (2010) Patellofemoral arthroplasty versus total knee arthroplasty in patients with isolated patellofemoral osteoarthritis. Am J Orthop (Belle Mead NJ) 39:487–491
52. Dahm DL, Kalisvaart MM, Stuart MJ, Slettedahl SW (2014) Patellofemoral arthroplasty: outcomes and factors associated with early progression of tibiofemoral arthritis. Knee Surg Sports Traumatol Arthrosc 22:2554–2559. https://doi.org/10.1007/s00167-014-3202-3
53. Davies AP (2013) High early revision rate with the FPV patello-femoral unicompartmental arthroplasty. Knee 20:482–484. https://doi.org/10.1016/j.knee.2013.07.005
54. deDeugd CM, Pareek A, Krych AJ et al (2017) Outcomes of patellofemoral arthroplasty based on radiographic severity. J Arthroplasty 32:1137–1142. https://doi.org/10.1016/j.arth.2016.11.006
55. Hernigou P, Caton J (2014) Design, operative technique and ten-year results of the Hermes™ patellofemoral arthroplasty. Int Orthop 38:437–442. https://doi.org/10.1007/s00264-013-2158-0
56. Konan S, Haddad FS (2016) Midterm outcome of Avon patellofemoral arthroplasty for posttraumatic unicompartmental osteoarthritis. J Arthroplast 31:2657–2659. https://doi.org/10.1016/j.arth.2016.06.005
57. Mont MA, Johnson AJ, Naziri Q, Kolisek FR, Leadbetter WB (2012) Patellofemoral arthroplasty: 7-year mean follow-up. J Arthroplast 27:358–361. https://doi.org/10.1016/j.arth.2011.07.010

58. Morris MJ, Lombardi AV Jr, Berend KR, Hurst JM, Adams JB (2013) Clinical results of patellofemoral arthroplasty. J Arthroplast 28:199–201. https://doi.org/10.1016/j.arth.2013.05.012
59. Odgaard A, Madsen F, Kristensen PW et al (2018) The mark coventry award: Patellofemoral arthroplasty results in better range of movement and early patient-reported outcomes than TKA. Clin Orthop Relat Res 476:87–100. https://doi.org/10.1007/s11999.0000000000000017
60. Odumenya M, Costa ML, Parsons N, Achten J, Dhillon M, Krikler SJ (2010) The Avon patellofemoral joint replacement: five-year results from an independent centre. J Bone Jt Surg Br 92:56–60. https://doi.org/10.1302/0301-620X.92B1.23135
61. Osarumwense D, Syed F, Nzeako O, Akilapa S, Zubair O, Waite J (2017) Patellofemoral joint arthroplasty: early results and functional outcome of the Zimmer gender solutions patello-femoral joint system. Clin Orthop Surg 9:295–302. https://doi.org/10.4055/cios.2017.9.3.295
62. Romagnoli S, Marullo M (2017) Mid-term clinical, functional, and radiographic outcomes of 105 gender-specific patellofemoral arthroplasties, with or without the association of medial unicompartmental knee arthroplasty. J Arthroplast 33:688–695. https://doi.org/10.1016/j.arth.2017.10.019
63. Sarda PK, Shetty A, Maheswaran SS (2011) Medium term results of Avon patellofemoral joint replacement. Indian J Orthop 45:439–444. https://doi.org/10.4103/0019-5413.83761
64. Starks I, Roberts S, White SH (2009) The Avon patellofemoral joint replacement: independent assessment of early functional outcomes. J Bone Jt Surg Br 91:1579–1582. https://doi.org/10.1302/0301-620X.91B12.23018
65. Ahearn N, Metcalfe AJ, Hassaballa MA et al (2016) The Journey patellofemoral joint arthroplasty: a minimum 5year follow-up study. Knee 23:900–904. https://doi.org/10.1016/j.knee.2016.03.004
66. Middleton SWF, Toms AD, Schranz PJ, Mandalia VI (2018) Mid-term survivorship and clinical outcomes of the Avon patellofemoral joint replacement. Knee 25:323–328. https://doi.org/10.1016/j.knee.2018.01.007
67. Sabatini L, Schirò M, Atzori F, Ferrero G, Massè A (2016) Patellofemoral joint arthroplasty: our experience in isolated patellofemoral and bicompartmental arthritic knees. Clin Med Insights Arthritis Musculoskelet Disord 9:189–193. https://doi.org/10.4137/CMAMD.S40498
68. Willekens P, Victor J, Verbruggen D, vande Kerckhove M, van der Straeten C (2015) Outcome of patellofemoral arthroplasty, determinants for success. Acta Orthop Belg 81:759–767
69. Williams DP, Pandit HG, Athanasou NA, Murray DW, Gibbons CL (2013) Early revisions of the Femoro-Patella Vialla joint replacement. Bone Joint J 95–B:793–797. https://doi.org/10.1302/0301-620X.95B6.31355
70. Meding JB, Wing JT, Keating EM, Ritter MA (2007) Total knee arthroplasty for isolated patellofemoral arthritis in younger patients. Clin Orthop Relat Res 464:78–82. https://doi.org/10.1097/BLO.0b013e3181576069

71. Mont MA, Haas S, Mullick T, Hungerford DS (2002) Total knee arthroplasty for patellofemoral arthritis. J Bone Jt Surg Am 84:1977–1981
72. Laskin RS, van Steijn M (1999) Total knee replacement for patients with patellofemoral arthritis. Clin Orthop Relat Res 367:89–95. https://doi.org/10.2106/00004623-200211000-00011
73. Parvizi J, Stuart MJ, Pagnano MW, Hanssen AD (2001) Total knee arthroplasty in patients with isolated patellofemoral arthritis. Clin Orthop Relat Res 392:147–152 https://doi.org/10.1097/00003086-200111000-00018
74. Dalury DF (2005) Total knee replacement for patellofemoral disease. J Knee Surg 18:274–277 https://doi.org/10.1055/s-0030-1248191
75. Saragaglia D, Mader R, Refaie R (2014) Are results of total knee arthroplasty for isolated patellofemoral OA as good as for medial compartment OA? A medium-term retrospective comparative study. Eur J Orthop Surg Traumatol 25:381–386. https://doi.org/10.1007/s00590-014-1516-y
76. Lonner JH (2017) Patellofemoral arthroplasty: an evolving science. Instr Course Lect 66:211–221
77. van Jonbergen HW, Poolman RW, van Kampen A (2010) Isolated patellofemoral osteoarthritis. A systematic review of treatment options using the GRADE approach. Acta Orthop 81:199–205. https://doi.org/10.3109/17453671003628756
78. Lonner JH (2010) Patellofemoral arthroplasty. Orthopedics. https://doi.org/10.3928/01477447-20100722-39
79. Collier MB, Eickmann TH, Sukezaki F, McAuley JP, Engh GA. Patient, implant, and alignment factors associated with revision of medial compartment unicondylar arthroplasty. J Arthroplasty. 2006;21(Suppl 2):108–15.
80. Bell SW, Anthony I, Jones B, et al. Improved accuracy of component positioning with robotic-assisted unicompartmental knee arthroplasty: data from a prospective, randomized controlled study. J Bone Joint Surg. 2016;98:627–35 (https://pubmed.ncbi.nlm.nih.gov/27098321/).
81. Cobb J, Henckel J, Gomes P, et al. Hands-on robotic unicompartmental knee replacement: a prospective, randomised controlled study of the acrobot system. J Bone Joint Surg. 2006;88-B:188–97 (https://pubmed.ncbi.nlm.nih.gov/16434522/).
82. Dunbar NJ, Roche MW, Park BH, et al. Accuracy of dynamic tactile-guided unicompartmental knee arthroplasty. J Arthroplasty. 2012;27:803–8 (https://pubmed.ncbi.nlm.nih.gov/22088782/).
83. Yip DK, Zhu YH, Chiu KY, Ng TP. Distal rotational alignment of the Chinese femur and its relevance in total knee arthroplasty. J Arthroplasty. 2004;19(5):613–9. https://doi.org/10.1016/j.arth.2003.11.008. PMID: 15284983.
84. Yue B, Varadarajan KM, Ai S, Tang T, Rubash HE, Li G. Differences of knee anthropometry between Chinese and white men and women. J Arthroplasty. 2011;26(1):124–30. https://doi.org/10.1016/j.arth.2009.11.020. Epub 2010 Feb 9. PMID: 20149574; PMCID: PMC3740371.

85. Oh-Ryong Kwon, Kyoung-Tak Kang,Juhyun Son, Dong-Suk Suh, Changhyun Baek, Yong-Gon Koh. Importance of joint line preservation in unicompartmental knee arthroplasty: finite element analysis. J Orthopaedic Res. https://doi.org/10.1002/jor.23279
86. Khow YZ, et al. The effect of tibial and femoral component coronal alignment on clinical outcomes and survivorship in unicompartmental knee arthroplasty. Bone Joint J. 2021;103-B(2):338–46. https://doi.org/10.1302/0301-620X.103B2.BJJ-2020-0959.R1.
87. Kim KT, Lee S, Lee JS, Kang MS, Koo KH (2018) Long-term clinical results of unicompartmental knee arthroplasty in patients younger than 60 years of age: minimum 10-year follow-up. Knee Surg Relat Res 30:28–33
88. Price AJ, Dodd CA, Svard UG, Murray DW (2005) Oxford medial unicompartmental knee arthroplasty in patients younger and older than 60 years of age. J Bone Joint Surg Br 87:1488–1492
89. Felts E, Parratte S, Pauly V, Aubaniac JM, Argenson JN (2010) Function and quality of life following medial unicompartmental knee arthroplasty in patients 60 years of age or younger. Orthop Traumatol Surg Res 96:861–867
90. Pennington DW, Swienckowski JJ, Lutes WB, Drake GN (2003) Unicompartmental knee arthroplasty in patients sixty years of age or younger. J Bone Joint Surg Am. 85-A:1968–1973
91. The Swedish National Board of Health And Welfare Swedish knee arthroplasty register. In: 2018. http://myknee.se/pdf/SVK_2018_Eng_1.0.pdf.
92. Riddle DL, Jiranek WA, McGlynn FJ (2008) Yearly incidence of unicompartmental knee arthroplasty in the United States. J Arthroplasty 23:408–412. https://doi.org/10.1016/j.arth.2007.04.012
93. National Joint Registry NJR report. https://reports.njrcentre.org.uk/knees-primary-procedures-components/K15v1NJR?reportid=5CF7C49E-FAEE-466C-89F0-4BEEFCFB2264defaults=DC__Reporting_Period__Date_Range=%22MAX%22,R__Filter__Implant_Type_Name=%22Knee-Bicondylar%22
94. Orthopaedic A, Association Australian Orthopaedic Association National Joint Replacement Registry. https://aoanjrr.sahmri.com/documents/10180/668596/Hip%2C+Knee+%26+Shoulder+Arthroplasty/c287d2a3-22df-a3bb-37a2-91e6c00bfcf0
95. Liddle AD, Pandit H, Judge A, Murray DW (2015) Optimal usage of unicompartmental knee arthroplasty: a study of 41 986 cases from the National Joint Registry for England and Wales. Bone Jt J 97-B(11):1506–1511
96. Badawy M, Espehaug B, Indrekvam K et al (2014) Higher revision risk for unicompartmental knee arthroplasty in low-volume hospitals. Acta Orthop 85:342–347. https://doi.org/10.3109/17453674.2014.920990
97. White SH, Ludkowski PF, Goodfellow JW (1991) Anteromedial osteoarthritis of the knee. J Bone Joint Surg Br 73-B:582–586
98. ZimmerBiomet Radiographic Assessment for Medial Oxford ® Partial Knee Replacement (PKR). https://www.oxfordpartialknee.net/content/dam/zb--minisites/oxford-partial-knee-hcp/documents/oxford-decision-aid-flyer.pdf

99. Hamilton TW, Pandit HG, Lombardi AV et al (2016) Radiological decision aid to determine suitability for medial unicompartmental knee arthroplasty: development and preliminary validation. Bone Joint J 98-B:3–10. https://doi.org/10.1302/0301-620X.98B10.BJJ-2016-0432.R1
100. Gibson PH, Goodfellow JW (1986) Stress radiography in degenerative arthritis of the knee. J Bone Jt Surg Br 68(4):608–609. https://doi.org/10.1302/0301-620X.68B4.3733839
101. Goodfellow J, O'Connor J, Murray DW (2002) The Oxford meniscal unicompartmental knee. J Knee Surg 15(4):240–246
102. Oosthuizen CR, Burger S, Vermaak DP, Goldschmidt P, Spangenberg R (2015) The X-ray knee instability and degenerative score (X-KIDS) to determine the preference for a partial or a total knee arthroplasty (PKA/TKA). South Afr Orthop J (SAOJ) 14(3):61–69. https://doi.org/10.17159/2309-8309/2015/v14n3a7
103. Bland JM, Altman DG (1986) Statistical methods for assessing agreement between two methods of clinical measurement. Lancet (London, England) 1(8476):307–310
104. Mortensen JF, Kappel A, Rasmussen LE, Ostgaard SE, Odgaard A (2021) The Rosenberg view and coronal stress radiographs give similar measurements of articular cartilage height in knees with osteoarthritis. Arch Orthop Trauma Surg. https://doi.org/10.1007/s00402-021-04136-z
105. Mont, M. A., Stuchin, S. A., Paley, D., Sharkey, P. F., Parvisi, J., Tria, A. J., Jr., Bonutti, P. M., and Etienne, G. (2004). Different surgical options for monocompartmental osteoarthritis of the knee: High tibial osteotomy versus unicompartmental knee arthroplasty versus total knee arthroplasty: Indications, techniques, results, and controversies. *Instructional Course Lectures, 53*, 265–283.
106. Broughton, N. S., Newman, J. H., and Baily, R. A. (1986). Unicompartmental replacement and high tibial osteotomy for osteoarthritis of the knee. A comparative study after 5–10 years' follow-up. *Journal of Bone and Joint Surgery. British Volume, 68*(3), 447–452. https://doi.org/10.1302/0301-620X.68B3.3733813
107. Ivarsson, I., and Gillquist, J. (1991). Rehabilitation after high tibial osteotomy and unicompartmental arthroplasty. A comparative study. *Clinical Orthopaedics and Related Research, 266*, 139–144.
108. Weale, A. E., and Newman, J. H. (1994). Unicompartmental arthroplasty and high tibial osteotomy for osteoarthrosis of the knee. A comparative study with a 12- to 17-year follow-up period. *Clinical Orthopaedics and Related Research, 302*, 134–137.
109. Stukenborg-Colsman, C., Wirth, C. J., Lazovic, D., and Wefer, A. (2001). High tibial osteotomy versus unicompartmental joint replacement in unicompartmental knee joint osteoarthritis: 7–10-year follow-up prospective randomised study. *The Knee, 8*(3), 187–194. https://doi.org/10.1016/s0968-0160(01)00097-7

110. Takeuchi, R., Umemoto, Y., Aratake, M., Bito, H., Saito, I., Kumagai, K., Sasaki, Y., Akamatsu, Y., Ishikawa, H., Koshino, T., and Saito, T. (2010). A mid term comparison of open wedge high tibial osteotomy vs unicompartmental knee arthroplasty for medial compartment osteoarthritis of the knee. *Journal of Orthopaedic Surgery and Research, 5*(1), 65. https://doi.org/10.1186/1749-799X-5-65
111. Rodriguez-Merchan, E. C. (2014). Medial unicompartmental osteoarthritis (MUO) of the knee: Unicompartmental knee replacement (UKR) or total knee replacement (TKR). *Archives of Bone and Joint Surgery, 2*(3), 137–140.
112. Zuiderbaan, H. A., van der List, J. P., Kleeblad, L. J., Appelboom, P., Kort, N. P., Pearle, A. D., and Rademakers, M. V. (2016). Modern indications, results, and global trends in the use of unicompartmental knee arthroplasty and high tibial osteotomy in the treatment of isolated medial compartment osteoarthritis. *American Journal of Orthopedics (Belle Mead, N.J.), 45*(6), E355–E361.
113. Petersen, W., and Metzlaff, S. (2016). Open wedge high tibial osteotomy (HTO) versus mobile bearing unicondylar medial joint replacement: Five years results. *Archives of Orthopaedic and Trauma Surgery, 136*(7), 983–989. https://doi.org/10.1007/s00402-016-2465-1
114. Nwachukwu, B. U., McCormick, F. M., Schairer, W. W., Frank, R. M., Provencher, M. T., and Roche, M. W. (2014). Unicompartmental knee arthroplasty versus high tibial osteotomy: United States practice patterns for the surgical treatment of unicompartmental arthritis. *Journal of Arthroplasty, 29*(8), 1586–1589. https://doi.org/10.1016/j.arth.2014.04.002
115. Yim, J. H., Song, E. K., Seo, H. Y., Kim, M. S., and Seon, J. K. (2013). Comparison of high tibial osteotomy and unicompartmental knee arthroplasty at a minimum follow-up of 3 years. *Journal of Arthroplasty, 28*(2), 243–247. https://doi.org/10.1016/j.arth.2012.06.011
116. Song, S. J., Bae, D. K., Kim, K. I., and Park, C. H. (2019). Long-term survival is similar between closed-wedge high tibial osteotomy and unicompartmental knee arthroplasty in patients with similar demographics. *Knee Surgery, Sports Traumatology, Arthroscopy, 27*(4), 1310–1319. https://doi.org/10.1007/s00167-019-05390-w
117. Krych, A. J., Reardon, P., Sousa, P., Pareek, A., Stuart, M., and Pagnano, M. (2017). Unicompartmental knee arthroplasty provides higher activity and durability than valgus-producing proximal tibial osteotomy at 5 to 7 years. *Journal of Bone and Joint Surgery. American Volume, 99*(2), 113–122. https://doi.org/10.2106/JBJS.15.01031
118. Cao, Z., Mai, X., Wang, J., Feng, E., and Huang, Y. (2018). Unicompartmental knee arthroplasty vs high tibial osteotomy for knee osteoarthritis: A systematic review and meta-analysis. *Journal of Arthroplasty, 33*(3), 952–959. https://doi.org/10.1016/j.arth.2017.10.025
119. Fu, D., Li, G., Chen, K., Zhao, Y., Hua, Y., and Cai, Z. (2013). Comparison of high tibial osteotomy and unicompartmental knee arthroplasty in the treat-

ment of unicompartmental osteoarthritis: A meta-analysis. *Journal of Arthroplasty, 28*(5), 759–765. https://doi.org/10.1016/j.arth.2013.02.010
120. Demey G, et al. Insufficient evidence to confirm benefits of custom partial knee arthroplasty: a systematic review. Knee Surg Sports Traumatol Arthrosc. 2022;30(12):3968–82.
121. Burger JA, et al. Mid-term survivorship and patient-reported outcomes of robotic-arm assisted partial knee arthroplasty. Bone Joint J. 2020;102-b(1):108–16.
122. Bray, R.; Macdonald-Taylor, K.; Miller, S.; Nugent, C. Medium term results of the cementless Oxford mobile bearing medial unicompartmental knee replacement. European Journal of Orthopaedic Surgery & Traumatology (2022). https://doi.org/10.1007/s00590-022-03289-w
123. Xie, Feng; Lo, Ngai-Nung; Tarride, Jean-Eric; O'Reilly, Daria; Goeree, Ron; Lee, Hin-Peng Total or partial knee replacement? Cost-utility analysis in patients with knee osteoarthritis based on a 2-year observational study. The European Journal of Health Economics (2009). https://doi.org/10.1007/s10198-009-0154-5
124. Smith, Stephanie; Alvand, Abtin; Locock, Louise; Ryan, Sara; Smith, James; Bayliss, Lee; Wilson, Hannah; Price, Andrew Partial or total knee replacement? Identifying patients' information needs on knee replacement surgery: a qualitative study to inform a decision aid. Quality of Life Research (2019). https://doi.org/10.1007/s11136-019-02381-9
125. D'Ambrosi, Riccardo; Valli, Federico; Nuara, Alessandro; Mariani, Ilaria; Di Feo, Fabrizio; Ursino, Nicola; Formica, Matteo; Mangiavini, Laura; Hantes, Michael; Migliorini, Filippo No difference in mobile and fixed bearing partial knee arthroplasty in octogenarians: a clinical trial. European Journal of Orthopaedic Surgery & Traumatology (2023). https://doi.org/10.1007/s00590-023-03537-7
126. Slamin, John; Parsley, Brian Evolution of customization design for total knee arthroplasty. Current Reviews in Musculoskeletal Medicine (2012). https://doi.org/10.1007/s12178-012-9141-z
127. Mertens, Joren; Floor, Valerie; Stuyts, Bart Functional outcome after bicompartmental knee replacement for medial and patellofemoral osteoarthritis. Archives of Orthopaedic and Trauma Surgery (2024). https://doi.org/10.1007/s00402-024-05543-8
128. Kulshrestha, Vikas; Sood, Munish; Kumar, Santhosh; Kharat, Kiran; Padhi, Prashanth P.; Kumar, Pardeep; Shrama, Saurabh; Stanley, Abin Early Outcomes of Modified Technique of Mobile Bearing Unicondylar Knee Replacement. Indian Journal of Orthopaedics (2023). 10.1007/s43465-023-00907-5
129. Elbardesy, Hany; McLeod, André; Gul, Rehan; Harty, James Midterm results of modern patellofemoral arthroplasty versus total knee arthroplasty for isolated patellofemoral arthritis: systematic review and meta-analysis of comparative studies. Archives of Orthopaedic and Trauma Surgery (2021). https://doi.org/10.1007/s00402-021-03882-4

130. Woon, Colin Y. L.; Christ, Alexander B.; Goto, Rie; Shanaghan, Kate; Shubin Stein, Beth E.; Gonzalez Della Valle, Alejandro Return to the operating room after patellofemoral arthroplasty versus total knee arthroplasty for isolated patellofemoral arthritis—a systematic review. International Orthopaedics (2019). https://doi.org/10.1007/s00264-018-04280-z
131. Yeung, Matthew H. Y.; Fu, Henry; Cheung, Amy; Kwan, Vincent Chan Wai; Cheung, Man Hong; Chan, Ping Keung; Chiu, Kwong Yuen; Yan, Chun Hoi Robotic arm-assisted unicondylar knee arthroplasty resulted in superior radiological accuracy: a propensity score-matched analysis. Arthroplasty (2023). https://doi.org/10.1186/s42836-023-00210-6
132. Walker, Tilman; Stupp, Julius; Reiner, Tobias; Panzram, Benjamin; Nees, Timo A.; Innmann, Moritz M.; Gotterbarm, Tobias; Merle, Christian Minimally invasive Oxford medial unicompartmental knee replacement in patients 50 years of age or younger. Archives of Orthopaedic and Trauma Surgery (2022). https://doi.org/10.1007/s00402-022-04539-6
133. Hiranaka, Takafumi; Furuhashi, Ryosuke; Takashiba, Kenichiro; Kodama, Takao; Michishita, Kazuhiko; Inui, Hiroshi; Togashi, Eita Agreement and accuracy of radiographic assessment using a decision aid for medial Oxford partial knee replacement: multicentre study. Knee Surgery & Related Research (2022). https://doi.org/10.1186/s43019-022-00140-8
134. van Langeveld, Stephan J.; Janssen, Stein J.; Oost, Iris Koenraadt-van; Terra, Maaike P.; van Geenen, Rutger C. I. Valgus stress radiographs have a minor additional value in detecting lateral cartilage wear when selecting patients for medial partial knee replacement. Archives of Orthopaedic and Trauma Surgery (2024). https://doi.org/10.1007/s00402-023-05187-0
135. Lee, Sun-Ho; Kim, Hae-Rim; Song, Eun-Kyoo; Seon, Jong-Keun Risk of Revision and Adverse Outcomes Following Partial Knee Replacement and High Tibial Osteotomy for Unicompartmental Knee Osteoarthritis: A Nationwide Cohort Study. Indian Journal of Orthopaedics (2021). https://doi.org/10.1007/s43465-021-00517-z

4.7 Constrained Knee

Machine Generated Summaries

Disclaimer: The summaries in this chapter were generated from Springer Nature publications using abstractive AI auto-summarization: An abstraction-based summarizer creates new text based on deep learning. New phrases are created to summarize the content. As the constituted sentences are machine selected, they may not fully reflect the body of the work, so we strongly advise that the original content is read and cited. The auto-generated summaries were curated by the editor to meet Springer Nature publication standards.

4.7.1 Results of Total Knee Arthroplasty with Nexgen Lps-Flex for Osteoarthritis in the Valgus Knee: A Study Of 26 Patients Followed for A Minimum of 2 Years [92]

This is a machine-generated summary of:

Nakano, Naoki; Matsumoto, Tomoyuki; Muratsu, Hirotsugu; Matsushita, Takehiko; Takayama, Koji; Matsuzaki, Tokio; Kuroda, Ryosuke; Kurosaka, Masahiro Results of total knee arthroplasty with NexGen LPS-Flex for osteoarthritis in the valgus knee: a study of 26 patients followed for a minimum of 2 years [92].

Published in: European Journal of Orthopaedic Surgery & Traumatology (2014).

Link to original: https://doi.org/10.1007/s00590-014-1505-1

If you want to cite the papers, please refer to the original.

For technical reasons we could not place the page where the original quote is coming from.

4.7.1.1 Research Highlights

Total knee arthroplasty (TKA) aims to provide painless walking and a good postoperative range of motion (ROM), which is particularly important for patients in Asian and Middle Eastern countries who often expect to perform activities requiring deep knee flexion, such as sitting cross-legged or kneeling. Postoperative ROM can be influenced by various factors, including the design of the prosthesis, which is often chosen based on the surgeon's preference. The NexGen Legacy posterior-stabilized (LPS) Flex system (Zimmer Biomet, Warsaw, IN) is a high-flexion prosthesis designed to enhance ROM by modifying the posterior condylar design. However, its effectiveness in patients with valgus knee deformities remains unclear. The study by Nakano et al. investigates the clinical and radiological outcomes of TKA using the NexGen LPS-Flex system in patients with valgus knee deformities.

The study involved primary TKA procedures performed on osteoarthritis patients with valgus knee deformities using the NexGen LPS-Flex fixed prosthesis. Patients with a femorotibial angle (FTA) less than 10° were included, while those requiring metal augmentation or extended stems were excluded. The surgical procedure involved precise bone cuts and soft tissue balancing to address deformities and achieve proper alignment. Postoperative care included active knee motion exercises and weight-bearing activities under supervision. Clinical outcomes were assessed using the Knee Society Knee Score (KSKS) and Function Score (KSFS), while radiological outcomes were evaluated through full-length weight-bearing radiographs. Statistical analysis was conducted to compare pre- and postoperative results.

The study found that TKA using the NexGen LPS-Flex implant resulted in generally good clinical outcomes for valgus knees, with significant improvements in

KSKS and KSFS scores postoperatively. Although the maximum flexion angle improved, it did not reach statistical significance compared to preoperative values. The mean postoperative FTA was near neutral alignment, indicating satisfactory correction of deformity. No cases of peroneal nerve palsy or revision surgery were reported during follow-up. Future study could involve larger cohorts and longer follow-up periods to further evaluate the long-term efficacy and potential advantages of high-flexion prostheses like the NexGen LPS-Flex compared to conventional designs in patients with valgus knee deformities.

4.7.2 Total Knee Arthroplasty in Valgus Knee Deformity: Is It Still a Challenge in 2021? [93]

This is a machine-generated summary of:

Alesi, D.; Meena, A.; Fratini, S.; Rinaldi, V. G.; Cammisa, E.; Lullini, G.; Vaccari, V.; Zaffagnini, S.; Marcheggiani Muccioli, G. M. Total knee arthroplasty in valgus knee deformity: is it still a challenge in 2021? [93].

Published in: MUSCULOSKELETAL SURGERY (2021).

Link to original: https://doi.org/10.1007/s12306-021-00695-x

If you want to cite the papers, please refer to the original.

For technical reasons we could not place the page where the original quote is coming from.

4.7.2.1 Research Highlights

Total knee arthroplasty (TKA) in patients with valgus knee deformities remains a significant challenge in orthopedic surgery. Valgus deformity, characterized by a lateral deviation of the knee, is often caused by osteoarthritis but can also result from conditions such as rheumatoid arthritis and post-traumatic arthritis. The complexity of this deformity is due to factors like hypoplastic lateral condyle, bone loss, and soft tissue contractures, which complicate achieving a well-balanced TKA. This study by Alesi et al. provides a comprehensive analysis of surgical techniques for correcting severe valgus deformity during TKA.

The study outlines various surgical approaches and techniques for managing valgus knee deformities during TKA. Preoperative planning is emphasized as crucial, involving clinical evaluation and radiological assessments to determine the extent of deformity and plan the surgical approach. The medial parapatellar approach is commonly used but may present challenges in accessing tight lateral structures. Alternatively, the lateral parapatellar approach offers better access for releasing tight lateral ligaments but comes with its own technical difficulties. The study also discusses mechanical alignment strategies, emphasizing the importance of correct bone resection and soft tissue balancing to achieve optimal outcomes. Techniques such as pie crusting for soft tissue release and medial reconstruction are explored to address severe deformities effectively.

The advances highlighted in this study include the detailed exploration of various surgical techniques tailored to different severities of valgus deformity. Future study could focus on refining these techniques to minimize complications such as instability and nerve injury while improving long-term outcomes. The choice of implant constraint remains a critical decision based on joint stability and bone defects, with recommendations leaning towards using the least constraint necessary for stability. This comprehensive review by Alesi et al. underscores the importance of a stepwise approach in managing valgus knee deformities during TKA, paving the way for improved surgical outcomes and patient satisfaction.

4.7.3 Slight Under-Correction Following Total Knee Arthroplasty for a Valgus Knee Results in Similar Clinical Outcomes [94]

This is a machine-generated summary of:

Lee, Sung-Sahn; Lee, Hyeon; Lee, Dae-Hee; Moon, Young-Wan Slight under-correction following total knee arthroplasty for a valgus knee results in similar clinical outcomes [94].

Published in: Archives of Orthopaedic and Trauma Surgery (2018).

Link to original: https://doi.org/10.1007/s00402-018-2957-2

If you want to cite the papers, please refer to the original.

For technical reasons we could not place the page where the original quote is coming from.

4.7.3.1 Research Highlights

Total knee arthroplasty (TKA) is traditionally considered successful when neutral limb alignment is restored, particularly aiming for a mechanical hip-knee-ankle (HKA) axis within 0° of neutral. However, recent studies have questioned the necessity of achieving neutral alignment, especially in cases of knee varus deformity, where slight under-correction has not led to inferior outcomes. Despite extensive research on varus deformities, the correlation between TKA outcomes and pre-operative valgus deformity remains unexplored. This study by Lee et al. investigates the relationship between post-operative HKA alignment and clinical outcomes in TKA patients with pre-operative valgus deformity.

The study was a retrospective review of prospectively collected data from TKAs performed by a single surgeon between January 2005 and November 2015. Patients with pre-operative valgus deformity and lateral compartment arthritis were included, resulting in 113 cases after applying exclusion criteria. The TKAs were categorized into three groups based on post-operative HKA alignment: neutral, mild valgus, and severe valgus. Surgical procedures aimed for neutral alignment using posterior-stabilized prostheses, with soft-tissue releases performed as needed to achieve balanced gaps. Clinical assessments such as range of motion (ROM) and the Western Ontario and McMaster Universities Osteoarthritis Index (WOMAC) were evaluated pre-operatively and at final follow-up. Radiographic assessments included measurements of HKA alignment, patellar tilt angle, and congruence angle.

The study found that slight under-correction of valgus deformity resulted in similar clinical outcomes to neutral alignment in TKA patients with pre-operative valgus deformity. However, significant under-correction was associated with increased patellofemoral incongruence. While the mild valgus group did not show superior outcomes compared to the neutral group, the severe valgus group exhibited a higher incidence of patellofemoral issues. Future studies could benefit from longer follow-up periods to assess implant longevity and incorporate post-operative CT scans to evaluate component rotation more accurately. Despite limitations such as its retrospective design and small sample size, this study contributes valuable insights into TKA outcomes for patients with pre-operative valgus deformity.

4.7.4 Effect of Total Knee Arthroplasty for Valgus Knee Correction on Clinical Outcome and Patellar Position [95]

This is a machine-generated summary of:

Zhou, Liang; Dai, Xuening; Zhou, Zhongyuan; Kong, Qian; Duan, Guoqing; Zhang, Yuanmin Effect of total knee arthroplasty for valgus knee correction on clinical outcome and patellar position [95].

Published in: International Orthopaedics (2023).

Link to original: https://doi.org/10.1007/s00264-023-05689-x

If you want to cite the papers, please refer to the original.

For technical reasons we could not place the page where the original quote is coming from.

4.7.4.1 Research Highlights

Total knee arthroplasty (TKA) is a widely used surgical intervention for end-stage knee disease, aiming to achieve optimal soft tissue balance and restore the neutral alignment of the lower limb. However, the impact of maintaining a neutral position on clinical outcomes remains unclear, with some studies suggesting that deviations from neutral alignment may not significantly affect post-operative satisfaction. This study by Zhou et al. investigates the effects of post-operative alignment on clinical efficacy and patellar tracking in patients with valgus knee deformity undergoing TKA.

The study retrospectively analysed patients who underwent TKA for knee osteoarthritis with valgus deformity at the Department of Orthopaedics, Affiliated Hospital of Tianjin University Medical University. Patients were divided into three groups based on post-operative hip-knee-ankle (HKA) alignment: neutral, mild valgus, and severe valgus. The surgical procedure involved standard techniques such as median knee incision, osteotomy, and soft tissue management. Clinical assessments included range of motion (ROM), Western Ontario and McMaster Universities Osteoarthritis Index (WOMAC), and Knee Society Score (KSS), while radiographic evaluations measured HKA alignment and patellar positioning indices. Statistical analyses were conducted to compare pre- and post-operative data across groups.

The study found that while slight undercorrection of valgus did not significantly impact short-term clinical outcomes, severe undercorrection was associated with poorer results and increased risk of patellar maltracking. The findings suggest that achieving a balance between correction and preservation of soft tissue integrity is crucial for optimal outcomes in TKA for valgus knees. Future study could focus on long-term effects and incorporate advanced imaging techniques like three-dimensional computed tomography to enhance measurement accuracy. Additionally, exploring individualized surgical approaches based on pre-operative deformity severity may further improve patient satisfaction and functional outcomes.

4.7.5 Severity of Valgus Knee Osteoarthritis Has No Effect on Clinical Outcomes After Total Knee Arthroplasty [96]

This is a machine-generated summary of:

Rueckl, Kilian; Runer, Armin; Jungwirth-Weinberger, Anna; Kasparek, Maximilian F.; Faschingbauer, Martin; Boettner, Friedrich Severity of valgus knee osteoarthritis has no effect on clinical outcomes after total knee arthroplasty [96].

Published in: Archives of Orthopaedic and Trauma Surgery (2021).

Link to original: https://doi.org/10.1007/s00402-021-03785-4

If you want to cite the papers, please refer to the original.

For technical reasons we could not place the page where the original quote is coming from.

4.7.5.1 Research Highlights

Total knee arthroplasty (TKA) is a common surgical procedure for patients with severe osteoarthritis (OA), where the decision to operate often considers factors such as pain, functional limitations, and radiographic evidence. Traditionally, it is believed that patients with more severe preoperative arthritis achieve better postoperative outcomes, leading to a tendency to delay surgery until OA progresses significantly. However, the correlation between joint space narrowing and postoperative results remains debated. This study by Rueckl et al. investigates whether the degree of mechanical deformity or OA severity at the time of surgery affects clinical outcomes in TKA for patients with valgus OA who have not responded to nonoperative treatments.

The study involved patients undergoing TKA with a minimum follow-up period of 1 year. Participants were selected based on advanced OA grades and minimal joint space width, with surgery indicated only after nonoperative treatments failed. All patients received standardized soft-tissue release procedures, and depending on post-release stability, either posterior stabilized inserts or constrained inlays were used. The study excluded cases lacking complete data, resulting in 100 knees from 85 patients being analysed. Pre- and postoperative evaluations included range of motion, flexion contracture, and various clinical outcome scores such as WOMAC and UCLA activity scores. Radiographic assessments determined mechanical and anatomical alignment using standardized views. Statistical analyses were conducted to compare outcomes across different degrees of deformity and OA severity.

The findings suggest that neither the degree of valgus deformity nor the severity of OA significantly impacts clinical outcomes in TKA for valgus OA patients who have failed nonoperative treatment. This challenges the notion that "bone-on-bone" arthritis is necessary for successful TKA outcomes. The study highlights that moderate OA with some joint space remaining can still result in favorable postoperative results. Future studies could explore long-term outcomes beyond the one-year follow-up and investigate specific knee-related outcome measures to further validate these findings. Additionally, understanding the implications of early versus delayed surgery could refine surgical decision-making for valgus OA patients.

4.7.6 Evaluation of the Rate of Post-Operative Dislocation in Patients with Ipsilateral Valgus Knee Deformity After Primary Total Hip Arthroplasty [97]

This is a machine-generated summary of:

Li, Hao; Xie, Jin-Wei; Ding, Zi-Chuan; Yuan, Ming-Cheng; Lai, Ya-Hao; Zhou, Zong-Ke Evaluation of the rate of post-operative dislocation in patients with ipsilateral valgus knee deformity after primary total hip arthroplasty [97].

Published in: International Orthopaedics (2022).

Link to original: https://doi.org/10.1007/s00264-022-05372-7

If you want to cite the papers, please refer to the original.

For technical reasons we could not place the page where the original quote is coming from.

4.7.6.1 Research Highlights

Total hip arthroplasty (THA) is a widely used surgical procedure to alleviate joint pain and correct deformities caused by end-stage hip diseases. Despite advancements in surgical techniques and prosthesis design, post-operative dislocation remains a prevalent complication, often necessitating costly revision surgeries. Identifying risk factors for dislocation is crucial to mitigate these outcomes. While factors such as advanced age, obesity, and surgical technique have been recognized, the impact of ipsilateral valgus knee deformity on dislocation rates after THA has not been thoroughly investigated. The study by Li et al. explores this relationship, hypothesizing that ipsilateral valgus knee deformity increases the risk of dislocation following THA.

The study involved a retrospective analysis of patients who underwent primary THA at a single institution between January 2010 and December 2015. Patients with ipsilateral valgus knee deformity were matched with those without the deformity based on sex, affected side, and surgery date. The researchers collected comprehensive pre-operative, intra-operative, and post-operative data, including demographics, surgical details, and radiographic measurements. Statistical analyses were conducted to compare dislocation rates between the two groups and identify independent risk factors for dislocation in patients with valgus knee deformity. The findings revealed that hips with ipsilateral valgus knee deformity had a significantly higher dislocation rate (6.7%) compared to those without (2.3%). Multivariate logistic regression analysis identified older age and malposition of the acetabular cup as independent risk factors for dislocation in this patient population.

The study's results suggest that ipsilateral valgus knee deformity poses additional challenges during THA, leading to increased dislocation risks. These findings underscore the importance of careful pre-operative planning and precise surgical execution in patients with this condition. The authors propose that if both THA and total knee arthroplasty (TKA) are necessary, performing TKA or corrective osteotomy before THA may be beneficial to reduce instability risks. Future studies with larger sample sizes could further validate these findings and explore optimal surgical strategies for managing patients with concurrent hip and knee deformities.

4.7.7 Total Knee Arthroplasty in the Varus Knee: Tips and Tricks [98]

This is a machine-generated summary of:

Rossi, Roberto; Cottino, Umberto; Bruzzone, Matteo; Dettoni, Federico; Bonasia, Davide Edoardo; Rosso, Federica Total knee arthroplasty in the varus knee: tips and tricks [98].

Published in: International Orthopaedics (2018).

Link to original: https://doi.org/10.1007/s00264-018-4116-3

If you want to cite the papers, please refer to the original.

For technical reasons we could not place the page where the original quote is coming from.

4.7.7.1 Research Highlights

Varus deformity of the knee is a prevalent angular deformity encountered in total knee arthroplasty (TKA), characterized by a mechanical axis deviation and associated bone and soft tissue abnormalities. This condition often involves medial joint line narrowing, proximal tibial deformity, and in severe cases, medial subluxation of the femur on the tibia. Despite its prevalence, the complexity of varus deformities, particularly those involving extra-articular components like femoral bowing or proximal tibial varus, poses significant challenges in achieving optimal surgical outcomes. The study by Rossi et al. explores comprehensive pre-operative planning and surgical techniques to address these challenges in TKA for varus knees.

The study employs a detailed methodology involving radiographic pre-operative planning to assess lower limb alignment and joint line obliquity. The authors emphasize the importance of individualized surgical approaches based on the severity and type of deformity. Techniques such as osteophyte removal, soft tissue balancing, and careful implant selection are highlighted as critical steps. The research outlines various procedures like tibial reduction osteotomy and medial epicondyle sliding osteotomy for severe cases where standard soft tissue balancing is insufficient. The study also discusses the use of different implant types, including posterior-stabilized (PS) implants and mid-level constraint (MLC) implants, tailored to specific deformities and patient needs.

The advancements presented by Rossi et al. contribute significantly to improving TKA outcomes in patients with varus knee deformities. By emphasizing meticulous pre-operative planning and individualized surgical strategies, the study enhances understanding of managing complex varus deformities effectively. Future study could focus on refining these techniques further or exploring long-term outcomes associated with different implant types and surgical approaches. The findings underscore the importance of tailored interventions to achieve optimal alignment, stability, and patient satisfaction in TKA procedures for varus knees.

4.7.8 Ankle and Hindfoot Alignment Changes in Advanced OA Varus Knees After Cruciate Retaining Total Knee Arthroplasty: A Prospective Cohort Study [99]

This is a machine-generated summary of:

Kapoor, Vikash; Ghosh, Mriganka M.; Chatterjee, Anirban; Debnath, Kaustav; Hasan, Gaji Mehdi Ankle and Hindfoot Alignment Changes in Advanced OA Varus Knees After Cruciate Retaining Total Knee Arthroplasty: A Prospective Cohort Study [99].

Published in: Indian Journal of Orthopaedics (2022).

Link to original: https://doi.org/10.1007/s43465-022-00754-w

Copyright of the summarized publication:

If you want to cite the papers, please refer to the original.

For technical reasons we could not place the page where the original quote is coming from.

4.7.8.1 Research Highlights

Knee deformity, particularly varus deformity, often results from the degenerative process of osteoarthritis and can lead to compensatory changes in the hip and ankle joints due to abnormal loading. Proper alignment during total knee arthroplasty (TKA) is crucial for implant survivorship and functional outcomes, but the impact of TKA on ankle and hindfoot alignment has not been extensively studied. The study by Kapoor et al. investigates the radiographic and functional changes in the ankle joint and hindfoot following TKA in patients with high-grade varus osteoarthritis of the knee in an Indian subcontinent population.

The study involved patients with advanced knee osteoarthritis who underwent TKA using a cruciate-retaining fixed-bearing prosthetic design. Pre- and post-operative full-leg standing radiographs were taken to assess changes in mechanical alignment, including the hip-knee-ankle angle, talar tilt, and other relevant angles. Functional outcomes were evaluated using the Knee Society Score (KSS) and the American Orthopaedic Foot and Ankle Score (AOFAS). The results showed significant improvements in these scores post-operatively, indicating better functional outcomes. Radiographic analysis revealed a decrease in hindfoot valgus post-TKA, although some valgus persisted. The study found a mild correlation between changes in knee varus deformity and hindfoot alignment angles.

The findings suggest that TKA not only corrects knee varus deformity but also induces compensatory changes in hindfoot alignment, reducing valgus without requiring direct intervention at the ankle level. This highlights the importance of considering lower limb alignment holistically during TKA to optimize outcomes. Future study could focus on developing predictive models for hindfoot alignment changes based on knee varus correction. However, limitations such as a small sample size, single-center design, and short follow-up period suggest that further research with larger cohorts is needed to validate these findings and explore long-term effects.

4.7.9 How Coronal Alignment Affects Distal Femoral Anatomy: An MRI-Based Comparison of Varus and Valgus Knees [100]

This is a machine-generated summary of:

Cohen, Daniel A; Gursel, Ali C; Low, Adrian K How coronal alignment affects distal femoral anatomy: an MRI-based comparison of varus and valgus knees [100].

Published in: Journal of Orthopaedic Surgery and Research (2019).

Link to original: https://doi.org/10.1186/s13018-019-1133-x

If you want to cite the papers, please refer to the original.

For technical reasons we could not place the page where the original quote is coming from.

4.7.9.1 Research Highlights

Total knee arthroplasty (TKA) success hinges on the precise alignment of femoral and tibial components to restore the mechanical axis and maintain soft tissue balance. The epicondylar axis (EA) is often used as a reference for femoral component rotation, but its intraoperative identification can be challenging. Consequently, the posterior condylar axis (PCA), which is more easily defined, is frequently used as a surrogate. However, recent studies suggest variability in the PCA-EA relationship, particularly in knees with valgus deformities. The study by Cohen et al. investigates how increasing coronal deformity affects the PCA-EA relationship using MRI data from arthritic knees.

The study analyzed MRIs from patients undergoing TKA to create patient-specific cutting blocks using the Biomet Signature system. MRIs of the ankle, hip, and knee were converted into 3D models to determine limb alignment and various axes, including EA and PCA. The researchers examined how coronal deformity influenced the PCA-EA relationship by categorizing knees into varus and valgus groups with varying degrees of deformity. Statistical analyses revealed that in valgus knees, there was greater external rotation of both EA and anterior-posterior (AP) axes relative to PCA compared to varus knees. However, no significant difference was found in PCA-EA relationships between different degrees of valgus deformity.

The study advances understanding by highlighting the heterogeneity in PCA-EA relationships across different knee deformities, challenging previous assumptions about consistent rotational alignment strategies in TKA. It suggests that relying solely on PCA for femoral component alignment may lead to malrotation, particularly in valgus knees when external rotation exceeds 3° from PCA. Future study could explore weight-bearing imaging modalities to better assess limb alignment and further investigate larger valgus deformities' impact on femoral component placement accuracy. These findings underscore the need for personalized approaches in TKA to optimize outcomes and reduce complications associated with rotational malalignment.

4.7.10 Is Medial Pivot Total Knee Arthroplasty Suitable for Patients with Valgus Knee Osteoarthritis? [101]

This is a machine-generated summary of:

Iwakiri, Kentaro; Ohta, Yoichi; Ohyama, Yohei; Minoda, Yukihide; Kobayashi, Akio; Nakamura, Hiroaki Is medial pivot total knee arthroplasty suitable for patients with valgus knee osteoarthritis? [101].

Published in: European Journal of Orthopaedic Surgery & Traumatology (2021).

Link to original: https://doi.org/10.1007/s00590-021-03007-y

If you want to cite the papers, please refer to the original.

For technical reasons we could not place the page where the original quote is coming from.

4.7.10.1 Research Highlights

Total knee arthroplasty (TKA) is a highly effective treatment for end-stage knee osteoarthritis, providing pain relief and improved function. While most TKA procedures address varus deformities, valgus deformities are less common and present unique challenges due to their distinct tibiofemoral articulation characteristics. The medial pivot-type TKA (MP-TKA) design, known for its stability and wear resistance, has shown promising long-term outcomes in varus knees. However, its efficacy in valgus knees remains unclear. The study by Iwakiri et al. investigates the mid-short-term postoperative outcomes of MP-TKA in patients with valgus knee osteoarthritis compared to those with varus deformities.

The study was a retrospective, single-center cohort analysis involving patients who underwent MP-TKA with a ceramic femoral component. Participants were selected based on specific criteria, including the ability to follow up for at least 2 years post-surgery. The surgical approach involved a standard medial parapatellar technique with modifications for gap balancing, including the pie crust technique for lateral soft tissue release in valgus knees. Outcomes were assessed through radiographic measurements, range of motion (ROM), and clinical scores such as the Western Ontario and McMaster Universities Arthritis Index (WOMAC). Statistical analyses compared results between the varus and valgus groups, focusing on ROM improvements and clinical outcomes.

The study found that MP-TKA provided equally favorable outcomes in both valgus and varus knee patients over the mid-term follow-up period. Despite initial concerns about medial conformity issues in valgus knees, the use of additional techniques like pie crusting allowed for effective alignment correction without extending surgical duration or increasing complications. Future study directions could explore larger sample sizes or different implant models to further validate these findings. The research suggests that MP-TKA is a viable option for patients with valgus knee deformity, expanding its applicability beyond traditional varus cases.

Bibliography

1. Sharkey PF, Hozack WJ, Rothman RH, Shastri S, Jacoby SM (2002) Insall award paper. Why are total knee arthroplasties failing today? Clin Orthop Relat Res 404:7–13. https://doi.org/10.1097/00003086-200211000-00003
2. Rodriguez-Merchan EC (2011) Instability following total knee arthroplasty. HSSJ 7(3):273–278
3. Vince KG, Abdeen A, Sugimori T (2006) The unstable total knee arthroplasty: causes and cures. J Arthroplasty 21(4 Suppl 1):44–49. https://doi.org/10.1016/j.arth.2006.02.101
4. Gonzalez MH, Mekhail AO. The failed total knee arthroplasty: evaluation and etiology. J Am Acad Orthop Surg. 2004;12:436–46.
5. Berend ME, Bertrand T. The role of implant constraint: not too little, not too much. Orthopedics. 2007;30(9):793.
6. Azzam K, Parvizi J, Kaufman D, Purtill JJ, Sharkey PF, Austin MS. Revision of the unstable total knee arthroplasty: outcome predictors. J Arthroplasty. 2011;26(8):1139–44. https://doi.org/10.1016/j.arth.2011.02.028.
7. Babis GC, Trousdale RT, Morrey BF. The effectiveness of isolated tibial insert exchange in revision total knee arthroplasty. J Bone Joint Surg Am. 2002;84-A(1):64.
8. Engh GA (1997) Bone loss classification. In: Engh GA, Rorabeck CH (eds) Revision total knee arthroplasty. Williams and Wilkins, Baltimore, pp 63–120
9. Mahomed NN, Barrett J, Katz JN, Baron JA, Wright J, Losina E (2005) Epidemiology of total knee replacement in the United States medicare population. J Bone Joint Surg Am 87:1222–1228

10. Johnson AJ, Sayeed SA, Naziri Q, Khanuja HS, Mont MA (2012) Minimizing dynamic knee spacer complications in infected revision arthroplasty. Clin Orthop Relat Res 470:220–227
11. Hwang SC, Kong JY, Nam DC, et al. Revision total knee arthroplasty with a cemented posterior stabilized, condylar constrained or fully constrained prosthesis: a minimum 2-year follow-up analysis. Clin Orthop Surg. 2010;2:112.
12. Kim YH, Kim JS. Revision total knee arthroplasty with use of a constrained condylar knee prosthesis. J Bone Joint Surg Am. 2009;91:1440.
13. Meijer MF, Reininga IH, Boerboom AL, Stevens M, Bulstra SK (2013) Poorer survival after a primary implant during revision total knee arthroplasty. Int Orthop 37:415–419
14. Radnay CS, Scuderi GR (2006) Management of bone loss. Augments, cones, offset stems. Clin Orthop Relat Res 446:83–92
15. Murray PB, Rand JA, Hanssen AD (1994) Cemented long-stem revision total knee arthroplasty. Clin Orthop Relat Res 309:116–123
16. Cram P, Lu X, Kates SL, Singh JA, Li Y, Wolf BR (2012) Total knee arthroplasty volume, utilization, and outcomes among Medicare beneficiaries, 1991–2010. JAMA 308:1227–1236
17. Learmonth ID, Young C, Rorabeck C (2007) The operation of the century: total hip replacement. Lancet Lond Engl 370:1508–1519
18. Romanini E, Decarolis F, Luzi I et al (2019) Total knee arthroplasty in Italy: reflections from the last fifteen years and projections for the next thirty. Int Orthop. https://doi.org/10.1007/s00264-018-4165-7
19. Chalmers BP, Matrka AK, Sems SA, Abdel MP, Sierra RJ, Hanssen AD, Pagnano MW, Mabry TM, Perry KI (2020) Two-stage arthrodesis for complex, failed, infected total knee arthroplasty. Bone Jt J 102-B: 170–175
20. Hungerer S, Kiechle M, von Rüden C, Militz M, Beitzel K, Morgenstern M (2017) Knee arthrodesis versus above-the-knee amputation after septic failure of revision total knee arthroplasty: comparison of functional outcome and complication rates. BMC Musculoskelet Disord 18:443
21. Postler A, Lützner C, Beyer F, Tille E, Lützner J. Analysis of total knee arthroplasty revision causes. BMC Musculoskelet Disord. 2018;19:55.
22. Cherian JJ, Bhave A, Harwin SF, Mont MA (2016) Outcomes and aseptic survivorship of revision total knee arthroplasty. Am J Orthop Belle Mead NJ 45:79–85
23. Sappey-Marinier E, Fratini S, Kremer H, Shatrov J, Batailler C, Servien E, Lustig S (2021) Similar outcomes to primary total knee arthroplasty achievable for aseptic revision using the same primary posterior-stabilised prosthesis at a mean follow-up of 49 months. Knee Surg Sports Traumatol Arthrosc 30(8):2854–2861. https://doi.org/10.1007/s00167-021-06716-3
24. Houfani F, Mainard D, Rubens-Duval B, Papin P-E, Pasquier G, Ehlinger M, French Society for Orthopaedic, Trauma Surgery (SoFCOT) (2021) Rotating-hinge prosthesis for aseptic revision knee arthroplasty: a multicentre retrospective study of 127 cases with a mean follow-up of five years. Orthop Traumatol Surg Res OTSR 107:102855

25. Scuderi GR, Bourne RB, Noble PC, Benjamin JB, Lonner JH, Scott WN. The new Knee Society Knee Scoring System. Clin Orthop Relat Res. 2012;470(1):3–19. https://doi.org/10.1007/s11999-011-2135-0.
26. Anouchi YS, McShane M, Kelly F Jr, Elting J, Stiehl J (1996) Range of motion in total knee replacement. Clin Orthop Relat Res 331:87–92
27. Ranawat CS (2003) Design may be counterproductive for optimizing flexion after TKR. Clin Orthop Relat Res 416:174–176
28. Ritter MA (2006) High-flexion knee designs: more hype than hope? In the affirmative. J Arthroplasty 21:40–41
29. Bin, S. I. and Nam, T. S. Early results of high-flex total knee arthroplasty: comparison study at 1 year after surgery. *Knee Surg. Sports Traumatol. Arthorosc. 15*, 350–355 (2007).
30. Huang HT, Su JY, Wang GJ (2005) The early results of high-flex total knee arthroplasty: a minimum of 2 years of follow-up. J Arthroplasty 20(5):674–679
31. Murphy M, Journeaux S, Russell T (2009) High-flexion total knee arthroplasty: a systematic review. Int Orthop 33(4):887–893
32. Elkus M, Ranawat CS, Rasquinha VJ et al (2004) Total knee arthroplasty for severe valgus deformity. Five to fourteen-year follow-up. J Bone Joint Surg Am 86:2671–2676. https://doi.org/10.2106/00004623-200412000-00013
33. McAuley JP, Collier MB, Hamilton WG et al (2008) Posterior cruciate-retaining total knee arthroplasty for valgus osteoarthritis. Clin Orthop Relat Res 466:2644–2649. https://doi.org/10.1007/s11999-008-0436-8
34. Rames RD, Mathison M, Meyer Z, Barrack RL, Nam D (2017) No impact of under-correction and joint line obliquity on clinical outcomes of total knee arthroplasty for the varus knee. Knee Surg Sports Traumatol Arthrosc. https://doi.org/10.1007/s00167-017-4507-9
35. Vanlommel L, Vanlommel J, Claes S, Bellemans J (2013) Slight undercorrection following total knee arthroplasty results in superior clinical outcomes in varus knees. Knee Surg Sports Traumatol Arthrosc 21(10):2325–2330. https://doi.org/10.1007/s00167-013-2481-4
36. Howell SM, Howell SJ, Kuznik KT, Cohen J, Hull ML. Does a kinematically aligned total knee athroplasty restore function without failure regardless of alignment category? *Clin Orthop Relat Res.* 2013;471:1000–1007.
37. Matziolis G, Adam J, Perka C (2010) Varus malalignment has no influence on clinical outcome in midterm follow-up after total knee replacement. Arch Orthop Trauma Surg 130(12):1487–1491. https://doi.org/10.1007/s00402-010-1064-9
38. Malghem J, Maldague B (1989) Patellofemoral joint: 30 degrees axial radiograph with lateral rotation of the leg. Radiology 170(2):566–567. https://doi.org/10.1148/radiology.170.2.2911687
39. Karachalios T, Sarangi PP, Newman JH (1994) Severe varus and valgus deformities treated by total knee arthroplasty. J Bone Joint Surg Br 76:938–942
40. Lording T, Lustig S, Neyret P (2017) Coronal alignment after total knee arthroplasty. EFORT Open Rev 1(1):12–17. https://doi.org/10.1302/2058-5241.1.000002

41. Smith CR, Vignos MF, Lenhart RL, Kaiser J, Thelen DG (2016) The influence of component alignment and ligament properties on tibiofemoral contact forces in total knee replacement. J Biomech Eng 138(2):021017. https://doi.org/10.1115/1.4032464
42. van Hamersveld KT, Marang-van de Mheen PJ, Nelissen RGHH (2019) The effect of coronal alignment on tibial component migration following total knee arthroplasty: a cohort study with long-term radiostereometric analysis results. J Bone Joint Surg Am 101(13):1203–1212. https://doi.org/10.2106/JBJS.18.00691
43. Keshmiri A, Dotzauer F, Baier C, Maderbacher G, Grifka J, Sendtner E (2017) Stability of capsule closure and postoperative anterior knee pain after medial parapatellar approach in TKA. Arch Orthop Trauma Surg 137(7):1019–1024. https://doi.org/10.1007/s00402-017-2706-y
44. Cerciello S, Robin J, Lustig S, Maccauro G, Heyse TJ, Neyret P (2016) The role of patelloplasty in total knee arthroplasty. Arch Orthop Trauma Surg 136(11):1607–1613. https://doi.org/10.1007/s00402-016-2577-7
45. Popovic N, Lemaire R (2003) Anterior knee pain with a posterior-stabilized mobile-bearing knee prosthesis: the effect of femoral component design. J Arthroplast 18(4):396–400
46. Buckland-Wright JC, Macfarlane DG, Williams SA, Ward RJ (1995) Accuracy and precision of joint space width measurements in standard and macroradiographs of osteoarthritic knees. Ann Rheum Dis 54(11):872–880
47. Peterfy C, Li J, Zaim S, Duryea J, Lynch J, Miaux Y, Yu W, Genant HK (2003) Comparison of fixed-flexion positioning with fluoroscopic semi-flexed positioning for quantifying radiographic joint-space width in the knee: test–retest reproducibility. Skelet Radiol 32(3):128–132. https://doi.org/10.1007/s00256-002-0603-z
48. Reichmann WM, Maillefert JF, Hunter DJ, Katz JN, Conaghan PG, Losina E (2011) Responsiveness to change and reliability of measurement of radiographic joint space width in osteoarthritis of the knee: a systematic review. Osteoarthr Carti/OARS Osteoarthr Res Soc 19(5):550–556. https://doi.org/10.1016/j.joca.2011.01.023
49. Mancuso CA, Ranawat CS, Esdaile JM, Johanson NA, Charlson ME (1996) Indications for total hip and total knee arthroplasties. Results of orthopaedic surveys. J Arthroplast 11(1):34–46
50. Liang MH, Cullen KE, Poss R (1982) Primary total hip or knee replacement: evaluation of patients. Ann Intern Med 97(5):735–739
51. Boettner F, Renner L, Arana Narbarte D, Egidy C, Faschingbauer M (2016) Total knee arthroplasty for valgus osteoarthritis: the results of a standardized soft-tissue release technique. Knee Surg Sports Traumatol Arthrosc 24(8):2525–2531. https://doi.org/10.1007/s00167-016-4054-9
52. Idusuyi OB, Morrey BF (1996) Peroneal nerve palsy after total knee arthroplasty. Assessment of predisposing and prognostic factors. J Bone Jt Surg Am Vol 78(2):177–184

53. Asp JP, Rand JA (1990) Peroneal nerve palsy after total knee arthroplasty. Clin Orthop Relat Res 261:233–237
54. Kellgren JH, Lawrence JS (1957) Radiological assessment of osteo-arthrosis. Ann Rheum Dis 16(4):494–502
55. Chang CB, Yoo JH, Koh IJ, Kang YG, Seong SC, Kim TK (2010) Key factors in determining surgical timing of total knee arthroplasty in osteoarthritic patients: age, radiographic severity, and symptomatic severity. J Orthop Traumatol Off J Italian Soc Orthop Traumatol 11(1):21–27. https://doi.org/10.1007/s10195-010-0086-y
56. Meding JB, Ritter MA, Faris PM, Keating EM, Harris W (2001) Does the preoperative radiographic degree of osteoarthritis correlate to results in primary total knee arthroplasty? J Arthroplast 16(1):13–16. https://doi.org/10.1054/arth.2001.16501
57. Maempel JF, Riddoch F, Calleja N, Brenkel IJ (2015) Longer hospital stay, more complications, and increased mortality but substantially improved function after knee replacement in older patients. Acta Orthop 86(4):451–456. https://doi.org/10.3109/17453674.2015.1040304
58. Stern SH, Moeckel BH, Insall JN (1991) Total knee arthroplasty in valgus knees. Clin Orthop Relat Res 273:5–8
59. Ritter MA, Davis KE, Davis P, Farris A, Malinzak RA, Berend ME, Meding JB (2013) Preoperative malalignment increases risk of failure after total knee arthroplasty. J Bone Joint Surg Am 95(2):126–131. https://doi.org/10.2106/JBJS.K.00607
60. Martin JR, Beahrs TR, Stuhlman CR, Trousdale RT (2016) Complex primary total knee arthroplasty: long-term outcomes. J Bone Jt Surg Am Vol 98(17):1459–1470. https://doi.org/10.2106/jbjs.15.01173
61. Gwam CU, Mistry JB, Mohamed NS, Thomas M, Bigart KC, Mont MA, Delanois RE (2017) Current epidemiology of revision total hip arthroplasty in the United States: national inpatient sample 2009 to 2013. J Arthroplasty 32(7):2088–2092
62. Ding ZC, Xu B, Liang ZM, Wang HY, Luo ZY, Zhou ZK (2020) Limited influence of comorbidities on length of stay after total hip arthroplasty: experience of enhanced recovery after surgery. Orthop Surg 12(1):153–161
63. Ding ZC, Zeng WN, Mou P, Liang ZM, Wang D, Zhou ZK (2020) Risk of dislocation after total hip arthroplasty in patients with crowe type iv developmental dysplasia of the hip. Orthop Surg 12(2):589–600
64. Lange J, Haas SB (2017) Correcting severe valgus deformity taking out the knock. Bone Joint J. https://doi.org/10.1302/0301-620X.99B1.BJJ-2016-0340.R1
65. Liu Q, Cheng X, Yan D, Zhou Y (2019) Plain radiography findings to predict dislocation after total hip arthroplasty. J Orthop Transl 18:1–6
66. Verdonk PC, Pernin J, Pinaroli A, Ait Si Selmi T, Neyret P (2009) Soft tissue balancing in varus total knee arthroplasty: an algorithmic approach. Knee Surg Sports Traumatol Arthrosc 17:660–666. https://doi.org/10.1007/s00167-009-0755-7

67. Thienpont E, Schwab PE, Cornu O, Bellemans J, Victor J (2017) Bone morphotypes of the varus and valgus knee. Arch Orthop Trauma Surg 137:393–400. https://doi.org/10.1007/s00402-017-2626-x
68. Gao F, Ma J, Sun W, Guo W, Li Z, Wang W (2016) The influence of knee malalignment on the ankle alignment in varus and valgus gonarthrosis based on radiographic measurement. Eur J Radiol 85:228–232. https://doi.org/10.1016/j.ejrad.2015.11.021
69. Norton AA, Callaghan JJ, Amendola A, Phisitkul P, Wongsak S, Liu SS, Fruehling-Wall C (2015) Correlation of knee and hindfoot deformities in advanced knee OA: compensatory hindfoot alignment and where it occurs. Clin Orthop Relat Res 473:166–174. https://doi.org/10.1007/s11999-014-3801-9
70. Mullaji AB, Shetty GM (2014) Correction of varus deformity during TKA with reduction osteotomy. Clin Orthop Relat Res 472:126–132. https://doi.org/10.1007/s11999-013-3077-5
71. Meftah M, Blum YC, Raja D, Ranawat AS, Ranawat CS (2012) Correcting fixed varus deformity with flexion contracture during total knee arthroplasty: the "inside-out" technique: AAOS exhibit selection. J Bone Joint Surg Am 94:e66. https://doi.org/10.2106/JBJS.K.01444
72. Rossi R, Rosso F, Cottino U, Dettoni F, Bonasia DE, Bruzzone M (2014) Total knee arthroplasty in the valgus knee. Int Orthop 38(2):273–283. https://doi.org/10.1007/s00264-013-2227-4
73. Pancio SI, Sousa PL, Krych AJ, Abdel MP, Levy BA, Dahm DL, Stuart MJ (2017) Increased risk of revision, reoperation, and implant constraint in TKA after multiligament knee surgery. Clin Orthop Relat Res 475:1618–1626. https://doi.org/10.1007/s11999-017-5230-z
74. Lachiewicz PF, Soileau ES (2006) Ten-year survival and clinical results of constrained components in primary total knee arthroplasty. J Arthroplasty 21:803–808. https://doi.org/10.1016/j.arth.2005.09.008
75. Mullaji A, Sharma A, Marawar S, Kanna R (2009) Quantification of effect of sequential posteromedial release on flexion and extension gaps: a computer-assisted study in cadaveric knees. J Arthroplast 24:795–805. https://doi.org/10.1016/j.arth.2008.03.018
76. Dixon MC, Parsch D, Brown RR, Scott RD (2004) The correction of severe varus deformity in total knee arthroplasty by tibial component downsizing and resection of uncapped proximal medial bone. J Arthroplast 19:19–22
77. Mullaji AB, Padmanabhan V, Jindal G (2005) Total knee arthroplasty for profound varus deformity: technique and radiological results in 173 knees with varus of more than 20 degrees. J Arthroplast 20:550–561. https://doi.org/10.1016/j.arth.2005.04.009
78. Ritter MA, Faris GW, Faris PM, Davis KE (2004) Total knee arthroplasty in patients with angular varus or valgus deformities of > or = 20 degrees. J Arthroplast 19:862–866

79. Mullaji A, Shetty GM (2011) Persistent hindfoot valgus causes lateral deviation of weightbearing axis after total knee arthroplasty. Clin Orthop Relat Res 469:1154–1160. https://doi.org/10.1007/s11999-010-1703-z
80. Chandler, J. T., and Moskal, J. T. (2004). Evaluation of knee and hindfoot alignment before and after total knee arthroplasty: a prospective analysis. *J Arthroplast, 19*(2), 211–216. https://doi.org/10.1016/j.arth.2003.09.007 PMID: 14973865.
81. Okamoto, Y., Otsuki, S., Jotoku, T., Nakajima, M., and Neo, M. (2017). Clinical usefulness of hindfoot assessment for total knee arthroplasty: persistent post-operative hindfoot pain and alignment in pre-existing severe knee deformity. *Knee Surgery, Sports Traumatology, Arthroscopy, 25*(8), 2632–2639. https://doi.org/10.1007/s00167-016-4122-1 Epub 2016 Apr 7 PMID: 27056693.
82. Berger RA, Rubash HE, Seel MJ, Thompson WH, Crossett LS. Determining the rotational alignment of the femoral component in total knee arthroplasty using the epicondylar axis. Clin Orthop Relat Res. 1993;286:40–7.
83. Griffin FM, Insall JN, Scuderi GR. The posterior condylar angle in osteoarthritic knees. J Arthroplast. 1998;13:812–5.
84. Yoshioka Y, Siu D, Cooke TD. The anatomy and functional axes of the femur. J Bone Jt Surg Am. 1987;69:873–80.
85. Victor J. Rotational alignment of the distal femur: a literature review. Orthop Traumatol Surg Res. 2009;95:365–72.
86. Matsuda S, Miura H, Nagamine R, Mawatari T, Tokunaga M, et al. Anatomical analysis of the femoral condyle in normal and osteoarthritic knees. J Orthop Res. 2004;22(1):104–9.
87. Ando G, Tsukimoto T (2002) Osteoarthritis of knee joint–standard concept and diagnosis. Clin Calcium 12(1):47–52
88. Krackow KA, Jones MM, Teeny SM, Hungerford DS (1991) Primary total knee arthroplasty in patients with fixed valgus deformity. Clin Orthop Relat Res 273:p9–18
89. Pritchett JW (2011) Patients prefer a bicruciate-retaining or the medial pivot total knee prosthesis. J Arthroplasty 26:224–228. https://doi.org/10.1016/j.arth.2010.02.012
90. Moro-oka TA, Shiraishi H, Iwamoto Y, Banks SA (2010) Modified gap-balancing technique in total knee arthroplasty: evaluation of the post-operative coronal laxity. Knee Surg Sports Traumatol Arthrosc 18(3):p375–380
91. Okuda M, Omokawa S, Tanaka Y, Okahashi K, Akahane M (2012) Validity and reliability of the Japanese orthopaedic association score for osteoarthritic knees. J Orthop Sci 17(6):p750–756XZ
92. Nakano, Naoki; Matsumoto, Tomoyuki; Muratsu, Hirotsugu; Matsushita, Takehiko; Takayama, Koji; Matsuzaki, Tokio; Kuroda, Ryosuke; Kurosaka, Masahiro Results of total knee arthroplasty with NexGen LPS-Flex for osteoarthritis in the valgus knee: a study of 26 patients followed for a minimum of 2 years. European Journal of Orthopaedic Surgery & Traumatology (2014). 10.1007/s00590-014-1505-1

93. Alesi, D.; Meena, A.; Fratini, S.; Rinaldi, V. G.; Cammisa, E.; Lullini, G.; Vaccari, V.; Zaffagnini, S.; Marcheggiani Muccioli, G. M. Total knee arthroplasty in valgus knee deformity: is it still a challenge in 2021?. MUSCULOSKELETAL SURGERY (2021). https://doi.org/10.1007/s12306-021-00695-x
94. Lee, Sung-Sahn; Lee, Hyeon; Lee, Dae-Hee; Moon, Young-Wan Slight undercorrection following total knee arthroplasty for a valgus knee results in similar clinical outcomes. Archives of Orthopaedic and Trauma Surgery (2018). https://doi.org/10.1007/s00402-018-2957-2
95. Zhou, Liang; Dai, Xuening; Zhou, Zhongyuan; Kong, Qian; Duan, Guoqing; Zhang, Yuanmin Effect of total knee arthroplasty for valgus knee correction on clinical outcome and patellar position. International Orthopaedics (2023). 10.1007/s00264-023-05689-x
96. Rueckl, Kilian; Runer, Armin; Jungwirth-Weinberger, Anna; Kasparek, Maximilian F.; Faschingbauer, Martin; Boettner, Friedrich Severity of valgus knee osteoarthritis has no effect on clinical outcomes after total knee arthroplasty. Archives of Orthopaedic and Trauma Surgery (2021). https://doi.org/10.1007/s00402-021-03785-4
97. Li, Hao; Xie, Jin-Wei; Ding, Zi-Chuan; Yuan, Ming-Cheng; Lai, Ya-Hao; Zhou, Zong-Ke Evaluation of the rate of post-operative dislocation in patients with ipsilateral valgus knee deformity after primary total hip arthroplasty. International Orthopaedics (2022). https://doi.org/10.1007/s00264-022-05372-7
98. Rossi, Roberto; Cottino, Umberto; Bruzzone, Matteo; Dettoni, Federico; Bonasia, Davide Edoardo; Rosso, Federica Total knee arthroplasty in the varus knee: tips and tricks. International Orthopaedics (2018). https://doi.org/10.1007/s00264-018-4116-3
99. Kapoor, Vikash; Ghosh, Mriganka M.; Chatterjee, Anirban; Debnath, Kaustav; Hasan, Gaji Mehdi Ankle and Hindfoot Alignment Changes in Advanced OA Varus Knees After Cruciate Retaining Total Knee Arthroplasty: A Prospective Cohort Study. Indian Journal of Orthopaedics (2022). https://doi.org/10.1007/s43465-022-00754-w
100. Cohen, Daniel A; Gursel, Ali C; Low, Adrian K How coronal alignment affects distal femoral anatomy: an MRI-based comparison of varus and valgus knees. Journal of Orthopaedic Surgery and Research (2019). https://doi.org/10.1186/s13018-019-1133-x
101. Iwakiri, Kentaro; Ohta, Yoichi; Ohyama, Yohei; Minoda, Yukihide; Kobayashi, Akio; Nakamura, Hiroaki Is medial pivot total knee arthroplasty suitable for patients with valgus knee osteoarthritis?. European Journal of Orthopaedic Surgery & Traumatology (2021). https://doi.org/10.1007/s00590-021-03007-y

Chapter 5
Surgical Approaches for Primary Total Knee Arthroplasty

Alfred J. Tria Jr. and Giles R. Scuderi

Introduction by the Editors

The surgical approach to the knee was originally a medial parapatellar technique that made visualization easier and allowed excellent exposure of the joint. For many years this was the standard for TKA. Follow up studies did show that there were some problems related to the patellar tracking and the quadriceps tendon. Multiple modifications were suggested over the past 50 years to improve the clinical symptoms without leading to complications related to a more limited access to the joint.

Insall proposed a midline technique directly over the patellar surface. This did improve tracking but presented the surgeon with a more difficult technique. Surgeons then looked at the vastus medialis and either divided it or lifted it laterally with the subvastus technique. The former proved to be quite acceptable, and the latter was again more challenging. The lateral arthrotomy moved to the other side of the joint but presented problems with closures and visualization.

Then, in the early 2000's attempts were made to limit the exposures to assist in a more rapid recovery. The mini-midvastus, the mini-subvastus, the quadriceps sparing, and the limited medial parapatellar all had supporters. While all these approaches did improve recovery time, there were more complications and some limitations to the long-term results.

Now, most approaches are more limited than in the past but the midvastus and the medial parapatellar are the main stay of the techniques. The references in this chapter go along with this outline and give a good overview of the present state of the art.

The midline skin incision is reviewed in the following. Calvert et al. favors a lateral approach for kneeling and this may be true but limits exposure. Nadeem et al.

A. J. Tria Jr. (✉)
Department of Orthopedics, Rutgers-Robert Wood Johnson Medical School, New Brunswick, NJ, USA

G. R. Scuderi
Department of Orthopedic Surgery, Northwell Health, Garden City, NY, USA

A. J. Tria Jr., G. R. Scuderi (eds.), *Total Knee Arthroplasty*,
https://doi.org/10.1007/978-3-032-00175-7_5

reviewed kneeling ability and favor MIS and lateral approaches but admit to greater difficulty with surgical exposure.. Pethes et al. evaluated gait patterns and favored the MIS approaches but admitted to the difficulties with exposure. There has always been discussion regarding the presence of multiple incisions and what is the best approach. Yeganeh et al. reported that the distance between incisions could be less than 5 cm but this may be a function of case choice and not applicable to all knees. Prabhu et al. confirmed that numbness around the knee joint is common but improves over time. Lecner et al. reported that that the midvastus and the medial parapatellar approaches afforded similar clinical results.

The midvastus approach has become an alternative popular approach to the knee. Maestro et al. and Flore et al. favor the mid vastus for its improved clinical results and less need for lateral releases.

When comparing the midvastus approach to the medial parapatellar arthrotomy, Zang et al. and Fetzko et al. found no difference in the clinical outcome, but Lin et al. favored the midvastus approach.

The medial parapatellar arthrotomy has been the most popular approach to the knee with the versality in all deformities and ability to be converted to a more extensile approach. Bellemans et al. reported that the valgus knee can be well approached using the medial parapatellar technique. Other approaches have been compared to the medial parapatellar arthrotomy for ability to expose the knee and ultimate outcome. Hirshcmann et al. showed that the tibial tubercle osteotomy was more extensile in the complex TKA with better function than the medial parapatellar arthrotomy but with a much higher complication rate related to the more osteotomy.

The subvastus articles report clinical results that are similar to other techniques. Scheibel et al. provides a detailed description of the anatomy of the vastus medialis and subvastus approach. Shah et al. reported the approach can be used for multiple scenarios including the stiff knee, the valgus knee, and the obese knee. While these reports do show technical abilities, the approach may not be that applicable in cases and other techniques have been reported to be much easier. Four articles compare the subvastus approach to the medial parapatellar. The long-term results are all very similar with some variations in the early post operative period.

The lateral approach has been favored by some for exposure of the valgus knee. Most reports found that the results of the lateral approach comparable to the medial approach. However there are technical issues with the lateral approach and Rajnish et al. report that the lateral approach can be more difficult for some surgeons. After correction of the valgus deformity with a lateral approach, there may be difficulties with closure and Jiang et al. offers a lateral approach defect closure for the valgus knee that may be useful in some difficult circumstances.

Minimally invasive approach, including the quadriceps sparing approach have been popularized. Yuan et al. reviewed the problems associated with the quadriceps sparing (QS) technique through a systematic review and metanalysis. The findings are well supported and should be considered when using the technique. Peng et al. compared the QS with the subvastus and show improved clinical results but with increased complications. Huang et al. found that the minimally invasive procedures did result in improved patellar alignment at 5 years but the actual clinical results were the same as in the medial parapatellar arthrotomy.

Difficult exposures do sometimes result in injury to the extensor mechanism. Oliva et al. addresses the complex problem of quadriceps tendon ruptures and favors the use of autografts versus either the allografts or synthetics but does agree that there really is no standardized protocol.

Each of the procedures in this review have merits and benefits. In most cases the long term results are all the same and the surgeon should choose the technique that is best in their hands understanding that some approaches do afford early benefits but with possible increase in the complications.

5.1 Midline

Machine Generated Summaries

Disclaimer: The summaries in this chapter were generated from Springer Nature publications using abstractive AI auto-summarization: An abstraction-based summarizer creates new text based on deep learning. New phrases are created to summarize the content. As the constituted sentences are machine selected, they may not fully reflect the body of the work, so we strongly advise that the original content is read and cited. The auto-generated summaries were curated by the editor to meet Springer Nature publication standards.

5.1.1 A Comparison of Kneeling Ability After Lateral or Midline Incisions in Total Knee Arthroplasty [93]

This is a machine-generated summary of:

Calvert, Nicholas; Milne, Lachlan; Kuster, Markus A comparison of kneeling ability after lateral or midline incisions in total knee arthroplasty [93].

Published in: European Journal of Orthopaedic Surgery & Traumatology (2016).

Link to original: https://doi.org/10.1007/s00590-016-1831-6

If you want to cite the papers, please refer to the original.

For technical reasons we could not place the page where the original quote is coming from.

5.1.1.1 Research Highlights

Kneeling is a crucial function of the knee joint, essential for various occupations and cultural practices. However, many patients have trouble kneeling after total knee arthroplasty (TKA), with factors such as scar position and skin hypoesthesia affecting their ability. Despite these challenges, there has been limited research on improving kneeling ability through incision placement or assessment methods. The study by Calvert et al. investigates the impact of incision placement on kneeling ability in TKA patients using a novel scoring system.

The study enrolled patients from a joint replacement assessment clinic, focusing on those with excellent Knee Society Scores one-year post-surgery. Participants were divided into two groups: those with a lateral skin incision performed by a single surgeon and those with a standard midline incision performed by two other surgeons. Both groups underwent medial parapatellar arthrotomy and received an LCS Primary Total Knee Replacement (DePuy- Synthes, Warsaw, IN, USA) without patella resurfacing. The researchers developed the Kneeling Ability Test (KAT) to quantify discomfort during kneeling at various flexion angles. Statistical analysis revealed no significant difference in Knee Society Scores between the groups, but those with lateral incisions had higher Forgotten Joint Scores and significantly better KAT results at higher flexion angles.

The study suggests that lateral skin incisions may enhance kneeling ability by preserving skin innervation and reducing discomfort associated with midline scars. This approach also appears to maintain better blood supply to the skin compared to midline incisions. While concerns about potential hematoma risks exist, the senior author reported no increased wound problems over years of using lateral incisions. The study's limitations include its small sample size and potential confounding factors from different surgeons. Future studies should be larger, randomized, and involve multiple surgeons to validate these findings further and explore ways to improve patient outcomes after TKA.

5.1.2 Surgery-Related Predictors of Kneeling Ability Following Total Knee Arthroplasty: A Systematic Review and Meta-analysis [94]

This is a machine-generated summary of:

Nadeem, Shaheer; Mundi, Raman; Chaudhry, Harman Surgery-related predictors of kneeling ability following total knee arthroplasty: a systematic review and meta-analysis [94].

Published in: Knee Surgery & Related Research (2021).

Link to original: https://doi.org/10.1186/s43019-021-00117-z

If you want to cite the papers, please refer to the original.

For technical reasons we could not place the page where the original quote is coming from.

5.1.2.1 Research Highlights

Total knee arthroplasty (TKA) is a common surgical procedure for alleviating pain and disability in patients with end-stage degenerative knee joint disease. Despite its general success, a significant number of patients remain dissatisfied after surgery, often due to persistent symptoms such as the inability to kneel. Kneeling is crucial for many daily activities and holds cultural, religious, and occupational significance. However, few studies have focused on kneeling ability as a primary outcome after TKA. The study by Nadeem et al. conducted a systematic review and meta-analysis to determine the prevalence of kneeling difficulties post-TKA and identify surgical approaches that may enhance kneeling ability.

The study followed the Preferred Reporting Items for Systematic Reviews and Meta-Analyses (PRISMA) guidelines, conducting a comprehensive literature search in MEDLINE and EMBASE databases. Eligible studies included those reporting postoperative kneeling outcomes in patients who underwent primary TKA. The researchers assessed kneeling ability based on patient-reported outcomes and categorized data from various scales. Statistical analyses were performed using a random effects model to pool data and determine odds ratios. The study included 36 articles featuring over 3000 TKA patients, with a mix of prospective cohort studies, cross-sectional studies, retrospective chart reviews, and randomized controlled trials (RCTs). The findings indicated that kneeling ability improved with longer follow-up durations, with significant differences observed between shorter and longer follow-up periods.

The study highlights that variations in surgical incision types significantly impact kneeling ability post-TKA. Minimally invasive surgery (MIS) showed improved outcomes compared to standard incisions, although it requires careful consideration due to its learning curve and potential stress on soft tissues. Anterolateral incisions were found to be superior to anteromedial ones in enhancing kneeling ability due to reduced risk of nerve damage. While prosthesis design variations showed limited impact on kneeling outcomes, further high-quality research is needed to explore perioperative interventions that could improve patient satisfaction regarding kneeling ability after TKA. Future study should also consider the role of rehabilitation programs and compare outcomes between different patient subsets.

5.1.3 *Variability of Gait in the Early Postoperative Period of Total Knee Arthroplasty with Different Surgical Technique [95]*

This is a machine-generated summary of:

Pethes, Ákos; Kiss, Rita M.; Szendrői, Miklós Variability of gait in the early postoperative period of total knee arthroplasty with different surgical technique [95].

Published in: International Orthopaedics (2013).

Link to original: https://doi.org/10.1007/s00264-013-2115-y

If you want to cite the papers, please refer to the original.

For technical reasons we could not place the page where the original quote is coming from.

5.1.3.1 Research Highlights

The number of knee replacements is increasing annually, with successful outcomes heavily reliant on appropriate rehabilitation and follow-up. Osteoarthritis (OA) of the knee joint and total knee arthroplasty (TKA) significantly affect gait parameters, including variability and stability. However, gait measurements on a treadmill are typically conducted 3 months post-TKA, leaving a knowledge gap regarding early postoperative gait patterns. The study by Pethes et al. investigates how different surgical techniques influence the variability of kinematical parameters during stepping in the early postoperative period.

The study involved 20 patients with gonarthrosis who underwent TKA at Semmelweis University, Budapest. Participants were randomly assigned to two groups: one receiving conventional surgery and the other undergoing minimally invasive surgery with computer-assisted navigation. Motion analysis was performed preoperatively and at 6 and 12 weeks postoperatively using a ZEBRIS ultrasound-based system (Zebris Medical, GmbH, Isny/Allgäu, Germany) on a PosturoMed© plate (Haider Bioswing Pullenreuth, Germany. This setup allowed for the measurement of kinematical parameters on both fixed and released platforms. The study focused on the coefficient of variation (CV) of cadence and angular parameters to assess dynamic stability. Results indicated that minimally invasive surgery led to faster recovery in stepping parameter variability compared to conventional techniques, although neither group reached normal values within 12 weeks.

The study advances understanding by highlighting the benefits of minimally invasive techniques in enhancing early postoperative recovery of gait stability after TKA. It underscores the importance of considering surgical technique when planning rehabilitation strategies. Future study could expand on these findings by analyzing a broader range of kinematical parameters over extended periods to further elucidate recovery trajectories. Additionally, this research provides a foundation for developing objective measurement techniques applicable in early postoperative assessments, potentially improving patient outcomes through tailored rehabilitation protocols.

5.1.4 The Distance Between New and Previous Incisions Does Not Affect Skin Necrosis in Total Knee Arthroplasty: A Parallel-Randomized Controlled Clinical Trial [96]

This is a machine-generated summary of:

Yeganeh, Ali; Moghtadaei, Mehdi; Ghaznavi, Alireza; Tavakoli, Nader; Soleimani, Mohammad; Cheraghiloohesara, Sahand; Taheri, Nima The distance between new and previous incisions does not affect skin necrosis in total knee arthroplasty: a parallel-randomized controlled clinical trial [96].

Published in: BMC Surgery (2022).

Link to original: https://doi.org/10.1186/s12893-022-01791-w

If you want to cite the papers, please refer to the original.

For technical reasons we could not place the page where the original quote is coming from.

5.1.4.1 Research Highlights

Wound complications are a significant concern following total knee arthroplasty (TKA), with poor healing potentially leading to severe outcomes such as limb amputation. Previous incision scars around the knee can complicate subsequent TKA procedures due to their susceptibility to skin complications like poor wound healing, sepsis, and necrosis. Traditionally, a minimum distance of 5 cm is recommended between new incisions and previous scars to mitigate these risks. However, this guideline can complicate surgical access to target structures in the knee. The study by Yeganeh et al. challenges this convention by investigating whether making a new incision closer than 5 cm from a previous scar increases the risk of skin complications.

The study was conducted as a randomized controlled trial at the Iran University of Medical Sciences, involving patients undergoing TKA with a single previous scar on the knee. Participants were randomly assigned to two groups: one where the new incision was made regardless of the previous scar's location and another where it adhered to the 5 cm distance guideline. The trial included strict inclusion and exclusion criteria to control for factors affecting wound healing, such as diabetes and smoking. All surgeries were performed by the same senior knee surgeon under standardized conditions. The primary outcome measured was the incidence of skin necrosis and other wound healing complications, while secondary outcomes included knee function assessed 6 months post-operation using the Knee Society Score.

The study found no significant difference in skin necrosis rates or other wound complications between the two groups, suggesting that making incisions closer than 5 cm from previous scars does not increase risk in otherwise healthy patients. This observation challenges the necessity of maintaining a strict distance from old scars during TKA procedures. However, limitations such as a short follow-up period and selective exclusion criteria suggest that further research is needed. Future studies with larger sample sizes and longer follow-up periods could provide more definitive evidence on this approach's safety and efficacy in TKA surgeries.

5.1.5 The Objective Measurement of Hypoaesthesia After Total Knee Arthroplasty and its Correlation with Skin Incision Length: A Prospective Study [97]

This is a machine-generated summary of:

Prabhu, Rudra; Kothari, Ronak; Keny, Swapnil A.; Kamble, Prashant; Rathod, Tushar; Mohanty, Shubhranshu S. The objective measurement of hypoaesthesia after Total Knee Arthroplasty and its correlation with skin incision length: a prospective study [97].

Published in: International Orthopaedics (2024).

Link to original: https://doi.org/10.1007/s00264-024-06316-z

If you want to cite the papers, please refer to the original.

For technical reasons we could not place the page where the original quote is coming from.

5.1.5.1 Research Highlights

With the increasing prevalence of end-stage knee arthritis, total knee arthroplasty (TKA) has become one of the most performed surgeries in orthopaedics. Despite its ability to improve quality of life, a significant percentage of patients report dissatisfaction post-surgery, often due to complications such as residual pain and functional limitations. A well-known complication of the standard midline approach in TKA is injury to the infrapatellar branch of the saphenous nerve, leading to hypoaesthesia around the knee. The study by Prabhu et al. investigates the correlation between the length of the midline skin incision and the area of numbness (AON) post-TKA, aiming to delineate the natural course of numbness and its impact on patient satisfaction.

The study was conducted in accordance with ethical guidelines and included patients 50 to 80 years of age undergoing unilateral primary TKA. Exclusion criteria were preoperative numbness or scars, postoperative complications other than peri-incisional numbness, and revision surgeries. Surgeries were performed using a standard midline incision, and postoperative numbness was assessed using monofilament testing. Patients marked areas of numbness on their skin, which were then traced onto paper for measurement using ImageJ software. The study found that most patients did not initially report numbness but identified it when questioned. The AON was larger in extension than in flexion immediately post-surgery but decreased over time, with no significant difference between flexion and extension at 6 months.

The findings suggest that while peri-incisional numbness is common after TKA with a midline incision, it tends to decrease over time. The study highlights the importance of informing patients about potential numbness to manage expectations and improve satisfaction rates. Future study could explore alternative incision techniques or methods to minimize nerve damage during TKA. Additionally, longer follow-up periods may be necessary to fully understand the duration and recovery process of hypoaesthesia post-surgery.

5.1.6 Does the Type of Surgical Approach Affect the Clinical Outcome of Total Knee Arthroplasty? [98]

This is a machine-generated summary of:

Lechner, Ricarda; Lazzeri, Matteo; Oberaigner, Wilhelm; Nardelli, Paul; Roth, Tobias; Köglberger, Paul; Krismer, Martin; Liebensteiner, Michael Christian Does the type of surgical approach affect the clinical outcome of total knee arthroplasty? [98].

Published in: Die Orthopädie (2021).

Link to original: https://doi.org/10.1007/s00132-021-04068-x

If you want to cite the papers, please refer to the original.

For technical reasons we could not place the page where the original quote is coming from.

5.1.6.1 Research Highlights

Total knee arthroplasty (TKA) is a common surgical procedure aimed at alleviating pain and restoring function in patients with severe knee arthritis. However, a significant percentage of patients report dissatisfaction post-surgery, often due to unexplained pain. Differentiating between implant-related, patient-related, and surgery-related factors is crucial in understanding these outcomes. Previous studies have explored the impact of different surgical approaches, particularly the medial midvastus (MMV) approach, on TKA outcomes. These studies have yielded mixed results, with some suggesting early postoperative benefits of the MMV approach in terms of quadriceps strength and patient-reported outcomes. The study by Lechner et al. investigates the MMV versus the medial parapatellar (MPP) approach using a larger sample size to assess differences in patient-reported knee scores, long-term postoperative range of motion (ROM), and prosthesis survival.

The study employed a retrospective comparative design using data from the state arthroplasty registry at the Medical University of Innsbruck, Austria. It included patients who underwent primary TKA with either the MMV or MPP approach. Exclusion criteria were applied to ensure consistency in surgical techniques and implant types. The researchers analyzed preoperative and postoperative data using the Western Ontario and McMaster Universities Osteoarthritis Index (WOMAC) to measure pain, stiffness, and physical function. ROM was assessed at various time points using goniometers. Statistical analyses were conducted to compare WOMAC scores and ROM between groups, while prosthesis survival was evaluated using Kaplan-Meier estimates. The study found no significant differences between the MMV and MPP groups in terms of WOMAC scores or ROM 1 year postoperatively. Additionally, prosthesis survival rates were similar for both approaches.

The findings suggest that both MMV and MPP approaches yield comparable clinical outcomes in primary TKA regarding early and late postoperative ROM, knee score outcomes, and prosthesis survival rates. This large-scale study provides robust evidence that neither approach negatively impacts long-term prosthesis longevity. Future study could focus on early postoperative parameters such as quadriceps strength or stair climbing ability to further elucidate any short-term benefits of the MMV approach. The strength of the study includes its large sample size and use of registry data, while limitations involve its retrospective nature and lack of early postoperative functional assessments. These results support the use of either surgical approach based on surgeon preference without compromising patient outcomes.

Bibliography

1. Holt G, Wheelan K, Gregori A (2006) The ethical implications of recent innovations in knee arthroplasty. J Bone Joint Surg 88(1):226–229
2. Harrell AG, Heniford BT (2005) Minimally invasive abdominal surgery: lux et veritas past, present, and future. Am J Surg 190(2):239–243
3. Seamon LG, Cohn DE, Henretta MS, Kim KH, Carlson MJ, Phillips GS, Fowler JM (2009) Minimally invasive comprehensive surgical staging for endometrial cancer: robotics or laparoscopy? Gynecol Oncol 113(1):36–41
4. Daouadi M, Zureikat AH, Zenati MS, Choudry H, Tsung A, Bartlett DL, Zeh HJ (2013) Robot-assisted minimally invasive distal pancreatectomy is superior to the laparoscopic technique. Ann Surg 257(1):128–132
5. Judet J, Judet R (1950) The use of an artificial femoral head for arthroplasty of the hip joint. J Bone Joint Surg Br 32B:166
6. Judet J (1952) Technique and results with the acrylic femoral head prosthesis. J Bone Joint Surg Br 34(2):173–180
7. Tria AJ Jr, Coon TM (2003) Minimal incision total knee arthroplasty: early experience. Clin Orthop Relat Res 416:185–190
8. Laskin RS (2003) Session IV: new techniques and concepts in total knee replacement. Clin Orthop Relat Res 416:151–153
9. Haas SB, Cook S, Beksac B (2004) Minimally invasive total knee replacement through a mini midvastus approach: a comparative study. Clin Orthop Relat Res 428:68–73

10. Repicci JA, Eberle RW (1999) Minimally invasive surgical technique for unicondylar knee arthroplasty. J South Orthop Assoc 8(1):20–27
11. Repicci JA, Hartman JF (2004) Minimally invasive unicondylar knee arthroplasty for the treatment of unicompartmental osteoarthritis: an outpatient arthritic bypass procedure. Orthop Clin 35(2):201–216
12. Tria AJ, Scuderi GR (2015) Minimally invasive knee arthroplasty: an overview. World J Orthop 6(10):804
13. Tenholder M, Clarke HD, Scuderi GR (2005) Minimal-incision total knee arthroplasty: the early clinical experience. Clin Orthop Relat Res 440:67–76
14. Tanavalee A, Thiengwittayaporn S, Itiravivong P (2007) Progressive quadriceps incision during minimally invasive surgery for total knee arthroplasty: the effect on early postoperative ambulation. J Arthroplasty 22(7):1013–1018
15. Reid JB III, Guttmann D, Ayala M, Lubowitz JH (2004) Minimally invasive surgery-total knee arthroplasty. Arthrosc J Arthrosc Relat Surg 20(8):884–889
16. Bonutti PM, Zywiel MG, Ulrich SD, Stroh DA, Seyler TM, Mont MA (2010) A comparison of subvastus and midvastus approaches in minimally invasive total knee arthroplasty. J Bone Joint Surg Am 92(3):575–582
17. Aglietti P, Baldini A, Sensi L (2006) Quadriceps-sparing versus mini-subvastus approach in total knee arthroplasty. Clin Orthop Relat Res 452:106–111
18. Alan RK, Tria AJ Jr (2006) Quadriceps-sparing total knee arthroplasty using the posterior stabilized TKA design. J Knee Surg 19(1):71–76
19. Lonner JH (2006) Minimally invasive approaches to TKA: results. Am J Orthop (Belle Mead NJ) 35(7 Suppl):27–29
20. Seon JK, Song EK (2006) Navigation-assisted less invasive total knee arthroplasty compared with conventional total knee arthroplasty: a randomized prospective trial. J Arthroplasty 21(6):777–782
21. Peng X, Zhang X, Cheng T, Cheng M, Wang J (2015) Comparison of the quadriceps-sparing and subvastus approaches versus the standard parapatellar approach in total knee arthroplasty: a meta-analysis of randomized controlled trials. BMC Musculoskelet Disord 31(16):327
22. Li C, Zeng Y, Shen B, Kang P, Yang J, Zhou Z, Pei F (2015) A meta-analysis of minimally invasive and conventional medial parapatella approaches for primary total knee arthroplasty. Knee Surg Sports Traumatol Arthrosc 23(7):1971–1985
23. Xu SZ, Lin XJ, Tong X, Wang XW (2014) Minimally invasive midvastus versus standard parapatellar approach in total knee arthroplasty: a meta-analysis of randomized controlled trials. PLoS ONE 9(5):e95311
24. Liu Z, Yang H (2011) Comparison of the minimally invasive and standard medial parapatellar approaches for total knee arthroplasty: systematic review and meta-analysis. J Int Med Res 39(5):1607–1617
25. Smith TO, King JJ, Hing CB (2012) A meta-analysis of randomised controlled trials comparing the clinical and radiological outcomes following minimally invasive to conventional exposure for total knee arthroplasty. Knee 19(1):1–7
26. Cheng T, Liu T, Zhang G, Peng X, Zhang X (2010) Does minimally invasive surgery improve short-term recovery in total knee arthroplasty? Clin Orthop Relat Res 468:1635–1648

27. Alcelik I, Sukeik M, Pollock R, Misra A, Shah P, Armstrong P, Dhebar MI (2012) Comparison of the minimally invasive and standard medial parapatellar approaches for primary total knee arthroplasty. Knee Surg Sports Traumatol Arthrosc 20(12):2502–2512
28. Reid MJ, Booth G, Khan RJ, Janes G (2014) Patellar eversion during total knee replacement: a prospective, randomized trial. J Bone Joint Surg 96(3):207–213
29. Dutton AQ, Yeo SJ, Yang KY, Lo NN, Chia KU, Chong HC (2008) Computer-assisted minimally invasive total knee arthroplasty compared with standard total knee arthroplasty: a prospective, randomized study. J Bone Joint Surg 90(1):2–9
30. Hafez MA, Chelule KL, Seedhom BB, Sherman KP (2006) Computer-assisted total knee arthroplasty using patient-specific templating. Clin Orthop Relat Res 444:184–192
31. Zhu M, Ang CL, Chong HC, Yeo SJ (2016) Computer-assisted minimally invasive total knee arthroplasty compared with conventional total knee arthroplasty: a prospective nine-year follow-up. Bone Joint J 98(SUPP 10):153
32. Hasegawa M, Miyazaki S, Yamaguchi T, Wakabayashi H, Sudo A (2017) Comparison of midterm outcomes of minimally invasive computer-assisted vs minimally invasive jig-based total knee arthroplasty. J Arthroplasty 32(1):43–46
33. Khakha RS, Chowdhry M, Norris M, Kheiran A, Patel N, Chauhan SK (2014) Five-year follow-up of minimally invasive computer assisted total knee arthroplasty (MICATKA) versus conventional computer assisted total knee arthroplasty (CATKA)—a population matched study. Knee 21(5):944–948
34. Klingenstein G, Porat M, Elsharkawy K, Reid J (2017) Evaluating the impact of morbid obesity on minimally invasive total knee replacement patients. Bone Joint J 99(SUPP 4):76–77
35. Hassaballa MA, Porteous AJ, Newman JH, Rogers CA (2003) Can knees kneel? Kneeling ability after total, unicompartmental and patellofemoral knee arthroplasty. Knee 10:155–160
36. Dawson J, Fitzpatrick R, Murray D et al (1998) Questionnaire on perceptions of patients about total knee replacement. J Bone Joint Surg Br Part B 80:63
37. Barrack R, Smith P, Munn B, Engh G, Rorabeck C (1998) A comparison of surgical approaches in total knee replacement. Ranawat Award Clin Orthop 356:16–21
38. Sharrad WJ (1964): Pressure effects on the knee in kneeling miners. In: Proceedings of annual meeting, England RCS
39. Berg P, Mjoberg B (1991) A lateral skin incision reduces peripatellar dysaesthesia after knee surgery. J Bone Joint Surg (Br) Part B 73:374–376
40. Borley NR, Edwards D, Villar RN (1995) Lateral skin flap numbness after total knee arthroplasty. J Arthroplasty 10(1):13–14
41. Hopton BP, Tommichan MC, Howell FR (2004) Reducing lateral skin flap numbness after total knee arthroplasty. Knee 11:289–291
42. de Achaval S, Kallen MA, Amick B, Landon G, Siff S, Edelstein D, Zhang H, Suarez-Almazor ME (2016) Patients' expectations about total knee arthroplasty outcomes. Health Expect 19(2):299–308. https://doi.org/10.1111/hex.12350

43. Sabeh KG, Hernandez VH, Cohen-Levy WB, Ong A, Orozco F, Bennett V, Post Z (2019) The effects of patient occupation, hobbies, and body mass index on kneeling after total knee arthroplasty. J Knee Surg. https://doi.org/10.1055/s-0039-3400740
44. Jain S, Pathak AC, Kalaivanan K (2016) Minimum 5-year follow-up results and functional outcome of rotating- platform high-flexion total knee arthroplasty: a prospective study of 701 knees. Arthroplast Today 2(3):127–132. https://doi.org/10.1016/j.artd.2016.01.006
45. Lenguerrand E, Wylde V, Gooberman-Hill R, Sayers A, Brunton L, Beswick AD, Dieppe P, Blom AW (2016) Trajectories of pain and function after primary hip and knee arthroplasty: the ADAPT Cohort Study. PLoS ONE 11(2):e0149306. https://doi.org/10.1371/journal.pone.0149306
46. Halket A, Stratford PW, Kennedy DM, Woodhouse LJ (2010) Using hierarchical linear modeling to explore predictors of pain after total hip and knee arthroplasty as a consequence of osteoarthritis. J Arthroplasty 25(2):254–262. https://doi.org/10.1016/j.arth.2009.01.007
47. Wood TJ, Petruccelli DT, Tushinski DM, Winemaker MJ, de Beer J (2020) Nuisance symptoms in total joint arthroplasty: prevalence and impact on patient satisfaction. J Arthroplasty 35(3):661–670. https://doi.org/10.1016/j.arth.2019.10.034
48. Ojima T, Yoshimura M, Katsuo S, Mizuno K, Yamakado K, Hayashi S, Tsuchiya H (2011) Transverse incision advantages for total knee arthroplasty. J Orthop Sci 16(5):524–530. https://doi.org/10.1007/s00776-011-0133-4
49. Hausdorff JM (2005) Gait variability. Methods, modeling and meaning. J Neuroeng Rehabil 20:19
50. McClelland JA, Webster KE, Feller JA (2009) Variability of walking and other daily activities in patients with total knee replacement. Gait Posture 30:288–295
51. Smith AJ, Lloyd DG, Wood DJ (2006) A kinematic and kinetic analysis of walking after total knee arthroplasty with and without patellar resurfing. Clin Biomech 21:379
52. Bejek Z, Paroczai R, Szendroi M, Kiss RM (2011) Gait analysis following TKA: comparison of conventional technique, computer-assisted navigation and minimally invasive technique combined with computer-assisted navigation. Knee Surg Sports Traumatol Arthrosc 19:285–291
53. Fuchs S, Floren M, Skwara A, Tibesku CO (2002) Quantitative gait analysis in unconstrained total knee arthroplasty patients. Int J Rehabil Res 25:65–70
54. Petersen MK, Andersen NT, Mogensen P, Voight M, Søballe K (2011) Gait analysis after total hip replacement with hip resurfacing implant or Mallory-head Exeter prosthesis: a randomised controlled trial. Int Orthop 35(5):667–674
55. Smith AJ, Lloyd DG, Wood DJ (2004) Pre-surgery knee joint loading pattern during walking predict the presence and severity of anterior knee pain after total knee arthroplasty. J Orthop Res 22:260–266
56. Hausdorff JM (2007) Gait dynamics, fractals and falls: finding meaning in the stride-to-stride fluctuations of human walking. Hum Mov Sci 26:555–589

57. Kiss RM (2011) Effect of severity of knee osteoarthritis on the variability of gait parameters. J Electromyogr Kinesiol 21:695–703
58. Kiss RM, Bejek Z, Szendroi M (2012) Variability of gait parameters in patients with total knee arthroplasty. J Electromyogr Kinesiol 20(7):1252–1260
59. Stergiou N, Moraiti C, Glakas G, Ristanis S, Georgoulis A (2004) The effect of walking speed on the stability of the anterior cruciate ligament deficient knee. Clin Biomech 19:57–63
60. Boeer J, Mueller O, Krauss I, Haupt G, Axmann D, Horstman T (2010) Effect of a sensory-motor exercise program for older adults with osteoarthritis or prosthesis of the hip using measurements made by Posturomed oscillatory platform. J Geriatr Phys Ther 33:10–15
61. Kiss RM (2011) A new parameter for characterizing balancing ability on an unstable oscillatory. Med Eng Phys. https://doi.org/10.1016/j.medengphy.2011.04.017
62. Müller O, Günther M, Krauß I, Horstman T (2004) Physical characterization of the therapeutic device Posturomed as a measuring device-Presentation of a procedure to characterize balancing ability. Biomed Tech 49:56–60, in German, Abstract in English
63. Dubost V, Kressig RW, Gonthier R, Herrmann FR, Aminian K, Najafi B, Beauchet O (2006) Relationship between dual task related changes in stride velocity and stride time variability in healthy older adults. Hum Mov Sci 25:372–382
64. Newel KM, Corcos DM (1993) Issues in variability and motor control. In: Newel KM, Corcos DM (eds) Variability and motor control. Human Kinetics Publishers, Champaign, pp 1–12
65. Yakhdani HRF, Bafgi HA, Meijer OG, Bruijn SM, van den Dikkenberg N, Stibbe AB, van Royen BJ, van Dieen JH (2010) Stability and variability of knee kinematics during gait in knee osteoarthritis before and after replacement surgery. Clin Biomech 25:230–236
66. van Zyl AA, van der Merwe JF, Snyman FPJ. Do previous scars around the knee matter in total knee arthroplasty? Orthop Proc. 2003;85B(SUPP_II):144.
67. Erivan R, Jacquet C, Villatte G, Ollivier M, Paprosky W. Epidemiology of painful knee after total knee arthroplasty in a tertiary care center: assessment by decision tree. Knee. 2020;27:1049–56.
68. Yu S, Saleh H, Bolz N, Buza J, Iorio R, Rathod PA, et al. Re-revision total hip arthroplasty: epidemiology and factors associated with outcomes. J Clin Orthop Trauma. 2020;11:43–6.
69. Ries MD. Skin necrosis after total knee arthroplasty. J Arthroplasty. 2002;17:74–7.
70. Shen Y, Han D, Qin F. Management of skin necrosis around incision following total knee arthroplasty. Zhongguo Xiu Fu Chong Jian Wai Ke Za Zhi. 2014;28:985–7.
71. Canovas F, Dagneaux L (2018) Quality of life after total knee arthroplasty. Orthop Traumatol Surg Res 104(1S). https://doi.org/10.1016/j.otsr.2017.04.017. p. S41-S46

72. Tsukada S, Kurosaka K, Nishino M, Hirasawa N (2018) Cutaneous hypesthesia and kneeling ability after total knee arthroplasty: a randomized controlled trial comparing anterolateral and anteromedial skin incision. J Arthroplasty 33(10):3174–3180. https://doi.org/10.1016/j.arth.2018.06.010
73. Mencia MM, Beharry A, Goalan R (2024) Skin numbness after total knee arthroplasty: complication or Side-Effect? Ortopedia, traumatologia, rehabilitacja. 26(1):363–368. https://doi.org/10.5604/01.3001.0054.4649
74. Laffosse JM, Potapov A, Malo M et al (2011) Hypesthesia after anterolateral versus midline skin incision in TKA: a randomized study. Clin Orthop Relat Res 469(11):3154–3163. https://doi.org/10.1007/s11999-011-1973-0
75. Skirven TM, Osterman AL, Fedorczyk J et al (2021) Rehabilitation of the hand and upper extremity, Elsevier Health Sciences, 7th edn., pp. 580–596
76. Gunst S, Villa V, Magnussen R et al (2016) Equivalent results of medial and lateral parapatellar approach for total knee arthroplasty in mild valgus deformities. Int Orthop 40:945–951
77. Huang AB, Wang HJ, Yu JK et al (2016) Optimal patellar alignment with minimally invasive approaches in total knee arthroplasty after a minimum five year follow-up. Int Orthop 40:487–492
78. Li Z, Cheng W, Sun L et al (2018) Mini-subvastus versus medial parapatellar approach for total knee arthroplasty: a prospective randomized controlled study. Int Orthop 42:543–549
79. Aslam MA, Sabir AB, Tiwari V et al (2017) Approach to total knee replacement: a randomized double blind study between medial parapatellar and midvastus approach in the early postoperative period in asian population. J Knee Surg 30:793–797
80. Bathis H, Perlick L, Blum C et al (2005) Midvastus approach in total knee arthroplasty: a randomized, double-blinded study on early rehabilitation. Knee Surg Sports Traumatol Arthrosc 13:545–550
81. Dalury DF, Jiranek WA (1999) A comparison of the midvastus and paramedian approaches for total knee arthroplasty. J Arthroplasty 14:33–37
82. Dalury DF, Snow RG, Adams MJ (2008) Electromyographic evaluation of the midvastus approach. J Arthroplasty 23:136–140
83. Engh GA, Holt BT, Parks NL (1997) A midvastus muscle-splitting approach for total knee arthroplasty. J Arthroplasty 12(3):322–331
84. Gelfer Y, Pinkas L, Horne T et al (2003) Symptomatic transient patellar ischemia following total knee replacement as detected by scintigraphy. A prospective, randomized, double-blind study comparing the mid-vastus to the medial para-patellar approach. Knee 10:341–345
85. Keating EM, Faris PM, Meding JB, Ritter MA (1999) Comparison of the midvastus muscle-splitting approach with the median parapatellar approach in total knee arthroplasty. J Arthroplasty 14(1):29–32
86. Layher F, Zipfel M, Sander K et al (2016) Functional comparison of the outcome after midvastus and medial parapatellar surgical approach in total knee arthroplasty. Z Orthop Unfall 154:50–57

87. Maestro A, Suarez MA, Rodriguez L et al (2000) The midvastus surgical approach in total knee arthroplasty. International Orthopaedics (SICOT) 24:104–107
88. Nutton RW, Wade FA, Coutts FJ et al (2014) Short term recovery of function following total knee arthroplasty: a randomised study of the medial parapatellar and midvastus approaches. Arthritis 2014:173857
89. Shukla R, Mahajan P, Singh M et al (2017) Outcome of total knee replacement via two approaches in Indian scenario. J Knee Surg 30:174–178
90. White RE Jr., Allman JK, Trauger JA et al (1999) Clinical comparison of the midvastus and medial parapatellar surgical approaches. Clin Orthop Relat Res 1999(367):117–122
91. Bellamy N, Buchanan WW, Goldsmith CH et al (1988) Validation study of WOMAC: a health status instrument for measuring clinically important patient relevant outcomes to antirheumatic drug therapy in patients with osteoarthritis of the hip or knee. J Rheumatol 15:1833–1840
92. Calvert, Nicholas; Milne, Lachlan; Kuster, Markus A comparison of kneeling ability after lateral or midline incisions in total knee arthroplasty. European Journal of Orthopaedic Surgery & Traumatology (2016). https://doi.org/10.1007/s00590-016-1831-6
93. Nadeem, Shaheer; Mundi, Raman; Chaudhry, Harman Surgery-related predictors of kneeling ability following total knee arthroplasty: a systematic review and meta-analysis. Knee Surgery & Related Research (2021). https://doi.org/10.1186/s43019-021-00117-z
94. Pethes, Ákos; Kiss, Rita M.; Szendrői, Miklós Variability of gait in the early postoperative period of total knee arthroplasty with different surgical technique. International Orthopaedics (2013). https://doi.org/10.1007/s00264-013-2115-y
95. Yeganeh, Ali; Moghtadaei, Mehdi; Ghaznavi, Alireza; Tavakoli, Nader; Soleimani, Mohammad; Cheraghiloohesara, Sahand; Taheri, Nima The distance between new and previous incisions does not affect skin necrosis in total knee arthroplasty: a parallel-randomized controlled clinical trial. BMC Surgery (2022). https://doi.org/10.1186/s12893-022-01791-w
96. Prabhu, Rudra; Kothari, Ronak; Keny, Swapnil A.; Kamble, Prashant; Rathod, Tushar; Mohanty, Shubhranshu S. The objective measurement of hypoaesthesia after Total Knee Arthroplasty and its correlation with skin incision length: a prospective study. International Orthopaedics (2024). https://doi.org/10.1007/s00264-024-06316-z
97. Lechner, Ricarda; Lazzeri, Matteo; Oberaigner, Wilhelm; Nardelli, Paul; Roth, Tobias; Köglberger, Paul; Krismer, Martin; Liebensteiner, Michael Christian Does the type of surgical approach affect the clinical outcome of total knee arthroplasty?. Die Orthopädie (2021). https://doi.org/10.1007/s00132-021-04068-x

5.2 Mid Vastus

Machine Generated Summaries
Disclaimer: The summaries in this chapter were generated from Springer Nature publications using abstractive AI auto-summarization: An abstraction-based summarizer creates new text based on deep learning. New phrases are created to summarize the content. As the constituted sentences are machine selected, they may not fully reflect the body of the work, so we strongly advise that the original content is read and cited. The auto-generated summaries were curated by the editor to meet Springer Nature publication standards.

5.2.1 The Midvastus Surgical Approach in Total Knee Arthroplasty [31]

This is a machine-generated summary of:

Maestro, A.; Suarez, M. A.; Rodriguez, L.; Guerra, C.; Murcia, A. The midvastus surgical approach in total knee arthroplasty [31].

Published in: International Orthopaedics (2000).

Link to original: https://doi.org/10.1007/s002640000116

If you want to cite the papers, please refer to the original.

For technical reasons we could not place the page where the original quote is coming from.

5.2.1.1 Research Highlights

Total knee arthroplasty (TKA) is commonly performed using the medial parapatellar approach, which involves dividing the medial patellar retinaculum and sometimes the quadriceps tendon. Alternative approaches, such as the sub-vastus and lateral approaches, have been developed to preserve the integrity of the quadriceps tendon and are particularly useful in specific cases like significant valgus deformity. However, these methods can lead to complications due to increased patellar forces during activities like walking or climbing stairs. The study by Maestro et al. from the Department of Orthopaedic Surgery at Hospital of Cabuenes in Gijon, Spain, explores a mid-vastus approach that aims to mitigate these issues by splitting the medial vastus in line with its fibers.

The retrospective study analyzed outcomes from total knee arthroplasties performed using either the mid-vastus or standard medial parapatellar approach. The same surgical team conducted all procedures using consistent implants and techniques, preserving the posterior cruciate ligament and employing cementation for fixation. The mid-vastus approach involved splitting the medial vastus muscle while preserving its attachment to the patella, allowing for better patellar mobilization without requiring lateral release. Patients were assessed preoperatively and postoperatively using clinical evaluations and radiographic analysis. The study found that patients who underwent the mid-vastus approach experienced fewer intra-operative lateral releases and demonstrated better early postoperative knee extension compared to those who had the parapatellar approach.

The findings suggest that the mid-vastus approach offers advantages in terms of early recovery and reduced need for lateral release, which can help maintain better patellar tracking without compromising vascular supply. This method may lead to fewer complications such as avascular necrosis or patellar fractures associated with traditional approaches that require lateral release. Future study could focus on long-term outcomes of this technique and its applicability across diverse patient populations with varying anatomical challenges. The research highlights a promising alternative for TKA that could improve patient recovery and reduce postoperative complications.

5.2.2 The Mini-Incision Mid-Vastus Approach for Total Knee Arthroplasty [32]

This is a machine-generated summary of:

Flören, Markus; Reichel, Heiko; Davis, Jack; Laskin, Richard S. The Mini-Incision Mid-Vastus Approach for Total Knee Arthroplasty [32].

Published in: Operative Orthopädie und Traumatologie (2008).

Link to original: https://doi.org/10.1007/s00064-008-1509-2

If you want to cite the papers, please refer to the original.

For technical reasons we could not place the page where the original quote is coming from.

5.2.2.1 Research Highlights

Total knee arthroplasty (TKA) is a common surgical procedure used to treat severe knee arthritis, with various approaches such as medial parapatellar, sub-vastus, and mid-vastus being employed. These techniques typically involve incisions of 15–25 cm to provide optimal exposure of the knee joint. While traditional methods have shown excellent long-term results, there is ongoing interest in less invasive techniques that may reduce soft-tissue trauma and enhance recovery. However, concerns remain about potential risks such as implant malalignment or poor fixation. The study by Flören et al. from the University of Ulm, Germany, and the Hospital for Special Surgery in New York explores the mini-incision mid-vastus (MMV) approach for TKA.

The study involved a retrospective analysis of patients who underwent TKA using the MMV approach compared to those who had the standard medial parapatellar arthrotomy. The MMV technique involves a smaller incision without patella eversion and aims to preserve the suprapatellar pouch, potentially reducing soft-tissue trauma. The researchers evaluated clinical outcomes using the Knee Society rating system and radiographic assessments over a minimum follow-up period of 1 year. The MMV group demonstrated significantly better flexion and stair-climbing ability at all evaluation points compared to the control group. The study also reported no major complications or implant malalignments in either group, suggesting that the MMV approach facilitates faster functional recovery without compromising implant positioning.

The findings indicate that the MMV approach offers significant advantages in terms of quicker recovery and improved knee function post-surgery. Future study could focus on long-term outcomes to further validate these benefits and assess any potential risks associated with this less invasive technique. Additionally, exploring patient-specific factors that may influence the success of the MMV approach could help refine patient selection criteria and optimize surgical outcomes. Overall, this study contributes valuable insights into enhancing recovery following TKA while maintaining safety and efficacy standards.

5.2.3 Mini-midvastus Versus Mini-medial Parapatellar Approach in Total Knee Arthroplasty: A Prospective, Randomized Study [33]

This is a machine-generated summary of:

Zhang, Zhenxiang; Zhu, Wei; Gu, Beibei; Zhu, Lixian; Chen, Chunmao Mini-midvastus versus mini-medial parapatellar approach in total knee arthroplasty: a prospective, randomized study [33].

Published in: Archives of Orthopaedic and Trauma Surgery (2012).

Link to original: https://doi.org/10.1007/s00402-012-1645-x

If you want to cite the papers, please refer to the original.

For technical reasons we could not place the page where the original quote is coming from.

5.2.3.1 Research Highlights

Total knee arthroplasty (TKA) has traditionally been performed using a standard approach that, while effective in the long term, involves significant soft-tissue disruption and patellar eversion, leading to a challenging and painful rehabilitation process. In contrast, minimally invasive surgery (MIS) techniques for knee arthroplasty, initially developed for unicondylar knee replacement, have shown promise in reducing recovery time and improving early outcomes. Despite these advancements, there has been a lack of prospective randomized studies comparing the short-term results of different MIS approaches for TKA. The study by Zhang et al. evaluates the early clinical and radiological outcomes of TKA using two minimally invasive techniques: the mini-midvastus and mini-medial parapatellar approaches.

In this study, patients with osteoarthritis of the knee were randomly assigned to undergo TKA using either the mini-midvastus or mini-medial parapatellar approach. The researchers employed a prospective randomized design with strict inclusion criteria to ensure consistency across patient groups. Surgical procedures were performed by a senior author using a posterior-stabilized prosthesis, with clinical data collected preoperatively and at various postoperative intervals. The study assessed parameters such as range of motion, pain levels using a visual analogue scale, skin incision length, blood loss, and complications. Radiological evaluations were conducted to assess alignment and component positioning. Statistical analyses were performed to compare outcomes between the two groups.

The study found no significant differences in short-term clinical recovery variables between the two approaches. Both techniques demonstrated similar benefits in terms of less invasion of the extensor mechanism and earlier return to function. The mini-medial parapatellar approach showed slightly higher rates of lateral retinacular release compared to the mini-midvastus approach; however, this difference was not statistically significant. The findings suggest that both minimally invasive approaches can achieve proper implant alignment without compromising patient outcomes. Future study could focus on long-term follow-up to confirm these results and further explore the learning curve associated with these techniques, ultimately guiding surgeons in selecting the most appropriate approach based on their experience and patient needs.

5.2.4 Computer-Assisted Total Knee Arthroplasty Using Mini Midvastus or Medial Parapatellar Approach Technique [34]

This is a machine-generated summary of:

Feczko, Peter; Engelmann, Lutz; Arts, Jacobus J.; Campbell, David Computer-assisted total knee arthroplasty using mini midvastus or medial parapatellar approach technique [34].

Published in: BMC Musculoskeletal Disorders (2016).
Link to original: https://doi.org/10.1186/s12891-016-0872-7

5.2.4.1 Research Highlights

Total knee arthroplasty (TKA) is a widely used surgical intervention for severe osteoarthritis of the knee, known for its long-term success in improving patients' functional capacity and quality of life. However, the conventional medial parapatellar approach can lead to significant tissue disruption and extended recovery times. Minimally invasive surgery (MIS) techniques have been developed to address these issues, focusing on minimizing tissue damage and improving recovery outcomes. Despite these advancements, comparative studies have not consistently shown one MIS approach to be superior. The study by Feczko et al. explores the potential benefits of combining computer-assisted surgery (CAS) with MIS techniques in TKA.

The study was a prospective, randomized multicenter trial involving 76 patients with end-stage knee osteoarthritis. Participants were randomly assigned to undergo TKA using either a mini-midvastus or medial parapatellar approach, both assisted by computer navigation. The primary outcomes measured were postoperative pain and range of motion (ROM), while secondary outcomes included surgery duration, blood loss, quadriceps strength, and functional scores such as the Knee Society Score (KSS) and WOMAC. The study utilized the Stryker Navigation System II (Stryker Orthopaedics, Kalamazoo, Michigan. USA) for precise component positioning and alignment assessments through radiological evaluations. Despite initial exclusions and some loss to follow-up, 69 patients completed the study period.

The findings revealed no significant differences in pain relief or ROM between the MIS and conventional approaches at various postoperative intervals. While the MIS approach resulted in longer surgery times and greater blood loss, it did not compromise implant positioning or limb alignment when combined with CAS. The study confirmed that CAS could mitigate alignment issues often associated with MIS techniques. Future study directions could focus on larger sample sizes or explore other potential benefits of CAS-MIS combinations in TKA. Overall, this research suggests that while CAS enhances surgical precision, the anticipated short-term benefits of MIS over conventional approaches remain unproven in this context.

5.2.5 *Mini-Midvastus Versus Medial Parapatellar Approach in Total Knee Arthroplasty: Difference in Patient-Reported Outcomes Measured with the Forgotten Joint Score [35]*

This is a machine-generated summary of:

Lin, Wei; Niu, Jinghui; Dai, Yike; Yang, Guangmin; Li, Ming; Wang, Fei Mini-midvastus versus medial parapatellar approach in total knee arthroplasty: difference in patient-reported outcomes measured with the Forgotten Joint Score [35].

Published in: Journal of Orthopaedic Surgery and Research (2020).

Link to original: https://doi.org/10.1186/s13018-020-01869-2

5.2.5.1 Research Highlights

Total knee arthroplasty (TKA) is a widely accepted treatment for end-stage osteoarthritis, known for restoring knee function, alleviating pain, and enhancing quality of life. Despite its success, the optimal surgical approach for TKA remains debated, with the medial parapatellar (MPP) and mini-midvastus (MMV) approaches being prominent options. The MPP approach provides excellent surgical visualization but may impair extensor function due to quadriceps tendon injury. Conversely, the MMV approach minimizes quadriceps damage and is associated with improved postoperative outcomes. However, few studies have assessed joint awareness post-TKA using different approaches. The study by Lin et al. investigates the functional outcomes of TKA via the MMV and MPP approaches using the Forgotten Joint Score (FJS), aiming to determine which method leads to better postoperative quality of life.

The study conducted a retrospective cohort analysis involving patients who underwent primary TKA via either the MMV or MPP approach. Patients were matched based on age, sex, body mass index, and follow-up time to ensure comparability. All surgeries were performed by a senior orthopaedic surgeon using standardized procedures and postoperative care protocols. The primary outcome measure was the FJS, which evaluates the patient's ability to forget their TKA in daily life—a key indicator of patient satisfaction. Secondary measures included operative time, tourniquet time, skin incision length, and time to straight leg raise. Data were collected at multiple intervals post-surgery and analyzed using statistical methods to assess differences between the two groups.

The study found that patients in the MMV group experienced better early postoperative outcomes in terms of pain relief and functional recovery compared to those in the MPP group. Notably, the FJS was consistently higher in the MMV group throughout follow-up, indicating greater patient satisfaction with this approach. The research suggests that preserving the extensor mechanism during surgery may contribute to these improved outcomes by reducing perioperative pain and facilitating quicker recovery. Future study could focus on prospective long-term evaluations to confirm these findings and explore minimal clinically important differences in FJS between surgical approaches. This research highlights the potential benefits of the MMV approach in achieving superior quality of life post-TKA by enhancing joint awareness outcomes.

Bibliography

1. Stern SH, Insall JN (1992) Posterior stabilized prosthesis: results after follow-up of nine to twelve years. J Bone Joint Surg Am 74:980–986
2. Keating EM, Meding JB, Faris PM, et al. Long-term followup of nonmodular total knee replacements. Clin Orthop 2002;404:34–39.
3. Scuderi GR, Tenholder M, Capeci C (2004) Surgical approaches in mini-incision total knee arthroplasty. Clin Orthop Relat Res 428:61–67
4. Tenholder M, Clarke HD, Scuderi GR (2005) Minimal-incision total knee arthroplasty: the early clinical experience. Clin Orthop Relat Res 440:67–76
5. Haas SB, Cook S, Beksac B (2004) Minimally invasive total knee replacement through a mini midvastus approach: a comparative study. Clin Orthop Relat Res 428:68–73
6. Karachalios Th, Giotikas D, Roidis N (2008) Total knee replacement performed with either a mini-midvastus or a standard approach: a prospective randomized clinical and radiological trial. J Bone Joint Surg Br 90:584–592

7. Kosilek FR, Bonutti PM, Hozack WJ et al (2007) Clinical experience using a minimally invasive surgical approach for total knee arthroplasty: early results of a prospective randomized study compared to a standard approach. J Arthroplasty 22:8–13
8. Dalury DF, Dennis DA (2005) Mini-incision total knee arthroplasty can increase risk of component malalignment. Clin Orthop Relat Res 440:77–81
9. Boerger TO, Aglietti P, Mondanelli N, Sensi L (2005) Mini-subvastus versus medial parapatellar approach in total knee arthroplasty. Clin Orthop Relat Res 440:82–87
10. Schroer WC, Diesfeld PJ, Reedy ME, LeMarr AR (2008) Mini-subvastus approach for total knee arthroplasty. J Arthroplasty 1:19–25
11. Tria AJ Jr, Coon TM (2003) Minimal incision total knee arthroplasty: early experience. Clin Orthop Relat Res 416:185–190
12. Tashiro Y, Miura H, Matsuda S et al (2007) Minimally invasive versus standard approach in total knee arthroplasty. Clin Orthop 463:144–150
13. Laskin RS, Beksac B, Phongjunakorn A, Pittors K, Davis J, Shim JC, Petersen M (2004) Minimally invasive total knee replacement through a mini-midvastus incision: an outcome study. Clin Orthop Relat Res 428:74–81
14. Kim JG, Lee SW, Ha JK, Choi HJ, Yang SJ, Lee MY. The effectiveness of minimally invasive total knee arthroplasty to preserve quadriceps strength: a randomized controlled trial. Knee. 2011;18:443–7.
15. Bauwens K, Matthes G, Wich M, Gebhard F, Hanson B, Ekkernkamp A, et al. Navigated total knee replacement. A meta-analysis. J Bone Joint Surg Am. 2007;89(2):261–9.
16. 16] Hernandez-Vaquero D, Noriega-Fernandez A, Fernandez-Carreira JM, Fernandez-Simon JM, Llorens de Los Rios J. Computer-assisted surgery improves rotational positioning of the femoral component but not the tibial component in total knee arthroplasty. Knee Surg Sports Traumatol Arthrosc. 2014;22(12):3127–34.
17. Dutton AQ, Yeo SJ. Computer-assisted minimally invasive total knee arthroplasty compared with standard total knee arthroplasty. Surgical technique. J Bone Joint Surg Am. 2009;91 Suppl 2 Pt 1:116–30.
18. Khakha RS, Chowdhry M, Norris M, Kheiran A, Patel N, Chauhan SK (2014) Five-year follow-up of minimally invasive computer assisted total knee arthroplasty (MICATKA) versus conventional computer assisted total knee arthroplasty (CATKA)—a population matched study. Knee 21(5):944–948
19. Tashiro Y, Miura H, Matsuda S, Okazaki K, Iwamoto Y. Minimally invasive versus standard approach in total knee arthroplasty. Clin Orthop Relat Res. 2007;463:144–50.
20. Gandhi R, Smith H, Lefaivre KA, Davey JR, Mahomed NN (2011) Complications after minimally invasive total knee arthroplasty as compared with traditional incision techniques: a meta-analysis. J Arthroplasty 26(1):29–35
21. Dayton MR, Bade MJ, Muratore T, Shulman BC, Kohrt WM, Stevens-Lapsley JE. Minimally invasive total knee arthroplasty: surgical implications for recovery. J Knee Surg. 2013;26(3):195–201.

22. Khanna A, Gougoulias N, Longo UG, Maffulli N. Minimally invasive total knee arthroplasty: a systematic review. Orthop Clin North Am. 2009;40(4):479–89.
23. Liu Z, Yang H (2011) Comparison of the minimally invasive and standard medial parapatellar approaches for total knee arthroplasty: systematic review and meta-analysis. J Int Med Res 39(5):1607–1617
24. Laskin RS, Beksac B, Phongjunakorn A, Petersen M. Minimally invasive total knee replacement through a mini-midvastus incision: an outcome study. Clin Orthop Relat Res. 2004;428:74–81.
25. Haas SB, Manitta MA, Burdick P. Minimally invasive total knee arthroplasty: the mini midvastus approach. Clin Orthop Relat Res. 2006;452:112–6.
26. Karachalios T, Giotikas D, Roidis N, Malizos KN. Total knee replacement performed with either a mini-midvastus or a standard approach: a prospective randomized clinical and radiological trial. J Bone Joint Surg (Br). 2008;90(5):584–91.
27. Liu H, Mei X, Zhang Z, Sun J. Mini-midvastus versus mini-medial parapatellar approach in simultaneous bilateral total knee arthroplasty with 24-month follow-up. Acta Orthop Traumatol Turc. 2015;49(6):586–92.
28. Behrend H, Giesinger K, Giesinger JM, Kuster MS. The "forgotten joint" as the ultimate goal in joint arthroplasty: validation of a new patient-reported outcome measure. J Arthroplast. 2012;27:430–6.e1.
29. Nestor MJ, Toulson CE, Backus SI, Lyman SL, Foote KL, Windsor RE. Mini–midvastus vs standard medial parapatellar approach: a prospective, randomised, double–blinded study in patients undergoing bilateral total knee arthroplasty. J Arthroplast. 2010;25(6 Suppl):5–11.
30. Karpman RR, Smith HL. Comparison of the early results of minimally invasive vs standard approaches to total knee arthroplasty: a prospective, randomised study. J Arthroplast. 2009;24:681–8.
31. Maestro, A.; Suarez, M. A.; Rodriguez, L.; Guerra, C.; Murcia, A. The midvastus surgical approach in total knee arthroplasty. International Orthopaedics (2000). https://doi.org/10.1007/s002640000116
32. Flören, Markus; Reichel, Heiko; Davis, Jack; Laskin, Richard S. The Mini-Incision Mid-Vastus Approach for Total Knee Arthroplasty. Operative Orthopädie und Traumatologie (2008). https://doi.org/10.1007/s00064-008-1509-2
33. Zhang, Zhenxiang; Zhu, Wei; Gu, Beibei; Zhu, Lixian; Chen, Chunmao Mini-midvastus versus mini-medial parapatellar approach in total knee arthroplasty: a prospective, randomized study. Archives of Orthopaedic and Trauma Surgery (2012). https://doi.org/10.1007/s00402-012-1645-x
34. Feczko, Peter; Engelmann, Lutz; Arts, Jacobus J.; Campbell, David Computer-assisted total knee arthroplasty using mini midvastus or medial parapatellar approach technique. BMC Musculoskeletal Disorders (2016). https://doi.org/10.1186/s12891-016-0872-7
35. Lin, Wei; Niu, Jinghui; Dai, Yike; Yang, Guangmin; Li, Ming; Wang, Fei Mini-midvastus versus medial parapatellar approach in total knee arthroplasty:

difference in patient-reported outcomes measured with the Forgotten Joint Score. Journal of Orthopaedic Surgery and Research (2020). https://doi.org/10.1186/s13018-020-01869-2

5.3 Medial Parapatellar

Machine Generated Summaries

Disclaimer: The summaries in this chapter were generated from Springer Nature publications using abstractive AI auto-summarization: An abstraction-based summarizer creates new text based on deep learning. New phrases are created to summarize the content. As the constituted sentences are machine selected, they may not fully reflect the body of the work, so we strongly advise that the original content is read and cited. The auto-generated summaries were curated by the editor to meet Springer Nature publication standards.

5.3.1 Comparison of Early Outcomes of Primary Total Knee Arthroplasties Performed Using Subvastus and Medial Parapatellar Approaches and Evaluation of Quadriceps Muscle Elastography [47]

This is a machine-generated summary of:

Güven, Mehmet Fatih; Özer, Mete; Özşahin, Mahmut Kürşat; Değer, Göker Utku; Adaletli, İbrahim; Aykan Kargin, Osman; Kaynak, Gökhan; Botanlıoğlu, Hüseyin Comparison of early outcomes of primary total knee arthroplasties performed using subvastus and medial parapatellar approaches and evaluation of quadriceps muscle elastography [47].

Published in: Archives of Orthopaedic and Trauma Surgery (2024).

Link to original: https://doi.org/10.1007/s00402-024-05570-5

If you want to cite the papers, please refer to the original.

For technical reasons we could not place the page where the original quote is coming from.

5.3.1.1 Research Highlights

In total knee arthroplasty (TKA) for treating knee osteoarthritis, the medial parapatellar (MP) approach is commonly used, involving an incision through the vastus medialis muscle. The subvastus approach (SV), however, preserves this muscle, potentially protecting the extensor mechanism and facilitating earlier recovery. Recent advancements in imaging, such as shear wave elastography (SWE), offer a novel method for evaluating tissue elasticity and monitoring postoperative recovery. Despite its potential, SWE is not yet a standard tool for assessing recovery after TKA. The study by Güven e al, compares the early outcomes of MP and SV approaches using SWE measurements focused on the vastus medialis muscle.

The study was conducted with 17 patients undergoing TKA due to primary osteoarthritis, divided into MP and SV groups. Preoperative SWE measurements of the vastus medialis and lateralis muscles were performed at rest and during contraction. Both groups followed identical exercise programs pre- and post-operation, with similar analgesic and anticoagulant treatments. The surgical procedures differed in incision techniques and prosthesis designs based on surgeon preferences. Postoperative assessments included Western Ontario and McMaster Universities Osteoarthritis Index (WOMAC) scores, Knee Society Scores (KSS), and SWE measurements at 3 months. Statistical analyses revealed no significant differences in clinical scores or SWE values between the two groups, although the SV group showed a slightly earlier straight leg raising time.

This study provides a novel perspective by isolating the vastus medialis for evaluation using SWE, distinguishing it from previous research that assessed overall quadriceps function. The findings suggest that both MP and SV approaches result in similar early-stage recovery outcomes as measured by KSS, WOMAC scores, and SWE values. Future study could include longer follow-up periods or larger patient groups to further explore differences between these surgical techniques. Additionally, incorporating measurements from non-operated knees might clarify anatomical influences on recovery outcomes. This research underscores the potential of SWE as a valuable tool for monitoring tissue healing in TKA patients.

5.3.2 A Prospective Comparative Study of the Midvastus and Medial Parapatellar Approaches for Total Knee Arthroplasty in the Early Postoperative Period [48]

This is a machine-generated summary of:

Maru, Michael; Akra, Gabriel; McMurtry, Ian; Port, Andy A prospective comparative study of the midvastus and medial parapatellar approaches for total knee arthroplasty in the early postoperative period [48].

Published in: European Journal of Orthopaedic Surgery & Traumatology (2009).

Link to original: https://doi.org/10.1007/s00590-009-0452-8

If you want to cite the papers, please refer to the original.

For technical reasons we could not place the page where the original quote is coming from.

5.3.2.1 Research Highlights

Total knee arthroplasty (TKA) has been a standard procedure for addressing severe knee joint issues, with significant advancements in knee biomechanics enhancing surgical techniques and implant longevity. Traditionally, the medial parapatellar approach has been the standard for TKA, offering excellent exposure but potentially compromising blood supply to the patella. To address these concerns, the midvastus approach was introduced, which preserves muscle integrity and may offer benefits such as reduced postoperative pain and improved muscle strength. The study by Maru e al. investigates whether the midvastus approach provides perioperative advantages over the medial parapatellar approach in TKA.

The study was a prospective observational cohort involving patients undergoing primary TKA with either the midvastus or medial parapatellar approach. Participants received spinal anesthesia with bupivacaine, and postoperative pain management was standardized. Exclusion criteria included previous arthrotomy and significant varus or valgus deformities. The study measured outcomes such as time to achieve straight leg raise (SLR), pain scores, hospital stay duration, and Oxford Knee Scores at various postoperative intervals. The midvastus group demonstrated a statistically significant shorter time to achieve SLR and hospital stay compared to the medial parapatellar group. However, differences in pain scores and other functional outcomes were not statistically significant.

The findings suggest that the midvastus approach may offer certain early postoperative benefits, such as quicker recovery of leg function and reduced hospital stay, which could be advantageous for both patients and healthcare systems. However, the study's lack of randomization and control group highlights the need for further research. Future studies could involve larger randomized controlled trials across multiple centers to validate these findings and determine the most effective surgical approach for TKA. This could lead to more tailored surgical strategies that optimize patient outcomes in knee arthroplasty.

5.3.3 Total Knee Arthroplasty in the Valgus Knee Using a Standard Medial Approach [49]

This is a machine-generated summary of:

Bellemans, J.; Vandenneucker, H.; Vanlauwe, J. Total knee arthroplasty in the valgus knee using a standard medial approach [49].

Published in: Interactive Surgery (2008).

Link to original: https://doi.org/10.1007/s11610-007-0046-2

If you want to cite the papers, please refer to the original.

For technical reasons we could not place the page where the original quote is coming from.

5.3.3.1 Research Highlights

The medial parapatellar approach is widely recognized among knee surgeons for performing standard total knee arthroplasty (TKA) due to its ability to provide a clear view of critical structures without compromising the extensor mechanism or soft tissue closure. This approach is particularly advantageous over the lateral approach, which often requires additional osteotomy and can lead to problematic soft tissue coverage, especially in valgus knees. However, the lateral approach allows easier access to shortened soft tissues, such as the iliotibial tract and lateral collateral ligament. The study by Bellemans et al. explores the surgical outcomes of valgus knees treated with TKA using a standard medial parapatellar approach combined with measured resection and differential ligament balancing.

The study retrospectively reviewed patients with valgus deformities exceeding five degrees who underwent TKA. Data were collected from a prospectively maintained database, including preoperative, intraoperative, and postoperative evaluations at regular intervals. The surgical technique involved a standard anteromedial approach with intramedullary alignment rods for both tibia and femur, measured bone resection, and differential ligament balancing in flexion and extension. The researchers assessed ligament tightness using spacer blocks or trial implants and performed necessary releases of structures like the iliotibial band or popliteus tendon based on specific tightness patterns. Postoperative alignment was corrected to neutral in most cases, with significant improvements in function scores and range of motion.

The study demonstrates that valgus knees can be effectively treated with TKA using a medial parapatellar approach when combined with a structured surgical algorithm focusing on matched resection and ligament balancing. The results align with existing literature on TKA outcomes for osteoarthritic patients, suggesting that releasing lateral structures from the medial side does not compromise technical execution or postoperative results. Future study directions could explore refining these techniques further or comparing them directly with alternative approaches to optimize patient outcomes in diverse clinical settings.

5.3.4 Biochemical Stress Evaluation After Medial Parapatellar and Subvastus Approach in Total Knee Replacement [50]

This is a machine-generated summary of:

Sabatini, L.; Nicolaci, G.; Atzori, F.; Oliva, A.; Aprato, A.; Terzolo, M.; Masse', A. Biochemical stress evaluation after medial parapatellar and subvastus approach in total knee replacement [50].

Published in: MUSCULOSKELETAL SURGERY (2017).

Link to original: https://doi.org/10.1007/s12306-017-0521-9

If you want to cite the papers, please refer to the original.

For technical reasons we could not place the page where the original quote is coming from.

5.3.4.1 Research Highlights

Total knee replacement (TKA) is a common recommendation for patients with severe osteoarthritis unresponsive to other treatments. The standard medial parapatellar approach, while effective, often results in significant intra-operative bleeding and post-operative pain, necessitating extensive physical therapy for recovery. Minimally invasive techniques, such as the subvastus approach, have been explored over the past two decades to mitigate these issues by avoiding damage to quadriceps fibers, potentially reducing pain and accelerating recovery. However, there is no consensus on the efficacy of the subvastus approach due to mixed results across studies. The study by Sabatini et al. investigates the biochemical and clinical outcomes of TKA using both standard and minimally invasive approaches, focusing on stress markers like salivary cortisol.

The study was conducted at San Luigi Gonzaga's Hospital in Turin, Italy, involving 15 patients who underwent TKA using either the medial parapatellar or mini-subvastus approach. Ethical approval was obtained, and patients were selected based on specific inclusion criteria such as age and BMI. The research employed both clinical assessments and biochemical markers to evaluate outcomes. Salivary cortisol levels were measured pre- and post-operatively to assess stress levels associated with each surgical technique. Blood samples were also collected to measure hematic cortisol, C-reactive protein (CRP), and creatine phosphokinase (CPK) levels. The study found that while there were no significant differences in tourniquet time or intra-operative bleeding between the two groups, the subvastus group showed a faster recovery trend in early post-operative periods.

The findings suggest that although the subvastus approach may lead to higher initial stress levels as indicated by salivary cortisol, this effect is acute and followed by a rapid decrease post-surgery. This could be attributed to the preservation of the extensor system in this minimally invasive technique. The study highlights salivary cortisol as a promising non-invasive marker for assessing surgical stress, potentially replacing blood samples in clinical practice. Future studies could expand on these findings by including a larger patient cohort and focusing on individuals with normal body weight to further evaluate stress markers like salivary cortisol and CPK levels under optimal conditions. Additionally, refining surgical techniques could enhance recovery outcomes by minimizing surgical stress even further.

5.3.5 Anterolateral Approach with Tibial Tubercle Osteotomy Versus Standard Medial Approach for Primary Total Knee Arthroplasty: Does It Matter? [51]

This is a machine-generated summary of:

Hirschmann, Michael T; Hoffmann, Mathias; Krause, Robert; Jenabzadeh, Reza-Amir; Arnold, Markus P; Friederich, Niklaus F Anterolateral approach with tibial tubercle osteotomy versus standard medial approach for primary total knee arthroplasty: does it matter? [51].

Published in: BMC Musculoskeletal Disorders (2010).

Link to original: https://doi.org/10.1186/1471-2474-11-167

If you want to cite the papers, please refer to the original.

For technical reasons we could not place the page where the original quote is coming from.

5.3.5.1 Research Highlights

Total knee arthroplasty (TKA) is a common surgical procedure for patients with severe osteoarthritis, typically performed using a medial parapatellar approach. However, this approach can lead to complications such as painful scarring and reduced extensor strength. An alternative is the lateral parapatellar subvastus approach with tibial tubercle osteotomy, which preserves the quadriceps muscle and patellar blood supply but is considered technically challenging and potentially riskier. The study by Hirschmann et al. investigates whether the choice of surgical approach affects early clinical and radiological outcomes in ligament balancing primary TKA.

The study was a prospective multicenter trial involving patients undergoing primary, ligament balancing, posterior cruciate-retaining TKA for tri-compartmental osteoarthritis. Patients were divided into two groups based on the surgical approach: medial parapatellar (MPA) or lateral parapatellar subvastus with tibial tubercle osteotomy (TubOT). Experienced surgeons performed the procedures across three centers, with standardized postoperative care and follow-up at 6 and 12 months. Clinical outcomes were assessed using pain scores, range of motion, and functional evaluations like the American Knee Society Score. Radiological assessments included implant positioning and mechanical alignment. Statistical analyses compared outcomes between the two groups.

The study found that patients treated with the lateral TubOT approach experienced better functional outcomes, less pain, and higher satisfaction at 2 years post-surgery compared to those who underwent the MPA approach. However, the TubOT group also had a higher early revision rate due to complications like tibial tubercle migration. Despite these complications, no significant differences in prosthetic alignment or radiolucencies were observed between groups. Future studies should focus on long-term outcomes to determine if the benefits of the TubOT approach outweigh its risks and whether it impacts prosthesis longevity compared to traditional methods.

5.3.6 Stability of Capsule Closure and Postoperative Anterior Knee Pain After Medial Parapatellar Approach in TKA [52]

This is a machine-generated summary of:

Keshmiri, Armin; Dotzauer, Fabian; Baier, Clemens; Maderbacher, Günther; Grifka, Joachim; Sendtner, Ernst Stability of capsule closure and postoperative anterior knee pain after medial parapatellar approach in TKA [52].

Published in: Archives of Orthopaedic and Trauma Surgery (2017).

Link to original: https://doi.org/10.1007/s00402-017-2706-y

If you want to cite the papers, please refer to the original.

For technical reasons we could not place the page where the original quote is coming from.

5.3.6.1 Research Highlights

Total knee arthroplasty (TKA) is a common surgical procedure for patients with knee osteoarthritis, but it often leads to complications such as anterior knee pain and patellar maltracking. Recent studies suggest that these issues may be linked to rotational malalignment of the femoral and/or tibial components, particularly the internal rotation of the femoral component, which affects patellofemoral kinematics. The medial patellofemoral ligament (MPFL) plays a crucial role in stabilizing the patella, and its dissection during TKA using a medial parapatellar approach may lead to instability and pain. However, the impact of MPFL dissection on postoperative outcomes has not been thoroughly investigated. The study by Keshmir et al. explores whether MPFL dissection in TKA contributes to patellar maltracking and medial joint capsule dehiscence, potentially resulting in anterior knee pain.

The study involved patients undergoing TKA for primary osteoarthritis, divided into two groups: one receiving a ligament-balanced technique using computer navigation and the other undergoing a conventional measured-resection technique. The researchers marked the joint capsule at standardized locations during surgery to ensure accurate closure and used titanium clips for postoperative radiological measurements. They assessed clinical outcomes using the Knee Society Score (KSS) and Feller Score preoperatively, as well as 10 days and 3 months post-surgery. Radiographic evaluations measured patellar tilt, shift, and capsule dehiscence. The study found that patients with more than 2 mm of capsule dehiscence showed significantly less improvement in Feller scores postoperatively. However, no significant differences were observed between the ligament-balanced and conventional groups regarding capsule dehiscence or clinical outcomes.

The findings suggest that MPFL dissection during TKA can lead to medial capsule dehiscence and poorer clinical outcomes, highlighting the importance of maintaining medial capsule tension regardless of surgical technique. While no significant differences were found between the two surgical approaches in terms of clinical outcomes or radiological measurements, future studies could explore alternative methods for setting femoral component rotation or consider MPFL augmentation to improve lateral restraining forces. Larger patient cohorts are needed to confirm these results and evaluate potential benefits of MPFL reconstruction or augmentation in TKA procedures.

5.3.7 Lateral Subvastus Approach with Tibial Tubercle Osteotomy for Primary Total Knee Arthroplasty: Clinical Outcome and Complications Compared to Medial Parapatellar Approach [53]

This is a machine-generated summary of:

Langen, Susanne; Gaber, Sonja; Zdravkovic, Vilijam; Giesinger, Karlmeinrad; Jost, Bernhard; Behrend, Henrik Lateral subvastus approach with tibial tubercle osteotomy for primary total knee arthroplasty: clinical outcome and complications compared to medial parapatellar approach [53].

Published in: European Journal of Orthopaedic Surgery & Traumatology (2015).
Link to original: https://doi.org/10.1007/s00590-015-1718-y

If you want to cite the papers, please refer to the original.

For technical reasons we could not place the page where the original quote is coming from.

5.3.7.1 Research Highlights

Total knee arthroplasty (TKA) is a common surgical procedure with generally positive outcomes and high patient satisfaction. Key factors influencing long-term success include anatomical leg alignment, ligament balancing, and precise prosthetic component positioning. The surgical approach also significantly impacts outcomes, with the medial parapatellar arthrotomy being the most common. However, the lateral subvastus approach (LSVA) with tibial tubercle osteotomy (TTO) is considered advantageous in certain cases, such as valgus deformities or patellar tracking abnormalities. The study by Langen et al. explores the functional outcomes of LSVA with TTO compared to the standard medial parapatellar approach (MPA), focusing on TTO-related complications.

The study was conducted retrospectively using data from a local knee arthroplasty registry, including patients who underwent primary TKA at a hospital over a specified period. Patients were divided into three groups: those who received the standard MPA, those with neutral leg alignment who underwent LSVA with TTO, and those with pronounced valgus alignment who also had LSVA with TTO. All patients received a cemented LCS® complete™ prosthesis (DePuy Orthopaedics, Warsaw, In., USA). The LSVA involved lateral release and step-cut osteotomy to prevent proximal migration of the tibial tubercle. Rehabilitation protocols were consistent across groups, involving continuous passive motion devices and physiotherapy. Outcomes were assessed using clinical examinations, radiographs, and questionnaires like the Western Ontario and McMaster Universities Osteoarthritis Index (WOMAC) and Knee Society Score (KSS). Statistical analyses revealed no significant differences in clinical outcomes between approaches after 1 year.

The study concludes that LSVA with TTO offers comparable functional outcomes to MPA 1 year postoperatively, supporting its use as an alternative in primary TKA when technical challenges with MPA are anticipated. Despite potential complications associated with TTO, such as intraoperative fractures or wound healing issues, these did not adversely affect patient outcomes in this study. Future study could focus on longer follow-up periods to assess long-term outcomes and further refine surgical techniques to minimize complications. The findings suggest that LSVA should be reserved for cases involving significant valgus deformities or patellar alignment issues, where it can be performed safely with precise surgical technique.

5.3.8 Comparison of the Modified Subvastus and Medial Parapatellar Approaches in Total Knee Arthroplasty [54]

This is a machine-generated summary of:

Jung, Young Bok; Lee, Yong Seuk; Lee, Eun Yong; Jung, Ho Joong; Nam, Chang Hyun Comparison of the modified subvastus and medial parapatellar approaches in total knee arthroplasty [54].

Published in: International Orthopaedics (2008).

Link to original: https://doi.org/10.1007/s00264-007-0510-y

If you want to cite the papers, please refer to the original.

For technical reasons we could not place the page where the original quote is coming from.

5.3.8.1 Research Highlights

Total knee arthroplasty (TKA) is commonly performed using the medial parapatellar approach, which provides a good surgical view but may impair blood supply to the patella, potentially leading to avascular necrosis and complications such as patella fracture or anterior knee pain. The subvastus approach, introduced by Hofmann et al., conserves blood supply and preserves quadriceps muscle function, reducing patella tracking issues. However, its clinical usefulness has been limited due to difficulties in subluxing the patella in muscular or obese patients. The study by Jung evaluates a modified subvastus approach designed to overcome these limitations and compares its clinical and radiological outcomes with the traditional medial parapatellar approach in TKA.

The study involved patients diagnosed with osteoarthritis undergoing their first TKA, randomly assigned to either the medial parapatellar or modified subvastus approach groups. The modified subvastus technique involved a vertical skin incision near the patella's midline, with careful dissection of the vastus medialis muscle to preserve blood vessels. This method aimed to facilitate patella suluxation while minimizing muscle damage. All surgeries were performed by the same surgeon using a posterior cruciate ligament-sacrificing design without patella resurfacing under specific conditions. Postoperative evaluations included range of motion assessments and radiographic analysis of patellar shift and tilt over a follow-up period of up to 2 years. Statistical analysis confirmed that the sample size was sufficient for comparing outcomes between groups.

The study found that patients undergoing the modified subvastus approach achieved active straight leg raising more quickly and demonstrated superior knee flexion up to 10 days post-surgery compared to those receiving the medial parapatellar approach. Although no significant differences were observed in long-term flexion range or radiographic measures of patellar alignment between groups, patient preference favored the modified subvastus approach in bilateral TKA cases. Future study could explore its application in different patient populations or refine techniques for challenging cases such as severely obese patients or those with prior surgeries affecting knee anatomy.

5.3.9 Sub-Vastus Approach Versus the Medial Parapatellar Approach in Primary Total Knee: A Randomised Controlled Trial [ISRCTN44544446] [55]

This is a machine-generated summary of:

Bridgman, Stephen; Walley, Gayle; MacKenzie, Gilbert; Clement, Darren; Griffiths, David; Maffulli, Nicola Sub-vastus approach versus the medial parapatellar approach in primary total knee: a randomised controlled trial [ISRCTN44544446] [55].

Published in: Trials (2006).

Link to original: https://doi.org/10.1186/1745-6215-7-23

If you want to cite the papers, please refer to the original.

For technical reasons we could not place the page where the original quote is coming from.

5.3.9.1 Research Highlights

Knee replacement surgery is widely recognized for its value, with numerous procedures performed annually in the UK. However, the optimal surgical approach to the knee joint remains uncertain. Traditionally, total knee replacements are conducted using a standard medial parapatellar arthrotomy, but the sub-vastus arthrotomy has been proposed as an alternative. Previous studies have suggested potential benefits of the sub-vastus approach, such as improved quadriceps strength and reduced hospital stay, but these studies were limited by small sample sizes and short follow-up periods. The study by Bridgman et al. aims to address these limitations through a randomized controlled trial comparing the standard medial parapatellar approach with the sub-vastus approach in total knee replacement.

The study involves a large sample population and includes long-term follow-up to evaluate both clinical and economic outcomes. Patients undergoing primary bi-compartmental knee replacement are recruited from North Staffordshire Hospital and randomized to either surgical approach on their day of admission. The primary outcome measure is the Knee Society Score, assessed at baseline and at 6, 12, and 26 weeks post-operatively by an independent assessor blinded to the surgical method used. Secondary outcomes include patient-reported measures such as quality-of-life indices (EuroQol-5D, WOMAC Osteoarthritis Index), time to return to normal activities, pain levels, and medical records data on complications and hospital stay length. The trial's design ensures rigorous data collection and analysis on an intention-to-treat basis.

This study represents a significant advance in evaluating surgical techniques for knee replacement by addressing previous methodological shortcomings. By involving a larger sample size and multiple surgeons, it enhances external validity and allows for subgroup analyses. Future study directions could include exploring variations in outcomes based on surgeon experience or patient demographics. The findings will provide valuable insights for orthopaedic surgeons seeking techniques that promote faster rehabilitation and shorter hospital stays, ultimately improving patient care in knee replacement surgery.

Bibliography

1. Shinohara M, Sabra K, Gennisson JL et al (2010) Real-time visualization of muscle stiffness distribution with ultrasound shear wave imaging during muscle contraction. Muscle Nerve 42:438–441. https://doi.org/10.1002/MUS.21723
2. Wang CZ, Li TJ, Zheng YP (2014) Shear modulus estimation on Vastus Intermedius of elderly and young females over the entire range of isometric contraction. PLoS ONE 9. https://doi.org/10.1371/JOURNAL.PONE.0101769
3. Eby SF, Cloud BA, Brandenburg JE et al (2015) Shear wave elastography of passive skeletal muscle stiffness: influences of sex and age throughout adulthood. Clin Biomech Elsevier Ltd 30:22–27. https://doi.org/10.1016/J.CLINBIOMECH.2014.11.011
4. Taljanovic MS, Gimber LH, Becker GW et al (2017) Shear-wave elastography: basic physics and musculoskeletal applications. Radiographics 37:855–870. https://doi.org/10.1148/RG.2017160116
5. Yoshida K, Itoigawa Y, Morikawa D et al (2023) Chronologic changes in the Elastic Modulus of a Healing Achilles Tendon rupture measured using Shear Wave Elastography. Foot Ankle Int 44:243–250. https://doi.org/10.1177/10711007221151083

6. Gulledge CM, Baumer TG, Juliano L et al (2019) Shear wave elastography of the healing human patellar tendon following ACL reconstruction. Knee 26:347–354. https://doi.org/10.1016/J.KNEE.2018.12.006
7. Engh GA, Parks NL (1998) Surgical technique of the midvastus arthrotomy. Clin Orthop 351:270–274
8. Hoppenfield S, deBoer P (1994) Surgical exposures in orthopaedics: the anatomic approach, 2nd edn. JB Lippincott, Philadelphia, pp 430–434
9. Dalury DF, Jiranek WA (1999) A comparison of the midvastus and paramedian approaches for total knee arthroplasty. J Arthroplasty 14:33–37
10. Keating EM, Faris PM, Meding JB, Ritter MA (1999) Comparison of the midvastus muscle-splitting approach with the median parapatellar approach in total knee arthroplasty. J Arthroplasty 14(1):29–32
11. Haas SB, Cook S, Beksac B (2004) Minimally invasive total knee replacement through a mini midvastus approach: a comparative study. Clin Orthop Relat Res 428:68–73
12. Buechel FF Sr. Long-term followup after mobile-bearing total knee replacement. Clin Orthop 2002;404:40–50.
13. Katz JN (2006) Total joint replacement in osteoarthritis. Best Pract Res Clin Rheumatol 20:145–153
14. Wylde V, Dieppe P, Hewlett S, Learmonth ID (2007) Total knee replacement: is it really an effective procedure for all? Knee 14:417–423
15. Hong-Wei L, Wei-Dong Gu, Nan-Wei Xu, Sun Jun-Ying (2014) Surgical approaches in total knee arthroplasty: a meta-analysis comparing the midvastus and subvastus to the medial peripatellar approach. J Arthroplast 29:2298–2304
16. Liu Z, Yang H (2011) Comparison of the minimally invasive and standard medial parapatellar approaches for total knee arthroplasty: systematic review and meta-analysis. J Int Med Res 39(5):1607–1617
17. Sanjeev J, Sandeep W, Mittal A, Hegde C (2013) Outcome of subvastus approach in elderly nonobese patients undergoing bilateral simultaneous total knee arthroplasty: a randomized controlled study. Indian J Orthop 47(1):45–49
18. Niki Y, Mochizuki T, Momohara S, Saito S, Toyama Y, Matsumoto H (2009) Is minimally invasive surgery in total knee arthroplasty really minimally invasive surgery? J Arthroplasty 24(4):499–504
19. Arnold MP, Friederich NF, Widmer H, Müller W: Lateral Approach to the Knee Combined with an Osteotomy of the Tibial Tuberosity. Its Use for Total Knee Replacement. [Lateraler Zugang zum Kniegelenk mit Osteotomie der Tuberositas tibiae. Oper Orthop Traumatol. 1999, 11: 223-232. https://doi.org/10.1007/BF02593984.
20. Piedade SR, Pinaroli A, Servien E, Neyret P: Tibial tubercle osteotomy in primary total knee arthroplasty: a safe procedure or not?. Knee. 2008, 15 (6): 439-446. https://doi.org/10.1016/j.knee.2008.06.006.
21. Insall JN, Dorr LD, Scott RD, Scott WN: Rationale of the Knee Society clinical rating system. Clin Orthop Relat Res. 1989, 13-14. 248

22. Bach CM, Nogler M, Steingruber IE, Ogon M, Wimmer C, Gobel G, Krismer M: Scoring systems in total knee arthroplasty. Clin Orthop Relat Res. 2002, 184-196. https://doi.org/10.1097/00003086-200206000-00022.399
23. Heesterbeek PJ, Jacobs WC, Wymenga AB (2009) Effects of the balanced gap technique on femoral component rotation in TKA. Clin Orthop Relat Res 467:1015–1022
24. Nikolaides AP, Kenanidis EI, Papavasiliou KA, Sayegh FE, Tsitouridis I, Kapetanos GA (2014) Measured resection versus gap balancing technique for femoral rotational alignment: a prospective study. J Ortho Surg 22:2
25. Karachalios T, Sarangi PP, Newman JH (1994) Severe varus and valgus deformities treated by total knee arthroplasty. J Bone Joint Surg 76(6):938–942
26. Stern SH, Moeckel BH, Insall JN (1991) Total knee arthroplasty in valgus knees. Clin Orthop Relat Res 273:5–8
27. Christian Z, Lukas L, van den Michel B, Peter N (2010) Tuberositas osteotomy for total knee arthroplasty: a review of the literature. J Knee Surg. https://doi.org/10.1055/s-0030-1267472
28. Whiteside L, Ohl M (1990) Tibial tubercle osteotomy for exposure of the difficult total knee arthroplasty. Clin Orthop Relat Res 260:6–9
29. Bellamy N, Buchanan WW, Goldsmith CH, Campbell J, Stitt LW (1988) Validation study of WOMAC: a health status instrument for measuring clinically important patient relevant outcomes to antirheumatic drug therapy in patients with osteoarthritis of the hip or knee. J Rheumatol 15(12):1833–1840
30. Insall JN, Dorr LD, Scott RD, Scott WN (1989) Rationale of the knee society clinical rating system. Clin Orthop Relat Res 248:13–14
31. Hay GC, Kampshoff J, Kuster MS (2010) Lateral subvastus approach with osteotomy of the tibial tubercle for total knee replacement: a two-year prospective, randomised, blinded controlled trial. J Bone Joint Surg Br 92(6):862–866
32. Nikolopoulos D, Polyzois I, Apostolopoulos A, Rossas C, Moutsios-Rentzos A, Michos I (2011) Total knee arthroplasty in severe valgus knee deformity: comparison of a standard medial parapatellar approach combined with tibial tubercle osteotomy. ESSKA 19(11):1834–1842. https://doi.org/10.1007/s00167-011-1474-4
33. Apostolopoulos A, Nikolopoulos D, Polyzois I, Nakos A, Liarokapis S, Stefanakis G, Michos I (2010) Total knee arthroplasty in severe valgus deformity: interest of combining a lateral approach with a tibial tubercle osteotomy. OTSR 96(7):777–784. https://doi.org/10.1016/j.otsr.2010.06.008
34. Chalidis BE, Ye K, Sachinis NP, Hawdon G, McMahon S (2013) Lateral parapatellar approach with tibial tubercle osteotomy for the treatment of non-correctable valgus knee osteoarthritis: a retrospective clinical study. Knee. https://doi.org/10.1016/j.knee.2013.05.008
35. Hofmann AA, Plaster RL, Murdock LE (1991) Subvastus (southern) approach for primary total knee arthroplasty. Clin Orthop Relat Res 269:70–77
36. In Y, Kim JM, Choi NY, Kim SJ (2007) Large Thigh girth is a relative contraindication for the subvastus approach in primary total knee arthroplasty. J Arthroplast 22:569–573

37. Pagnano MW, Meneghini RM (2006) Minimally invasive total knee arthroplasty with an optimized subvastus approach. J Arthroplasty 21:22–26
38. Matsueda M, Gustilo RB (2000) Subvastus and medial parapatellar approaches in total knee arthroplasty. Clin Orthop Relat Res 371:161–168
39. Fauré BT, Benjamin JB, Lindsey B, Volz RG, Schutte D (1993) Comparison of the subvastus and paramedian surgical approaches in bilateral knee arthroplasty. J Arthroplasty 8:511–516
40. Insall JN, Dorr LD, Scott RD, Scott NW: Rationale for the Knee Society Clinical Rating System. Clinical Orthopaedics and Related Research. 1989, 248: 13-14.
41. Fauré BT, Benjamin JB, Lindsey B, Volz RG, Schutte D (1993) Comparison of the subvastus and paramedian surgical approaches in bilateral knee arthroplasty. J Arthroplasty 8(5):511–516
42. EuroQol Group: EuroQol EQ-5D. user guide. 1996
43. Bellamy N: WOMAC Osteoarthritis Index. A users Guide. 1996, London, Ontario
44. Barrack RL: Resurfacing of the patellar in total knee arthroplasty. Journal of Bone and Joint Surgery. 1997, 79-A (8): 1121-1120.
45. Roysam GS, Oakley MJ (2001) Subvastus approach for total knee arthroplasty: a prospective, randomized, and observer-blinded trial. J Arthroplasty 16(4):454–457
46. Maric Z, Ott DM, Karpman RR: The standard versus the subvastus (southern) approach for total knee arthroplasty: a randomised prospective study. Orthop Trans. 1991, 15: 43-
47. Güven, Mehmet Fatih; Özer, Mete; Özşahin, Mahmut Kürşat; Değer, Göker Utku; Adaletli, İbrahim; Aykan Kargin, Osman; Kaynak, Gökhan; Botanlıoğlu, Hüseyin Comparison of early outcomes of primary total knee arthroplasties performed using subvastus and medial parapatellar approaches and evaluation of quadriceps muscle elastography. Archives of Orthopaedic and Trauma Surgery (2024). https://doi.org/10.1007/s00402-024-05570-5
48. Maru, Michael; Akra, Gabriel; McMurtry, Ian; Port, Andy A prospective comparative study of the midvastus and medial parapatellar approaches for total knee arthroplasty in the early postoperative period. European Journal of Orthopaedic Surgery & Traumatology (2009). https://doi.org/10.1007/s00590-009-0452-8
49. Bellemans, J.; Vandenneucker, H.; Vanlauwe, J. Total knee arthroplasty in the valgus knee using a standard medial approach. Interactive Surgery (2008). https://doi.org/10.1007/s11610-007-0046-2
50. Sabatini, L.; Nicolaci, G.; Atzori, F.; Oliva, A.; Aprato, A.; Terzolo, M.; Masse', A. Biochemical stress evaluation after medial parapatellar and subvastus approach in total knee replacement. MUSCULOSKELETAL SURGERY (2017). https://doi.org/10.1007/s12306-017-0521-9
51. Hirschmann, Michael T; Hoffmann, Mathias; Krause, Robert; Jenabzadeh, Reza-Amir; Arnold, Markus P; Friederich, Niklaus F Anterolateral approach with tibial tubercle osteotomy versus standard medial approach for primary

total knee arthroplasty: does it matter?. BMC Musculoskeletal Disorders (2010). https://doi.org/10.1186/1471-2474-11-167
52. Keshmiri, Armin; Dotzauer, Fabian; Baier, Clemens; Maderbacher, Günther; Grifka, Joachim; Sendtner, Ernst Stability of capsule closure and postoperative anterior knee pain after medial parapatellar approach in TKA. Archives of Orthopaedic and Trauma Surgery (2017). https://doi.org/10.1007/s00402-017-2706-y
53. Langen, Susanne; Gaber, Sonja; Zdravkovic, Vilijam; Giesinger, Karlmeinrad; Jost, Bernhard; Behrend, Henrik Lateral subvastus approach with tibial tubercle osteotomy for primary total knee arthroplasty: clinical outcome and complications compared to medial parapatellar approach. European Journal of Orthopaedic Surgery & Traumatology (2015). https://doi.org/10.1007/s00590-015-1718-y
54. Jung, Young Bok; Lee, Yong Seuk; Lee, Eun Yong; Jung, Ho Joong; Nam, Chang Hyun Comparison of the modified subvastus and medial parapatellar approaches in total knee arthroplasty. International Orthopaedics (2008). https://doi.org/10.1007/s00264-007-0510-y
55. Bridgman, Stephen; Walley, Gayle; MacKenzie, Gilbert; Clement, Darren; Griffiths, David; Maffulli, Nicola Sub-vastus approach versus the medial parapatellar approach in primary total knee: a randomised controlled trial [ISRCTN44544446]. Trials (2006). https://doi.org/10.1186/1745-6215-7-23

5.4 Subvastus

Machine Generated Summaries

Disclaimer: The summaries in this chapter were generated from Springer Nature publications using abstractive AI auto-summarization: An abstraction-based summarizer creates new text based on deep learning. New phrases are created to summarize the content. As the constituted sentences are machine selected, they may not fully reflect the body of the work, so we strongly advise that the original content is read and cited. The auto-generated summaries were curated by the editor to meet Springer Nature publication standards.

5.4.1 Total Knee Arthroplasty Using Subvastus Approach in Stiff Knee [20]

This is a machine-generated summary of:

Shah, Nilen A.; Patil, Hitendra Gulabrao; Vaishnav, Vinod O.; Savale, Abhijit Total knee arthroplasty using subvastus approach in stiff knee [20].

Published in: Indian Journal of Orthopaedics (2016).
Link to original: https://doi.org/10.4103/0019-5413.177582

If you want to cite the papers, please refer to the original.
For technical reasons we could not place the page where the original quote is coming from.

5.4.1.1 Research Highlights

Total knee arthroplasty (TKA) is a widely recognized procedure for improving quality of life by alleviating pain and enhancing knee function. However, achieving deep flexion post-surgery is crucial for certain populations due to cultural and religious practices. Preoperative range of motion (ROM) is a significant determinant of postoperative outcomes, yet limited ROM poses challenges in surgical exposure and increases complication risks. The subvastus approach, known for facilitating early recovery, is often avoided in cases with restricted ROM due to exposure difficulties. The study by Shah et al. explores the efficacy of the subvastus approach in TKA for patients with limited preoperative ROM, presenting their findings in the Indian Journal of Orthopaedics.

The study involved a retrospective analysis of patients who underwent TKA using the subvastus approach between 2010 and 2015. Patients with preoperative knee flexion less than 90 degrees were included, and data on demographics, radiographs, deformities, and knee society scores were collected prospectively. The surgical technique involved careful dissection to expose the knee joint while minimizing trauma to surrounding tissues. Postoperative care included early mobilization exercises to enhance recovery. The authors reported significant improvements in knee flexion post-surgery, with mean flexion increasing from 70 degrees preoperatively to 110 degrees postoperatively. Complications were minimal, with only one case of partial patellar tendon avulsion successfully managed intraoperatively.

The study demonstrates that the subvastus approach can yield satisfactory outcomes in TKA for knees with limited preoperative ROM, challenging previous contraindications associated with this technique. The authors suggest that addressing etiological factors such as tight quadriceps mechanisms and osteophytes can enhance surgical success. Future study could focus on larger sample sizes and long-term follow-up to validate these findings further. This research contributes valuable insights into optimizing surgical approaches for complex TKA cases, potentially influencing clinical practice guidelines for managing stiff knees in arthroplasty procedures.

5.4.2 Total Knee Arthroplasty in Valgus Knees Using Minimally Invasive Medial-Subvastus Approach [21]

This is a machine-generated summary of:

Shah, Nilen Amulak; Jain, Nimesh Prakash Total knee arthroplasty in valgus knees using minimally invasive medial-subvastus approach [21].

Published in: Indian Journal of Orthopaedics (2016).

Link to original: https://doi.org/10.4103/0019-5413.173517

If you want to cite the papers, please refer to the original.

For technical reasons we could not place the page where the original quote is coming from.

5.4.2.1 Research Highlights

Angular deformities around the knee joint, such as valgus knees, require careful consideration during total knee arthroplasty (TKA) to restore normal alignment. Valgus knees, characterized by a mechanical tibiofemoral angle greater than 10 degrees, can result from bony deformities or soft tissue contractures. Traditional approaches to TKA in valgus knees often involve lateral capsular approaches, which may lead to complications like quadriceps muscle function deficits and reduced patient satisfaction. The study by Shah et al. explores the efficacy of a minimally invasive medial-subvastus approach for TKA in valgus knees, aiming to improve functional outcomes with fewer complications.

The study was conducted retrospectively on patients with valgus deformity who underwent primary TKA using the subvastus approach between January 2010 and December 2015. The researchers included patients without previous knee arthrotomy or neurological issues and obtained informed consent from all participants. The surgical procedure involved a mini-subvastus approach without using a pneumatic tourniquet, with careful dissection and minimal medial ligament release. Postoperative management included early mobilization and pain control through continuous femoral nerve block. The study evaluated preoperative and postoperative clinical status using the American Knee Society scores and radiographic assessments of mechanical alignment.

The findings suggest that the mini-subvastus approach provides satisfactory exposure for TKA in valgus knees, resulting in early functional recovery and minimal complications. The study reported significant improvements in functional scores and mechanical alignment postoperatively. Future studies could focus on long-term outcomes and comparisons with other surgical approaches to further validate these findings. The mini-subvastus approach shows promise as an effective technique for TKA in valgus knees, potentially offering better patient satisfaction due to its muscle-sparing nature and reduced postoperative pain.

5.4.3 Mini-Subvastus Approach for Total Knee Arthroplasty in Obese Patients [22]

This is a machine-generated summary of:

Shah, Nilen; G, Nilesh; Patel, Narendra Mini-subvastus approach for total knee arthroplasty in obese patients [22].

Published in: Indian Journal of Orthopaedics (2010).

Link to original: https://doi.org/10.4103/0019-5413.65157

If you want to cite the papers, please refer to the original.

For technical reasons we could not place the page where the original quote is coming from.

5.4.3.1 Research Highlights

Obesity is a well-documented risk factor for degenerative osteoarthritis of the knee, often leading to total knee arthroplasty (TKA) due to increased joint load. The standard medial parapatellar approach for TKA in obese patients is associated with higher complication rates and inferior outcomes compared to non-obese patients. The study by Shah et al. explores the efficacy of the mini-subvastus approach for TKA in obese patients, hypothesizing that this method could overcome the challenges posed by obesity without compromising surgical outcomes.

The study included obese patients diagnosed with primary osteoarthritis who underwent TKA using the mini-subvastus approach between January 2006, and July 2007. The researchers documented patient demographics, including thigh girth, and performed preoperative assessments such as hematological tests and imaging. During surgery, a tourniquet was used in some cases, while tranexamic acid was administered to minimize bleeding in others. The mini-subvastus approach involved a smaller incision and preserved quadriceps integrity, allowing for early postoperative rehabilitation. The surgical technique emphasized careful dissection and retraction to achieve adequate exposure without patellar eversion until necessary. Postoperative care included pain management with femoral nerve catheters and early mobilization exercises.

The study found that the mini-subvastus approach provided satisfactory exposure in all cases, including those with large thigh girth or severe deformities. The average surgical time was 90 minutes, with minimal blood loss and no need for lateral release. Patients experienced significant improvements in Knee Society scores postoperatively, with early quadriceps recovery and high rates of unaided walking by day three. Complications were minimal, with only one case each of partial medial ligament injury and patellar tendon avulsion. Future study could focus on comparing this approach directly with traditional methods to further validate its benefits in obese populations.

5.4.4 A Detailed Anatomical Description of the Subvastus Region and its Clinical Relevance for the Subvastus Approach in Total Knee Arthroplasty [23]

This is a machine-generated summary of:

Scheibel, M.; Schmidt, W.; Thomas, M.; von Salis-Soglio, G. A detailed anatomical description of the subvastus region and its clinical relevance for the subvastus approach in total knee arthroplasty [23].

Published in: Surgical and Radiologic Anatomy (2002).

Link to original: https://doi.org/10.1007/s00276-002-0004-y

If you want to cite the papers, please refer to the original.

For technical reasons we could not place the page where the original quote is coming from.

5.4.4.1 Research Highlights

Total knee arthroplasty (TKA) is a common surgical procedure, and the subvastus approach is one technique used to perform it. This approach is favored for preserving the integrity of the extensor mechanism, potentially leading to quicker recovery and less postoperative pain. However, it presents challenges in terms of exposure, particularly in the lateral patellofemoral compartment. The study by Scheibel et al. from the University of Leipzig and ATOS-Clinic Heidelberg provides a detailed anatomical description of the subvastus region, focusing on its vascular and neural structures to aid in determining safe incision limits during TKA.

The study involved dissecting 32 embalmed human cadaver thighs to map out the anatomical structures within the subvastus region. The researchers carefully removed skin, subcutaneous fat, and superficial fascia before mobilizing the sartorius muscle to expose the subvastus region. They identified key vascular structures such as the descending genicular artery and its branches, as well as the saphenous nerve. The team documented variations in these structures across specimens, noting differences in origin and branching patterns. This detailed mapping aims to guide surgeons in making safer incisions by understanding where critical blood vessels and nerves are located.

The study provides valuable insights into the anatomical variations within the subvastus region that can impact surgical outcomes. By identifying nine different vascular patterns, this research highlights the importance of tailoring surgical approaches based on individual anatomy to minimize neurovascular injury risks. Future study could focus on correlating these anatomical variations with clinical outcomes to further refine surgical techniques for TKA using the subvastus approach. This work underscores the need for continued exploration into optimizing surgical methods while maintaining patient safety and improving recovery times.

5.4.5 Outcome of Subvastus Approach in Elderly Nonobese Patients Undergoing Bilateral Simultaneous Total Knee Arthroplasty: A Randomized Controlled Study [24]

This is a machine-generated summary of:

Jain, Sanjeev; Wasnik, Sandeep; Mittal, Amber; Hegde, Chintan Outcome of subvastus approach in elderly nonobese patients undergoing bilateral simultaneous total knee arthroplasty: A randomized controlled study [24].

Published in: Indian Journal of Orthopaedics (2013).

Link to original: https://doi.org/10.4103/0019-5413.106900

If you want to cite the papers, please refer to the original.

For technical reasons we could not place the page where the original quote is coming from.

5.4.5.1 Research Highlights

Total knee arthroplasty (TKA) is a common procedure for patients with osteoarthritis but concerns about postoperative pain and recovery time remain significant. The standard medial parapatellar approach, while effective, often results in a longer recovery period, which can be disappointing for patients eager to return to full activity. Although long-term outcomes of the subvastus and medial parapatellar approaches are similar, early functional outcomes vary across studies. Few randomized controlled trials have directly compared these approaches in terms of early recovery. The study by Jain et al. at Dr. L. H. Hiranandani Hospital in Mumbai, India investigates the early functional outcomes of the subvastus versus medial parapatellar approach in elderly, non-obese patients undergoing bilateral simultaneous TKA.

In this study, 100 elderly patients with minimal knee deformity undergoing bilateral simultaneous TKA were randomized into two groups: one receiving the subvastus approach and the other the medial parapatellar approach. The surgeries were performed by a single experienced surgeon using computer navigation for alignment, with consistent anesthesia and physiotherapy protocols across both groups. Key parameters such as Visual Analog Scale (VAS) scores for pain, time to straight leg raise, ability to use a commode chair, stair climbing ability, and discharge timing were assessed postoperatively. The study found that while initial VAS scores were similar between groups, the subvastus group experienced significantly less pain from day two onwards and achieved earlier functional milestones like straight leg raising and stair climbing.

The findings suggest that the subvastus approach may offer advantages in terms of faster rehabilitation and reduced hospital stay compared to the medial parapatellar approach. This could lead to increased patient satisfaction due to less postoperative pain and quicker mobilization. Future study could focus on objectively measuring quadriceps strength postoperatively to further validate these results. Despite its technical demands and longer learning curve, the subvastus approach appears promising for non-obese elderly patients where early rehabilitation is crucial.

5.4.6 Better Outcomes after Mini-Subvastus Approach for Primary Total Knee Arthroplasty: A Bayesian Network Meta-analysis [25]

This is a machine-generated summary of:

Migliorini, Filippo; Aretini, Paolo; Driessen, Arne; El Mansy, Yasser; Quack, Valentin; Tingart, Markus; Eschweiler, Jörg Better outcomes after mini-subvastus approach for primary total knee arthroplasty: a Bayesian network meta-analysis [25].

Published in: European Journal of Orthopaedic Surgery & Traumatology (2020).

Link to original: https://doi.org/10.1007/s00590-020-02648-9

If you want to cite the papers, please refer to the original.

For technical reasons we could not place the page where the original quote is coming from.

5.4.6.1 Research Highlights

Total knee arthroplasty (TKA) is a widely accepted procedure for treating end-stage knee joint disease, yet the optimal surgical approach remains debated. The traditional medial parapatellar (MPP) approach, introduced by Von Langenbeck, is favored for its excellent exposure of knee surfaces but criticized for causing significant damage to surrounding tissues. Minimally invasive techniques, such as the mini-subvastus (MSV), mini-midvastus (MMV), and quadriceps-sparing (QS) approaches, have been developed to minimize this damage and preserve the extensor mechanism. However, no comprehensive study has compared these approaches to determine the most effective one. The study by Migliorini et al. conducts a Bayesian network meta-analysis to evaluate these surgical techniques based on perioperative data, clinical scores, and functional outcomes.

The study followed PRISMA guidelines (Preferred Reporting Items for Systematic reviews and Meta-Analyses) for systematic reviews and included clinical trials with levels I and III evidence. A thorough literature search was conducted across major databases using specific keywords related to TKA approaches. Articles were screened based on eligibility criteria, focusing on perioperative data such as surgery duration and blood loss, as well as functional outcomes like range of motion and clinical scores. The analysis involved 28 studies comprising randomized clinical trials and retrospective cohort studies. A Bayesian hierarchical random-effects model was used to compare the approaches, ensuring methodological quality through the PEDro (Physiotherapy Evidence Database) appraisal score. The MSV approach showed superior results in terms of hospital stay duration, functional outcomes like flexion and range of motion, and clinical scores such as the Knee Society Score.

The findings suggest that the MSV approach offers significant advantages over other techniques in TKA by reducing hospital stay length and improving functional recovery while maintaining satisfactory surgical outcomes. However, challenges remain in terms of execution difficulty and learning curve associated with minimally invasive techniques. Future study should address implant positioning accuracy and complication rates to further validate these findings. Despite its limitations, this meta-analysis provides valuable insights into optimizing surgical strategies for TKA, highlighting the potential benefits of adopting minimally invasive approaches like MSV in clinical practice.

5.4.7 Mini-Subvastus Versus Medial Parapatellar Approach for Total Knee Arthroplasty: A Prospective Randomized Controlled Study [26]

This is a machine-generated summary of:

Li, Ziyu; Cheng, Wendan; Sun, Liangye; Yao, Yunfeng; Cao, Qiliang; Ye, Shuming; Qi, Lei; Xu, Shenglin; Wu, Xiaosan; Jing, Juehua Mini-subvastus versus medial parapatellar approach for total knee arthroplasty: a prospective randomized controlled study [26].

Published in: International Orthopaedics (2017).

Link to original: https://doi.org/10.1007/s00264-017-3703-z

If you want to cite the papers, please refer to the original.

For technical reasons we could not place the page where the original quote is coming from.

5.4.7.1 Research Highlights

Total knee arthroplasty (TKA) is a well-established surgical intervention for osteoarthritis, traditionally performed using the medial parapatellar approach, which provides excellent surgical field exposure but can damage the extensor mechanism. Minimally invasive techniques, such as the mini-subvastus approach, have been developed to reduce soft tissue injury and potentially enhance recovery. However, concerns remain about whether these techniques can maintain proper mechanical alignment and prosthesis positioning. The study by Li et al. compares the early clinical and radiological outcomes of the mini-subvastus approach with the traditional medial parapatellar approach in a prospective, randomized trial.

The study involved patients diagnosed with primary unilateral knee osteoarthritis who were randomly assigned to undergo TKA via either the mini-subvastus or medial parapatellar approach. Both groups received the same type of knee prosthesis and anesthesia, with surgeries performed by experienced joint surgeons. The mini-subvastus group utilized a smaller incision and preserved the vastus medialis without dissection, employing specialized alignment techniques for prosthetic placement. Outcomes measured included operation time, incision length, hospital stay duration, pain levels, range of motion (ROM), and radiographic alignment. Data collection was blinded to ensure unbiased results.

The findings revealed that patients in the mini-subvastus group experienced faster recovery times, less postoperative pain, and shorter hospital stays compared to those in the medial parapatellar group. Despite longer operation times for the mini-subvastus approach, there was no significant difference in blood loss or tourniquet time between groups. Importantly, both approaches achieved comparable prosthesis positioning and limb alignment without increased complication rates. Future study could focus on larger sample sizes to confirm these results and explore long-term outcomes of minimally invasive TKA techniques. This research suggests that the mini-subvastus approach offers significant early postoperative benefits without compromising surgical precision or safety.

5.4.8 Comparing the Sub-Vastus and Medial Parapatellar Approaches in Total Knee Arthroplasty: A Meta-analysis of Short-Term Outcomes [27]

This is a machine-generated summary of:

Sukeik, Mohamed; Sohail, Mohammad Zain; Hossain, Fahad Siddique; AlShryda, Sattar; Powell, James Comparing the Sub-Vastus and Medial Parapatellar Approaches in Total Knee Arthroplasty: A Meta-Analysis of Short-Term Outcomes [27].

Published in: Dr. Sulaiman Al Habib Medical Journal (2021).

Link to original: https://doi.org/10.2991/dsahmj.k.210203.001

If you want to cite the papers, please refer to the original.

For technical reasons we could not place the page where the original quote is coming from.

5.4.8.1 Research Highlights

Total knee arthroplasty (TKA) is a common procedure for alleviating pain and restoring function in patients with severe knee arthritis. Traditional approaches, such as the medial parapatellar (MPP) approach, have been widely used due to their simplicity and effectiveness in providing surgical exposure. However, alternative techniques like the subvastus(SV) approach have been developed to potentially improve postoperative recovery by preserving the quadriceps muscle and reducing trauma to the extensor mechanism. Despite these theoretical benefits, there is ongoing debate about whether the SV approach offers significant advantages over the MPP approach, particularly concerning postoperative pain, knee flexion, and overall functional outcomes. The study by Sukeik et al. provides a comprehensive systematic review and meta-analysis of randomized controlled trials (RCTs) to evaluate these approaches.

The study followed the guidelines from the Cochrane Handbook for Systematic Reviews and included 25 RCTs comparing the SV and MPP approaches in primary TKA. The researchers focused on key outcomes such as postoperative knee flexion, pain scores, days to straight leg raise (SLR), functional knee scores, lateral releases, duration of surgery, hospital stay length, blood loss, and complications. The analysis revealed that the SV approach resulted in improved knee flexion and reduced pain scores on the first day postoperatively compared to the MPP approach. However, these benefits were not sustained at later follow-up points such as weeks or months post-surgery. Additionally, while the SV approach led to fewer lateral releases and quicker SLR achievement, it was associated with longer operation times without an increase in complication rates.

The findings suggest that while the SV approach may offer some short-term advantages in terms of early postoperative recovery, these do not translate into long-term benefits over the MPP approach. The study highlights significant heterogeneity among trials and potential biases that could affect results. Future studies should focus on well-designed RCTs with longer follow-up periods to better assess medium- and long-term outcomes of these surgical techniques. This research underscores the need for careful consideration of patient-specific factors when choosing between surgical approaches for TKA.

5.4.9 SMOC Approach for Total Knee Arthroplasty in Valgus Knees [28]

This is a machine-generated summary of:

Li, Tao; Liu, Yikai; Li, Chenkai; Zhang, Haining SMOC approach for total knee arthroplasty in valgus knees [28].

Published in: Journal of Orthopaedic Surgery and Research (2022).

Link to original: https://doi.org/10.1186/s13018-022-03002-x

If you want to cite the papers, please refer to the original.

For technical reasons we could not place the page where the original quote is coming from.

5.4.9.1 Research Highlights

Total knee arthroplasty (TKA) is a well-established surgical procedure for alleviating pain and enhancing function in patients with advanced knee osteoarthritis. The utilization of TKA has significantly increased, with projections indicating millions of procedures annually in the near future. However, the standard medial parapatellar (MP) approach often yields unsatisfactory outcomes, particularly in valgus knees, due to issues like incomplete axis restoration and joint instability. Recently, the subvastus approach has been explored for its potential benefits in minimally invasive surgery. The study by Li et al. evaluates the clinical and radiological outcomes of the subvastus with minimal oblique cut (SMOC) approach in valgus knees, focusing on functional recovery, tibiofemoral alignment, and postoperative complications.

The study involved patients undergoing primary TKA using either the MP or SMOC approach, with posterior-stabilized implants. Exclusion criteria included varus knees and special prostheses. Both approaches followed similar perioperative procedures, including femoral nerve block anesthesia and multimodal drug cocktails for pain relief. The SMOC approach involved a midline incision and careful handling of the vastus medialis oblique (VMO) to minimize tissue damage. Data from 100 knees were analyzed for preoperative parameters like age and valgus angle, perioperative parameters such as operative time and drainage amount, and postoperative outcomes including range of motion (ROM) and Hospital for Special Surgery (HSS) scores. Statistical analyses revealed that while operative time was longer for SMOC, it resulted in less drainage, lower pain scores post-operation, and faster recovery times compared to MP.

The study's findings suggest that the SMOC approach offers advantages over the traditional MP method in terms of short-term recovery without increasing complication rates. Notably, there were no cases of postoperative patellar subluxation in the SMOC group compared to five cases in the MP group. This could be attributed to less extensive lateral soft tissue release in SMOC procedures. Future study directions could explore long-term outcomes of the SMOC approach or its application in more complex knee deformities. Overall, this research indicates that the SMOC technique may enhance early postoperative recovery for patients undergoing TKA for valgus knees while maintaining satisfactory alignment and stability.

5.4.10 Subvastus Versus Medial Parapatellar Approach in Total Knee Arthroplasty [29]

This is a machine-generated summary of:

Cila, Erdal; Güzel, Volkan; Özalay, Metin; Tan, Jale; Şimşek, Aykın S.; Kanatlı, Ulunay; Öztürk, Akif Subvastus versus medial parapatellar approach in total knee arthroplasty [29].

Published in: Archives of Orthopaedic and Trauma Surgery (2002).

Link to original: https://doi.org/10.1007/s004020100319

If you want to cite the papers, please refer to the original.

For technical reasons we could not place the page where the original quote is coming from.

5.4.10.1 Research Highlights

Total knee arthroplasty (TKA) techniques have evolved significantly, leading to high patient satisfaction rates. The standard medial parapatellar approach, as described by Insall, is widely used due to its excellent exposure of the knee joint. However, complications involving the extensor mechanism remain a common cause for re-operations in aseptic knees. The study by Cila et al. from Gazi University, Ankara, Turkey, compares the standard medial parapatellar approach with the subvastus approach in TKA to assess differences in quadriceps strength and knee scores.

In this prospective randomized study, 22 knees from patients with primary degenerative joint disease were treated with TKA using either the medial parapatellar or subvastus approach. The study employed the Hospital for Special Surgery knee scoring system and isometric and isokinetic quadriceps strength tests to evaluate outcomes. Patients were randomly assigned to one of the two surgical approaches and underwent surgery under regional anesthesia with prophylactic measures against infection and thrombosis. Postoperative evaluations were conducted at various intervals up to 6 months after surgery. The results indicated that while both groups showed significant improvements in knee scores over time, the subvastus group demonstrated superior quadriceps strength at 6 weeks post-surgery compared to the medial parapatellar group.

The study suggests that the subvastus approach may offer early postoperative advantages in terms of quadriceps strength and rehabilitation. However, by 6 months post-surgery, both groups achieved similar outcomes in terms of muscle strength and knee scores. Future study could explore long-term benefits of the subvastus approach or investigate its applicability in patients with specific conditions such as obesity or preoperative flexion contractures. Despite its early advantages, the subvastus approach's long-term benefits remain comparable to those of the standard medial parapatellar approach, which continues to be a reliable method for achieving successful TKA outcomes.

5.4.11 Early Results of Subvastus Versus Medial Parapatellar Approach in Primary Total Knee Arthroplasty [30]

This is a machine-generated summary of:

Weinhardt, C.; Barisic, M.; Bergmann, E. G.; Heller, K. D. Early results of subvastus versus medial parapatellar approach in primary total knee arthroplasty [30].

Published in: Archives of Orthopaedic and Trauma Surgery (2004).

Link to original: https://doi.org/10.1007/s00402-004-0692-3

If you want to cite the papers, please refer to the original.

For technical reasons we could not place the page where the original quote is coming from.

5.4.11.1 Research Highlights

Total knee arthroplasty (TKA) is a common surgical procedure for patients with severe osteoarthritis, but it often results in complications such as severe knee pain and reduced quadriceps strength. The conventional medial parapatellar arthrotomy, which involves splitting the quadriceps tendon, has been implicated in these issues due to the potential formation of painful scar tissue. The subvastus approach, which preserves the extensor mechanism of the knee, has shown favorable long-term outcomes compared to the parapatellar approach. However, early rehabilitation results remain inconclusive. The study by Weinhardt et al. investigates the immediate postoperative outcomes of TKA using either the parapatellar or subvastus approach.

In this randomized prospective study, patients diagnosed with osteoarthritis were assigned to undergo TKA using either the parapatellar or subvastus approach. The surgical procedures were identical except for the approach used. All patients received a cemented Genesis II knee prosthesis (Smith and Nephew, Memphis, Tenn., USA) with a patella inlay. Postoperative care included a daily gait rehabilitation program allowing full weight-bearing until discharge. Clinical and radiographic data were collected preoperatively, immediately postoperatively, and before discharge to assess parameters such as leg axis correction and tibial component inclination. The study found no significant differences between groups in terms of gender distribution, pain levels, or range of motion at discharge. However, patients in the subvastus group demonstrated earlier passive range of motion and active straight leg raising compared to those in the parapatellar group.

The study suggests that while both surgical approaches result in significant improvements in pain and function post-TKA, the subvastus approach may offer advantages in early rehabilitation by allowing quicker recovery of muscle strength and slightly less postoperative pain. Future study could explore long-term functional outcomes and further refine patient selection criteria to optimize surgical approach choice. Additionally, understanding factors influencing range of motion could enhance postoperative care strategies for TKA patients. The findings support wider use of the subvastus approach due to its potential benefits in preserving quadriceps integrity and improving patellofemoral alignment without prolonging surgery duration.

5.4.12 The Midvastus Approach for Total Knee Arthroplasty [31]

This is a machine-generated summary of:

Hube, Robert; Sotereanos, Nicholas G.; Reichel, Heiko The midvastus approach for total knee arthroplasty [31].

Published in: Orthopaedics & Traumatology Surgery & Research (2002).

Link to original: https://doi.org/10.1007/s00065-002-1052-x

If you want to cite the papers, please refer to the original.

For technical reasons we could not place the page where the original quote is coming from.

5.4.12.1 Research Highlights

Total knee arthroplasty (TKA) is a common surgical procedure aimed at alleviating pain and restoring function in patients with severe knee arthritis. However, complications related to the patellofemoral joint, such as lateral patellar tracking and anterior knee pain, can compromise the success of TKA. These issues are often attributed to surgical errors, including rotational malalignments and improper component placement. The study by Hube et al. from the Orthopedic Clinic and Policlinic at Martin Luther University Halle-Wittenberg, Germany, and the Department of Orthopedic Surgery at Allegheny General Hospital, USA, explores the midvastus approach for TKA,

The study details the midvastus approach, which preserves the continuity between the quadriceps tendon and vastus medialis by partially splitting the vastus medialis muscle in line with its fibers. This technique aims to reduce postoperative lateral patellar tracking and minimize interference with knee extension. The researchers conducted surgeries on patients using this approach between 1995 and 1998, with average follow-ups of 34 months. The method involved meticulous surgical techniques such as subperiosteal dissection and careful handling of soft tissues to ensure optimal exposure of the knee joint while avoiding damage to critical structures. The study reported that all patellae glided freely without lateral tracking post-surgery, eliminating the need for lateral release procedures.

The findings suggest that the midvastus approach offers significant advantages over traditional methods by reducing patellofemoral complications and preserving quadriceps function. Future study could focus on long-term outcomes and comparisons with other surgical approaches in diverse patient populations. The reduced incidence of complications like avascular necrosis and fractures highlights its potential as a preferred technique for TKA. Further research may explore refining this approach to enhance visualization in obese patients or address other relative contraindications identified in this study.

Bibliography

1. Boerger TO, Aglietti P, Mondanelli N, Sensi L (2005) Mini-subvastus versus medial parapatellar approach in total knee arthroplasty. Clin Orthop Relat Res 440:82–87
2. Laskin RS, Beksac B, Phongjunakorn A, Pittors K, Davis J, Shim JC, Petersen M (2004) Minimally invasive total knee replacement through a mini-midvastus incision: an outcome study. Clin Orthop Relat Res 428:74–81
3. Hofmann AA, Plaster RL, Murdock LE (1991) Subvastus (Southern) approach for primary total knee arthroplasty. Clin Orthop Relat Res 269:70–77
4. Urban LM (1981) The straight-leg-raising test: a review. J Orthop Sports Phys Ther 2(3):117–133. https://doi.org/10.2519/jospt.1981.2.3.117
5. Migliorini F, Eschweiler J, Tingart M, Rath B (2019) Posterior-stabilized versus cruciate-retained implants for total knee arthroplasty: a meta-analysis of clinical trials. Eur J Orthop Surg Traumatol 29(4):937–946. https://doi.org/10.1007/s00590-019-02370-1
6. Dayton MR, Bade MJ, Muratore T, Shulman BC, Kohrt WM, Stevens-Lapsley JE. Minimally invasive total knee arthroplasty: surgical implications for recovery. J Knee Surg. 2013;26(3):195–201.
7. Lin SY, Chen CH, Fu YC, Huang PJ, Lu CC, Su JY, et al. Comparison of the clinical and radiological outcomes of three minimally invasive techniques for total knee replacement at two years. Bone Joint J. 2013;95-B(7):906–10.
8. Lin WP, Lin J, Horng LC, Chang SM, Jiang CC (2009) Quadriceps-sparing, minimal-incision total knee arthroplasty: a comparative study. J Arthroplasty 24(7):1024–1032. https://doi.org/10.1016/j.arth.2008.07.005
9. Thiengwittayaporn S, Fusakul Y, Kangkano N, Jarupongprapa C, Charoenphandhu N (2015) Hand-held navigation may improve accuracy in minimally invasive total knee arthroplasty: a prospective randomized controlled trial. Int Orthop 40(1):51–57

10. Pan WM, Li XG, Tang TS, Qian ZL, Zhang Q, Zhang CM. Mini-subvastus versus a standard approach in total knee arthroplasty: a prospective, randomized controlled study. J Int Med Res. 2010;38(3):890–900.
11. Lai Z, Shi S, Fei J, Wei W. Total knee arthroplasty performed with either a mini-subvastus or a standard approach: a prospective randomized controlled study with a minimum follow-up of 2 years. Arch Orthop Trauma Surg. 2014;134(8):1155–62.
12. Thiengwittayaporn S, Kanjanapiboonwong A, Junsee D (2013) Midterm outcomes of electromagnetic computer-assisted navigation in minimally invasive total knee arthroplasty. J Orthop Surg Res 8(1):37
13. Canovas F, Dagneaux L (2018) Quality of life after total knee arthroplasty. Orthop Traumatol Surg Res 104(1S). https://doi.org/10.1016/j.otsr.2017.04.017. p. S41-S46
14. Barnett R. Osteoarthritis. Lancet. 2018;391(10134):1985. https://doi.org/10.1016/S0140-6736(18)31064-X.
15. Koninckx A, Schwab PE, Deltour A, Thienpont E. The minimally invasive far medial subvastus approach for total knee arthroplasty in valgus knees. Knee Surg Sports Traumatol Arthrosc 2014;22:1765–70.
16. Hanssen AD (2002) The subvastus approach for total knee arthroplasty resulted in better short-term outcomes than did the parapatellar approach. J Bone Joint Surg Am 84:325
17. Hofmann AA, Plaster RL, Murdock LE (1991) Subvastus (Southern) approach for primary total knee arthroplasty. Clin Orthop 269:70–77
18. Roysam GS, Oakley MJ (2001) Subvastus approach for total knee arthroplasty: a prospective, randomized, and observer-blinded trial. J Arthroplasty 16:454–457
19. Matsueda M, Gustilo RB (2000) Subvastus and medial parapatellar approaches in total knee arthroplasty. Clin Orthop 371:161–168
20. Shah, Nilen A.; Patil, Hitendra Gulabrao; Vaishnav, Vinod O.; Savale, Abhijit Total knee arthroplasty using subvastus approach in stiff knee. Indian Journal of Orthopaedics (2016). https://doi.org/10.4103/0019-5413.177582
21. Shah, Nilen Amulak; Jain, Nimesh Prakash Total knee arthroplasty in valgus knees using minimally invasive medial-subvastus approach. Indian Journal of Orthopaedics (2016). https://doi.org/10.4103/0019-5413.173517
22. Shah, Nilen; G, Nilesh; Patel, Narendra Mini-subvastus approach for total knee arthroplasty in obese patients. Indian Journal of Orthopaedics (2010). https://doi.org/10.4103/0019-5413.65157
23. Scheibel, M.; Schmidt, W.; Thomas, M.; von Salis-Soglio, G. A detailed anatomical description of the subvastus region and its clinical relevance for the subvastus approach in total knee arthroplasty. Surgical and Radiologic Anatomy (2002). https://doi.org/10.1007/s00276-002-0004-y
24. Jain, Sanjeev; Wasnik, Sandeep; Mittal, Amber; Hegde, Chintan Outcome of subvastus approach in elderly nonobese patients undergoing bilateral simultaneous total knee arthroplasty: A randomized controlled study. Indian Journal of Orthopaedics (2013). https://doi.org/10.4103/0019-5413.106900

25. Migliorini, Filippo; Aretini, Paolo; Driessen, Arne; El Mansy, Yasser; Quack, Valentin; Tingart, Markus; Eschweiler, Jörg Better outcomes after mini-subvastus approach for primary total knee arthroplasty: a Bayesian network meta-analysis. European Journal of Orthopaedic Surgery & Traumatology (2020). https://doi.org/10.1007/s00590-020-02648-9
26. Li, Ziyu; Cheng, Wendan; Sun, Liangye; Yao, Yunfeng; Cao, Qiliang; Ye, Shuming; Qi, Lei; Xu, Shenglin; Wu, Xiaosan; Jing, Juehua Mini-subvastus versus medial parapatellar approach for total knee arthroplasty: a prospective randomized controlled study. International Orthopaedics (2017). https://doi.org/10.1007/s00264-017-3703-z
27. Sukeik, Mohamed; Sohail, Mohammad Zain; Hossain, Fahad Siddique; AlShryda, Sattar; Powell, James Comparing the Sub-Vastus and Medial Parapatellar Approaches in Total Knee Arthroplasty: A Meta-Analysis of Short-Term Outcomes. Dr. Sulaiman Al Habib Medical Journal (2021). https://doi.org/10.2991/dsahmj.k.210203.001
28. Li, Tao; Liu, Yikai; Li, Chenkai; Zhang, Haining SMOC approach for total knee arthroplasty in valgus knees. Journal of Orthopaedic Surgery and Research (2022). https://doi.org/10.1186/s13018-022-03002-x
29. Cila, Erdal; Güzel, Volkan; Özalay, Metin; Tan, Jale; Şimşek, Aykın S.; Kanatlı, Ulunay; Öztürk, Akif Subvastus versus medial parapatellar approach in total knee arthroplasty. Archives of Orthopaedic and Trauma Surgery (2002). https://doi.org/10.1007/s004020100319
30. Weinhardt, C.; Barisic, M.; Bergmann, E. G.; Heller, K. D. Early results of subvastus versus medial parapatellar approach in primary total knee arthroplasty. Archives of Orthopaedic and Trauma Surgery (2004). https://doi.org/10.1007/s00402-004-0692-3
31. Hube, Robert; Sotereanos, Nicholas G.; Reichel, Heiko The midvastus approach for total knee arthroplasty. Orthopaedics & Traumatology Surgery & Research (2002). https://doi.org/10.1007/s00065-002-1052-x

5.5 Lateral

Machine Generated Summaries

Disclaimer: The summaries in this chapter were generated from Springer Nature publications using abstractive AI auto-summarization: An abstraction-based summarizer creates new text based on deep learning. New phrases are created to summarize the content. As the constituted sentences are machine selected, they may not fully reflect the body of the work, so we strongly advise that the original content is read and cited. The auto-generated summaries were curated by the editor to meet Springer Nature publication standards.

5.5.1 Comparative Analysis of Outcomes of Lateral Versus Medial Approach in the Total Knee Arthroplasty for Valgus Deformity: A Systematic Review and Meta-analysis [29]

This is a machine-generated summary of:

Rajnish, Rajesh Kumar; Srivastava, Amit; Yadav, Sandeep Kumar; Elhence, Abhay; Gahlot, Nitesh; Kumar, Prasoon; Gupta, Saurabh; Aggarwal, Sameer Comparative Analysis of Outcomes of Lateral Versus Medial Approach in the Total Knee Arthroplasty for Valgus Deformity: A Systematic Review and Meta-analysis [29].

Published in: Indian Journal of Orthopaedics (2024).

Link to original: https://doi.org/10.1007/s43465-024-01211-6

If you want to cite the papers, please refer to the original.

For technical reasons we could not place the page where the original quote is coming from.

5.5.1.1 Research Highlights

Total knee arthroplasty (TKA) is a common surgical procedure for end-stage knee osteoarthritis, particularly in cases of varus knee deformity. However, a subset of patients presents with valgus knee deformity, which complicates the procedure due to the need for precise soft tissue balancing and implant positioning. The medial approach is traditionally used for TKA in valgus knees, but its effectiveness compared to the lateral approach remains uncertain. The study by Rajnish et al. provides a comprehensive systematic review and meta-analysis comparing the medial and lateral approaches for TKA in valgus knees.

The study conducted an extensive literature search across multiple databases, adhering to Preferred Reporting Items for Systematic Reviews and Meta-Analyses (PRISMA) guidelines, to identify relevant randomized controlled trials (RCTs) and non-RCTs comparing the two surgical approaches. The authors included studies that reported on outcomes such as postoperative knee function, complications, range of motion, coronal alignment, surgery duration, blood loss, pain score, and patellar tilt. Data extraction was performed independently by two authors to minimize bias. The meta-analysis utilized both fixed and random effects models based on statistical heterogeneity assessed by the I^2 test. The study found that while the medial approach resulted in a better Knee Society Score (KSS), both approaches showed comparable results in terms of overall complications, knee flexion range of motion (ROM), postoperative alignment, surgery duration, blood loss, pain scores, and patellar tilt.

The findings suggest that while the medial approach may offer superior KSS outcomes due to surgeon familiarity and exposure challenges with the lateral approach, both techniques are largely equivalent in other critical measures. Future study could focus on high-quality RCTs with standardized implants and longer follow-up periods to further validate these findings. Additionally, exploring factors such as implant selection and soft tissue management could enhance understanding of optimal surgical strategies for valgus knee TKA.

5.5.2 A Lateral Approach Defect Closure Technique with Deep Fascia Flap for Valgus Knee TKA [30]

This is a machine-generated summary of:

Jiang, Jun; C Fernandes, Julio A lateral approach defect closure technique with deep fascia flap for valgus knee TKA [30].

Published in: Journal of Orthopaedic Surgery and Research (2015).

Link to original: https://doi.org/10.1186/s13018-015-0316-3

If you want to cite the papers, please refer to the original.

For technical reasons we could not place the page where the original quote is coming from.

5.5.2.1 Research Highlights

In total knee arthroplasty (TKA) for valgus knee deformities, surgeons often choose between medial and lateral parapatellar approaches. The lateral approach is favored for its superior visualization of lateral structures and the ability to perform lateral releases directly, which some studies suggest leads to better clinical outcomes. However, a significant challenge with the lateral approach is the creation of a lateral capsular defect that is difficult to close due to high tissue tension, leading to potential complications such as prosthetic exposure and infection. The study by Jiang et al. introduces an innovative surgical technique using a deep fascia flap to effectively close this defect in valgus knee TKA performed through a lateral parapatellar approach.

The study involved nine TKA surgeries on eight patients with varying degrees of valgus deformity. The researchers employed a midline skin incision combined with a lateral parapatellar capsular approach to avoid interference with future revision surgeries and reduce infection risk. The surgical procedure included sequential soft tissue releases to correct the valgus deformity, followed by the placement of knee prostheses. To address the midportion defect in the lateral capsular incision, the team developed a technique using a deep fascia flap dissected from over the patella and quadriceps tendon. This flap was flipped laterally and sutured into place, providing coverage for the defect while maintaining tension resistance during knee flexion.

The introduction of this deep fascia flap technique represents a significant advancement in managing lateral capsular defects in valgus knee TKA. The study reported no postoperative complications such as hematoma or infection, and patients showed improved valgus angles and patellar tilt post-surgery. Future study could explore long-term outcomes of this technique and its application in more severe cases or other types of knee surgeries. This method offers an effective solution for enhancing joint seal integrity and reducing postoperative complications associated with traditional closure techniques.

5.5.3 Equivalent Results of Medial and Lateral Parapatellar Approach for Total Knee Arthroplasty in Mild Valgus Deformities [31]

This is a machine-generated summary of:

Gunst, Stanislas; Villa, Vincent; Magnussen, Robert; Servien, Elvire; Lustig, Sebastien; Neyret, Philippe Equivalent results of medial and lateral parapatellar approach for total knee arthroplasty in mild valgus deformities [31].

Published in: International Orthopaedics (2015).

Link to original: https://doi.org/10.1007/s00264-015-2893-5

If you want to cite the papers, please refer to the original.

For technical reasons we could not place the page where the original quote is coming from.

5.5.3.1 Research Highlights

Total knee arthroplasty (TKA) is a widely accepted procedure for treating knee osteoarthritis, with the medial parapatellar approach being the standard technique. However, in cases of valgus osteoarthritis, achieving proper soft tissue balance can be challenging due to the contracture of lateral structures. The lateral parapatellar approach, as recommended by Keblish, offers direct access to these structures and may facilitate better ligament balance. Despite its potential benefits, the lateral approach is less familiar to many surgeons, and concerns about exposure and tissue coverage remain. The study by Gunst et al. compares the medial and lateral parapatellar approaches in TKA for knees with moderate valgus deformity.

The study was conducted at a single center and involved a review of a prospectively collected knee arthroplasty registry. Patients with a pre-operative hip-knee-ankle angle indicating moderate valgus deformity were included. The surgical technique was consistent across all cases, with variations in incision placement based on the approach used. In the lateral approach, additional techniques such as Z-plasty and tibial tuberosity osteotomy (TTO) were employed when necessary to improve exposure and facilitate closure. Post-operative outcomes were assessed through radiographic data and clinical scores, with no significant differences found between the two groups in terms of complication rates or functional outcomes.

The study's findings suggest that both approaches yield comparable results in terms of function and radiological outcomes without increasing operative time or complication risk. The lateral approach may offer advantages in visualizing tight lateral tissues without necessitating extensive releases, potentially reducing the need for TTO over time. Future study could focus on long-term outcomes and further refine patient selection criteria to optimize surgical techniques for specific deformities. Despite its technical challenges, the lateral parapatellar approach appears to be a viable option for TKA in moderately valgus knees, providing an effective alternative to the traditional medial approach.

5.5.4 A Prospective Randomized Study in 20 Patients Undergoing Bilateral TKA Comparing Midline Incision to Anterolateral Incision [32]

This is a machine-generated summary of:

Maniar, Rajesh N.; Singhi, Tushar; Nanivadekar, Arun; Maniar, Parul R.; Singh, Jaivardhan A prospective randomized study in 20 patients undergoing bilateral TKA comparing midline incision to anterolateral incision [32].

Published in: Journal of Orthopaedics and Traumatology (2017).

Link to original: https://doi.org/10.1007/s10195-017-0444-0

If you want to cite the papers, please refer to the original.

For technical reasons we could not place the page where the original quote is coming from.

5.5.4.1 Research Highlights

Total knee arthroplasty (TKA) commonly employs a midline incision, but this approach often results in lateral flap numbness due to surgical trauma to the infrapatellar branches of the saphenous nerve. This numbness can persist for weeks to years postoperatively, leading to patient dissatisfaction. Previous studies have suggested that an anterolateral incision might reduce this numbness by sparing the infrapatellar nerve division. However, these studies compared different patients, introducing variability in anatomical and subjective responses. The study by Maniar et al. addresses these limitations by comparing midline and anterolateral incisions in the same patients undergoing simultaneous bilateral TKA.

In this prospective randomized study, female osteoarthritis patients with bilateral varus deformity underwent TKA with one knee receiving a midline incision and the other an anterolateral incision. The incisions were randomized using sealed envelopes, and all other surgical steps remained identical. Sensory assessments were conducted preoperatively and at 6, 12, and 24 weeks postoperatively using various tests such as touch, pain, vibration, and two-point discrimination across six quadrants of each knee. Subjective patient preferences were recorded using Wald's Sequential Probability Ratio Test (SPRT), while objective sensation scores were analyzed using paired t-tests. The study found that knees with anterolateral incisions had significantly lower sensation loss scores compared to those with midline incisions at all follow-up points.

The study concludes that anterolateral incisions offer advantages in reducing lateral flap numbness without compromising surgical outcomes or scar quality at one-year post-surgery. While both incision types showed improved sensation over time, the recovery was notably better with anterolateral incisions. Future study could explore the long-term implications of these findings on revision surgeries and further refine techniques to optimize patient outcomes in TKA procedures. The research highlights the potential for anterolateral incisions to become a standard practice in reducing postoperative sensory deficits in TKA patients.

5.5.5 Lateral Versus Medial Approach for Total Knee Arthroplasty for Valgus Knee Deformity Shows Comparable Functional Outcomes, Hip–Knee–Ankle Angle Values, and Complication Rates: A Meta-analysis of Comparative Studies [33]

This is a machine-generated summary of:

Mercurio, Michele; Gasparini, Giorgio; Galasso, Olimpio; Familiari, Filippo; Cofano, Erminia; Sanzo, Valentina; Ciolli, Gianluca; Corona, Katia; Cerciello, Simone Lateral versus medial approach for total knee arthroplasty for valgus knee deformity shows comparable functional outcomes, hip–knee–ankle angle values, and complication rates: a meta-analysis of comparative studies [33].

Published in: Archives of Orthopaedic and Trauma Surgery (2023).

Link to original: https://doi.org/10.1007/s00402-023-05088-2

If you want to cite the papers, please refer to the original.

For technical reasons we could not place the page where the original quote is coming from.

5.5.5.1 Research Highlights

Valgus knee deformity is a significant condition affecting patients requiring total knee arthroplasty (TKA), characterized by complex anatomical challenges. TKA is a well-established procedure for alleviating pain and improving function in patients with end-stage knee osteoarthritis, but the optimal surgical approach for valgus knees remains debated. The medial parapatellar approach has traditionally been the gold standard yet concerns about excessive release of medial structures and inconsistent restoration of the anatomical axis persist. The study by Mercurio et al.

conducts a meta-analysis to compare the functional and radiographic outcomes, as well as complications, between medial and lateral approaches for TKA in valgus knees.

The study employed a systematic review and meta-analysis methodology, adhering to the Preferred Reporting Items for Systematic Reviews and Meta-Analyses (PRISMA) guidelines. Researchers searched multiple databases, including PubMed and Cochrane Central, to identify relevant studies without date restrictions. Two authors independently screened articles based on predefined inclusion criteria focusing on comparative outcomes of medial versus lateral approaches in TKA for valgus deformity. Data extraction included patient demographics, surgical details, and outcomes such as Knee Society Score (KSS), range of motion (ROM), surgical time, and complications. The quality of studies was assessed using the modified Newcastle–Ottawa Scale and Cochrane risk-of-bias tool. Statistical analyses were performed using random- or fixed-effect models depending on heterogeneity levels.

The meta-analysis revealed that both medial and lateral approaches yield comparable functional outcomes in terms of KSS and ROM, with no significant differences in surgical time or postoperative hip-knee-ankle angle values. Complication rates, including periprosthetic joint infection, fracture, and peroneal nerve injury, were also similar between the two approaches. Future study directions could involve larger patient cohorts with standardized implant types evaluated over long-term follow-up periods to validate these findings further. This comprehensive analysis provides valuable insights into surgical decision-making for TKA in valgus knees but highlights the need for continued research to refine these approaches.

Bibliography

1. Keblish, P. A. (1991). The lateral approach to the valgus knee. Surgical technique and analysis of 53 cases with over two-year follow-up evaluation. *Clinical Orthopaedics and Related Research., 271*, 52–62.
2. Xu, G., Fu, X., Tian, P., Bahat, D., Huang, Y., and Li, Z. (2020). The lateral and medial approach in total arthroplasty for valgus knee: A meta-analysis of current literature. *Journal of Comparative Effectiveness Research, 9*(1), 35–44. https://doi.org/10.2217/cer-2019-0111
3. Wang, B., Xing, D., Li, J. J., Zhu, Y., Dong, S., and Zhao, B. (2019). Lateral or medial approach for valgus knee in total knee arthroplasty—which one is better? A systematic review. *Journal of International Medical Research, 47*(11), 5400–5413. https://doi.org/10.1177/0300060519882208
4. Nikolopoulos D, Polyzois I, Apostolopoulos A, Rossas C, Moutsios-Rentzos A, Michos I (2011) Total knee arthroplasty in severe valgus knee deformity: comparison of a standard medial parapatellar approach combined with tibial tubercle osteotomy. ESSKA 19(11):1834–1842. https://doi.org/10.1007/s00167-011-1474-4
5. Dudek, P., Marczak, D., Okoń, T., Grzelecki, D., Szneider, J., and Kowalczewski, J. (2022). Lateral or medial parapatellar surgical approach to the valgus osteoarthritic knee? A retrospective single-center study. *Journal of Clinical Medicine, 11*(19), 5953. https://doi.org/10.3390/jcm11195953

6. Gunst S, Villa V, Magnussen R et al (2016) Equivalent results of medial and lateral parapatellar approach for total knee arthroplasty in mild valgus deformities. Int Orthop 40:945–951
7. Guo CJ, Liu J, Niu DS, et al. Clinical application of different operative approach of total knee replacement in knee valgus patients. Retrospective cohort study. Int J Surg. 2018;49:80–3. https://doi.org/10.1016/j.ijsu.2017.12.008.
8. Sekiya H, Takatoku K, Takada H, Sugimoto N, Hoshino Y. Lateral approach is advantageous in total knee arthroplasty for valgus deformed knee. Eur J Orthop Surg Traumatol 2014;24:111–5.
9. Kornilov, N., Kulyaba, T., Petukhov, A., Ignatenko, V., and Thienpont, E. (2015). Computer navigation helps achieving appropriate gap balancing and restoration of alignment in total knee arthroplasty for fixed valgus knee osteoarthritis irrespective of the surgical approach. *Acta Orthopaedica Belgica, 81*(4), 673–681.
10. Niki Y, Matsumoto H, Hakozaki A, Kanagawa H, Toyama Y, Suda Y. Clinical and radiographic outcomes of minimally invasive total knee arthroplasty through a lateral approach. Knee Surg Sports Traumatol Arthrosc 2011;19:973–9.
11. Fidddian NJ, Blakeway C, Kumar A. Replacement arthroplasty of valgus knee—a modified lateral capsular approach with repositioning of vastus lateralis. J Bone Joint Surg[Br]. 1998;80B:859–61.
12. Bassaine M, Jeanrot C, Gagey O, Huten D. The composite meniscal-capsular-fat pad flap in a lateral approach to the fixed valgus knee: an anatomical study. J Arthroplasty. 2007;22(4):601–4.
13. Buechel EF. A sequencial three-step lateral release for correcting fixed valgus knee deformities during total knee arthroplasty. Clin Orthop Relat Res. 1991;260:170–5.
14. Keblish PA. The lateral approach for total knee arthroplasty. Journal of knee surgery. 2003;16(1):62–8.
15. Seebacher JR, Inglis AE, Marshall JL, Warren RF. The structure of the posterolateral aspect of the knee. J Bone Joint Surg Am. 1982;64(4):536–41.
16. Keblish PA (1991) Surgical Technique and Analysis of 53 Cases With Over Two-Year Follow-Up Evaluation. Clin Orthop Relat Res 271:52
17. Insall JN, Dorr LD, Scott RD, Scott WN (1989) Rationale of the Knee Society clinical rating system. Clin Orthop Relat Res
18. Satish BR, Ganesan JC, Chandran P, Basanagoudar PL, Balachandar D. Efficacy and mid term results of lateral parapatellar approach without tibial tubercle osteotomy for primary total knee arthroplasty in fixed valgus knees. J Arthroplasty 2013;28:1751–6.
19. Kerver ALA, Leliveld MS, den Hartog D, Verhofstad MHJ, Kleinrensink GJ (2013) The surgical anatomy of the infrapatellar branch of the saphenous nerve in relation to incisions for anteromedial knee surgery. J Bone Joint Surg Am 95:2119–2125
20. Tennent TD, Birch NC, Holmes MJ, Birch R, Goddard NJ (1998) Knee pain and the infrapatellar branch of the saphenous nerve. J R Soc Med 91:573–575

21. Laffosse JM, Potapov A, Malo M et al (2011) Hypesthesia after anterolateral versus midline skin incision in TKA: a randomized study. Clin Orthop Relat Res 469(11):3154–3163. https://doi.org/10.1007/s11999-011-1973-0
22. DePeretti F, Argenson C, Beracassat R, Bourgeon Y. Problèmes artériels et nerveux posés par les incisions cutanées antérieures au niveau de l'articulation du genou (in French) (1987) [Arterial and neurologic problems posed by anterior cutaneous incisions at the level of the knee joint. Rev Chir Orthop Reparatrice Appar Mot73 (suppl 2):231–233
23. Johnson DP, Eastwood DM, Bader DL (1991) Biomechanical factors in wound healing following knee arthroplasty. J Med Eng Technol 5:8–14
24. Johnson DP (1988) Midline or parapatellar incision for knee arthroplasty: a comparative study of wound viability. J Bone Joint Surg Br 70:656–658
25. Schiapparelli F-F, Amsler F, Hirschmann MT (2018) Medial parapatellar approach leads to internal rotation of tibial component in total knee arthroplasty. Knee Surg Sports Traumatol Arthrosc 26:1564–1570. https://doi.org/10.1007/s00167-017-4586-7
26. Karachalios T, Sarangi PP, Newman JH. Severe varus and valgus deformities treated by total knee arthroplasty. J Bone Joint Surg Br 1994;76:938–42.
27. Greenberg, A., Kandel, L., Liebergall, M., Mattan, Y., and Rivkin, G. (2020). Total knee arthroplasty for valgus deformity via a lateral approach: Clinical results, comparison to medial approach, and review of recent literature. *Journal of Arthroplasty, 35*(8), 2076–2083. https://doi.org/10.1016/j.arth.2020.03.037
28. Kornilov N, Kulyaba T, PetuKhov A et al (2015) Computer navigation helps achieving appropriate gap balancing and restoration of alignment in total knee arthroplasty for fixed valgus knee osteoarthritis irrespective of the surgical approach. Acta Orthop 81:673–681
29. Rajnish, Rajesh Kumar; Srivastava, Amit; Yadav, Sandeep Kumar; Elhence, Abhay; Gahlot, Nitesh; Kumar, Prasoon; Gupta, Saurabh; Aggarwal, Sameer Comparative Analysis of Outcomes of Lateral Versus Medial Approach in the Total Knee Arthroplasty for Valgus Deformity: A Systematic Review and Meta-analysis. Indian Journal of Orthopaedics (2024). https://doi.org/10.1007/s43465-024-01211-6
30. Jiang, Jun; C Fernandes, Julio A lateral approach defect closure technique with deep fascia flap for valgus knee TKA. Journal of Orthopaedic Surgery and Research (2015). https://doi.org/10.1186/s13018-015-0316-3
31. Gunst, Stanislas; Villa, Vincent; Magnussen, Robert; Servien, Elvire; Lustig, Sebastien; Neyret, Philippe Equivalent results of medial and lateral parapatellar approach for total knee arthroplasty in mild valgus deformities. International Orthopaedics (2015). https://doi.org/10.1007/s00264-015-2893-5
32. Maniar, Rajesh N.; Singhi, Tushar; Nanivadekar, Arun; Maniar, Parul R.; Singh, Jaivardhan A prospective randomized study in 20 patients undergoing bilateral TKA comparing midline incision to anterolateral incision. Journal of Orthopaedics and Traumatology (2017). https://doi.org/10.1007/s10195-017-0444-0

33. Mercurio, Michele; Gasparini, Giorgio; Galasso, Olimpio; Familiari, Filippo; Cofano, Erminia; Sanzo, Valentina; Ciolli, Gianluca; Corona, Katia; Cerciello, Simone Lateral versus medial approach for total knee arthroplasty for valgus knee deformity shows comparable functional outcomes, hip–knee–ankle angle values, and complication rates: a meta-analysis of comparative studies. Archives of Orthopaedic and Trauma Surgery (2023). https://doi.org/10.1007/s00402-023-05088-2

5.6 Quadriceps Sparing and MIS Procedures

Machine Generated Summaries

Disclaimer: The summaries in this chapter were generated from Springer Nature publications using abstractive AI auto-summarization: An abstraction-based summarizer creates new text based on deep learning. New phrases are created to summarize the content. As the constituted sentences are machine selected, they may not fully reflect the body of the work, so we strongly advise that the original content is read and cited. The auto-generated summaries were curated by the editor to meet Springer Nature publication standards.

5.6.1 Minimally Invasive Total Knee Replacement: Techniques and Results [59]

This is a machine-generated summary of:

Picard, Frederic; Deakin, Angela; Balasubramanian, Navin; Gregori, Alberto Minimally invasive total knee replacement: techniques and results [59].

Published in: European Journal of Orthopaedic Surgery & Traumatology (2018).

Link to original: https://doi.org/10.1007/s00590-018-2164-4

If you want to cite the papers, please refer to the original.

For technical reasons we could not place the page where the original quote is coming from.

5.6.1.1 Research Highlights

The MIS approach for total knee replacement (TKR) emerged in the early twenty-first century, driven by advancements in computer-assisted technology. Early studies indicated that MIS TKR could reduce post-operative pain and blood loss while improving recovery times. However, concerns have been raised about potential complications such as component malalignment and nerve damage. The study by Picard et al. reviews the current state of MIS TKR, including mini-medial parapatellar, mini-midvastus, mini-subvastus, and quadriceps-sparing techniques.

Each approach is assessed for its impact on surgical outcomes and potential complications. The authors highlight that while MIS techniques can offer benefits like reduced incision size and quicker recovery, they also present challenges such as restricted visual fields during surgery. The review discusses how new technologies like computer-assisted navigation and patient-specific instrumentation have been developed to address these challenges. However, the study notes that despite these advancements, there is still no consensus on the superiority of MIS over conventional TKR in terms of long-term outcomes.

The review underscores the need for careful patient selection when considering MIS TKR, suggesting that it may be best suited for non-obese patients with minimal joint deformity. The authors also emphasize the importance of surgeon experience and training in achieving successful outcomes with MIS techniques. Future study directions include further investigation into the long-term safety and efficacy of MIS TKR compared to conventional methods. The study suggests that while MIS has driven innovation in knee replacement surgery, its widespread adoption may be limited until more conclusive evidence is available regarding its benefits over traditional approaches.

5.6.2 Malalignment and Malposition of Quadriceps-Sparing Approach in Primary Total Knee Arthroplasty: A Systematic Review and Meta-analysis [53]

This is a machine-generated summary of:

Yuan, Fu-Zhen; Wang, Shao-Jie; Zhou, Zhu-Xing; Yu, Jia-Kuo; Jiang, Dong Malalignment and malposition of quadriceps-sparing approach in primary total knee arthroplasty: a systematic review and meta-analysis [53].

Published in: Journal of Orthopaedic Surgery and Research (2017).

Link to original: https://doi.org/10.1186/s13018-017-0627-7

If you want to cite the papers, please refer to the original.

For technical reasons we could not place the page where the original quote is coming from.

5.6.2.1 Research Highlights

Total knee arthroplasty (TKA) is a widely used procedure for alleviating pain and restoring function in patients with advanced knee arthritis. Recently, minimally invasive surgery (MIS) techniques, such as the quadriceps-sparing (QS) approach, have gained attention for their potential to reduce recovery time and pain by minimizing soft tissue damage. However, concerns have been raised about the accuracy of component positioning and limb alignment with these techniques. The study by Yuan et al. conducts a meta-analysis to compare the traditional medial parapatellar (MP) approach with the QS approach in terms of limb alignment and prosthesis positioning.

The study involved a comprehensive search of databases including PubMed, Embase, and the Cochrane Collaboration Library to identify relevant literature from January, 2006, until March, 2017. The researchers included randomized controlled trials and retrospective comparative studies that evaluated limb alignment and prosthesis position outcomes in MP and QS approaches for TKA. Data extraction was performed independently by two reviewers, focusing on factors such as sample size, follow-up duration, and prosthesis type. The quality of the studies was assessed using tools recommended by the Cochrane Collaboration and the Newcastle-Ottawa Scale. Statistical analysis was conducted using Review Manager software to calculate odds ratios and assess heterogeneity. The meta-analysis found that the MP approach resulted in fewer outliers in hip-knee-ankle angle, coronal tibial component angle, and femoral notch compared to the QS approach.

The study highlights that while the MP approach offers superior radiological outcomes in terms of alignment and component positioning, it is associated with longer rehabilitation times. The QS approach may lead to more outliers due to limited visualization but offers benefits in terms of reduced postoperative pain. Future study could focus on improving surgical instruments and techniques to enhance the accuracy of QS procedures while maintaining their minimally invasive advantages. The authors note that further large-scale, well-designed randomized controlled trials are needed to confirm these findings and address limitations such as potential bias from retrospective studies and varying levels of surgical expertise among included studies.

5.6.3 Comparison of the Quadriceps-Sparing and Subvastus Approaches Versus the Standard Parapatellar Approach in Total Knee Arthroplasty: A Meta-analysis of Randomized Controlled Trials [54]

This is a machine-generated summary of:

Peng, Xiaochun; Zhang, Xianlong; Cheng, Tao; Cheng, Mengqi; Wang, Jiaxing Comparison of the quadriceps-sparing and subvastus approaches versus the standard parapatellar approach in total knee arthroplasty: a meta-analysis of randomized controlled trials [54].

Published in: BMC Musculoskeletal Disorders (2015).

Link to original: https://doi.org/10.1186/s12891-015-0783-z

If you want to cite the papers, please refer to the original.

For technical reasons we could not place the page where the original quote is coming from.

5.6.3.1 Research Highlights

Total knee arthroplasty (TKA) is a widely successful procedure for patients with end-stage knee diseases, traditionally performed using the medial parapatellar approach. This standard approach, while providing excellent visualization, compromises the peripatellar blood supply and quadriceps muscle, potentially leading to complications such as avascular necrosis and anterior knee pain. In recent years, minimally invasive techniques like the quadriceps-sparing and subvastus approaches have emerged, promising better clinical outcomes by preserving the quadriceps tendon and vastus medialis insertion. However, studies comparing these techniques with the standard approach have yielded conflicting results. The study by Peng et al. conducts a meta-analysis of randomized controlled trials to quantitatively assess the efficacy and safety of these approaches in TKA.

The study followed the Preferred Reporting Items for Systematic Reviews and Meta-Analyses (PRISMA) guidelines to include randomized controlled trials comparing the subvastus or quadriceps-sparing approaches with the standard parapatellar approach in TKA. The researchers searched multiple databases for relevant studies published between January, 1982, until July, 2014ultimately including 19 RCTs in their analysis. The primary outcomes assessed were Knee Society Scores (KSS) and Visual Analog Scale (VAS) scores for pain, while secondary outcomes included range of motion (ROM), operative time, and postoperative complications. The meta-analysis revealed that the quadriceps-sparing approach significantly improved KSS at certain postoperative intervals but required longer operative time compared to the standard approach. The subvastus approach showed advantages in VAS scores, ROM, straight leg raise, and lateral retinacular release without increasing operative time.

The findings suggest that both minimally invasive approaches offer specific benefits over the standard parapatellar technique; however, they also present challenges such as increased operative time for the quadriceps-sparing method. Future study could focus on multi-center RCTs with larger sample sizes to further validate these results. Additionally, while these approaches show promise in improving certain clinical outcomes, they do not meet all criteria for an ideal TKA technique. Surgeons should weigh these factors when considering surgical options for TKA patients.

5.6.4 Complex Ruptures of the Quadriceps Tendon: A Systematic Review of Surgical Procedures and Outcomes [55]

This is a machine-generated summary of:

Oliva, Francesco; Marsilio, Emanuela; Migliorini, Filippo; Maffulli, Nicola Complex ruptures of the quadriceps tendon: a systematic review of surgical procedures and outcomes [55].

Published in: Journal of Orthopaedic Surgery and Research (2021).

Link to original: https://doi.org/10.1186/s13018-021-02696-9

If you want to cite the papers, please refer to the original.

For technical reasons we could not place the page where the original quote is coming from.

5.6.4.1 Research Highlights

Quadriceps tendon rupture (QTR) is a rare but challenging condition, often affecting middle-aged males and associated with systemic conditions like diabetes and chronic renal failure. The multi-layered structure of the quadriceps tendon can be compromised in chronic ruptures, leading to tendon retraction and loss of function. While acute QTRs are typically managed with primary repair, chronic cases, especially those following total knee arthroplasty (TKA), present significant treatment challenges due to the lack of consensus on optimal surgical techniques. This study by Oliva et al. systematically reviews the literature to evaluate the epidemiology, treatment strategies, and outcomes of chronic QTRs, QTRs post-TKA, and re-ruptures.

The study conducted a comprehensive literature search following the Preferred Reporting Items for Systematic Reviews and Meta-Analyses (PRISMA) guidelines focusing on complex QTRs and their surgical interventions. The authors included clinical studies reporting on incidence, risk factors, treatment methods, and complications associated with these injuries. They categorized patients into three groups: chronic QTRs, QTRs after primary TKA, and re-ruptures. Various surgical techniques were analyzed, including end-to-end sutures, V-Y lengthening, tendon grafts, and synthetic mesh augmentation. The review found that synthetic augmentation was frequently used for QTRs post-TKA, while tendon grafts were preferred for chronic ruptures and re-ruptures. Despite the variety of techniques employed, all patients regained active knee extension post-surgery; however, some experienced extension lag or decreased flexion.

The study highlights that while autografts tend to yield better functional outcomes with fewer complications compared to allografts or synthetic materials, there remains no standardized protocol for managing complex QTRs. Future study should focus on comparing surgical procedures to establish evidence-based guidelines for treating these injuries effectively. The authors emphasize the importance of surgeon experience in selecting appropriate techniques due to the current lack of consensus in the literature. Further research is needed to refine rehabilitation protocols and improve long-term outcomes for patients with complex quadriceps tendon ruptures.

5.6.5 Quadriceps-Sparing Versus Traditional Medial Parapatellar Approaches for Total Knee Arthroplasty: A Meta-analysis [56]

This is a machine-generated summary of:

Yuan, Fu-Zhen; Zhang, Ji-Ying; Jiang, Dong; Yu, Jia-Kuo Quadriceps-sparing versus traditional medial parapatellar approaches for total knee arthroplasty: a meta-analysis [56].

Published in: BMC Musculoskeletal Disorders (2019).

Link to original: https://doi.org/10.1186/s12891-019-2482-7

If you want to cite the papers, please refer to the original.

For technical reasons we could not place the page where the original quote is coming from.

5.6.5.1 Research Highlights

Total knee arthroplasty (TKA) is a widely used surgical procedure for patients with end-stage knee arthritis, known for its effectiveness in alleviating pain and improving function. Traditionally, the medial parapatellar (MP) approach has been the gold standard technique for TKA. However, the quadriceps-sparing (QS) approach has emerged as a popular alternative, theoretically offering faster muscle recovery by minimizing disruption to the extensor mechanism and suprapatellar pouch. Despite numerous studies comparing these approaches, conclusions remain controversial, with some research indicating no significant differences between them. The study by Yuan et al. compares the efficacy and safety of the QS versus MP approaches through a comprehensive meta-analysis.

The study conducted a systematic search of multiple databases, including PubMed and EMBase, to identify relevant studies without restrictions on region or language. The authors included both randomized controlled trials (RCTs) and retrospective comparative studies that met specific criteria, focusing on adult patients undergoing primary TKA. Data extraction was performed using a predesigned sheet, and methodological quality was assessed using established guidelines such as the Cochrane Handbook for RCTs and the Newcastle-Ottawa Scale for non-RCTs. Statistical analysis was carried out using Review Manager software, with significance set at $P < 0.05$. The meta-analysis included 17 studies comprising eight RCTs and found that while the QS approach improved range of motion (ROM) postoperatively and reduced incision length, it also increased surgical and tourniquet time compared to the MP approach.

The findings suggest that the QS approach may offer advantages in terms of early recovery and cosmetic outcomes without increasing surgical risks. However, it requires longer surgical time, which could lead to higher hospital costs. The study highlights that while QS may improve certain postoperative outcomes like ROM and incision length, it does not significantly differ from MP in terms of complications or prosthesis alignment. Future study could focus on long-term outcomes beyond 10 years to better understand the implications of mechanical axis alignment and prosthesis positioning on functional scores. Additionally, ensuring surgeons are skilled in both approaches is crucial for optimal patient outcomes.

5.6.6 Optimal Patellar Alignment with Minimally Invasive Approaches in Total Knee Arthroplasty after a Minimum Five Year Follow-Up [57]

This is a machine-generated summary of:

Huang, Ai-Bing; Wang, Hai-Jun; Yu, Jia-Kuo; Yang, Bo; Ma, Dong; Zhang, Ji-Ying Optimal patellar alignment with minimally invasive approaches in total knee arthroplasty after a minimum 5 year follow-up [57].

Published in: International Orthopaedics (2015).

Link to original: https://doi.org/10.1007/s00264-015-2896-2

If you want to cite the papers, please refer to the original.

For technical reasons we could not place the page where the original quote is coming from.

5.6.6.1 Research Highlights

Patellofemoral syndrome is a prevalent complication following total knee arthroplasty (TKA), with proper patellar alignment being a significant challenge. Factors such as pre-operative deformity, prosthesis design, and surgical approach influence post-operative patellofemoral articulation, with the surgical approach being a primary factor. Minimally invasive surgical techniques, such as the mini-medial parapatellar (MMP) and quadriceps-sparing (QS) approaches, have been associated with benefits like reduced post-operative pain and quicker recovery compared to the traditional medial parapatellar (MPP) approach. However, clinical data on post-operative patellar alignment outcomes among these approaches are lacking. The study by Huang et al. investigates the long-term effects of these three surgical techniques on patellar alignment in TKA patients.

The study was designed as a retrospective comparative analysis involving patients with osteoarthritis who underwent primary TKA using one of the three approaches: MPP, MMP, or QS. Patients were followed for a minimum of 5 years post-surgery. The inclusion criteria ensured a consistent patient profile across groups, excluding those with inflammatory arthritis or prior lateral retinacular release. All surgeries were performed by an experienced surgeon using standardized procedures for each approach. Radiographic evaluations assessed patellar tilt (PT) and patellar displacement (PD) before surgery and at final follow-up. Clinical outcomes were measured using various scoring systems like VAS, KSS, and WOMAC. Statistical analyses compared outcomes across groups to determine differences in patellar alignment and clinical scores.

The study found that minimally invasive approaches (MMP and QS) resulted in better patellar alignment than the traditional MPP approach after 5 years. The QS approach showed the most favorable outcomes in terms of PT and PD correction. Despite these differences in alignment, no significant correlation was found between post-operative patellar alignment and clinical scores such as VAS or WOMAC. The study suggests that while minimally invasive techniques may improve patellar tracking, they do not necessarily translate to better clinical outcomes. Future study could involve prospective trials with longer follow-up periods to validate these findings further and explore other factors influencing TKA outcomes.

5.6.7 Minimally Invasive Medial Femoral Approach to Total Knee Arthroplasty Improves Short-Term Outcomes Compared to the Standard Medial Parapatellar Approach: A Systematic Review and Meta-analysis [58]

This is a machine-generated summary of:

Yang, Xin; Cheng, Qing-hao; Yang, Yong-ze; Zhang, An-ren; Fan, Hua; Guo, Hong-zhang Minimally invasive medial femoral approach to total knee arthroplasty improves short-term outcomes compared to the standard medial parapatellar approach: a systematic review and meta-analysis [58].

Published in: Journal of Orthopaedic Surgery and Research (2023).

Link to original: https://doi.org/10.1186/s13018-023-04136-2

If you want to cite the papers, please refer to the original.

For technical reasons we could not place the page where the original quote is coming from.

5.6.7.1 Research Highlights

Total knee arthroplasty (TKA) is a widely used treatment for advanced knee osteoarthritis, with the medial parapatellar (MP) approach being the most common surgical method. However, this approach can lead to complications such as patellar subluxation and aseptic necrosis, affecting knee extensor function recovery. Minimally invasive surgery (MIS) techniques have been developed to improve short-term recovery and reduce complications. Despite their benefits, MIS techniques face criticism for potentially compromising prosthesis positioning and force alignment due to limited exposure. The study by Yang et al. compares the mini-midvastus (MMV) approach with the standard MP approach through a systematic review and meta-analysis of randomized controlled trials.

The study conducted a comprehensive literature search across multiple databases, including PubMed and Cochrane Library, focusing on randomized controlled trials comparing MMV and MP approaches in TKA. The researchers included studies that met strict inclusion criteria, excluding semi-randomized trials and those with inconsistent baselines or unscientific methods. Data extraction and quality assessment were performed by two independent researchers using the Cochrane Collaboration tool. Statistical analysis was conducted using Review Manager software, employing random or fixed effect models based on heterogeneity tests. The results indicated that the MMV approach showed superior early-stage outcomes in terms of Knee Society Scores (KSS), Visual Analog Scale (VAS) scores for pain, and range of motion (ROM), although no significant differences were observed in mid- to long-term outcomes compared to the MP approach.

The study highlights that while the MMV approach offers better early postoperative outcomes, it requires longer surgical times and higher technical skills from surgeons. The findings suggest that MMV may be more beneficial for early recovery but does not significantly differ from MP in long-term efficacy or complication rates. Future study could focus on long-term clinical evidence and include outcome indicators like lower limb alignment to provide a more comprehensive evaluation of these surgical approaches. Despite some limitations, such as potential biases in included studies, this research provides valuable insights into optimizing surgical methods for TKA.

Bibliography

1. Tria AJ Jr, Coon TM (2003) Minimal incision total knee arthroplasty: early experience. Clin Orthop Relat Res 416:185–190
2. Floren M, Reichel H, Davis J, Laskin RS. The mini-incision mid-vastus approach for total knee arthroplasty. Oper Orthop Traumatol. 2008;20:534–43.
3. Laskin RS, Beksac B, Phongjunakorn A, Pittors K, Davis J, Shim JC, Petersen M (2004) Minimally invasive total knee replacement through a mini-midvastus incision: an outcome study. Clin Orthop Relat Res 428:74–81
4. Higgins JP, Altman DG, Gotzsche PC, Juni P, Moher D, Oxman AD, Savovic J, Schulz KF, Weeks L, Sterne JA (2011) The Cochrane Collaboration's tool for assessing risk of bias in randomised trials. BMJ 343:d5928. https://doi.org/10.1136/bmj.d5928
5. Wells GA, Shea B, O'Connell D, Peterson J, Welch V, Losos M, et al. The Newcastle-Ottawa Scale (NOS) for assessing the quality of nonrandomised studies in meta-analyses. http://www.ohri.ca/programs/clinical_epidemiology/oxford.asp. Accessed 24 Mar 2017.
6. Higgins J, Thomas J, Churchill R, Lasserson T, Li TJ, Page M, et al. Cochrane Handbook for Systematic Reviews of Interventions.2017. http://handbook.cochrane.org/front_page.htm. Accessed 21 Mar 2017.
7. King J, Stamper DL, Schaad DC, Leopold SS. Minimally invasive total knee arthroplasty compared with traditional total knee arthroplasty. Assessment of the learning curve and the postoperative recuperative period. J Bone Joint Surg Am. 2007;89:1497–503.
8. Chin PL, Foo LS, Yang KY, Yeo SJ, Lo NN. Randomized controlled trial comparing the radiologic outcomes of conventional and minimally invasive techniques for total knee arthroplasty. J Arthroplast. 2007;22:800–6.
9. Huang HT, Su JY, Chang JK, Chen CH, Wang GJ. The early clinical outcome of minimally invasive quadriceps-sparing total knee arthroplasty: Report of a 2-year followup. J Arthroplasty 2007;22:1007–12.
10. Shen H, Zhang XL, Wang Q, Shao JJ, Jiang Y. Minimally invasive total knee arthroplasty through a quadriceps sparing approach: a comparative study. Zhonghua Wai Ke Za Zhi. 2007;45:1083–6.
11. Tashiro Y, Miura H, Matsuda S, Okazaki K, Iwamoto Y. Minimally invasive versus standard approach in total knee arthroplasty. Clin Orthop Relat Res. 2007;463:144–50.
12. Kim YH, Sohn KS, Kim JS. Short-term results of primary total knee arthroplasties performed with a mini-incision or a standard incision. J Arthroplast. 2006;21:712–8.

13. Kim YH, Kim JS, Kim DY (2007) Clinical outcome and rate of complications after primary total knee replacement performed with quadriceps-sparing or standard arthrotomy. J Bone Joint Surg Br 89(4):467–470
14. Karpman RR, Smith HL (2009) Comparison of the early results of minimally invasive vs standard approaches to total knee arthroplasty: a prospective, randomized study. J Arthroplasty 24(5):681–688. https://doi.org/10.1016/j.arth.2008.03.011
15. Chen AF, Alan RK, Redziniak DE, Tria AJ (2006) Quadriceps sparing total knee replacement. J Bone Joint Surg 88(11):1448–1453
16. Hofmann AA, Plaster RL, Murdock LE. Subvastus (Southern) approach for primary total knee arthroplasty. Clin Orthop Relat Res. 1991;269:70–7.
17. Lin TC, Wang HK, Chen JW, Chiu CM, Chou HL, Chang CH. Minimally invasive knee arthroplasty with the subvastus approach allows rapid rehabilitation: A prospective, biomechanical and observational study. J Phys Ther Sci 2013;25:557–62.
18. Lin WP, Lin J, Horng LC, Chang SM, Jiang CC (2009) Quadriceps-sparing, minimal-incision total knee arthroplasty: a comparative study. J Arthroplasty 24(7):1024–1032. https://doi.org/10.1016/j.arth.2008.07.005
19. Chiang H, Lee CC, Lin WP, Jiang CC (2012) Comparison of quadriceps-sparing minimally invasive and medial parapatellar total knee arthroplasty: a 2-year follow-up study. J Formos Med Assoc 111(12):698–704. https://doi.org/10.1016/j.jfma.2011.11.025
20. Wegrzyn J, Parratte S, Coleman-Wood K, Kaufman KR, Pagnano MW (2013) The John Insall award: no benefit of minimally invasive TKA on gait and strength outcomes: a randomized controlled trial. Clin Orthop Relat Res 471(1):46–55. https://doi.org/10.1007/s11999-012-2486-1
21. Moher D, Liberati A, Tetzlaff J, Altman DG, Group P. Preferred reporting items for systematic reviews and meta-analyses: the PRISMA statement. J Clin Epidemiol. 2009;10:1006–12.
22. Higgins. JPT, Green. S. Cochrane Handbook for Systematic Reviews of Interventions Version 5.1.0 [updated March 2011]. The Cochrane Collaboration. Available at: www.cochrane-handbookorg. Accessed 2 June 2014
23. Teng Y, Du W, Jiang J et al (2012) Subvastus versus medial parapatellar approach in total knee arthroplasty: meta-analysis. Orthopedics 35. https://doi.org/10.3928/01477447-20121120-16
24. Ilan DI, Tejwani N, Keschner M, Leibman M. Quadriceps tendon rupture. J Am Acad Orthop Surg. 2003;11(3):192–200. https://doi.org/10.5435/00124635-200305000-00006.
25. Clayton RA, Court-Brown CM. The epidemiology of musculoskeletal tendinous and ligamentous injuries. Injury. 2008;39(12):1338–44. https://doi.org/10.1016/j.injury.2008.06.021.
26. Yepes H, Tang M, Morris SF, Stanish WD. Relationship between hypovascular zones and patterns of ruptures of the quadriceps tendon. J Bone Joint Surg Am. 2008;90(10):2135–41. https://doi.org/10.2106/JBJS.G.01200.

27. Elattar O, McBeth Z, Curry EJ, Parisien RL, Galvin JW, Li X. Management of chronic quadriceps tendon rupture: a critical analysis review. JBJS Rev. 2021;9(5). https://doi.org/10.2106/JBJS.RVW.20.00096.
28. Burnett RS, Berger RA, Paprosky WG, et al. Extensor mechanism allograft reconstruction after total knee arthroplasty A comparison of two techniques. J Bone Joint Surg Am. 2004;86(12):2694–9. https://doi.org/10.2106/00004623-200412000-00016.
29. Forslund J, Gold S, Gelber J. Allograft reconstruction of a chronic quadriceps tendon rupture with use of a novel technique. JBJS Case Connect. 2014;4(2):e42. https://doi.org/10.2106/JBJS.CC.M.00230.
30. Lim CT, Amanatullah DF, Huddleston JI 3rd, et al. Reconstruction of disrupted extensor mechanism after total knee arthroplasty. J Arthroplasty. 2017;32(10):3134–40. https://doi.org/10.1016/j.arth.2017.05.005.
31. Wise BT, Erens G, Pour AE, Bradbury TL, Roberson JR. Long-term results of extensor mechanism reconstruction using Achilles tendon allograft after total knee arthroplasty. Int Orthop. 2018;42(10):2367–73. https://doi.org/10.1007/s00264-018-3848-4.
32. Abdel MP, Pagnano MW, Perry KI, Hanssen AD. Extensor mechanism reconstruction with use of Marlex mesh. JBJS Essent Surg Tech. 2019;9(2):e21. https://doi.org/10.2106/JBJS.ST.18.00106.
33. Nodzo SR, Rachala SR. Polypropylene mesh augmentation for complete quadriceps rupture after total knee arthroplasty. Knee. 2016;23(1):177–80. https://doi.org/10.1016/j.knee.2015.09.007.
34. Niki Y, Mochizuki T, Momohara S, Saito S, Toyama Y, Matsumoto H (2009) Is minimally invasive surgery in total knee arthroplasty really minimally invasive surgery? J Arthroplasty 24(4):499–504
35. Moher D, Liberati A, Tetzlaff J, Altman DG, for the PRISMA Group. Preferred reporting items for systematic reviews and meta-analyses: the PRISMA statement. BMJ. 2009;339(jul21 1):b2535. https://doi.org/10.1136/bmj.b2535.
36. Shamseer L, Moher D, Clarke M, Ghersi D, Liberati A, Petticrew M, Shekelle P, Stewart LA. Preferred reporting items for systematic review and meta-analysis protocols (PRISMA-P) 2015: elaboration and explanation. BMJ. 2015;349:g7647.
37. Higgins JPT GS. Cochrane handbook for systematic reviews of interventions, vol. 2017. The Cochrane Collaboration; 2011. Available: http://handbook.cochrane.org/front_page.htm.
38. Varela-Egocheaga JR, Suárez-Suárez MA, Fernández-Villán M, González-Sastre V, Varela-Gómez JR, Rodríguez-Merchán C (2010) Minimally invasive subvastus approach: improving the results of total knee arthroplasty: a prospective, randomized trial. Clin Orthop Relat Res 468(5):1200–1208
39. Wulker N, Lambermont JP, Sacchetti L, Lazaro JG, Nardi J (2010) A prospective randomized study of minimally invasive total knee arthroplasty compared with conventional surgery. J Bone Jt Surg Am 92(7):1584–1590. https://doi.org/10.2106/JBJS.H.01070

40. Bracey DN, Brown ML, Beard HR, Mannava S, Nazir OF, Seyler TM, Lang JE (2015) Effects of patellofemoral overstuffing on knee flexion and patellar kinematics following total knee arthroplasty: a cadaveric study. Int Orthop. https://doi.org/10.1007/s00264-015-2715-9
41. Župan A, Snoj Ž, Antolič V, Pompe B (2014) Better results with patelloplasty compared to traditional total knee arthroplasty. Int Orthop 38:1621–1625. https://doi.org/10.1007/s00264-014-2366-2
42. Pongcharoen B, Yakampor T, Charoencholvanish K. Patellar tracking and anterior knee pain are similar after medial parapatellar and midvastus approaches in minimally invasive TKA. Clin Orthop Relat Res. 2013;471(5):1654–60.
43. Liu J, Sun ZH, Tian WW, Sun YB, Wang L, Cao JG, et al. Primary observation and study of total knee arthroplasty with medial inferior femoral approach. Chin J Orthod Surg. 2008;09:649–52.
44. Nestor BJ, Toulson CE, Backus SI et al (2010) Mini-midvastus vs. standard medial parapatellar approach: a prospective, randomized, double-blinded study in patients undergoing bilateral total knee arthroplasty. J Arthroplasty 25:5–11
45. Walter F, Haynes MB, Markel DC. A randomized prospective study evaluating the effect of patellar eversion on the early functional outcomes in primary total knee arthroplasty. J Arthroplasty. 2007;22(4):509–14.
46. Fu PL, Li XH, Wu YL, Xie QY, Sun JY, Wu HS. Comparison of the advantages of initial total knee arthroplasty in the placement of the prosthesis by the medial approach and the medial bypass approach of the femoral muscles. Tissue Eng Res Clin Rehabil China. 2008;09:1793–6.
47. Cho KY, Kim KI, Umrani S, Kim SH (2014) Better quadriceps recovery after minimally invasive total knee arthroplasty. Knee Surg Sports Traumatol Arthrosc 22(8):1759–1764. https://doi.org/10.1007/s00167-013-2556-2
48. Karachalios Th, Giotikas D, Roidis N (2008) Total knee replacement performed with either a mini-midvastus or a standard approach: a prospective randomized clinical and radiological trial. J Bone Joint Surg Br 90:584–592
49. Guy SP, Farndon MA, Conroy JL, Bennett C, Grainger AJ, London NJ. A prospective randomized study of minimally invasive midvastus total knee arthroplasty compared with standard total knee arthroplasty. Knee. 2012;19(6):866–71.
50. Juosponis R, Tarasevicius S, Smailys A, Kalesinskas RJ (2009) Functional and radiological outcome after total knee replacement performed with mini-midvastus or conventional arthrotomy: controlled randomised trial. Int Orthop 33(5):1233–1237. https://doi.org/10.1007/s00264-008-0630-z
51. Zora H, Gungor HR, Bayrak G, Savkin R, Buker N. Does mini-midvastus approach have an advantageous effect on rapid recovery protocols over medial parapatellar approach in total knee arthroplasty? Jt Dis Relat Surg. 2020;31(3):571–81.
52. Zhang Z, Zhu W, Gu B, Zhu L, Chen C. Mini-midvastus versus mini-medial parapatellar approach in total knee arthroplasty: a prospective, randomized study. Arch Orthop Trauma Surg. 2013;3:389–95.

53. Yuan, Fu-Zhen; Wang, Shao-Jie; Zhou, Zhu-Xing; Yu, Jia-Kuo; Jiang, Dong Malalignment and malposition of quadriceps-sparing approach in primary total knee arthroplasty: a systematic review and meta-analysis. Journal of Orthopaedic Surgery and Research (2017). https://doi.org/10.1186/s13018-017-0627-7
54. Peng, Xiaochun; Zhang, Xianlong; Cheng, Tao; Cheng, Mengqi; Wang, Jiaxing Comparison of the quadriceps-sparing and subvastus approaches versus the standard parapatellar approach in total knee arthroplasty: a meta-analysis of randomized controlled trials. BMC Musculoskeletal Disorders (2015). 10.1186/s12891-015-0783-z
55. Oliva, Francesco; Marsilio, Emanuela; Migliorini, Filippo; Maffulli, Nicola Complex ruptures of the quadriceps tendon: a systematic review of surgical procedures and outcomes. Journal of Orthopaedic Surgery and Research (2021). https://doi.org/10.1186/s13018-021-02696-9
56. Yuan, Fu-Zhen; Zhang, Ji-Ying; Jiang, Dong; Yu, Jia-Kuo Quadriceps-sparing versus traditional medial parapatellar approaches for total knee arthroplasty: a meta-analysis. BMC Musculoskeletal Disorders (2019). https://doi.org/10.1186/s12891-019-2482-7
57. Huang, Ai-Bing; Wang, Hai-Jun; Yu, Jia-Kuo; Yang, Bo; Ma, Dong; Zhang, Ji-Ying Optimal patellar alignment with minimally invasive approaches in total knee arthroplasty after a minimum five year follow-up. International Orthopaedics (2015). https://doi.org/10.1007/s00264-015-2896-2
58. Yang, Xin; Cheng, Qing-hao; Yang, Yong-ze; Zhang, An-ren; Fan, Hua; Guo, Hong-zhang Minimally invasive medial femoral approach to total knee arthroplasty improves short-term outcomes compared to the standard medial parapatellar approach: a systematic review and meta-analysis. Journal of Orthopaedic Surgery and Research (2023). https://doi.org/10.1186/s13018-023-04136-2
59. Picard, Frederic; Deakin, Angela; Balasubramanian, Navin; Gregori, Alberto Minimally invasive total knee replacement: techniques and results. European Journal of Orthopaedic Surgery & Traumatology (2018). https://doi.org/10.1007/s00590-018-2164-4

Chapter 6
Surgical Techniques for Primary Total Knee Arthroplasty

Alfred J. Tria Jr. and Giles R. Scuderi

Introduction by the Editors

Since the initiation of modern total knee arthroplasty (TKA) in the 1970s, the surgical technique has continued to evolve. It became evident that the desired surgery needed to produce a reproducible result that mimicked the normal anatomy and kinematics of the knee. TKA needed to have an anatomic goal, which would need to be thoroughly defined from which the desired surgical plan would be established. Restoration of a neutral mechanical axis has been a long-standing principle of total knee arthroplasty (TKA). This alignment is based upon the precept that post-operative alignment following TKA should be within 3^0 of a neutral mechanical axis or "coronal safe zone." Recently, there has been some debate over the acceptable mechanical alignment and alternative alignment techniques have emerged offering innovative solutions tailored to the unique anatomical and biomechanical characteristics of each patient. These approaches leverage advanced technologies to enhance precision and personalization. Among the prominent individualized techniques are kinematic alignment, unrestricted kinematic alignment, restricted kinematic alignment, inverse kinematic alignment, and functional alignment. These strategies aim to replicate natural knee kinematics and improve patient-reported outcomes by preserving or reconstructing the individual's native joint alignment. Despite their promise, these techniques come with unique challenge. As TKA evolves, the balance between achieving natural knee kinematics and maintaining durable implant performance remains at the forefront.

This chapter reviews the various surgical techniques that are being used with attention to alignment options. With our editorial prerogative, we reviewed each of

A. J. Tria Jr. (✉)
Department of Orthopedics, Rutgers-Robert Wood Johnson Medical School, New Brunswick, NJ, USA

G. R. Scuderi
Department of Orthopedic Surgery, Northwell Health, Garden City, NY, USA

A. J. Tria Jr., G. R. Scuderi (eds.), *Total Knee Arthroplasty*,
https://doi.org/10.1007/978-3-032-00175-7_6

the referenced articles and summarized our own conclusions, as detailed below. As you read each of the computer-generated summaries that follow in this chapter you can draw your own conclusions.

Mechanical alignment continues to be the most popular technique. Liow et al. looked at functional outcomes using stereotaxic navigation and Gao et al. used a accelerometer-based navigation to produce the mechanical alignment. Both articles indicate that the results were more accurate, but they did not improve clinical results and required more time and greater expense. Patil et al. looked functional outcome and concluded that a 3-degree deviation from the neutral mechanical axis was best but the data to support this is not totally clear. In a desire to establish a preoperative plan, Wen et al. used radiologic measurements for planning purposes. It is not clear how the operating surgeon can incorporate these into the standard surgery. Palasamy et al. studied Indian knees and noted a preponderance of tibial varus deformity. The surgical results with the knees aligned mechanically were significantly improved but he does open the discussion to using kinematic alignment. Thongpulssawasdi et al. concluded that a threshold angle of 3.5 degrees was predictive of the need for a MCL release. While this may be statistically indicated, it does not seem to be required especially if the surgery is based on kinematic alignment.

Numerous reports have shown good results with kinematic alignment and surgeons are considering it as an alternative technique. Ragunandhan et al. reported on the results of kinematic alignment in an Indian population with good to excellent results. Concern that kinematic alignment may result in internal rotation of the femoral component, Nedopil et al. evaluated patellofemoral instability after kinematic TKA with results that appear to be secondary to the position of the femoral component, especially with increased flexion and tended to occur without trauma about 5-months postoperatively. This stresses the importance of surgical technique. Hsu et al. observed, as one would suspect, that kinematic alignment is influenced by preoperative planning. Understanding the concept of kinematic alignment, Hutt et al. just documented that kinematic alignment often results in a varus tibial cut. This is concerning especially as there are no established guidelines as to how much tibial varus is acceptable.

Advocates of the gap balancing technique for TKA, stress the importance of the supporting soft tissues and need for releases when correcting fixed deformity. Migliorini et al. and Adel et al. compared gap balancing to measured resection each showing that the techniques both produce similar results. Knowing that there are nuances to gap balanicing, several of the articles present nuances on the gap balancing technique. Fickert et al., Hu et al., Valpiano et al., Hananuchi et al., Zhang et al., Grifka et al., Sriphiram et al., Nowakowski et al. Matsui et al. Hommel et al. Xuequan et al., and Tsai et al. These articles illustrate modifications and slight additions that improve the technique.

The one unresolved issue in TKA is to resurface the patella or not and is a persistent topic of discussion over the years. Beaupre et al. did a randomized controlled study of retention versus resurfacing at 5–10 years and showed similar results but an 8% reoperation rate in the unresurfaced group. This is similar to what has been previously reported. Trying to develop a rationalized approach Palanisamy et al.

developed an algorithm for decision making for resurfacing that will have to be validated in the future. Choi et al. compared the two approaches in a bilateral setting and showed that the patients did not perceive any difference in the results. The remainder of the articles review various aspects of resurfacing and Dogruoz et al. studied circumferential denervation of the patella and showed that this approach was no different than when it was not performed.

These papers illustrate the benefits of each technique and show that in the hands of experienced surgeons the results are all similar. Therefore, surgeons should choose the operative technique that they fully understand and are most comfortable with the approach.

6.1 Mechanical Alignment

Machine Generated Summaries

Disclaimer: The summaries in this chapter were generated from Springer Nature publications using abstractive AI auto-summarization: An abstraction-based summarizer creates new text based on deep learning. New phrases are created to summarize the content. As the constituted sentences are machine selected, they may not fully reflect the body of the work, so we strongly advise that the original content is read and cited. The auto-generated summaries were curated by the editor to meet Springer Nature publication standards.

6.1.1 Computer-Assisted Stereotaxic Navigation Improves the Accuracy of Mechanical Alignment and Component Positioning in Total Knee Arthroplasty [38]

This is a machine-generated summary of:

Liow, Ming Han Lincoln; Goh, Graham Seow-Hng; Pang, Hee-Nee; Tay, Darren Keng Jin; Lo, Ngai Nung; Yeo, Seng Jin Computer-assisted stereotaxic navigation improves the accuracy of mechanical alignment and component positioning in total knee arthroplasty [38].

Published in: Archives of Orthopaedic and Trauma Surgery (2016).

Link to original: https://doi.org/10.1007/s00402-016-2483-z

If you want to cite the papers, please refer to the original.

For technical reasons we could not place the page where the original quote is coming from.

6.1.1.1 Research Highlights

Total knee arthroplasty (TKA) is a widely accepted treatment for advanced knee arthritis, yet the optimal mechanical alignment and component positioning remain subjects of debate due to their potential impact on implant longevity. Traditional TKA techniques often lack precision in achieving ideal mechanical alignment, prompting interest in technologies like computer-assisted surgery (CAS) that promise enhanced accuracy without compromising surgical efficiency. The study by Liow et al.c explores the efficacy of the iASSIST (Zimmer-Biomet, Warsaw, Indiana, USA) knee computer-assisted stereotaxic navigation system in improving mechanical alignment and component positioning in TKA.

The study involved patients with tricompartmental osteoarthritis undergoing TKA using either conventional methods or the iASSIST system at a single institution. Two senior surgeons performed the surgeries, with one using the conventional technique and the other employing the CASN (Computer Assisted Stereotaxic Navigation) method. The iASSIST system utilizes disposable electronic stereotaxic pods for alignment feedback, eliminating the need for large consoles or navigation arrays. The study assessed post-operative outcomes through radiological evaluations and clinical assessments at 6 months. Results indicated that while both groups showed significant improvements in clinical scores, the CASN group achieved superior mechanical alignment and component positioning compared to the conventional group. However, surgeries using CASN were longer, and no significant differences in clinical outcomes were observed between the two groups.

The findings suggest that while CASN systems like iASSIST offer improved alignment accuracy, they do not necessarily translate into better short-term clinical outcomes compared to conventional TKA methods. Future study could focus on long-term outcomes to determine if improved alignment leads to enhanced implant survivorship or patient satisfaction over time. Additionally, considerations regarding cost-effectiveness and surgical duration remain critical as these factors influence the broader adoption of CAS technologies in orthopedic practice. The study highlights the need for further research to establish definitive clinical benefits before widespread implementation of new navigation systems in TKA procedures.

6.1.2 The Accelerometer-Based Navigation System Demonstrated Superior Radiological Outcomes in Restoring Mechanical Alignment and Component Sagittal Positioning in Total Knee Arthroplasty [39]

This is a machine-generated summary of:

Gao, Jiaxiang; Hou, Yunfei; Li, Rujun; Ke, Yan; Li, Zhichang; Lin, Jianhao The accelerometer-based navigation system demonstrated superior radiological outcomes in restoring mechanical alignment and component sagittal positioning in total knee arthroplasty [39].

Published in: BMC Musculoskeletal Disorders (2021).
Link to original: https://doi.org/10.1186/s12891-021-04213-9

If you want to cite the papers, please refer to the original.
For technical reasons we could not place the page where the original quote is coming from.

6.1.2.1 Research Highlights

Total knee arthroplasty (TKA) outcomes are significantly influenced by the precise positioning of components, as malalignment can lead to increased polyethylene wear and higher revision rates. Conventional techniques for bone resection may be limited in cases with extra-articular deformities or excessive anterior femoral bowing, resulting in high outlier ratios. Computer-assisted surgery (CAS) has been developed to improve accuracy in limb alignment and component positioning, with handheld accelerometer-based navigation (ABN) systems emerging as a cost-effective alternative to large-console CAS. The study by Gao et al. investigates the postoperative radiological and clinical outcomes of TKA using the ABN system compared to conventional techniques.

The study conducted a retrospective review of patients who underwent primary TKA using either the ABN system or conventional methods at Peking University People's Hospital. The researchers collected preoperative demographic data and assessed clinical outcomes using Knee Society scores and range of motion (ROM). Radiological evaluations were performed using standardized postoperative radiographs, analysed by independent observers. Propensity score matching was employed to minimize confounding factors, ensuring comparable groups for analysis. The study found that the ABN group had significantly higher proportions of TKAs within a ± 3° deviation in most radiological variables, indicating improved accuracy in component positioning compared to the conventional group.

The findings suggest that while both ABN and conventional techniques resulted in significant clinical improvements postoperatively, the ABN system provided superior radiological outcomes, particularly in sagittal alignment. Future study could explore long-term effects on prosthesis survivorship and functional outcomes. The study highlights potential advantages of ABN in cases with complex anatomical challenges and suggests strategies to minimize technical errors during navigation TKA. Despite some limitations, such as its retrospective nature and short follow-up period, this research underscores the value of ABN systems in enhancing surgical precision in TKA.

6.1.3 Effect of Joint Line Orientation Parameters on Initial Bone Resection in Mechanically Aligned Total Knee Arthroplasty: A Retrospective Clinicoradiological Correlation Study [40]

This is a machine-generated summary of:

Wen, Liang; Yu, Yang; Ma, Desi; Wang, Zhiwei Effect of joint line orientation parameters on initial bone resection in mechanically aligned total knee arthroplasty: a retrospective clinicoradiological correlation study [40].

Published in: BMC Musculoskeletal Disorders (2023).

Link to original: https://doi.org/10.1186/s12891-023-06299-9

If you want to cite the papers, please refer to the original.

For technical reasons we could not place the page where the original quote is coming from.

6.1.3.1 Research Highlights

In mechanically aligned total knee arthroplasty (MA-TKA), discrepancies in bone resection between the medial and lateral compartments of the knee are common due to the perpendicular alignment of components to the mechanical axes of the femur and tibia. This approach often disregards variations in joint line orientation, leading to imbalances in the extension gap. Recent classifications incorporating joint linc orientation suggest that MA significantly alters native joint line orientation in most individuals. The study by Wen et a. investigates how native joint line orientation affects initial bone resection in MA-TKA and whether preoperative measurements can predict intraoperative adjustments.

The study conducted a correlation analysis using retrospective radiological measurements and virtual bone resection simulations. Joint line orientation parameters, such as the mechanical lateral distal femoral angle (mLDFA) and medial proximal tibial angle (MPTA), were measured on full-length weight-bearing radiographs. The researchers evaluated the relationship between these parameters and bone resection thickness to assess their impact on initial bone resection and potential intraoperative adjustments. The study included patients with Kellgren-Lawrence grade III-IV knee osteoarthritis, excluding those with conditions that could affect measurement accuracy. Statistical analyses revealed that mLDFA and MPTA were positively correlated with maximum resection thickness in varus knees, with mLDFA having a more significant impact.

The study advances understanding by highlighting the importance of preoperative assessment of joint line orientation parameters, such as mLDFA and MPTA, in predicting bone resection during MA-TKA. It suggests that attention to these parameters could help avoid unnecessary intraoperative adjustments or bone loss. Future study could explore larger patient cohorts or incorporate additional factors like soft tissue laxity to refine predictive models further. The findings underscore the potential for improved surgical planning through routine preoperative radiographic evaluations, ultimately enhancing patient outcomes in total knee arthroplasty.

6.1.4 Coronal Plane Alignment Classification of Arthritic Knees in a South Indian Population and Functional Outcome Comparison Post-Mechanical Alignment Total Knee Arthroplasty [41]

This is a machine-generated summary of:

Palanisamy, Yuvarajan; Natarajan, Sugumar; Prasad, Arjun R.; Rajan, David V. Coronal Plane Alignment Classification of Arthritic Knees in a South Indian Population and Functional Outcome Comparison Post-mechanical Alignment Total Knee Arthroplasty [41].

Published in: Indian Journal of Orthopaedics (2024).

Link to original: https://doi.org/10.1007/s43465-024-01154-y

If you want to cite the papers, please refer to the original.

For technical reasons we could not place the page where the original quote is coming from.

6.1.4.1 Research Highlights

Primary total knee arthroplasty (TKA) is a widely performed and successful surgical procedure, with its prevalence expected to increase significantly in the coming years. Traditionally, the mechanical alignment strategy has been the gold standard for TKA, validated by numerous studies for its role in promoting implant longevity. However, the introduction of the constitutional varus concept by Bellemans challenged this conventional approach, leading to the development of various alignment strategies aimed at improving patient satisfaction by enhancing native knee kinematics. The study by Palanisamy et al. addresses this issue in the Indian population by classifying arthritic knees based on coronal plane alignment of the knee (CPAK) types in South India and comparing functional outcomes following TKA using traditional mechanical alignment.

The study was conducted over 2 years (September 2021 to August 2023), at an orthopedic specialty center, involving South Indian patients with degenerative knee osteoarthritis scheduled for TKA. Excluding those with inflammatory arthritis or previous limb deformities, the researchers used hip-to-ankle standing full-length radiographs to classify knees into nine CPAK types based on medial proximal tibial angle (MPTA) and lateral distal femoral angle (LDFA). The study included 200 patients for classification analysis and 100 patients for post-operative functional outcome assessment. Functional outcomes were measured using the Oxford Knee Score and Visual Analog Scale for pain at 6 months and 1-year post-TKA. The results showed significant improvements in these scores across all CPAK types, indicating effective pain relief and enhanced knee function following mechanically aligned TKA.

The study highlights that despite morphometric variations between South and North Indian populations, CPAK distribution in South India is comparable to that of the entire Indian population. This finding suggests a predominance of varus arthritic knees in India, contrasting with neutral knees in Western populations. While mechanical alignment remains effective across CPAK types, future studies could explore kinematic alignment's potential advantages in functional outcomes. The study's limitations include a small sample size for certain CPAK types and a focus solely on mechanical alignment. Nonetheless, it provides a foundation for future research on larger cohorts with extended follow-up periods to further investigate optimal alignment strategies in TKA.

6.1.5 Revisiting the Tibial Crest as Reference for the Mechanical Alignment of the Tibial Component in Total Knee Arthroplasty: A Cadaveric Study on Caucasian Tibiae [42]

This is a machine-generated summary of:

Cinotti, Gianluca; Ripani, Francesca Romana; Sinno, Ennio; Sarti, Sara; LaTorre, Giuseppe; Giannicola, Giuseppe Revisiting the tibial crest as reference for the mechanical alignment of the tibial component in total knee arthroplasty: a cadaveric study on Caucasian tibiae [42].

Published in: MUSCULOSKELETAL SURGERY (2020).

Link to original: https://doi.org/10.1007/s12306-020-00639-x

If you want to cite the papers, please refer to the original.

For technical reasons we could not place the page where the original quote is coming from.

6.1.5.1 Research Highlights

Total knee arthroplasty (TKA) failures can arise from various conditions, with aseptic loosening being the most prevalent cause for revision surgeries years after the initial procedure. While factors such as micromovement, stress shielding, and high joint fluid pressure are known contributors to aseptic loosening, the role of implant alignment remains contentious. Finite element analysis suggests that varus alignment of the tibial component can significantly alter load distribution, accelerating wear and leading to early loosening. The study by Cinotti et al. investigates whether the tibial crest (TC) can serve as a reliable anatomical landmark for aligning the tibial component with the mechanical axis (MA) during TKA in Caucasian patients.

The study analysed 92 dried Caucasian tibiae to explore the relationship between the TC and MA. Excluding specimens with deformities or degenerative changes, researchers identified anatomical axes and used guidewires and metal markers to map the TC's course. Radiographs were taken in different positions to assess how well the TC aligned with the MA. The TC exhibited three distinct patterns: a curved course, a straight course, and a combination of both. Quantitative analysis revealed that while some TC courses intersected with the MA at specific points, variability in these intersections was significant, particularly in the distal tibia. Statistical tests confirmed these findings, showing that while some TC courses could align with the MA, they were not consistent enough to serve as primary landmarks.

The study concludes that due to its variable morphology and inconsistent relationship with the MA, the TC is not a reliable primary anatomical landmark for coronal alignment of the tibial component in standard TKA for Caucasian patients. However, an axis connecting specific points along the TC may serve as an additional reference in challenging cases where traditional landmarks are difficult to identify due to patient anatomy or high BMI. Future study could explore larger sample sizes or different populations to validate these findings further and potentially refine surgical techniques for improved outcomes in TKA procedures.

6.1.6 Predictive Factors for Deep Medial Collateral Ligament Release in Adjusted Mechanical Alignment Total Knee Arthroplasty [43]

This is a machine-generated summary of:

Thongpulsawasdi, Nimit; Achawakulthep, Chaiwat; Intiyanaravut, Tawan; Anusitviwat, Chirathit; Yuenyongviwat, Varah Predictive factors for deep medial collateral ligament release in adjusted mechanical alignment total knee arthroplasty [43].

Published in: Journal of Orthopaedic Surgery and Research (2024).

Link to original: https://doi.org/10.1186/s13018-024-05046-7

6.1.6.1 Research Highlights

Total knee arthroplasty (TKA) is a critical procedure for managing severe knee arthritis, requiring precise alignment, implant placement, and soft tissue balance to ensure successful outcomes. Achieving optimal alignment and stability is crucial for both clinical functionality and the long-term success of TKA. In cases of medial compartment osteoarthritis, medial soft tissue release is sometimes necessary to maintain joint stability and improve postoperative results. However, finding the right balance in medial soft tissue release is challenging; excessive release can lead to joint instability, while insufficient release may cause discomfort and stiffness post-surgery. The study by Thongpulsawasdi et al. investigates the factors influencing medial collateral ligament (MCL) release during adjusted mechanical alignment robotic-assisted TKA.

The study was conducted as a retrospective analysis at a tertiary hospital, focusing on patients who underwent primary TKA with robotic assistance for medial compartment osteoarthritis. The researchers utilized a standardized procedural sequence with the robotic surgical assistant ROSA (Zimmer Biomet, Warsaw, IN, USA), employing cemented posterior-stabilized TKA prostheses through a standard medial parapatellar approach. The study involved assessing alignment and soft tissue laxity through various stress tests and intra-operative planning to achieve mechanical alignment with a Hip-Knee-Ankle (HKA) angle of 0 degrees. Adjustments were made to femoral and tibial cuts to ensure gap balance, with MCL release performed based on specific criteria related to gap measurements. Statistical analysis was conducted using R-program software to determine the optimal threshold for predicting MCL release necessity.

The study identified several parameters associated with the need for medial soft tissue release, including the initial HKA angle and stress test angles in extension positions. A threshold HKA angle of 3.5 degrees was found to be predictive of the necessity for MCL release, demonstrating high sensitivity and specificity. This finding suggests that not all patients with medial compartment osteoarthritis require soft tissue release, potentially reducing surgical invasiveness and improving recovery outcomes. Future study could focus on validating these findings in larger populations and exploring long-term clinical implications of MCL release decisions in TKA procedures. The study highlights the importance of preoperative knee alignment in determining surgical approaches for optimal patient outcomes.

6.1.7 Functional Outcome of Mechanical Alignment in Total Knee Arthroplasty Surgery: A Short-Term Cohort Study at an Indian Tertiary Care Hospital [44]

This is a machine-generated summary of:

Patil, Vishwajit V.; Sancheti, Parag K.; Patil, Kailash; Gugale, Sunny; Shyam, Ashok Functional Outcome of Mechanical Alignment in Total Knee Arthroplasty Surgery: A Short-Term Cohort Study at an Indian Tertiary Care Hospital [44].

Published in: Indian Journal of Orthopaedics (2023).
Link to original: https://doi.org/10.1007/s43465-023-01016-z

If you want to cite the papers, please refer to the original.
For technical reasons we could not place the page where the original quote is coming from.

6.1.7.1 Research Highlights

The optimal alignment of knee components during TKA remains debated, with mechanical alignment traditionally favored for its association with implant longevity and patient satisfaction. The study by Patil et al. at the Sancheti Institute for Orthopaedics and Rehabilitation in Pune, India, investigates the importance of neutral anatomical component alignment in TKA patients using long-standing radiographs.

The study employed a retrospective and prospective cohort design to evaluate short-term outcomes of TKA in patients with OA or rheumatoid arthritis. Conducted between June 2019 and September 2020, it included patients who met specific inclusion criteria while excluding those with post-operative complications like implant loosening or fractures. Preoperative and postoperative assessments involved clinical examinations, radiological evaluations using long-leg X-rays, and functional measures such as the Oxford Knee Score and Knee Society Score. The study analysed changes in the hip-knee-ankle (HKA) axis post-surgery, revealing significant improvements in functional outcomes and pain reduction. Statistical analyses demonstrated that achieving a neutral mechanical alignment postoperatively correlated with better functional scores.

The findings suggest that restoring a neutral mechanical alignment in TKA can enhance implant durability and patient function. While the study focused on mechanical alignment, it highlights the need for future research incorporating kinematic alignment and rotational measurements through advanced imaging techniques like CT scans. The authors emphasize that achieving a postoperative neutral mechanical alignment of ±3 degrees should be standard practice in TKA procedures to optimize outcomes. Further long-term studies from Indian centers could validate these findings and refine surgical techniques for improved patient care.

Bibliography

1. Mason JB, Fehring TK, Estok R, Banel D, Fahrbach K (2007) Meta-analysis of alignment outcomes in computer-assisted total knee arthroplasty surgery. J Arthroplasty 22(8):1097–1106. https://doi.org/10.1016/j.arth.2007.08.001
2. Anderson KC, Buehler KC, Markel DC (2005) Computer assisted navigation in total knee arthroplasty: comparison with conventional methods. J Arthroplasty 20(7 Suppl 3):132–138. https://doi.org/10.1016/j.arth.2005.05.009
3. Ensini A, Catani F, Leardini A, Romagnoli M, Giannini S (2007) Alignments and clinical results in conventional and navigated total knee arthroplasty. Clin Orthop Relat Res 457:156–162. https://doi.org/10.1097/BLO.0b013e3180316c92
4. Lutzner J, Dexel J, Kirschner S (2013) No difference between computer-assisted and conventional total knee arthroplasty: five-year results of a prospective randomised study. Knee Surg Sports Traumatol Arthrosc 21(10):2241–2247. https://doi.org/10.1007/s00167-013-2608-7
5. Laskin RS, Beksaç B. Computer-assisted navigation in TKA: where we are and where we are going. Clin Orthop Relat Res. 2006;1:452127–31. https://doi.org/10.1097/01.blo.0000238823.78895.dc.
6. Gao X, Sun Y, Chen ZH, Dou TX, Liang QW, Li X. Comparison of the accelerometer-based navigation system with conventional instruments for total knee arthroplasty: a propensity score-matched analysis. J Orthop Surg Res. 2019;14(1):223. https://doi.org/10.1186/s13018-019-1258-y.
7. Kinney MC, Cidambi KR, Severns DL, Gonzales FB. Comparison of the iAssist handheld guidance system to conventional instruments for mechanical Axis restoration in Total knee arthroplasty. J Arthroplast. 2018;33(1):61–6. https://doi.org/10.1016/j.arth.2017.06.004.
8. Liow MH, Goh GS, Pang HN, Tay DK, Lo NN, Yeo SJ. Computer-assisted stereotaxic navigation improves the accuracy of mechanical alignment and component positioning in total knee arthroplasty. Arch Orthop Trauma Surg. 2016;136(8):1173–80. https://doi.org/10.1007/s00402-016-2483-z.
9. Moo IH, Chen JYQ, Chau DHH, Tan SW, Lau ACK, Teo YS. Similar radiological results with accelerometer-based navigation versus conventional technique in total knee arthroplasty. J Orthop Surg (Hong Kong). 2018;26(2):2309499018772374. https://doi.org/10.1177/2309499018772374.
10. Nam D, Cody EA, Nguyen JT, Figgie MP, Mayman DJ (2014) Extramedullary guides versus portable, accelerometer-based navigation for tibial alignment in total knee arthroplasty: a randomized, controlled trial: winner of the 2013 HAP PAUL award. J Arthroplasty 29(2):288–294. https://doi.org/10.1016/j.arth.2013.06.006
11. Kim YH, Park JW, Kim JS, Park SD. The relationship between the survival of total knee arthroplasty and postoperative coronal, sagittal and rotational alignment of knee prosthesis. Int Orthop. 2014;38(2):379–85. https://doi.org/10.1007/s00264-013-2097-9.

12. Hirschmann MT, Moser LB, Amsler F, Behrend H, Leclerq V, Hess S. Functional knee phenotypes: a novel classification for phenotyping the coronal lower limb alignment based on the native alignment in young non-osteoarthritic patients. Knee Surg sports Traumatol arthroscopy: official J ESSKA. 2019;27(5):1394–402.
13. Schnurr C, Csécsei G, Nessler J, Eysel P, König DP. How much tibial resection is required in total knee arthroplasty? Int Orthop. 2010;35(7):989–94.
14. Pagan, C. A., Karasavvidis, T., Lebrun, D. G., Jang, S. J., MacDessi, S. J., and Vigdorchik, J. M. (2023). Geographic variation in knee phenotypes based on the coronal plane alignment of the knee classification: A systematic review. *Journal of Arthroplasty, 38*(9), 1892-1899.e1.
15. Tarassoli, P., Wood, J. A., Chen, D. B., Griffiths-Jones, W., Bellemans, J., and MacDessi, S. J. (2022). Arithmetic hip-knee-ankle angle and stressed hip-knee-ankle angle: Equivalent methods for estimating constitutional lower limb alignment in kinematically aligned total knee arthroplasty. *Knee Surgery, Sports Traumatology, Arthroscopy, 30*(9), 2980–2990.
16. Toyooka, S., Osaki, Y., Masuda, H., Arai, N., Miyamoto, W., Ando, S., et al. (2023). Distribution of coronal plane alignment of the knee classification in patients with knee osteoarthritis in Japan. *The Journal of Knee Surgery, 36*(7), 738–743.
17. Hsu, C. E., Chen, C. P., Wang, S. P., Huang, J. T., Tong, K. M., and Huang, K. C. (2022). Validation and modification of the coronal plane alignment of the knee classification in the Asian population. *Bone and Joint Open, 3*(3), 211–217.
18. Sappey-Marinier, E., Batailler, C., Swan, J., Schmidt, A., Cheze, L., MacDessi, S. J., et al. (2022). Mechanical alignment for primary TKA may change both knee phenotype and joint line obliquity without influencing clinical outcomes: A study comparing restored and unrestored joint line obliquity. *Knee Surgery, Sports Traumatology, Arthroscopy, 30*(8), 2806–2814.
19. Mulpur, P., Desai, K. B., Mahajan, A., Masilamani, A. B. S., Hippalgaonkar, K., and Reddy, A. V. G. (2022). Radiological Evaluation of the phenotype of indian osteoarthritic knees based on the coronal plane alignment of the knee classification (CPAK). *Indian Journal of Orthopaedics, 56*(12), 2066–2076.
20. Steele, J. R., Jang, S. J., Brilliant, Z. R., Mayman, D. J., Sculco. P. K., Jerabek, S.A., et al. (2023) Deep learning phenotype automation and cohort analyses of 1,946 knees using the coronal plane alignment of the knee classification. *The Journal of Arthroplasty, 38*(6S), S215–S221.e1.
21. MacDessi, S. J., Griffiths-Jones, W., Harris, I. A., Bellemans, J., and Chen, D. B. (2021) Coronal plane alignment of the knee (CPAK) classification. *The Bone and Joint Journal, 103-B*(2), 329–337.
22. Parker Vail T, Lang JE (2006) Surgical techniques and instrumentation in total knee arthroplasty. In: Scott WN (ed) Insall and scott surgery of the knee, vol 1. Churchill Livingstone Elsevier, Philadelphia, pp 1455–1521
23. Schneider M, Heisel C, Aldinger PR et al (2007) Use of palpable tendons for extramedullary tibial alignment in total knee arthroplasty. J Arthroplasty 22:219–226

24. Cinotti G, Sessa P, D'Arino A et al (2015) Improving tibial component alignment in total knee arthroplasty. Knee Surg Sports Traumatol Arthrosc 23:3563–3570
25. Osvald MH, Jakob RP, Schneider ES et al (1993) Radiological analysis of normal axial alignment of femur and tibia in view of total knee arthroplasty. J Arthroplasty 8:419–426
26. Rivière C, Villet L, Jeremic D, Vendittoli P-A. What you need to know about kinematic alignment for total knee arthroplasty. Orthop Traumatol Surg Res OTSR. 2021;107:102773. https://doi.org/10.1016/j.otsr.2020.102773.
27. Selvanathan N, Ayeni FE, Sorial R. Incidence of soft tissue releases in robotic assisted cementless TKA with mechanical alignment and flexion gap balancing. Arthroplasty Lond Engl. 2023;5:28. https://doi.org/10.1186/s42836-023-00188-1.
28. Wada K, Hamada D, Tamaki S, Higashino K, Fukui Y, Sairyo K. Influence of Medial Collateral Ligament Release for Internal Rotation of Tibia in posterior-stabilized total knee arthroplasty: a cadaveric study. J Arthroplasty. 2017;32:270–3. https://doi.org/10.1016/j.arth.2016.06.013.
29. Herschmiller T, Grosso MJ, Cunn GJ, Murtaugh TS, Gardner TR, Geller JA. Step-wise medial collateral ligament needle puncturing in extension leads to a safe and predictable reduction in medial compartment pressure during TKA. Knee Surg Sports Traumatol Arthrosc off J ESSKA. 2018;26:1759–66. https://doi.org/10.1007/s00167-017-4777-2.
30. Ahn JH, Lee SH, Yang TY. Varus-valgus stress radiograph as a predictor for extensive medial release in total knee arthroplasty. Int Orthop. 2016;40:1639–46. https://doi.org/10.1007/s00264-015-3018-x.
31. Rivière C, Iranpour F, Auvinet E, Howell S, Vendittoli PA, Cobb J, Parratte S. Alignment options for total knee arthroplasty: a systematic review. Orthop Traumatol Surg Res. 2017;103(7):1047–56. https://doi.org/10.1016/j.otsr.2017.07.010.
32. Hernandez-Vaquero D, Noriega-Fernandez A, Roncero-Gonzalez S, Ruete-Gil GL, Fernandez-Carreira JM. Can the need for soft tissue release in total knee replacement be predicted pre-operatively? A study based on surgical navigation. Int Orthop. 2022;46:815–21. https://doi.org/10.1007/s00264-021-05263-3.
33. Sajjadi MM, Okhovatpour MA, Safaei Y, Faramarzi B, Zandi R. Is standing coronal Long-Leg Alignment View Effective in Predicting the Extent of Medial Soft tissue release in Varus deformity during total knee arthroplasty? J Knee Surg. 2022;35:1192–8. https://doi.org/10.1055/s-0040-1721787.
34. Lee YS, Howell SM, Won YY, Lee OS, Lee SH, Vahedi H, et al. Kinematic alignment is a possible alternative to mechanical alignment in total knee arthroplasty. Knee Surg Sports Traumatol Arthrosc. 2017;25(11):3467–79. https://doi.org/10.1007/s00167-017-4558-y.
35. Sekiya, H., Takatoku, K., Takada, H., Sasanuma, H., and Sugimoto, N. (2009). Postoperative lateral ligamentous laxity diminishes with time after TKA in the varus knee. *Clinical Orthopaedics and Related Research, 467*(6), 1582–1586.

36. Karachalios, T., Sarangi, P. P., and Newman, J. H. (1994). Severe varus and valgus deformities treated by total knee arthroplasty. *Journal of Bone and Joint Surgery. British Volume, 76*(6), 938–942.
37. Howell, S. M., Papadopoulos, S., Kuznik, K., Ghaly, L. R., and Hull, M. L. (2015). Does varus alignment adversely affect implant survival and function six years after kinematically aligned total knee arthroplasty? *International Orthopaedics, 39*(11), 2117–2124.
38. Liow, Ming Han Lincoln; Goh, Graham Seow-Hng; Pang, Hee-Nee; Tay, Darren Keng Jin; Lo, Ngai Nung; Yeo, Seng Jin Computer-assisted stereotaxic navigation improves the accuracy of mechanical alignment and component positioning in total knee arthroplasty. Archives of Orthopaedic and Trauma Surgery (2016). 10.1007/s00402-016-2483-z
39. Gao, Jiaxiang; Hou, Yunfei; Li, Rujun; Ke, Yan; Li, Zhichang; Lin, Jianhao The accelerometer-based navigation system demonstrated superior radiological outcomes in restoring mechanical alignment and component sagittal positioning in total knee arthroplasty. BMC Musculoskeletal Disorders (2021). 10.1186/s12891-021-04213-9
40. Wen, Liang; Yu, Yang; Ma, Desi; Wang, Zhiwei Effect of joint line orientation parameters on initial bone resection in mechanically aligned total knee arthroplasty: a retrospective clinicoradiological correlation study. BMC Musculoskeletal Disorders (2023). https://doi.org/10.1186/s12891-023-06299-9
41. Palanisamy, Yuvarajan; Natarajan, Sugumar; Prasad, Arjun R.; Rajan, David V. Coronal Plane Alignment Classification of Arthritic Knees in a South Indian Population and Functional Outcome Comparison Post-mechanical Alignment Total Knee Arthroplasty. Indian Journal of Orthopaedics (2024). https://doi.org/10.1007/s43465-024-01154-y
42. Cinotti, Gianluca; Ripani, Francesca Romana; Sinno, Ennio; Sarti, Sara; LaTorre, Giuseppe; Giannicola, Giuseppe Revisiting the tibial crest as reference for the mechanical alignment of the tibial component in total knee arthroplasty: a cadaveric study on Caucasian tibiae. MUSCULOSKELETAL SURGERY (2020). https://doi.org/10.1007/s12306-020-00639-x
43. Thongpulsawasdi, Nimit; Achawakulthep, Chaiwat; Intiyanaravut, Tawan; Anusitviwat, Chirathit; Yuenyongviwat, Varah Predictive factors for deep medial collateral ligament release in adjusted mechanical alignment total knee arthroplasty. Journal of Orthopaedic Surgery and Research (2024). https://doi.org/10.1186/s13018-024-05046-7
44. Patil, Vishwajit V.; Sancheti, Parag K.; Patil, Kailash; Gugale, Sunny; Shyam, Ashok Functional Outcome of Mechanical Alignment in Total Knee Arthroplasty Surgery: A Short-Term Cohort Study at an Indian Tertiary Care Hospital. Indian Journal of Orthopaedics (2023). https://doi.org/10.1007/s43465-023-01016-z

6.2 Kinematic Approach and Alternative Alignments

Machine Generated Summaries

Disclaimer: The summaries in this chapter were generated from Springer Nature publications using abstractive AI auto-summarization: An abstraction-based summarizer creates new text based on deep learning. New phrases are created to summarize the content. As the constituted sentences are machine selected, they may not fully reflect the body of the work, so we strongly advise that the original content is read and cited. The auto-generated summaries were curated by the editor to meet Springer Nature publication standards.

6.2.1 Outcomes of Kinematically Aligned Total Knee Arthroplasty in Indian Population—Case Series with Three Year Clinical Results [55]

This is a machine-generated summary of:

Ragunandhan, Narayanasamy; Jeya Venkatesh, Palanisamy Outcomes of Kinematically Aligned Total Knee Arthroplasty in Indian Population—Case Series with Three Year Clinical Results [55].

Published in: Indian Journal of Orthopaedics (2021).

Link to original: https://doi.org/10.1007/s43465-021-00521-3

If you want to cite the papers, please refer to the original.

For technical reasons we could not place the page where the original quote is coming from.

6.2.1.1 Research Highlights

Proper knee alignment is crucial for the long-term success of total knee arthroplasty (TKA), with mechanically aligned TKA being the current standard. However, a significant percentage of patients remain dissatisfied post-surgery, potentially due to the imposition of a uniform mechanical alignment that does not consider individual anatomical variations. The study by Ragunandhan et al. investigates the effectiveness of kinematically aligned TKA in improving patient satisfaction and functional outcomes in an Indian population with osteoarthritis, using the Oxford Knee Score as a measure.

The study involved patients who underwent kinematically aligned TKA between February 2018 and February 2020. Excluding those with inflammatory arthritis or previous knee surgeries, the researchers used full-length weight-bearing radiographs for preoperative planning. The surgical procedure involved precise bone resections based on cartilage wear and bone loss, using conventional instruments modified for kinematic alignment. Postoperative care included early weight-bearing and standardized pain management protocols. The outcomes were assessed using the Oxford Knee Score, with statistical analysis performed to compare preoperative and postoperative scores.

The study found significant improvements in functional scores postoperatively, with no catastrophic failures observed over a 3-year follow-up period. While the results suggest that kinematically aligned TKA can achieve good to excellent patient satisfaction, the study's limitations include its small sample size and lack of direct comparison with mechanically aligned TKA. Future studies should involve larger randomized trials to establish definitive conclusions about the benefits of kinematic alignment in diverse populations. The pilot data from this study could aid in designing such trials, potentially leading to more personalized approaches in knee arthroplasty.

6.2.2 What Clinical Characteristics and Radiographic Parameters Are Associated with Patellofemoral Instability After Kinematically Aligned Total Knee Arthroplasty? [57]

This is a machine-generated summary of:

Nedopil, Alexander J.; Howell, Stephen M.; Hull, Maury L. What clinical characteristics and radiographic parameters are associated with patellofemoral instability after kinematically aligned total knee arthroplasty? [57].

Published in: International Orthopaedics (2016).

Link to original: https://doi.org/10.1007/s00264-016-3287-z

If you want to cite the papers, please refer to the original.

For technical reasons we could not place the page where the original quote is coming from.

6.2.2.1 Research Highlights

Patellofemoral instability, characterized by subluxation and dislocation of the patella, is a significant concern for patients undergoing total knee arthroplasty (TKA), leading to pain and functional impairment. This condition is particularly problematic in mechanically aligned TKA, where complications such as anterior knee pain and patellar issues often necessitate revision surgery. Kinematically aligned TKA has emerged as a promising alternative, offering better pain relief and function. However, concerns remain about its potential to increase the risk of patellofemoral instability due to the use of femoral components designed for mechanical alignment. The study by Nedopil et al. investigates the clinical characteristics and radiographic parameters associated with patellofemoral instability in kinematically aligned TKA.

The study conducted a case-control analysis over 9 years, examining patients who underwent kinematically aligned TKA and presented with patellofemoral instability. Researchers identified patients with this complication and matched them with a control group of patients without instability based on surgery date, sex, and knee deformity. The study utilized both patient-specific instrumentation and manual techniques to set the femoral component's alignment. Radiographic assessments were performed post-operatively to evaluate component positioning. The findings revealed that patellofemoral instability typically presented without a traumatic event around 5 months post-operatively, with symptoms most pronounced during activities like stair descent. The study found that greater flexion of the femoral component was associated with instability, while internal-external malrotation of the tibial component was not a significant factor.

The research highlights that limiting the flexion of the femoral component could reduce the risk of patellofemoral instability in kinematically aligned TKA. The study suggests that using improved surgical techniques and instrumentation could mitigate this risk, potentially lowering reoperation rates and enhancing patient outcomes as measured by the Oxford Knee score. Future study directions may include refining surgical methods to further minimize component malalignment and exploring alternative implant designs tailored specifically for kinematic alignment to enhance stability and patient satisfaction post-TKA.

6.2.3 Total Knee Arthroplasty According to the Original Knee Phenotypes with Kinematic Alignment Surgical Technique—Early Clinical and Functional Outcomes [58]

This is a machine-generated summary of:

Hsu, Cheng-En; Huang, Jen-Ting; Tong, Kwok-Man; Huang, Kui-Chou Total knee arthroplasty according to the original knee phenotypes with kinematic alignment surgical technique—early clinical and functional outcomes [58].

Published in: BMC Musculoskeletal Disorders (2020).

Link to original: https://doi.org/10.1186/s12891-020-03862-6

If you want to cite the papers, please refer to the original.

For technical reasons we could not place the page where the original quote is coming from.

6.2.3.1 Research Highlights

Total knee arthroplasty (TKA) is a common surgical intervention for advanced osteoarthritis of the knee, yet dissatisfaction rates remain high, even in uncomplicated cases. This has led to questions about whether mechanical alignment, which aims for a neutral alignment by cutting bones perpendicular to the mechanical axis, is the best approach. An alternative method, kinematic alignment (KA), seeks to restore the knee's pre-disease joint line, potentially improving ligament balance and patient satisfaction. The study by Hsu et al. investigates a phenotype-oriented KA-TKA approach that sets individualized alignment targets based on patients' knee phenotypes to improve functional and radiographic outcomes.

The study was conducted as a prospective series involving patients with advanced osteoarthritis who underwent TKA at a single hospital. Patients were categorized into five knee phenotypes based on their preoperative mechanical alignment of the femur and tibia. The surgical technique involved setting specific alignment targets for each phenotype and using bone cut thickness as a reference during surgery. Postoperative evaluations included radiographic measurements and functional assessments at various follow-up intervals. The results showed significant improvements in functional outcomes across all phenotypes, with no significant differences in outcomes such as Oxford Knee Score (OKS), Combined Knee Society Score (CKSS), and range of motion (ROM) between different phenotypes.

The study advances the understanding of KA-TKA by demonstrating that individualized alignment targets based on knee phenotype can lead to excellent functional outcomes and implant survival rates over 3 years. This approach may be particularly beneficial when patient-specific instrumentation or computer navigation is unavailable. Future study could focus on longer follow-up periods to assess long-term complications such as aseptic loosening and further validate these findings in larger populations. The phenotype-oriented KA method offers a practical alternative for achieving optimal surgical outcomes while preserving natural knee kinematics.

6.2.4 Modified Kinematic Alignment Better Restores Plantar Pressure Distribution Than Mechanical Alignment in Total Knee Arthroplasty: A Randomized Controlled Trial [59]

This is a machine-generated summary of:

Wang, Guiguan; Zhang, Yue; Chen, Long; Yu, Guoyu; Luo, Fenqi; Xu, Jie Modified kinematic alignment better restores plantar pressure distribution than mechanical alignment in total knee arthroplasty: a randomized controlled trial [59].

Published in: Scientific Reports (2024).

Link to original: https://doi.org/10.1038/s41598-024-79566-x

6.2.4.1 Research Highlights

Gait function is closely linked to knee health and biomechanics, with knee osteoarthritis (KOA) significantly impacting gait mechanics and mobility. Total knee arthroplasty (TKA) is a key intervention for end-stage KOA, yet the optimal alignment strategy—mechanical alignment (MA) versus kinematic alignment

(KA)—remains debated. While MA aims for even load distribution by aligning the prosthesis perpendicularly to mechanical axes, KA tailors prosthesis placement to individual anatomy for potentially better outcomes. Despite numerous gait analysis studies comparing KA and MA, results are inconsistent, particularly regarding plantar pressure distribution post-TKA. The study by Wang et al. focuses on the impact of KA and MA on plantar pressure distribution.

The study was a secondary analysis of a randomized controlled trial involving patients with unilateral TKA at a single institution. Participants were divided into KA and MA groups, with preoperative varus knees and contralateral native knees as controls. The surgical procedures differed in alignment techniques: KA used modified kinematic alignment with specific osteotomy angles, while MA employed mechanical alignment strategies. Pedobarographic analysis was conducted using pressure-sensitive insoles to assess plantar pressure distribution during walking at one- and two-year follow-ups. Statistical analyses compared clinical outcomes, radiographic metrics, and plantar pressure distributions between the groups.

The study found that KA more effectively restored natural plantar pressure distribution in both forefoot and rearfoot compared to MA, aligning more closely with the contralateral native knee. This suggests that KA may lead to more physiologic gait mechanics and better functional outcomes post-TKA. While both groups showed significant improvements in clinical scores, the trend favored KA in terms of patient satisfaction and functional outcomes. Future study could focus on larger sample sizes and longer follow-up periods to confirm these findings and evaluate long-term durability of KA in TKA.

6.2.5 Postoperative Clinical Outcomes for Kinematically, Restricted Kinematically, or Mechanically Aligned Total Knee Arthroplasty: A Systematic Review and Network Meta-Analysis of Randomized Controlled Trials [60]

This is a machine-generated summary of:

Miura, Takanori; Takahashi, Tsuneari; Watanabe, Jun; Kataoka, Yuki; Ae, Ryusuke; Saito, Hidetomo; Takeshita, Katsushi; Miyakoshi, Naohisa Postoperative clinical outcomes for kinematically, restricted kinematically, or mechanically aligned total knee arthroplasty: a systematic review and network meta-analysis of randomized controlled trials [60].

Published in: BMC Musculoskeletal Disorders (2023).

Link to original: https://doi.org/10.1186/s12891-023-06448-0

If you want to cite the papers, please refer to the original.

For technical reasons we could not place the page where the original quote is coming from.

6.2.5.1 Research Highlights

Total knee arthroplasty (TKA) is a well-established surgical procedure for alleviating pain and improving function in patients with end-stage knee osteoarthritis. While mechanically aligned TKA (MATKA) is the gold standard, some patients remain dissatisfied post-surgery, prompting interest in alternative approaches like kinematically aligned TKA (KATKA), which aims to restore the knee's pre-arthritic anatomy. However, concerns about component loosening, particularly in the tibia due to varus placement, persist. The study by Miura et al. explores the clinical outcomes of MATKA, KATKA, and a modified version called restricted KATKA (rKATKA), using a network meta-analysis to compare these techniques.

The study conducted a network meta-analysis of randomized controlled trials (RCTs) to evaluate the clinical outcomes of MATKA, KATKA, and rKATKA. The researchers included both published and unpublished studies without language or country restrictions to minimize publication bias. Adult patients who underwent primary TKA for knee osteoarthritis were considered, with surgical techniques defined by specific alignment criteria. The primary outcomes assessed were postoperative range of motion and revision surgeries, while secondary outcomes included component alignment and adverse events. Data from 11 RCTs involving 1200 knees were analyzed using a frequentist model to synthesize effect sizes and rank treatments based on P-scores.

The analysis revealed that KATKA and rKATKA showed comparable postoperative range of motion and patient-reported outcome measures (PROMs) to MATKA. However, no significant differences in revision rates or adverse events were observed between MATKA and KATKA. The study highlighted slight variations in postoperative coronal component alignments between the techniques but found similar hip-knee-ankle angles across all methods. Although KATKA showed potential for improved PROMs over MATKA, the effect size was small with low confidence ratings. Future studies with long-term follow-up are needed to assess the safety and effectiveness of these surgical techniques further, especially in patients with severe varus deformities.

6.2.6 Functional Joint Line Obliquity After Kinematic Total Knee Arthroplasty [61]

This is a machine-generated summary of:

Hutt, Jonathan; Massé, Vincent; Lavigne, Martin; Vendittoli, Pascal-André Functional joint line obliquity after kinematic total knee arthroplasty [61].

Published in: International Orthopaedics (2015).

Link to original: https://doi.org/10.1007/s00264-015-2733-7

If you want to cite the papers, please refer to the original.

For technical reasons we could not place the page where the original quote is coming from.

6.2.6.1 Research Highlights

The optimal alignment of components in total knee arthroplasty (TKA) is a topic of ongoing debate. Traditionally, surgeons aim for a neutral lower limb axis, which has shown long-term success but can alter the joint line orientation compared to the patient's natural anatomy. This approach does not always restore normal knee function, leading to dissatisfaction in some patients. An alternative method, kinematic alignment, seeks to preserve the knee's natural anatomy by aligning components according to the patient's original joint orientation. However, concerns exist about whether this approach might negatively impact implant survivorship due to potential varus alignment of tibial components. The study by Hutt et al. explores whether kinematic TKA maintains a joint line parallel to the floor during weight-bearing, despite varying obliquity to mechanical axes.

The study involved 55 patients who underwent kinematic TKA performed by a single surgeon using optical computer navigation. The procedure aimed to recreate the patient's native joint orientation by adjusting bone cuts for cartilage wear and bone loss. Postoperative coronal orientation was assessed using long-leg standing radiographs, measuring angles such as the hip-knee-ankle (HKA) angle and medial proximal tibial angle (MPTA). Statistical analysis revealed that while many TKAs had tibial components in varus relative to the mechanical axis, only a small percentage showed excessive varus when weight-bearing. This suggests that kinematic alignment may better represent functional loading conditions compared to traditional methods.

The study's findings indicate that kinematically aligned TKAs often result in a joint line angle in varus relative to the mechanical axis but align more favorably during weight-bearing. This could explain why kinematic alignment has not led to higher failure rates despite concerns about varus alignment. Future study should focus on evaluating joint line orientation in three dimensions during functional activities and exploring dynamic imaging techniques. These advancements could provide deeper insights into how different alignment strategies affect implant fixation and wear over time, potentially improving clinical outcomes and patient satisfaction with TKA procedures.

6.2.7 Effect of Inverse Kinematic Alignment Total Knee Arthroplasty on Coronal Alignment of the Ankle Joint in Patients with Varus Knee Deformity [62]

This is a machine-generated summary of:

Shichman, Ittai; Hallak, Amer; Ashkenazi, Itay; Warschwaski, Yaniv; Gold, Aviram; Snir, Nimrod Effect of inverse kinematic alignment total knee arthroplasty on coronal alignment of the ankle joint in patients with varus knee deformity [62].

Published in: Archives of Orthopaedic and Trauma Surgery (2024).

Link to original: https://doi.org/10.1007/s00402-024-05549-2

If you want to cite the papers, please refer to the original.

For technical reasons we could not place the page where the original quote is coming from.

6.2.7.1 Research Highlights

Total knee arthroplasty (TKA) has long been the standard surgical intervention for end-stage knee osteoarthritis, yet a significant percentage of patients remain dissatisfied post-surgery. Enhancing patient satisfaction often involves optimizing native knee alignment, with modern approaches focusing on restoring coronal alignment to improve clinical outcomes. Inverse Kinematic Alignment (iKA) is a patient-specific technique that considers individual preoperative and intraoperative parameters to preserve indigenous alignment and joint line inclination. However, there is no consensus on the optimal technique for patient-specific alignment, and the impact of coronal knee alignment adjustments on hip and ankle alignment remains underexplored. The study by Shichman et al. investigates the postoperative outcomes in ankle joint coronal alignment relative to the knee in patients undergoing robotic TKA using iKA techniques.

The study involved querying electronic medical records to identify patients who underwent iKA TKA with imageless robotic arm assistance between January 2022, and August 2023. Patients included were diagnosed with primary osteoarthritis of the knee and underwent elective primary TKA. Exclusions were made for secondary osteoarthritis diagnoses, post-traumatic arthritis, pathologic knee lesions, revision TKA, or any past ankle trauma or surgical hardware. Radiographic assessments were conducted preoperatively and 6 months postoperatively using full-body low-dose imaging. Radiographic measurements were performed by experienced orthopedic surgeons to assess changes in lower limb alignment. The study found significant changes in ankle alignment in patients with severe varus correction ($\geq 5°$), particularly in terms of talar inclination and tibial plafond inclination (TPI), while no significant changes were observed in neutral varus/valgus corrections.

The findings suggest that correcting severe varus knee deformity can significantly influence postoperative ankle joint alignment, highlighting the importance of considering ankle morphology when planning TKA procedures. While iKA appears to preserve or minimize substantial coronal alignment changes in patients with neutral preoperative knee deformities, further research is needed to explore these effects in valgus knee deformities and assess clinical ankle symptoms postoperatively. Future studies could focus on evaluating sub-talar joint compensation mechanisms and incorporating three-dimensional imaging techniques to provide a more comprehensive understanding of the biomechanical impacts of TKA on lower limb alignment.

Bibliography

1. Liu, D., Dan, M., et al. (2016). Blood management strategies in total knee arthroplasty. *Knee Surgery and Related Research, 28*, 179–187.
2. Hirschmann, M. T., Becker, R., Tandogan, R., et al. (2019). Alignment in TKA: what has been clear is not anymore! *Knee Surgery, Sports Traumatology, Arthroscopy, 27*, 2037–2039.

3. Sappey-Marinier, E., Pauvert, A., Batailler, C., et al. (2020). Kinematic versus mechanical alignment for primary total knee arthroplasty with minimum 2 years follow-up: a systematic review. *SICOT-J, 6*, 18.
4. Young, S. W., Sullivan, N. P. T., Walker, M. L., et al. (2020). No difference in 5-year clinical or radiographic outcomes between kinematic and mechanical alignment in TKA. A randomized controlled trial. *Clinical Orthopaedics and Related Research®, 478*, 1271–1279.
5. Bourne, R. B., Chesworth, B. M., Davis, A. M., et al. (2010). Patient satisfaction after total knee arthroplasty: who is satisfied and who is not? *Clinical Orthopaedics and Related Research, 468*, 57–63.
6. Petersen, C. L., Kjærsgaard, J. B., Kjærgaard, N., et al. (2017). Thresholds for Oxford Knee Score after total knee replacement surgery: a novel approach to post-operative evaluation. *Journal of Orthopaedic Surgery and Research, 12*, 89.
7. Kahlenberg CA, Nwachukwu BU, McLawhorn AS, Cross MB, Cornell CN, Padgett DE. Patient satisfaction after total knee replacement: a systematic review. HSS Journal®. 2018;14(2):192–201.
8. Price AJ, Alvand A, Troelsen A, Katz JN, Hooper G, Gray A, et al. Knee replacement. Lancet. 2018;392(10158):1672–82.
9. Vendittoli P-A, Martinov S, Blakeney WG. Restricted kinematic alignment, the fundamentals, and clinical applications. Front Surg. 2021;8:697020.
10. Blakeney W, Clément J, Desmeules F, Hagemeister N, Rivière C, Vendittoli PA. Kinematic alignment in total knee arthroplasty better reproduces normal gait than mechanical alignment. Knee Surg Sports Traumatol Arthrosc. 2019;27(5):1410–7. https://doi.org/10.1007/s00167-018-5174-1.
11. Winnock de Grave P, Luyckx T, Claeys K, Tampere T, Kellens J, Müller J, et al. Higher satisfaction after total knee arthroplasty using restricted inverse kinematic alignment compared to adjusted mechanical alignment. Knee Surg Sports Traumatol Arthrosc. 2022;30(2):488–99.
12. Gao Zx L, Nj Z, Sy, Yu W, Dai Yx, Xiao C. Comparison of kinematic alignment and mechanical alignment in total knee arthroplasty: a meta-analysis of randomized controlled clinical trials. Orthop Surg. 2020;12(6):1567–78.
13. Clatworthy M. Patient-specific TKA with the Velys™ robotic-assisted solution. Surg Technol Int. 2022;40:315–20.
14. Aflatooni JO, Wininger AE, Park KJ, Incavo SJ. Alignment options and robotics in total knee arthroplasty. Front Surg. 2023;10:1106608.
15. Anouchi YS, Whiteside LA, Kaiser AD, Milliano MT (1993) The effects of axial rotational alignment of the femoral component on knee stability and patellar tracking in total knee arthroplasty demonstrated on autopsy specimens. Clin Orthop Relat Res 287:170–177
16. Brar AS, Howell SM, Hull ML (2016) What are the bias, imprecision, and limits of agreement for finding the flexion-extension plane of the knee with five tibial reference lines? Knee 23(3):406–411. https://doi.org/10.1016/j.knee.2016.01.005
17. Calliess T, Bauer K, Stukenborg-Colsman C, Windhagen H, Budde S, Ettinger M (2016) PSI kinematic versus non-PSI mechanical alignment in total knee

arthroplasty: a prospective, randomized study. Knee Surg, Sports Traumatol, Arthrosc: Off J ESSKA. https://doi.org/10.1007/s00167-016-4136-8
18. Nam, D., Nunley, R. M., and Barrack, R. L. (2014). Patient dissatisfaction following total knee replacement. *The Bone and Joint Journal, 96-B*, 96–100.
19. Ishikawa M, Kuriyama S, Ito H, Furu M, Nakamura S, Matsuda S (2015) Kinematic alignment produces near-normal knee motion but increases contact stress after total knee arthroplasty: a case study on a single implant design. Knee 22(3):206–212. https://doi.org/10.1016/j.knee.2015.02.019
20. Howell, S. M., Papadopoulos, S., Kuznik, K. T., et al. (2013). Accurate alignment and high function after kinematically aligned TKA performed with generic instruments. *Knee Surgery Sports Traumatology Arthroscopy, 21*, 2271–2280.
21. Nedopil AJ, Howell SM, Hull ML (2016) Does malrotation of the tibial and femoral components compromise function in kinematically aligned total knee arthroplasty? Orthop Clin North Am 47(1):41–50. https://doi.org/10.1016/j.ocl.2015.08.006
22. Nedopil AJ, Howell SM, Rudert M, Roth J, Hull ML (2013) How frequent is rotational mismatch within 0 degrees +/−10 degrees in kinematically aligned total knee arthroplasty? Orthopedics 36(12):e1515–e1520
23. Howell SM, Kuznik K, Hull ML, Siston RA (2010) Longitudinal shapes of the tibia and femur are unrelated and variable. Clin Orthop Relat Res 468(4):1142–1148. https://doi.org/10.1007/s11999-009-0984-6
24. MacDessi SJ, Griffiths-Jones W, Chen DB, Griffiths-Jones S, Wood JA, Diwan AD, Harris IA. Restoring the constitutional alignment with a restrictive kinematic protocol improves quantitative soft-tissue balance in total knee arthroplasty: a randomized controlled trial. Bone Joint J. 2020;102-B(1):117–24.
25. Lin, Y. H., Chang, F. S., Chen, K. H., Huang, K. C., and Su, K. C. (2018). Mismatch between femur and tibia coronal alignment in the knee joint: Classification of five lower limb types according to femoral and tibial mechanical alignment. *BMC Musculoskeletal Disorders, 19*(1), 411.
26. Higano Y, Hayami T, Omori G, Koga Y, Endo K, Endo N. The varus alignment and morphologic alterations of proximal tibia affect the onset of medial knee osteoarthritis in rural Japanese women: case control study from the longitudinal evaluation of Matsudai knee osteoarthritis survey. J Orthop Sci. 2016;21(2):166–71.
27. Kang, K. T., Koh, Y. G., Nam, J. H., Kwon, S. K. and Park, K. K. Kinematic Alignment in Cruciate retaining implants improves the biomechanical function in total knee arthroplasty during gait and Deep Knee Bend. *J. Knee Surg. 33*, 284–293 (2020).
28. McNair, P. J. et al. A comparison of walking Gait following mechanical and Kinematic Alignment in total knee joint replacement. *J. Arthroplasty. 33*, 560–564 (2018).
29. Niki, Y., Nagura, T., Nagai, K., Kobayashi, S. and Harato, K. Kinematically aligned total knee arthroplasty reduces knee adduction moment more than

mechanically aligned total knee arthroplasty. *Knee Surg. Sports Traumatol. Arthrosc. 26*, 1629–1635 (2018).
30. Almaawi AM, Hutt JRB, Masse V, Lavigne M, Vendittoli PA. The impact of mechanical and restricted kinematic alignment on knee anatomy in Total knee Arthroplasty. J Arthroplast. 2017;32(7):2133–40.
31. Hiyama S, Takahashi T, Takeshita K. Kinematically aligned total knee arthroplasty did not show superior patient-reported outcome measures: an updated meta-analysis of randomized controlled trials with at least 2-year follow-up. J Knee Surg. 2022;35:634–9.
32. Risitano S, Cacciola G, Sabatini L, Capella M, Bosco F, Giustra F, et al. Restricted kinematic alignment in primary total knee arthroplasty: a systematic review of radiographic and clinical data. J Orthop. 2022;33:37–43.
33. Luo, Z., Zhou, K., Peng, L., et al. (2020). Similar results with kinematic and mechanical alignment applied in total knee arthroplasty. *Knee Surgery Sports Traumatology Arthroscopy, 28*, 1720–1735.
34. Liu, B., Feng, C. and Tu, C. Kinematic alignment versus mechanical alignment in primary total knee arthroplasty: an updated meta-analysis of randomized controlled trials. *J. Orthop. Surg. Res. 17*, 201 (2022).
35. Page MJ, McKenzie JE, Bossuyt PM, Boutron I, Hoffmann TC, Mulrow CD, et al. The PRISMA 2020 statement: an updated guideline for reporting systematic reviews. BMJ. 2021;372:n71.
36. Hutton B, Salanti G, Caldwell DM, Chaimani A, Schmid CH, Cameron C, et al. The PRISMA extension statement for reporting of systematic reviews incorporating network meta-analyses of health care interventions: checklist and explanations. Ann Intern Med. 2015;162:777–84.
37. Dossett, H. G., Estrada, N. A., Swartz, G. J., et al. (2014). A randomised controlled trial of kinematically and mechanically aligned total knee replacements: two-year clinical results. *The Bone and Joint Journal, 96-B*, 907–913.
38. Waterson, H. B., Clement, N. D., Eyres, K. S., Mandalia, V. I., and Toms, A. D. (2016). The early outcome of kinematic versus mechanical alignment in total knee arthroplasty: a prospective randomised control trial. *Bone Joint J, 98-B*(10), 1360–1368. https://doi.org/10.1302/0301-620X.98B10.36862
39. McEwen PJ, Dlaska CE, Jovanovic IA, Doma K, Brandon BJ. Computer-assisted kinematic and mechanical Axis Total knee arthroplasty: a prospective randomized controlled trial of bilateral simultaneous surgery. J Arthroplast. 2020;35(2):443–50. https://doi.org/10.1016/j.arth.2019.08.064.
40. Young, S. W., Walker, M. L., Bayan, A., et al. (2017). The Chitranjan S. Ranawat Award. No difference in 2-year functional outcomes using kinematic versus mechanical alignment in tka: a randomized controlled clinical trial. *Clinical Orthopaedics and Related Research, 475*, 9–20.
41. Matsumoto, T. et al. Radiological and clinical comparison of kinematically versus mechanically aligned total knee arthroplasty. *Bone Joint J. 99-b*, 640–646 (2017).
42. Yeo JH, Seon JK, Lee DH, Song EK. No difference in outcomes and gait analysis between mechanical and kinematic knee alignment methods using robotic

total knee arthroplasty [published correction appears in Knee Surg Sports Traumatol Arthrosc. 2019 Jul; 27(7):2385]. Knee Surg Sports Traumatol Arthrosc. 2019;27:1142–7.
43. Bellemans J, Colyn W, Vandenneucker H, Victor J (2012) The Chitranjan Ranawat award: is neutral mechanical alignment normal for all patients? The concept of constitutional varus. Clin Orthop Relat Res 470(1):45–53. https://doi.org/10.1007/s11999-011-1936-5
44. Victor JM, Bassens D, Bellemans J, Gursu S, Dhollander AA, Verdonk PC. Constitutional varus does not affect joint line orientation in the coronal plane. Clin Orthop Relat Res. 2014;472(1):98–104.
45. Howell SM, Howell SJ, Kuznik KT, Cohen J, Hull ML. Does a kinematically aligned total knee arthroplasty restore function without failure regardless of alignment category? Clin Orthop Relat Res. 2013;471(3):1000–7.
46. Dossett HG, Swartz GJ, Estrada NA, LeFevre GW, Kwasman BG (2012) Kinematically versus mechanically aligned total knee arthroplasty. Orthopedics 35(2):e160–e169. https://doi.org/10.3928/01477447-20120123-04
47. Gu, Y., Roth, J. D., Howell, S. M., et al. (2014). How frequently do four methods for mechanically aligning a total knee arthroplasty cause collateral ligament imbalance and change alignment from normal in white patients? AAOS exhibit selection. *The Journal of Bone and Joint Surgery, 96*, e101.
48. Lee JH, Jeong BO (2012) Radiologic changes of ankle joint after total knee arthroplasty. Foot Ankle Int. https://doi.org/10.3113/FAI.2012.1087
49. Ariyawatkul T, Pornrattanamaneewong C, Narkbunnam R, Chareancholvanich K (2014) Talar coronal malalignment as a consequence after high tibial osteotomy in osteoarthritic knee patients. J Med Assoc Thai. ;97
50. Winnock de Grave P, Luyckx T, Van Criekinge T et al (2023) Inverse kinematic alignment accommodates native coronal knee alignment better in comparison to adjusted mechanical alignment and restricted kinematic alignment. Knee Surg Sports Traumatol Arthrosc 31. https://doi.org/10.1007/s00167-023-07326-x
51. Winnock de Grave P, Van Criekinge T, Luyckx T et al (2023) Restoration of the native tibial joint line obliquity in total knee arthroplasty with inverse kinematic alignment does not increase knee adduction moments. Knee Surg Sports Traumatol Arthrosc 31. https://doi.org/10.1007/s00167-023-07464-2
52. Murgier J, Clatworthy M (2022) Variable rotation of the femur does not affect outcome with patient specific alignment navigated balanced TKA. Knee Surg Sports Traumatol Arthrosc 30. https://doi.org/10.1007/s00167-020-06226-8
53. Gao F, Ma J, Sun W et al (2017) Radiographic assessment of knee–ankle alignment after total knee arthroplasty for varus and valgus knee osteoarthritis. Knee 24. https://doi.org/10.1016/j.knee.2016.09.023
54. Chang CB, Chung CY, Park MS et al (2020) Aggravation of ankle varus incongruency following total knee replacement correcting ≥ 10° of genu varum deformity: a radiographic assessment. J Arthroplasty 35. https://doi.org/10.1016/j.arth.2020.06.027

55. Ragunandhan, Narayanasamy; Jeya Venkatesh, Palanisamy Outcomes of Kinematically Aligned Total Knee Arthroplasty in Indian Population—Case Series with Three Year Clinical Results. Indian Journal of Orthopaedics (2021). 10.1007/s43465-021-00521-3
56. Nedopil, Alexander J.; Howell, Stephen M.; Hull, Maury L. What clinical characteristics and radiographic parameters are associated with patellofemoral instability after kinematically aligned total knee arthroplasty?. International Orthopaedics (2016). https://doi.org/10.1007/s00264-016-3287-z
57. Hsu, Cheng-En; Huang, Jen-Ting; Tong, Kwok-Man; Huang, Kui-Chou Total knee arthroplasty according to the original knee phenotypes with kinematic alignment surgical technique—early clinical and functional outcomes. BMC Musculoskeletal Disorders (2020). https://doi.org/10.1186/s12891-020-03862-6
58. Wang, Guiguan; Zhang, Yue; Chen, Long; Yu, Guoyu; Luo, Fenqi; Xu, Jie Modified kinematic alignment better restores plantar pressure distribution than mechanical alignment in total knee arthroplasty: a randomized controlled trial. Scientific Reports (2024). https://doi.org/10.1038/s41598-024-79566-x
59. Miura, Takanori; Takahashi, Tsuneari; Watanabe, Jun; Kataoka, Yuki; Ae, Ryusuke; Saito, Hidetomo; Takeshita, Katsushi; Miyakoshi, Naohisa Postoperative clinical outcomes for kinematically, restricted kinematically, or mechanically aligned total knee arthroplasty: a systematic review and network meta-analysis of randomized controlled trials. BMC Musculoskeletal Disorders (2023). https://doi.org/10.1186/s12891-023-06448-0
60. Hutt, Jonathan; Massé, Vincent; Lavigne, Martin; Vendittoli, Pascal-André Functional joint line obliquity after kinematic total knee arthroplasty. International Orthopaedics (2015). https://doi.org/10.1007/s00264-015-2733-7
61. Shichman, Ittai; Hallak, Amer; Ashkenazi, Itay; Warschwaski, Yaniv; Gold, Aviram; Snir, Nimrod Effect of inverse kinematic alignment total knee arthroplasty on coronal alignment of the ankle joint in patients with varus knee deformity. Archives of Orthopaedic and Trauma Surgery (2024). https://doi.org/10.1007/s00402-024-05549-2

6.3 Ligament Gap Balancing Approach

Machine Generated Summaries

Disclaimer: The summaries in this chapter were generated from Springer Nature publications using abstractive AI auto-summarization: An abstraction-based summarizer creates new text based on deep learning. New phrases are created to summarize the content. As the constituted sentences are machine selected, they may not fully reflect the body of the work, so we strongly advise that the original content is read and cited. The auto-generated summaries were curated by the editor to meet Springer Nature publication standards.

6.3.1 Precision of Ci-Navigated Extension and Flexion Gap Balancing in Total Knee Arthroplasty and Analysis of Potential Predictive Variables [96]

This is a machine-generated summary of:

Fickert, S.; Jawhar, A.; Sunil, P.; Scharf, H.-P Precision of Ci-navigated extension and flexion gap balancing in total knee arthroplasty and analysis of potential predictive variables [96].

Published in: Archives of Orthopaedic and Trauma Surgery (2011).

Link to original: https://doi.org/10.1007/s00402-011-1419-x

If you want to cite the papers, please refer to the original.

For technical reasons we could not place the page where the original quote is coming from.

6.3.1.1 Research Highlights

Total knee arthroplasty (TKA) success hinges on precise joint line creation, limb alignment, and soft tissue balancing. Malalignment and improper ligamentous balancing can lead to postoperative pain, instability, and long-term complications such as loosening and failure. While computer-assisted navigation in TKA has shown improvements in component positioning and limb alignment, the accuracy of ligament balancing remains underexplored. The study by Fickert et al. evaluates the accuracy of limb alignment and gap balancing in computer-navigated TKA using intraoperative measurements.

The study involved 225 patients with primary osteoarthritis undergoing computer-navigated TKA using the DePuy Ci system (DePuy Orthopedics, Ray**nham, Massachusetts, USA)**. Excluding other arthritis causes and previous surgeries, the research focused on achieving accurate limb alignment and medial-lateral gap balancing. The Ci Navigation system, a nonimage-based optical wireless system, facilitated precise bone morphing and ligament balancing through data acquisition and tracking. The surgical process included tibial resection followed by femoral adjustments to achieve optimal extension and flexion gaps. Statistical analysis was conducted on various alignment parameters to assess the accuracy of the navigation system.

The study demonstrated that computer-assisted navigation significantly improves gap balancing accuracy in TKA. Over 90% of knees achieved coronal alignment within ±3°, with minimal variance in extension and flexion gaps. The findings suggest that factors such as age, sex, preoperative deformity, and osteoarthritis grade do not influence gap balancing accuracy. Future study could explore the impact of femoral rotation and component flexion on flexion gaps further. This research underscores the potential of navigation systems to enhance surgical precision in TKA while highlighting areas for continued investigation into optimizing ligament balancing techniques.

6.3.2 Spacer-Based Gap Balancing Is Useful in Total Knee Arthroplasty: A 3-Year Follow-Up of a Retrospective Study [97]

This is a machine-generated summary of:

Hu, Yanhui; Song, Da; Liu, Yi; Zhao, Yong; Ma, Wenpu; Yang, Yiqun; Yuan, Zhenfeng Spacer-based gap balancing is useful in total knee arthroplasty: a 3-year follow-up of a retrospective study [97].

Published in: Journal of Orthopaedic Surgery and Research (2021).

Link to original: https://doi.org/10.1186/s13018-021-02788-6

If you want to cite the papers, please refer to the original.

For technical reasons we could not place the page where the original quote is coming from.

6.3.2.1 Research Highlights

Total knee arthroplasty (TKA) is a well-established surgical intervention for severe knee osteoarthritis, offering significant clinical benefits. However, a subset of patients continues to experience poor joint balance postoperatively, leading to pain and dissatisfaction. Achieving precise prosthesis alignment and soft tissue balance is crucial for optimal recovery. Two primary techniques, measured resection (MR) and gap balancing (GB), are employed to achieve this goal. The MR technique uses anatomical landmarks for femoral component rotation but can be variable due to individual anatomical differences. Conversely, the GB technique focuses on soft tissue tension to balance extension and flexion gaps but requires specific tools for implementation. The study by Hu et al. investigates the efficacy of a modified spacer block-assisted GB technique compared to the traditional MR technique in TKA.

The study involved patients undergoing primary TKA with either the GB or MR technique, with ethical approval and informed consent obtained. The GB group utilized a modified spacer block to achieve ligament balance by sequentially inserting spacers into the joint space until optimal tension was achieved. This determined the femoral rotation resection angle. In contrast, the MR group used a posterior condylar referencing jig set to a standard external rotation angle. Both groups underwent similar surgical procedures post-resection, including tibial keel processing and patella management. Postoperative care included prophylactic antibiotics and anticoagulants, with early mobilization encouraged. Outcomes were assessed through clinical scores, radiographic evaluations, and complication monitoring over an average follow-up period of 24 months.

The study found no significant differences in functional outcomes or clinical scores between the GB and MR groups at 2 years post-surgery. Both techniques resulted in similar ranges of motion and patient satisfaction levels. However, the GB technique required greater external rotation resection angles and more posterior femoral condyle resections than the MR technique. Despite these differences, no cases of postoperative flexion instability were observed in the GB group. Future study could explore the application of this modified spacer block tool in cases with severe deformities or over longer follow-up periods to assess prosthesis survival rates comprehensively. The findings suggest that while both techniques are viable, the modified spacer block offers a cost-effective and straightforward approach for surgeons favoring gap balancing methods in TKA procedures.

6.3.3 Gap Balancing Versus Measured Resection for Primary Total Knee Arthroplasty: A Meta-Analysis Study [98]

This is a machine-generated summary of:

Migliorini, Filippo; Eschweiler, Jörg; Mansy, Yasser El; Quack, Valentin; Schenker, Hanno; Tingart, Markus; Driessen, Arne Gap balancing versus measured resection for primary total knee arthroplasty: a meta-analysis study [98].

Published in: Archives of Orthopaedic and Trauma Surgery (2020).

Link to original: https://doi.org/10.1007/s00402-020-03478-4

If you want to cite the papers, please refer to the original.

For technical reasons we could not place the page where the original quote is coming from.

6.3.3.1 Research Highlights

Total knee arthroplasty (TKA) is a widely performed procedure that aims to restore joint biomechanics and improve patient quality of life. The surgical techniques for TKA, particularly gap balancing (GB) and measured resection (MR), are highly standardized, yet debates persist regarding their comparative effectiveness. The GB technique involves initial soft tissue release followed by bone resection to achieve balance, while the MR technique focuses on direct bony resection using anatomical landmarks. Despite numerous studies, there remains a lack of consensus on which technique offers superior implant alignment and surgical outcomes. The study by Migliorini et al. conducts a meta-analysis to update current evidence and explore potential advantages of GB over MR in terms of clinical scores, radiological measurements, and complications.

The study employed a comprehensive literature search across major databases such as PubMed, Google Scholar, Scopus, and Embase, adhering to the Preferred Reporting Items for Systematic Reviews and Meta-Analyses (PRISMA) guidelines. Two independent authors conducted the search and data extraction, focusing on clinical studies comparing MR and GB techniques for primary TKA. The analysis included randomized clinical trials and cohort studies published in the last few years, excluding reviews, case reports, and non-clinical studies. Data from 1000 TKAs were analysed for post-operative clinical scores, operating time, radiological measurements, and complications like infections and aseptic loosening. Statistical analysis was performed using Review Manager Software (Cochrane Review) to assess continuous and dichotomous variables. The study found no significant differences in clinical scores or complication rates between the two techniques but noted that the GB group had a higher joint line position and required longer operating time.

The findings suggest that both GB and MR techniques are comparable in terms of safety and feasibility for TKA. While the GB technique showed a higher joint line position, it did not translate into significant differences in clinical outcomes or complication rates compared to MR. Future study could focus on long-term survivorships of these techniques to provide more definitive conclusions. The study highlights the need for further high-quality research with larger sample sizes to address existing heterogeneities and explore potential benefits of each technique more thoroughly.

6.3.4 Asymmetric Gap Balancing Improves Knee Kinematics Following Primary Total Knee Arthroplasty [99]

This is a machine-generated summary of:

Valpiana, Pieralberto; Salvi, Andrea Giordano; Ghirardelli, Stefano; Bernardi, Matteo; Petralia, Giuseppe; Aloisi, Giuseppe; Schaller, Christian; Indelli, Pier Francesco Asymmetric gap balancing improves knee kinematic following primary total knee arthroplasty [99].

Published in: Arthroplasty (2024).

Link to original: https://doi.org/10.1186/s42836-024-00243-5

If you want to cite the papers, please refer to the original.

For technical reasons we could not place the page where the original quote is coming from.

6.3.4.1 Research Highlights

Historically, achieving normal knee kinematics after total knee arthroplasty (TKA) has been challenging, even with cruciate-sparing designs and mechanical alignment techniques. Traditional surgical methods aimed for symmetric balancing between the lateral and medial knee compartments, but this approach does not replicate the native knee's kinematic profile. The study by Valpiana et al.explores the potential benefits of a robot-assisted surgical technique that introduces slight mediolateral gap asymmetry during TKA to improve postoperative knee kinematics.

The study involved two retrospectively matched groups of patients who underwent medially stabilized TKA due to isolated knee disease. Group A received traditional symmetric gap balancing, while Group B underwent a robot-assisted "simplified" kinematic alignment with slight mediolateral asymmetry in flexion and extension gaps. The surgeries were performed under spinal anesthesia using a tourniquet, and all patients were evaluated radiologically before undergoing gait analysis. The gait analysis utilized an instrumented treadmill to assess spatiotemporal parameters and kinematic variables. Statistical analysis was conducted using Statistical Package for Social Sciences (SPSS) software (IBM, Chicago, IL, USA) to compare outcomes between the groups. The results indicated no significant differences in spatiotemporal parameters between the healthy controls and TKA groups, but notable differences in kinematic parameters were observed between the two TKA groups.

The study highlights that slightly asymmetric intercompartmental gap balancing during TKA may offer kinematic advantages over traditional symmetric approaches. Despite these findings, significant differences remain between normal knees and those treated with TKA. Future study could focus on further refining these techniques and exploring their clinical benefits through larger cohort studies. Additionally, defining optimal intercompartmental gap differences remains an area for further research. This study underscores the potential of advanced technologies in enhancing surgical precision but also emphasizes the need for continued investigation into achieving normal knee kinematics post-TKA.

6.3.5 Sagittal Gap Balancing with the Concept of a Single Radius Femoral Component in Posterior Cruciate Sacrificing Total Knee Arthroplasty with Patient-Specific Instrumentation [100]

This is a machine-generated summary of:

Hananouchi, Takehito Sagittal gap balancing with the concept of a single radius femoral component in posterior cruciate sacrificing total knee arthroplasty with patient-specific instrumentation [100].

Published in: International Orthopaedics (2014).

Link to original: https://doi.org/10.1007/s00264-014-2536-2

If you want to cite the papers, please refer to the original.

For technical reasons we could not place the page where the original quote is coming from.

6.3.5.1 Research Highlights

Total knee arthroplasty (TKA) requires precise soft tissue balance to ensure optimal outcomes, with intra-operative gap measurements being a key method for evaluating this balance. Traditionally, the goal has been to achieve equal flexion and extension gaps, but recent studies suggest that this may not always be feasible due to factors like posterior capsule tightness and anterior muscle tension. The study by

Hananouchi et al. explores whether three-dimensional pre-operative planning using patient-specific instrumentation (PSI) can achieve equal sagittal flexion and extension gaps in TKA.

The study involved 11 patients diagnosed with osteoarthritis who underwent TKA using PSI. Pre-operative CT scans were used to plan the placement of a single-radius femoral component, aligning it with the knee's flexion-extension axis. The PSI guided the surgical procedure, ensuring precise bone cuts and component placement. Intra-operative gap measurements were taken using a tensor device under a constant distraction force, both at full extension and at 90 degrees of flexion. Postoperative CT scans assessed the accuracy of component alignment compared to pre-operative plans.

The findings revealed that the flexion gap was consistently larger than the extension gap, indicating that equal sagittal gaps were not achieved despite precise pre-operative planning and execution. This suggests that aiming for equal flexion and extension gaps in PS-TKA may not be realistic when using a single-radius femoral component. Future study could focus on refining pre-operative planning techniques to better account for anatomical variations and soft tissue influences on gap measurements. Additionally, further research is needed to explore the long-term clinical implications of these findings and whether alternative strategies might improve sagittal gap balancing in TKA procedures.

6.3.6 Prediction of Gap Balancing Based on 2-D Radiography in Total Knee Arthroplasty for Knee Osteoarthritis Patients [101]

This is a machine-generated summary of:

Zhang, Zhuo; Luo, Yang; Zhang, Chong; Wang, Xin; Zhang, Tianwei; Zhang, Guoqiang Prediction of gap balancing based on 2-D radiography in total knee arthroplasty for knee osteoarthritis patients [101].

Published in: Arthroplasty (2023).

Link to original: https://doi.org/10.1186/s42836-023-00218-y

If you want to cite the papers, please refer to the original.

For technical reasons we could not place the page where the original quote is coming from.

6.3.6.1 Research Highlights

Total knee arthroplasty (TKA) is a widely used surgical intervention for knee osteoarthritis, yielding generally favorable outcomes. Preoperative planning is crucial for successful TKA, with digital planning systems and three-dimensional imaging enhancing precision. A critical step in TKA is gap balancing, which ensures stable and balanced medial-lateral and flexion-extension gaps. Traditionally, this process relies heavily on the surgeon's experience and manual techniques. However, quantifying a balanced gap post-osteophyte removal remains challenging. The study by Zhang et al. introduces a novel approach using computer-assisted methods to predict the influence of osteophytes on postoperative gap balancing in TKA.

The study involved reviewing radiographic data from 110 patients who underwent primary TKA From January 2021 to December 2021. The researchers developed a three-dimensional planning system incorporating an algorithm to predict joint gaps based on preoperative plain films of the knee. They calculated the area of osteophytes using trapeziform measurements on radiographs and assessed the impact of osteophyte removal on joint gaps. The team employed statistical analyses, including univariable and multivariable linear regression, to establish relationships between predictive variables and joint gaps. A tenfold cross-validation was conducted to ensure model robustness, resulting in an equation that predicts joint gap changes based on osteophyte size and bone cuts.

The study advances preoperative planning for TKA by providing a quantitative method to estimate soft tissue release requirements using plain films. This approach allows surgeons to calculate targeted joint gaps preoperatively, potentially improving surgical outcomes. Future study could focus on refining the model by incorporating additional variables such as implant dimensions or conducting prospective studies with larger sample sizes to enhance accuracy. The integration of machine learning in this context demonstrates its potential utility in optimizing surgical planning and execution in orthopedic procedures.

6.3.7 Improved Femoral Component Rotation in Total Knee Arthroplasty: An Anatomical Study with Optimized Gap Balancing [102]

This is a machine-generated summary of:

Grifka, Joachim; Baier, Clemens; Maderbacher, Günther Improved femoral component rotation in total knee arthroplasty: an anatomical study with optimized gap balancing [102].

Published in: Archives of Orthopaedic and Trauma Surgery (2020).

Link to original: https://doi.org/10.1007/s00402-020-03557-6

If you want to cite the papers, please refer to the original.

For technical reasons we could not place the page where the original quote is coming from.

6.3.7.1 Research Highlights

Total knee arthroplasty (TKA) is a widely successful orthopedic procedure, with computer-assisted surgery often used to achieve optimal alignment of the knee joint. Achieving a balanced flexion and extension gap is crucial for the success of TKA, as it ensures proper knee function and patient satisfaction. Traditional methods for determining femoral component rotation rely on anatomical landmarks, which can vary significantly among individuals. The study by Grifka et al. investigates the effectiveness of these anatomical landmarks in achieving a balanced flexion gap during TKA.

The study involved ten cadaveric knees from Thiel-fixated bodies, ensuring no prior injuries or osteoarthritis through CT scans. Using a CT-free navigation device, the researchers assessed various anatomical landmarks and performed tibial cuts perpendicular to the mechanical axis. A double tensiometer was used to evaluate ligament status, and adjustments were made to achieve symmetric flexion and extension gaps. The femoral component rotation was measured relative to the posterior condylar line, with results compared against traditional anatomical landmarks like the Whiteside line and surgical transepicondylar axis. The study found significant deviations between ligament-balanced femoral component rotation and those determined by anatomical landmarks, indicating that these traditional methods may not be suitable for achieving a well-balanced flexion gap.

The findings suggest that relying solely on anatomical landmarks for femoral component rotation in TKA may not ensure a balanced flexion gap, as these do not account for individual variations in ligament status. The study highlights the importance of using gap balancing techniques that consider both bony anatomy and ligamentous conditions. Future study could focus on refining navigational techniques to improve accuracy in achieving balanced knee arthroplasties. Additionally, exploring alternative methods or technologies that integrate real-time assessment of ligament tension could further enhance surgical outcomes in TKA procedures.

6.3.8 Effects of Posterior Condylar Osteophytes on Gap Balancing in Computer-Assisted Total Knee Arthroplasty with Posterior Cruciate Ligament Sacrifice [103]

This is a machine-generated summary of:

Sriphirom, Pornpavit; Siramanakul, Chaiyaporn; Chanopas, Boonyawat; Boonruksa, Sirisuk Effects of posterior condylar osteophytes on gap balancing in computer-assisted total knee arthroplasty with posterior cruciate ligament sacrifice [103].

Published in: European Journal of Orthopaedic Surgery & Traumatology (2018).

Link to original: https://doi.org/10.1007/s00590-017-2118-2

If you want to cite the papers, please refer to the original.

For technical reasons we could not place the page where the original quote is coming from.

6.3.8.1 Research Highlights

Total knee arthroplasty (TKA) aims to achieve balanced extension and flexion gaps while restoring neutral limb alignment. Computer-assisted surgery (CAS) in TKA has improved gap balancing and prosthesis positioning, but challenges remain, particularly with patient-specific instrument (PSI) planning. PSI-based templates have shown limitations in calculating factors contributing to gaps, such as osteophytes, which are typically removed before gap planning. However, tight soft tissues can complicate osteophyte removal. The study by Sriphirom et al. investigates the impact of posterior condylar osteophytes on gap balancing during CAS TKA and examines how osteophyte thickness affects gap changes.

The study was conducted on varus osteoarthritic knees with posterior condylar osteophytes undergoing primary TKA using a navigation system. Exclusion criteria included severe varus deformity, valgus knee deformity, significant bony defects, and knee instability. Preoperative imaging assessed osteophyte position, and a mini-midvastus approach was used for surgery. The tibial cut was performed first under navigation guidance, followed by measurement of extension and flexion gaps using a knee balancer. Posterior condylar osteophytes were removed with a curved osteotome, and their thickness was measured with a vernier caliper. Gap widths were measured before and after osteophyte removal to assess changes. Statistical analyses revealed significant increases in both extension and flexion gaps post-removal, with the flexion gap showing a greater increase.

The study advances understanding of how posterior condylar osteophyte removal affects gap balancing in CAS TKA. It highlights the relationship between osteophyte thickness and changes in lateral extension and flexion gaps but not the medial extension gap. The findings suggest that removing these osteophytes can lead to unintended increases in gap sizes, potentially affecting surgical outcomes. Future study could focus on refining CAS TKA software and PSI templates to account for these changes more accurately, enhancing precision in gap planning for better patient outcomes.

6.3.9 Influence of Tibial Slope on Extension and Flexion Gaps in Total Knee Arthroplasty: Increasing the Tibial Slope Affects Both Gaps [104]

This is a machine-generated summary of:

Nowakowski, Andrej Maria; Kamphausen, Marcus; Pagenstert, Geert; Valderrabano, Victor; Müller-Gerbl, Magdalena Influence of tibial slope on extension and flexion gaps in total knee arthroplasty: increasing the tibial slope affects both gaps [104].

Published in: International Orthopaedics (2014).

Link to original: https://doi.org/10.1007/s00264-014-2373-3

If you want to cite the papers, please refer to the original.

For technical reasons we could not place the page where the original quote is coming from.

6.3.9.1 Research Highlights

In total knee arthroplasty, achieving optimal implant alignment in flexion and extension is crucial for ensuring proper ligament tension and postoperative function. Surgeons often aim to create equal and symmetrical flexion and extension gaps, which are influenced by factors such as deformities, osteolysis, and surgical approach. The preparation of these gaps can be affected by bony resections, which in turn influence capsular and ligamentous tension. Previous studies have suggested that increasing the tibial slope can improve knee flexion by equalizing the flexion and extension gaps. However, the extent of this effect, particularly on the osseous resection gap without distraction, remains unclear. The study by Nowakowski et al. investigates how increasing the tibial slope affects the osseous resection gaps in both flexion and extension using tibiofemoral contact points for measurement.

The study utilized formalin-fixed knee joint specimens from a university-level anatomy course to assess changes in osseous resection gaps with varying tibial slopes. The researchers performed virtual bone resections on these specimens using CT scans to simulate different tibial slopes ranging from 0° to 6°. A customized frame was used to secure the specimens during imaging, allowing for precise measurements of tibiofemoral contact points in both full extension and 90° flexion. The data were analysed using a standardized coordinate system and high-precision visualization software. Linear regression analysis was employed to evaluate the relationship between tibial slope adjustments and changes in osseous resection gaps. The results indicated that increasing the tibial slope led to a significant widening of the lateral compartment gap during flexion compared to the medial compartment.

The findings of this study suggest that while increasing the tibial slope can affect both flexion and extension osseous resection gaps, it may not be advisable to use this method alone for equilibrating narrow flexion gaps when both extension gap and tibial slope are appropriately adjusted. Instead, ligament balancing procedures should be considered to achieve optimal alignment without additional bony resections. Future study could explore alternative methods for gap equilibration that do not rely solely on altering bony structures, potentially improving surgical outcomes in total knee arthroplasty.

6.3.10 The Knee Position at Tourniquet Inflation Does Not Affect the Gap Balancing During Total Knee Arthroplasty [105]

This is a machine-generated summary of:

Matsui, Yoshio; Matsuura, Masanori; Hidaka, Noriaki The knee position at tourniquet inflation does not affect the gap balancing during total knee arthroplasty [105].

Published in: Archives of Orthopaedic and Trauma Surgery (2021).

Link to original: https://doi.org/10.1007/s00402-021-04017-5

If you want to cite the papers, please refer to the original.
For technical reasons we could not place the page where the original quote is coming from.

6.3.10.1 Research Highlights

Soft tissue balance is crucial for the success of total knee arthroplasty (TKA), as improper balancing can lead to knee instability, prolonged pain, and early failure. Various methods have been developed to achieve precise soft tissue balancing, including the use of special tensors that measure intraoperative gap balances under conditions similar to the postoperative state. However, the impact of air tourniquet use during TKA on gap measurement remains controversial, with concerns about its effects on muscle strength and potential for deep vein thrombosis. The study by Matsui et al. investigates whether the knee position at tourniquet inflation affects intraoperative gap measurement during TKA.

In this prospective study, approved by an institutional review board, two senior surgeons performed TKAs on patients using Vanguard PS and Persona PS systems (Zimmer-Biomet, Warsaw, Indiana, USA). The study involved inflating a tourniquet to 300 mmHg in either a fully flexed or extended knee position. Gap measurements were taken using two types of tensors—the True Tensor® and Offset Repo-Tensor®—after completing bone cuts and soft-tissue releases. The researchers measured the gap twice: once under tourniquet inflation and once after release, comparing the differences between flexion and extension positions using statistical analysis. The results showed that all mean gap differences were clinically insignificant (<1 mm and < 1°), regardless of whether the tourniquet was inflated in a flexed or extended position.

The study's findings suggest that knee position at tourniquet inflation does not significantly affect gap measurements during TKA, allowing surgeons to measure gaps without considering knee position at inflation. This research provides valuable insights for surgical practice, especially when navigation systems are unavailable due to cost constraints. Future study could explore other types of prostheses beyond the fixed posterior stabilized implants used in this research to determine if these findings are generalizable across different TKA systems. Additionally, further investigation into optimal tourniquet pressure settings could enhance surgical outcomes while minimizing potential neurovascular risks.

6.3.11 Kinematic Femoral Alignment with Gap Balancing and Patient-Specific Instrumentation in Total Knee Arthroplasty: A Randomized Clinical Trial [106]

This is a machine-generated summary of:

Hommel, Hagen; Abdel, Matthew P.; Perka, Carsten Kinematic femoral alignment with gap balancing and patient-specific instrumentation in total knee arthroplasty: a randomized clinical trial [106].

Published in: European Journal of Orthopaedic Surgery & Traumatology (2016).

Link to original: https://doi.org/10.1007/s00590-016-1865-9

If you want to cite the papers, please refer to the original.

For technical reasons we could not place the page where the original quote is coming from.

6.3.11.1 Research Highlights

Given the aging population and the rising prevalence of obesity, the incidence of gonarthrosis and the subsequent demand for total knee arthroplasty (TKA) are increasing. Complications such as instability, malalignment, and malrotation after TKA contribute to patient dissatisfaction, with many experiencing limited function and residual pain. Optimal implant alignment and rotation are crucial to improving outcomes. While patient-specific instrumentation (PSI) has shown promise in addressing these issues, inconsistencies remain in achieving precise femoral component rotation. The study by Hommel et al. explores the efficacy of combining PSI with a gap balancing technique to enhance clinical outcomes in TKA.

The study was a randomized controlled trial involving 50 patients scheduled for unilateral primary TKA due to gonarthrosis. Participants were randomized into two groups: one using standard PSI with conventional measured resection techniques, and the other employing PSI with a gap balancing approach. Preoperative planning involved creating a three-dimensional model of the knee from MRI data to establish anatomical landmarks for PSI production. The surgeries were performed by a single surgeon using a medial parapatellar approach, with specific attention to achieving neutral mechanical axes and appropriate femoral rotation. Postoperative assessments included range of motion (ROM), stability, and various clinical scores at 6- and 12-month follow-ups.

The study found that the PSI gap balancing group demonstrated significantly superior functional scores compared to the standard PSI group at both follow-up intervals. Although differences in ROM were not statistically significant, the gap balancing technique showed potential benefits in minimizing anterior knee pain and postoperative stiffness. The study highlights that while PSI combined with gap balancing offers promising results, further research is needed to confirm these findings' clinical relevance over longer-term outcomes. Future study could explore optimizing tibial cuts to enhance alignment accuracy further and assess the generalizability of these results across different surgical settings.

6.3.12 Measured Resection Versus Gap Balancing for Total Knee Arthroplasty [107]

This is a machine-generated summary of:

Abdel, Matthew P. Measured Resection Versus Gap Balancing for Total Knee Arthroplasty [107].

Published in: Clinical Orthopaedics and Related Research® (2014).

Link to original: https://doi.org/10.1007/s11999-014-3524-y

If you want to cite the papers, please refer to the original.

For technical reasons we could not place the page where the original quote is coming from.

6.3.12.1 Research Highlights

Total knee arthroplasty (TKA) is a common surgical procedure expected to increase significantly in the United States over the next two decades, particularly among younger and more active patients. While radiographic alignment is often emphasized, achieving proper soft-tissue balance is crucial for successful outcomes. There is ongoing debate among surgeons regarding the best approach to achieve optimal alignment and soft-tissue tensioning, with some favoring a measured resection technique and others advocating for a gap-balancing technique. Matthew Abdel explores these two approaches through discussions with Bryan D. Springer and Sébastien Parratte, highlighting their respective experiences and insights.

The study delves into the methodologies of both techniques, examining their advantages and limitations. The gap-balancing technique, as explained by Dr. Springer, involves progressively releasing ligaments to create equal flexion and extension gaps, relying on ligament tension rather than fixed bony landmarks to set femoral component rotation. This method aims to achieve better femoral component rotation and stability compared to measured resection techniques. Conversely, Dr. Parratte discusses the measured resection technique, which uses bony landmarks to set femoral rotation but may not always ensure midflexion stability due to potential inaccuracies in landmark identification during surgery. Both surgeons acknowledge that factors such as implant selection and preoperative coronal alignment influence the choice of technique, with surgeon experience playing a significant role.

The article suggests that while neither technique has been definitively proven superior in terms of patient-reported outcomes or survivorship, combining elements from both approaches may offer the most reliable results. Future study could focus on hybrid techniques that integrate aspects of gap balancing and measured resection to optimize alignment and soft-tissue balance while minimizing complications such as joint line elevation or femoral component malrotation. The authors emphasize that understanding individual anatomy and utilizing advanced imaging technologies could further enhance TKA outcomes by allowing for more personalized surgical approaches.

6.3.13 Measurement for Gap Balancing Technique in Patients Undergoing Total Knee Arthroplasty: A Large Retrospective Observational Study [108]

This is a machine-generated summary of:

Xuequan, Zhao; Bin, Zhao; Shuzhang, Yao; Kanduo, Cao; Chongxi, Ren Measurement for gap balancing technique in patients undergoing total knee arthroplasty: a large retrospective observational study [108].

Published in: Journal of Orthopaedic Surgery and Research (2022).

Link to original: https://doi.org/10.1186/s13018-022-03104-6

For technical reasons we could not place the page where the original quote is coming from.

6.3.13.1 Research Highlights

Total knee arthroplasty (TKA) is a widely used surgical procedure for alleviating pain and restoring function in patients with advanced osteoarthritis or rheumatoid arthritis. A critical aspect of TKA is achieving proper axial alignment of the lower limb, which enhances patient satisfaction and extends the lifespan of the prosthesis. Despite high survivorship rates reported in previous studies, issues with limb alignment post-TKA can lead to chronic pain, posing a significant health burden. The study by Xuequan et al. introduces an innovative method for measuring osteotomy location during TKA, demonstrating promising imaging outcomes and clinical results.

The study involved a retrospective review of patients who underwent TKA using a novel osteotomy measurement technique between January 1, 2012 and December 31, 2015. Patients were divided into two groups: one receiving the new method and the other undergoing traditional procedures as a control. The researchers employed a detailed surgical approach involving precise measurements of the extension gap and flexion gap using custom-designed modules to ensure balanced osteotomies. This method aimed to achieve optimal rotational alignment of the femoral component, thereby reducing complications such as anterior knee pain and prosthesis loosening. Post-operative rehabilitation included exercises to enhance joint mobility and strength, with outcomes assessed through various scoring systems over several years.

The study's findings suggest that this new osteotomy measurement technique offers significant advantages in achieving balanced flexion-extension gaps, potentially improving surgical precision and reducing unnecessary trauma. While both the measurement osteotomy technique and gap balance technique yielded satisfactory results in patients with mild knee disease, the latter showed promise in addressing complex deformities by prioritizing gap balancing. Future study could focus on multicenter trials with comprehensive imaging assessments to further validate these findings and explore their implications for improving TKA outcomes across diverse patient populations.

6.3.14 A New Gap Balancing Technique with Functional Alignment in Total Knee Arthroplasty Using the MAKO Robotic Arm System: A Preliminary Study [109]

This is a machine-generated summary of:

Tsai, Hung-Kang; Bao, Zhengyuan; Wu, Dengxian; Han, Jing; Jiang, Qing; Xu, Zhihong A new gap balancing technique with functional alignment in total knee arthroplasty using the MAKO robotic arm system: a preliminary study [109].

Published in: BMC Surgery (2024).

Link to original: https://doi.org/10.1186/s12893-024-02524-x

If you want to cite the papers, please refer to the original.

For technical reasons we could not place the page where the original quote is coming from.

6.3.14.1 Research Highlights

Traditional mechanical alignment in total knee arthroplasty (TKA) aims for neutral alignment by adjusting bone resections perpendicular to the femoral and tibial mechanical axes, which has shown good implant survivorship but lower patient satisfaction due to soft tissue release. Kinematic alignment (KA) and functional alignment (FA) are newer techniques that aim to improve outcomes by preserving individual anatomical structures and minimizing soft tissue impact, respectively. However, concerns about KA include potential risks of aseptic loosening due to unrestricted alignment. The study by Tsai et al. describes a spacer-based gap balancing technique with FA using the MAKO (Stryker, Mahwah, New Jersey, USA) robotic arm system, aiming to enhance precision in TKA procedures.

The study involved 22 patients undergoing primary TKA with the MAKO robotic arm system, performed by a single experienced orthopedic surgeon. The researchers utilized a patented modified spacer-based gap tool under the supervision of a MAKO product specialist. Pre-operative assessments included measuring the hip-knee-ankle angle and recording knee function scores. During surgery, osteophytes were removed to improve gap measurement accuracy, and tibial resections were adjusted to achieve balanced extension-flexion gaps. The modified gap plate instrument was used for ligament tension assessment, allowing fine-tuning of medial and lateral gaps. Post-operative management included routine analgesia and rehabilitation guidance. Clinical outcomes including lower limb alignment, Knee Society Score (KSS) and Western Ontario and McMaster Universities Arthritis Index (WOMAC) were recorded before surgery, 3 months and 1 year after surgery.

The study demonstrated that the new technique achieved controlled limb alignment and satisfied clinical outcomes without requiring soft tissue release in most cases. The mean post-operative hip-knee-ankle angle indicated more neutral alignment compared to traditional methods. Future study could focus on larger populations and longer follow-ups to verify the technique's effectiveness and reliability further. Additionally, developing quantifiable gap tension assessments could enhance the tool's utility for beginners in TKA procedures. Overall, this spacer-based gap balancing technique with FA using the MAKO robotic arm system shows promise in improving patient satisfaction and functional outcomes after TKA.

Bibliography

1. Bottros J, Gad B, Krebs V, Barsoum WK (2006) Gap balancing in total knee arthroplasty. J Arthroplasty 21(4 Suppl 1):11–15. https://doi.org/10.1016/j.arth.2006.02.084
2. Bolognesi M, Hofmann A (2005) Computer navigation versus standard instrumentation for TKA: a single-surgeon experience. Clin Orthop Relat Res 440:162–169 (pii:00003086-200511000-00029)
3. Matziolis G, Krocker D, Weiss U, Tohtz S, Perka C (2007) A prospective, randomized study of computer-assisted and conventional total knee arthroplasty. Three-dimensional evaluation of implant alignment and rotation. J Bone Joint Surg Am 89(2):236–243. https://doi.org/10.2106/JBJS.F.00386
4. Lee DH, Padhy D, Park JH, Jeong WK, Han SB The impact of a rectangular or trapezoidal flexion gap on the femoral component rotation in TKA. Knee Surg Sports Traumatol Arthrosc 19(7):1141–1147. https://doi.org/10.1007/s00167-011-1422-3
5. Sheth NP, Husain A, Nelson CL. Surgical techniques for total knee arthroplasty: measured resection, gap balancing, and hybrid. J Am Acad Orthop Surg. 2017;25(7):499–508. https://doi.org/10.5435/JAAOS-D-14-00320.
6. Mercuri, J. J., Pepper, A. M., Werner, J. A. and Vigdorchik, J. M. Gap balancing, measured resection, and Kinematic Alignment: how, when, and why? *JBJS Rev.* 7, e2 (2019).
7. Daines BK, Dennis DA. Gap balancing vs. measured resection technique in total knee arthroplasty. Clin Orthop Surg. 2014;6(1):1–8. https://doi.org/10.4055/cios.2014.6.1.1.
8. Springer BD, Parratte S, Abdel MP. Measured resection versus gap balancing for total knee arthroplasty. Clin Orthop Relat Res. 2014;472(7):2016–22. https://doi.org/10.1007/s11999-014-3524-y.
9. Castelli CC, Falvo DA, Iapicca ML, Gotti V. Rotational alignment of the femoral component in total knee arthroplasty. Ann Transl Med. 2016;4(1):4. https://doi.org/10.3978/j.issn.2305-5839.2015.12.66.

10. Yau WP, Chiu KY, Tang WM. How precise is the determination of rotational alignment of the femoral prosthesis in total knee arthroplasty: an in vivo study. J Arthroplasty. 2007;22(7):1042–8. https://doi.org/10.1016/j.arth.2006.12.043.
11. Grifka J, Baier C, Maderbacher G. Improved femoral component rotation in total knee arthroplasty: an anatomical study with optimized gap balancing. Arch Orthop Trauma Surg. 2020;141:1669–75. https://doi.org/10.1007/s00402-020-03557-6.
12. Babazadeh S, Dowsey MM, Stoney JD, Choong PF. Gap balancing sacrifices joint-line maintenance to improve gap symmetry: a randomized controlled trial comparing gap balancing and measured resection. J Arthroplasty. 2014;29(5):950–4. https://doi.org/10.1016/j.arth.2013.09.036.
13. Lavoie F. Spacer-based gap balancing in total knee arthroplasty: clinical success with a reproducible technique. J Knee Surg. 2017;30(8):798–806. https://doi.org/10.1055/s-0036-1597970.
14. Nagai K, Muratsu H, Matsumoto T, Miya H, Kuroda R, Kurosaka M. Soft tissue balance changes depending on joint distraction force in total knee arthroplasty. J Arthroplasty. 2014;29(3):520–4. https://doi.org/10.1016/j.arth.2013.07.025.
15. Bercovy M, Kerboull L, Müller JH, Saffarini M, Sailhan F. Satisfactory mid-to long-term outcomes of TKA aligned using conventional instrumentation for flexion gap balancing with minimal soft tissue release. Knee Surg Sports Traumatol Arthrosc. 2020; https://doi.org/10.1007/s00167-020-06360-3.
16. Gungor HR, Ok N. Use of a spacer block tool for assessment of joint line position during revision knee arthroplasty. J Knee Surg. 2021; https://doi.org/10.1055/s-0040-1722628.
17. Tapasvi SR, Shekhar A, Patil SS, Dipane MV, Chowdhry M, McPherson EJ. Comparison of gap balancing vs measured resection technique in patients undergoing simultaneous bilateral total knee arthroplasty: one technique per knee. J Arthroplasty. 2020;35(3):732–40. https://doi.org/10.1016/j.arth.2019.10.002.
18. Hernandez-Hermoso JA, Nescolarde-Selva L, Rodriguez-Montserrat D, Martinez-Pastor JC, Garcia-Oltra E, Lopez-Marne S (2019) Different femoral rotation with navigated flexion-gap balanced or measured resection in total knee arthroplasty does not lead to different clinical outcomes. Knee Surg Sports Traumatol Arthrosc. https://doi.org/10.1007/s00167-019-05591-3
19. Dennis DA, Komistek RD, Kim RH, Sharma A. Gap balancing versus measured resection technique for total knee arthroplasty. Clin Orthop Relat Res. 2010;468(1):102–7. https://doi.org/10.1007/s11999-009-1112-3.
20. Mantas JP, Bloebaum RD, Skedros JG, Hofmann AA (1992) Implications of reference axes used for rotational alignment of the femoral component in primary and revision knee arthroplasty. J Arthroplasty 7(4):531–535. https://doi.org/10.1016/s0883-5403(06)80075-6
21. Katz MA, Beck TD, Silber JS, Seldes RM, Lotke PA (2001) Determining femoral rotational alignment in total knee arthroplasty: reliability of techniques. J Arthroplasty 16(3):301–305. https://doi.org/10.1054/arth.2001.21456

22. Howell SM, Hull ML, Nedopil AJ, Rivière C. Caliper-verified kinematically aligned total knee arthroplasty: rationale, targets, accuracy, balancing, implant survival, and outcomes. Instr Course Lect. 2023;72:241–59.
23. Dennis DA. Measured resection: an outdated technique in total knee arthroplasty. Orthopedics. 2008;31(9):940, 943–4.
24. Vajapey SP, Pettit RJ, Li M, Chen AF, Spitzer AI, Glassman AH. Risk factors for mid-flexion instability after total knee arthroplasty: a systematic review. J Arthroplasty. 2020;35(10):3046–54. (Epub 2020 May 21).
25. Valpiana P, Ghirardelli S, Valtanen RS, Risitano S, Iannotti F, Schaller C, Zepeda K, Engl M, Indelli PF. Biomechanical considerations for an easily-restricted robot-assisted kinematic alignment: a surgical technique note. Arthroplasty. 2023;5(1):29.
26. Koo S, Andriacchi TP. The knee joint center of rotation is predominantly on the lateral side during normal walking. J Biomech. 2008;41(6):1269–73.
27. Mikashima Y, Harman MK, Coburn J, Hodge WA, Banks SA. In vivo kinematics of an Acl-substituting knee arthroplasty during gait and stair activities. Orthop Proc. 2010;92-B(SUPP_I):120–1.
28. Insall J, Ranawat CS, Scott WN, Walker P (1976) Total condylar knee replacement: preliminary report. Clin Orthop Relat Res 120:149–154
29. Tanzer M, Smith K, Burnett S (2002) Posterior-stabilized versus cruciate-retaining total knee arthroplasty. Balancing the gap. J Arthroplasty 17:813–819
30. Matsumoto T, Muratsu H, Tsumura N, Mizuno K, Kurosaka M, Kuroda R (2009) Soft tissue balance measurement in posterior-stabilized total knee arthroplasty with a navigation system. J Arthroplasty 24(3):358–364
31. Hananouchi T, Yamamoto K, Ando W, Fudo K, Ohzono K (2012) The intraoperative gap difference (flexion gap minus extension gap) is altered by insertion of the trial femoral component. Knee 19(5):601–605
32. Hananouchi T, Nakamura N, Kakimoto A, Yohsikawa H, Sugano N (2008) CT-based planning of a single-radius femoral component in total knee arthroplasty using the ROBODOC system. Comput Aided Surg 13(1):23–29
33. Okamoto S, Mizu-uchi H, Okazaki K, Hamai S, Tashiro Y, Nakahara H, et al. Two-dimensional planning can result in internal rotation of the femoral component in total knee arthroplasty. Knee Surg Sports Traumatol Arthrosc. 2016;24(1):229–35 (Epub 20141009).
34. Tanzer M, Makhdom AM. Preoperative planning in primary total knee arthroplasty. J Am Acad Orthop Surg. 2016;24(4):220–30 (Epub 2016/03/19).
35. Wu PH, Zhang ZQ, Gu MH, Zhao XY, Kang Y, Liao WM, et al. Radiographic measurement of femoral lateral bowing and distal femoral condyle resection thickness: variances and effects on total knee arthroplasty planning. Chin Med J (Engl). 2017;130(21):2557–62.
36. Kobayashi A, Ishii Y, Takeda M, Noguchi H, Higuchi H, Toyabe S. Comparison of analog 2D and digital 3D preoperative templating for predicting implant size in total knee arthroplasty. Comput Aided Surg. 2012;17(2):96–101 (Epub 20120206).

37. Hyer JM, White S, Cloyd J, Dillhoff M, Tsung A, Pawlik TM, et al. Can We Improve Prediction of Adverse Surgical Outcomes? Development of a Surgical Complexity Score Using a Novel Machine Learning Technique. J Am Coll Surg. 2020;230(1):43–52 e1 (Epub 2019/11/02).
38. Groot OQ, Bongers MER, Ogink PT, Senders JT, Karhade AV, Bramer JAM, et al. Does artificial intelligence outperform natural intelligence in interpreting musculoskeletal radiological studies? A systematic review. Clin Orthop Rclat Res. 2020;478(12):2751–64 (Epub 2020/08/03).
39. Picard F, Deakin AH, Riches PE, Deep K, Baines J. Computer assisted orthopaedic surgery: past, present and future. Med Eng Phys. 2019;72:55–65 (Epub 2019/09/27).
40. Jamshidi A, Pelletier JP, Martel-Pelletier J. Machine-learning-based patient-specific prediction models for knee osteoarthritis. Nat Rev Rheumatol. 2019;15(1):49–60.
41. Karnuta JM, Navarro SM, Haeberle HS, Helm JM, Kamath AF, Schaffer JL, et al. Predicting Inpatient Payments Prior to Lower Extremity Arthroplasty Using Deep Learning: Which Model Architecture Is Best? J Arthroplasty. 2019;34(10):2235–41 e1 Epub 2019/06/25.
42. Ramkumar PN, Karnuta JM, Navarro SM, Haeberle HS, Scuderi GR, Mont MA, et al. Deep learning preoperatively predicts value metrics for primary total knee arthroplasty: development and validation of an artificial neural network model. J Arthroplasty. 2019;34(10):2220–7 e1 (Epub 2019/07/10).
43. Victor J (2009) Rotational alignment of the distal femur: a literature review. Orthop Traumatol Surg Res 95(5):365–372
44. Lombardi AV Jr, Berend KR, Aziz-Jacobo J, Davis MB (2008) Balancing the flexion gap: relationship between tibial slope and posterior cruciate ligament release and correlation with range of motion. J Bone Joint Surg Am 90(Suppl 4):121–132. https://doi.org/10.2106/JBJS.H.00685
45. Peters CL, Jimenez C, Erickson J, Anderson MB, Pelt CE (2013) Lessons learned from selective soft-tissue release for gap balancing in primary total knee arthroplasty: an analysis of 1216 consecutive total knee arthroplasties: AAOS exhibit selection. J Bone Joint Surg Am 95(20):e152. https://doi.org/10.2106/JBJS.L.01686
46. Gu, Y., Roth, J. D., Howell, S. M., et al. (2014). How frequently do four methods for mechanically aligning a total knee arthroplasty cause collateral ligament imbalance and change alignment from normal in white patients? AAOS exhibit selection. *The Journal of Bone and Joint Surgery, 96*, e101.
47. Whiteside LA, Arima J (1995) The anteroposterior axis for femoral rotational alignment in valgus total knee arthroplasty. Clin Orthop Relat Res 321:168–172
48. Akagi M, Oh M, Nonaka T, Tsujimoto H et al (2004) An anteroposterior axis of the tibia for total knee arthroplasty. Clin Orthop Relat Res 420:213–219
49. Clemens U, Miehke RK (2005) Advanced navigation planning including soft tissue management. Orthopedics. 28(Suppl):s1259–s1262

50. Vail TP, Lang JE (2006) Surgical techniques and instrumentation in total knee arthroplasty. In: Windsor RE, Scott WN (eds) Surgery of the knee, 4th edn. Churchill Livingstone, New York, p 1516
51. Sriphirom P, Raungthong N, Chutchawan P, Thiranon C, Sukandhavesa N (2012) Influence of a secondary downsizing of the femoral component on the extension gap: a cadaveric study. Orthopedics 35(10 Suppl):56–59. https://doi.org/10.3928/01477447-20120919-59
52. Chaiyakit P, Meknavin S, Hongku N (2009) Effects of posterior cruciate ligament resection in total knee arthroplasty using computer assisted surgery. J Med Assoc Thai 92(Suppl 6):S80–S84
53. Baldini A, Scuderi GR, Aglietti P, Chalnick D, Insall JN (2004) Flexion–extension gap changes during total knee arthroplasty. Effect of posterior cruciate ligament and posterior Osteophytes removal. J Knee Surg 17(2):69–72
54. Minoda Y, Sakawa A, Aihara M, Tada K, Kadoya Y, Kobayashi A (2007) Flexion gap preparation opens the extension gap in posterior cruciate ligament-retaining TKA. Knee Surg Sports Traumatol Arthrosc 15(11):1321–1325. https://doi.org/10.1007/500167-007-0394-9
55. Seo SS, Kim CW, Seo JH, Kim DH, Kim OG, Lee CR (2017) Effects of resection of posterior condyles of femur on extension gap of knee joint in total knee arthroplasty. J Arthroplast 32(60):1819–1823. https://doi.org/10.1016/j.arth.2017.01.042
56. Griffin FM, Insall JN, Scuderi GR (2000) Accuracy of soft tissue balancing in total knee arthroplasty. J Arthroplasty 15(8):970–973. https://doi.org/10.1054/arth.2000.6503
57. Nowakowski AM, Majewski M, Muller-Gerbl M, Valderrabano V (2012) Measurement of knee joint gaps without bone resection: "physiologic" extension and flexion gaps in total knee arthroplasty are asymmetric and unequal and anterior and posterior cruciate ligament resections produce different gap changes. J Orthop Res 30(4):522–527
58. Freeman MA, Pinskerova V. The movement of the normal tibio-femoral joint. J Biomech. 2005;38(2):197–208.
59. Matsumoto T, Muratsu H, Tsumura N, Mizuno K, Kuroda R, Yoshiya S, Kurosaka M (2006) Joint gap kinematics in posterior-stabilized total knee arthroplasty measured by a new tensor with the navigation system. J Biomech Eng 128(6):867–871. https://doi.org/10.1115/1.2354201
60. Matsumoto T, Kuroda R, Kubo S, Muratsu H, Mizuno K, Kurosaka M (2009) The intra-operative joint gap in cruciate-retaining compared with posterior-stabilised total knee replacement. J Bone Joint Surg (Br) 91(4):475–480
61. Liu D, Graham D, Gillies K, Gillies RM (2014) Effects of tourniquet use on quadriceps function and pain in total knee arthroplasty. Knee Surg Relat Res 26:207–213. https://doi.org/10.5792/ksrr.2014.26.4.207
62. Dennis DA, Kittelson AJ, Yang CC, Miner TM, Kim RH, Stevens-Lapsley JE (2016) Does tourniquet use in TKA affect recovery of lower extremity strength and function? A randomized trial. Clin Orthop Relat Res 474:69–77. https://doi.org/10.1007/s11999-015-4393-8

63. Ejaz A, Laursen AC, Kappel A, Laursen MB, Jakobsen T, Rasmussen S, Nielsen PT (2014) Faster recovery without the use of a tourniquet in total knee arthroplasty. Acta Orthop 85:422–426. https://doi.org/10.3109/17453674.2014.931197
64. Liu Y, Si H, Zeng Y, Li M, Xie H, Shen B (2020) More pain and slower functional recovery when a tourniquet is used during total knee arthroplasty. Knee Surg Sports Traumatol Arthrosc 28:1842–1860. https://doi.org/10.1007/s00167-019-05617-w
65. Kubosaka M, Ishida K, Sasaki H, Shibanuma N, Kuroda R, Matsumoto T (2017) Effect of suture and tourniquet on intraoperative kinematics in navigated total knee arthroplasty. J Arthroplasty 32(6):1824–1828. https://doi.org/10.1016/j.arth.2017.01.033
66. Nakano N, Matsumoto T, Muratsu H, Takayama K, Kuroda R, Kurosaka M (2016) Postoperative knee flexion angle is affected by lateral laxity in cruciate-retaining total knee arthroplasty. J Arthroplasty 31(2):401–405. https://doi.org/10.1016/j.arth.2015.09.028
67. Yoon JR, Yang JH (2018) Satisfactory short-term results of navigation-assisted gap-balancing total knee arthroplasty using ultracongruent insert. J Arthroplasty 33(3):723–728. https://doi.org/10.1016/j.arth.2017.09.049
68. Jang SW, Koh IJ, Kim MS, Kim JY, In Y (2016) Semimembranosus release for medial soft tissue balancing does not weaken knee flexion strength in patients undergoing varus total knee arthroplasty. J Arthroplasty 31(11):2481–2486. https://doi.org/10.1016/j.arth.2016.04.022
69. Jawhar A, Hutter K, Scharf HP (2016) Outcome in total knee arthroplasty with a medial-lateral balanced versus unbalanced gap. J Orthop Surg (Hong Kong) 24(3):298–301. https://doi.org/10.1177/1602400305
70. Matsuzaki T, Matsumoto T, Kubo S, Muratsu H, Matsushita T, Kawakami Y, Ishida K, Oka S, Kuroda R, Kurosaka M (2014) Tibial internal rotation is affected by lateral laxity in cruciate-retaining total knee arthroplasty: an intraoperative kinematic study using a navigation system and offset-type tensor. Knee Surg Sports Traumatol Arthrosc 22(3):615–620. https://doi.org/10.1007/s00167-013-2627-4
71. Matziolis G, Pfiel S, Wassilew G, Boenicke H, Perka C (2011) Kinematic analysis of the flexion axis for correct femoral component placement. Knee Surg Sports Traumatol Arthrosc 19(9):1504–1509
72. Victor J, Dujardin J, Vandenneucker H, Arnout N, Bellemans J (2014) Patient-specific instrumentations do not improve accuracy in total knee arthroplasty: a prospective randomized controlled trial. Clin Orthop Relat Res 472(1):263–271
73. Fitz W, Jager S, Rieger JS, Seebach E, Bitsch RG (2015) Femoral rotation in total knee arthroplasty: a comparison of patient individualized jigs with gap balancing in relation to anatomic landmarks. Knee Surg Sports Traumatol Arthrosc. https://doi.org/10.1007/s00167-015-3836-9

74. Sassoon A, Nam D, Nunley R, Barrack R (2015) Systematic review of patient-specific instrumentation in total knee arthroplasty: new but not improved. Clin Orthop Relat Res 473(1):151–158
75. Becker R, Malzdorf M, Starke C, Randolf P, Lohmann C (2012) No difference between tibia-first and femur-first techniques in TKA using computer-assisted surgery. Knee Surg Sports Traumatol Arthrosc 20(10):2011–2016. https://doi.org/10.1007/s00167-012-1928-3
76. Pang HN, Yeo SJ, Chong HC, Chin PL, Ong J, Lo NN (2011) Computer-assisted gap balancing technique improves outcome in total knee arthroplasty, compared with conventional measured resection technique. Knee Surg Sports Traumatol Arthrosc 19(9):1496–1503. https://doi.org/10.1007/s00167-011-1483-3
77. Dossett HG, Swartz GJ, Estrada NA, LeFevre GW, Kwasman BG (2012) Kinematically versus mechanically aligned total knee arthroplasty. Orthopedics 35(2):e160–e169
78. Dennis DA. Measured resection: an outdated technique in total knee arthroplasty. Orthopedics. 2008;31(940):43–4.
79. Blakeney W, Beaulieu Y, Puliero B, Kiss MO, Vendittoli PA. Bone resection for mechanically aligned total knee arthroplasty creates frequent gap modifications and imbalances. Knee Surg Sports Traumatol Arthrosc. 2020;28:1532–41.
80. Koskinen E, Eskelinen A, Paavolainen P, Pulkkinen P, Remes V. Comparison of survival and cost-effectiveness between unicondylar arthroplasty and total knee arthroplasty in patients with primary osteoarthritis: a follow-up study of 50,493 knee replacements from the Finnish Arthroplasty Register. Acta Orthop. 2008;79:499–507.
81. Akizuki S, Horiuchi H. Measured (anatomical reference) resection technique for cruciate-retaining total knee arthroplasty. In: Matsuda S, Lustig S, Van Der Merwe W, editors. Soft tissue balancing in total knee arthroplasty. Berlin: Springer; 2017. p. 49–57.
82. Wood AR, Rabbani TA, Sheffer B, Wagner RA, Sanchez HB. Protecting the PCL during total knee arthroplasty using a bone island technique. J Arthroplasty. 2018;33:102–6.
83. Kobayashi H, Akamatsu Y, Kumagai K, Kusayama Y, Ishigatsubo R, Muramatsu S, Saito T. The surgical epicondylar axis is a consistent reference of the distal femur in the coronal and axial planes. Knee Surg Sports Traumatol Arthrosc. 2014;22:2947–53.
84. Lee JK, Lee S, Chun SH, Kim KT, Lee MC. Rotational alignment of femoral component with different methods in total knee arthroplasty: a randomized, controlled trial. BMC Musculoskelet Disord. 2017;18:1–7.
85. Insall JN, Binazzi R, Soudry M, Mestriner LA. Total knee arthroplasty. Clin Orthop Relat Res. 1985(192):13–22.
86. Oussedik S, Abdel MP, Victor J, Pagnano MW, Haddad FS. Alignment in total knee arthroplasty. Bone Joint J. 2020;102–b(3):276–9.

87. Clark GW, Esposito CI, Wood D. Individualized functional knee alignment in total knee arthroplasty: a robotic-assisted technique. Techniques Orthop. 2022;37(3):185–91.
88. Shatrov J, Battelier C, Sappey-Marinier E, Gunst S, Servien E, Lustig S. Functional alignment philosophy in total knee arthroplasty - rationale and technique for the varus morphotype using a CT based robotic platform and individualized planning. Sicot j. 2022;8:11.
89. Deckey DG, Rosenow CS, Verhey JT, Brinkman JC, Mayfield CK, Clarke HD et al. Robotic-assisted total knee arthroplasty improves accuracy and precision compared to conventional techniques. Bone Joint J. 2021;103-b(6 Supple A):74–80.
90. Rossi SMP, Benazzo F. Individualized alignment and ligament balancing technique with the ROSA® robotic system for total knee arthroplasty. Int Orthop. 2023;47(3):755–62.
91. Murphy GT, Shatrov J, Duong J, Fritsch BA. How does the use of quantified gap-balancing affect component positioning and limb alignment in robotic total knee arthroplasty using functional alignment philosophy? A comparison of two robotic platforms. Int Orthop. 2023;47(5):1221–32.
92. Mancino F, Rossi SMP, Sangaletti R, Caredda M, Terragnoli F, Benazzo F. Increased accuracy in component positioning using an image-less robotic arm system in primary total knee arthroplasty: a retrospective study. Arch Orthop Trauma Surg. 2024;144(1):393–404.
93. Bollars P, Meshram P, Al Thani S, Schotanus MGM, Albelooshi A. Achieving functional alignment in total knee arthroplasty: early experience using a second-generation imageless semi-autonomous handheld robotic sculpting system. Int Orthop. 2023;47(2):585–93.
94. Almaawi AM, Hutt JRB, Masse V, Lavigne M, Vendittoli PA. The impact of mechanical and restricted kinematic alignment on knee anatomy in Total knee Arthroplasty. J Arthroplast. 2017;32(7):2133–40.
95. Aunan E, Kibsgård TJ, Diep LM, Röhrl SM. Intraoperative ligament laxity influences functional outcome 1 year after total knee arthroplasty. Knee Surg Sports Traumatol Arthrosc. 2015;23(6):1684–92.
96. Fickert, S.; Jawhar, A.; Sunil, P.; Scharf, H.-P Precision of Ci-navigated extension and flexion gap balancing in total knee arthroplasty and analysis of potential predictive variables. Archives of Orthopaedic and Trauma Surgery (2011). https://doi.org/10.1007/s00402-011-1419-x
97. Hu, Yanhui; Song, Da; Liu, Yi; Zhao, Yong; Ma, Wenpu; Yang, Yiqun; Yuan, Zhenfeng Spacer-based gap balancing is useful in total knee arthroplasty: a 3-year follow-up of a retrospective study. Journal of Orthopaedic Surgery and Research (2021). https://doi.org/10.1186/s13018-021-02788-6
98. Migliorini, Filippo; Eschweiler, Jörg; Mansy, Yasser El; Quack, Valentin; Schenker, Hanno; Tingart, Markus; Driessen, Arne Gap balancing versus measured resection for primary total knee arthroplasty: a meta-analysis study. Archives of Orthopaedic and Trauma Surgery (2020). 10.1007/s00402-020-03478-4

99. Valpiana, Pieralberto; Salvi, Andrea Giordano; Ghirardelli, Stefano; Bernardi, Matteo; Petralia, Giuseppe; Aloisi, Giuseppe; Schaller, Christian; Indelli, Pier Francesco Asymmetric gap balancing improves knee kinematic following primary total knee arthroplasty. Arthroplasty (2024). https://doi.org/10.1186/s42836-024-00243-5
100. Hananouchi, Takehito Sagittal gap balancing with the concept of a single radius femoral component in posterior cruciate sacrificing total knee arthroplasty with patient-specific instrumentation. International Orthopaedics (2014). https://doi.org/10.1007/s00264-014-2536-2
101. Zhang, Zhuo; Luo, Yang; Zhang, Chong; Wang, Xin; Zhang, Tianwei; Zhang, Guoqiang Prediction of gap balancing based on 2-D radiography in total knee arthroplasty for knee osteoarthritis patients. Arthroplasty (2023). https://doi.org/10.1186/s42836-023-00218-y
102. Grifka, Joachim; Baier, Clemens; Maderbacher, Günther Improved femoral component rotation in total knee arthroplasty: an anatomical study with optimized gap balancing. Archives of Orthopaedic and Trauma Surgery (2020). https://doi.org/10.1007/s00402-020-03557-6
103. Sriphirom, Pornpavit; Siramanakul, Chaiyaporn; Chanopas, Boonyawat; Boonruksa, Sirisuk Effects of posterior condylar osteophytes on gap balancing in computer-assisted total knee arthroplasty with posterior cruciate ligament sacrifice. European Journal of Orthopaedic Surgery & Traumatology (2018). https://doi.org/10.1007/s00590-017-2118-2
104. Nowakowski, Andrej Maria; Kamphausen, Marcus; Pagenstert, Geert; Valderrabano, Victor; Müller-Gerbl, Magdalena Influence of tibial slope on extension and flexion gaps in total knee arthroplasty: increasing the tibial slope affects both gaps. International Orthopaedics (2014). https://doi.org/10.1007/s00264-014-2373-3
105. Matsui, Yoshio; Matsuura, Masanori; Hidaka, Noriaki The knee position at tourniquet inflation does not affect the gap balancing during total knee arthroplasty. Archives of Orthopaedic and Trauma Surgery (2021). https://doi.org/10.1007/s00402-021-04017-5
106. Hommel, Hagen; Abdel, Matthew P.; Perka, Carsten Kinematic femoral alignment with gap balancing and patient-specific instrumentation in total knee arthroplasty: a randomized clinical trial. European Journal of Orthopaedic Surgery & Traumatology (2016). https://doi.org/10.1007/s00590-016-1865-9
107. Abdel, Matthew P. Measured Resection Versus Gap Balancing for Total Knee Arthroplasty. Clinical Orthopaedics and Related Research® (2014). https://doi.org/10.1007/s11999-014-3524-y
108. Xuequan, Zhao; Bin, Zhao; Shuzhang, Yao; Kanduo, Cao; Chongxi, Ren Measurement for gap balancing technique in patients undergoing total knee arthroplasty: a large retrospective observational study. Journal of Orthopaedic Surgery and Research (2022). https://doi.org/10.1186/s13018-022-03104-6
109. Tsai, Hung-Kang; Bao, Zhengyuan; Wu, Dengxian; Han, Jing; Jiang, Qing; Xu, Zhihong A new gap balancing technique with functional alignment in total knee arthroplasty using the MAKO robotic arm system: a preliminary study. BMC Surgery (2024). https://doi.org/10.1186/s12893-024-02524-x

6.4 The Patella—Resurface or Not

Machine Generated Summaries

Disclaimer: The summaries in this chapter were generated from Springer Nature publications using abstractive AI auto-summarization: An abstraction-based summarizer creates new text based on deep learning. New phrases are created to summarize the content. As the constituted sentences are machine selected, they may not fully reflect the body of the work, so we strongly advise that the original content is read and cited. The auto-generated summaries were curated by the editor to meet Springer Nature publication standards.

6.4.1 Patellar Resurfacing Complications in Total Knee Arthroplasty [149]

This is a machine-generated summary of:

Schiavone Panni, Alfredo; Cerciello, Simone; Del Regno, Chiara; Felici, Alessandro; Vasso, Michele Patellar resurfacing complications in total knee arthroplasty [149].

Published in: International Orthopaedics (2013).

Link to original: https://doi.org/10.1007/s00264-013-2244-3

If you want to cite the papers, please refer to the original.

For technical reasons we could not place the page where the original quote is coming from.

6.4.1.1 Research Highlights

Total knee arthroplasty (TKA) is a widely performed procedure for treating advanced knee joint arthritis, offering satisfactory long-term outcomes. However, early designs without patellar replacement were linked to complications such as anterior knee pain and patellar maltracking. These issues led to the development of tricompartmental replacements that included patellar resurfacing, though this approach also introduced new complications. The study by Panni et al. examines the outcomes of patellar resurfacing in TKA, aiming to address the ongoing debate over its necessity and effectiveness.

The study retrospectively analysed a series of total knee prostheses implanted using a consistent technique with posterior-stabilized NexGen Zimmer prostheses(Zimmer Biomet, Warsaw, Indiana, USA). The researchers reviewed patient charts to determine the percentage of patellar resurfacing and conducted follow-up examinations, including physical assessments, Hospital for Special Surgery scores, X-ray analyses, and computed tomography scans in selected cases. Out of 280 patients available for follow-up at an average FU of 96 (58–144) months post-operatively, the study found that while most patients had satisfactory outcomes, some experienced anterior knee pain and patellofemoral complications. In cases where conservative treatment was insufficient, further surgical interventions were performed to address issues like patellar maltracking or instability.

The findings suggest that while patellar resurfacing can reduce the risk of reoperation compared to retaining the native patella, it does not necessarily eliminate anterior knee pain or improve patient satisfaction significantly. The study highlights the importance of precise surgical technique and careful patient selection to minimize complications associated with patellar resurfacing. Future study could focus on refining surgical methods and exploring alternative approaches to improve outcomes for patients undergoing TKA. The results contribute to the ongoing discussion about the best practices for managing the patella during knee arthroplasty, emphasizing that decisions should be tailored to individual patient needs and circumstances.

6.4.2 Patellar Resurfacing as a Second Stage Procedure for Persistent Anterior Knee Pain After Primary Total Knee Arthroplasty [150]

This is a machine-generated summary of:

Daniilidis, Kiriakos; Vogt, Bjoern; Gosheger, Georg; Henrichs, Marcel; Dieckmann, Ralf; Schulz, Dino; Hoell, Steffen Patellar resurfacing as a second stage procedure for persistent anterior knee pain after primary total knee arthroplasty [150].

Published in: International Orthopaedics (2012).

Link to original: https://doi.org/10.1007/s00264-011-1463-8

If you want to cite the papers, please refer to the original.

For technical reasons we could not place the page where the original quote is coming from.

6.4.2.1 Research Highlights

Total knee arthroplasty (TKA) is a widely used and effective procedure for treating primary osteoarthritis of the knee. However, the management of persistent anterior knee pain (AKP) following TKA remains a significant challenge, with rotational alignment of the tibial and femoral components playing a crucial role in patellar tracking and clinical outcomes. Despite numerous studies on TKA, there is limited information on the treatment of AKP, particularly regarding the long-term outcomes of secondary patellar resurfacing. The study by Daniilidis et al. aims to evaluate the clinical outcomes of secondary patellar resurfacing in patients experiencing persistent AKP after TKA.

The study retrospectively reviewed patients who underwent secondary isolated patellar resurfacing using Genesis I/II components (Smith and Nephew, Memphis, Tenn., USA). The average age of participants was 68 years, with a mean follow-up period of 24 months. Inclusion criteria required persistent AKP post-TKA without improvement from conservative therapy. Pre- and postoperative X-rays were conducted to assess patellar alignment, and patients with mechanical disorders or infections were excluded. Surgical procedures were performed using standard techniques, allowing full weight-bearing postoperatively. Clinical outcomes were assessed using the Knee Society Score (KSS) and a custom-made satisfaction questionnaire. Results indicated significant improvements in both KSS and functional scores; however, patient satisfaction varied, with eight patients satisfied and six dissatisfied due to persistent AKP.

The study highlights that while secondary patellar resurfacing can improve clinical scores, patient satisfaction is not guaranteed, as some continue to experience pain without identifiable causes. The findings suggest that the decision to perform patellar resurfacing should be carefully considered on an individual basis. Future study could focus on identifying specific criteria for patient selection to optimize outcomes and further investigate the potential benefits of primary patellar resurfacing during initial TKA procedures to prevent revision surgeries for AKP.

6.4.3 A Prospective Evaluation of a Largely Cementless Total Knee Arthroplasty Cohort without Patellar Resurfacing: 10-Year Outcomes and Survivorship [151]

This is a machine-generated summary of:

Napier, Richard J.; O'Neill, Christopher; O'Brien, Seamus; Doran, Emer; Mockford, Brian; Boldt, Jens; Beverland, David E. A prospective evaluation of a largely cementless total knee arthroplasty cohort without patellar resurfacing: 10-year outcomes and survivorship [151].

Published in: BMC Musculoskeletal Disorders (2018).

Link to original: https://doi.org/10.1186/s12891-018-2128-1

If you want to cite the papers, please refer to the original.

For technical reasons we could not place the page where the original quote is coming from.

6.4.3.1 Research Highlights

The theoretical benefits of a rotating platform design in Total Knee Arthroplasty (TKA) are well-documented, with the aim of increasing articular surface congruity to reduce polyethylene wear and using a mobile bearing to minimize constraint forces, potentially leading to greater long-term survivorship. Despite these theoretical advantages, such benefits have not been conclusively demonstrated in the literature. Additionally, while cemented fixation for TKA is known for excellent long-term survivorship, cementless fixation offers benefits like shorter surgical time and reduced infection rates. A recent Cochrane review suggested that good early fixation could significantly reduce the risk of later aseptic loosening. The study by Napier et al. evaluates the performance of a rotating platform TKA using predominantly cementless fixation without patellar resurfacing over a minimum 5-year follow-up period.

The study was conducted prospectively at a regional orthopedic center, recruiting patients scheduled for primary TKA between March 2010 and January 2012. Exclusion criteria included previous knee surgery or inability to give informed consent. All patients received an LCS Complete Rotating Platform TKA (DePuy Syntheses, Johnson and Johnson, Warsaw, Indiana, USA) without patellar resurfacing, performed under the care of the senior author. The surgical approach focused on achieving a balanced knee through bone cuts rather than soft tissue releases. Hybrid fixation with a cemented tibia was initially used in female patients with valgus deformities due to concerns about early post-operative tibial insufficiency fractures. Patients were mobilized full weight-bearing on the first post-operative day and reviewed at regular intervals post-operatively for clinical and radiographic assessments. The study assessed clinical outcomes using Oxford Knee Scores and Bartlett Patellar Scores, alongside quality-of-life measures.

The study found significant improvements in all outcome measures from pre-operative to 5-year follow-up, including patellar scores and pain scores. Radiographic analysis showed no progressive radiolucent lines (RLLs) in femoral zones, indicating excellent femoral component fixation. While some RLLs were observed in cementless tibial components, they were non-progressive and often resolved over time. The cumulative implant survivorship was 97% at 5 years when excluding revisions due to infection. This study supports the use of non-cemented porous coated fixation without patellar resurfacing using a non-posterior stabilized mobile bearing TKA, suggesting excellent medium-term survivorship with potential for superior long-term outcomes compared to cemented TKA. Future studies could further explore the long-term benefits and cost-effectiveness of cementless versus cemented TKA approaches.

6.4.4 Isolated Effects of Patellar Resurfacing in Total Knee Arthroplasty and Their Relation to Native Patellar Geometry [152]

This is a machine-generated summary of:

Sauer, Adrian; Thorwaechter, Christoph; Dupraz, Ingrid; Maas, Allan; Steinbrueck, Arnd; Grupp, Thomas M.; Woiczinski, Matthias Isolated effects of patellar resurfacing in total knee arthroplasty and their relation to native patellar geometry [152].

Published in: Scientific Reports (2022).

Link to original: https://doi.org/10.1038/s41598-022-16810-2

If you want to cite the papers, please refer to the original.

For technical reasons we could not place the page where the original quote is coming from.

6.4.4.1 Research Highlights

In total knee arthroplasty (TKA), the decision to resurface the patella remains a contentious issue, with evidence suggesting that resurfacing can enhance clinical outcomes and reduce the likelihood of revision surgery. However, understanding the isolated effects of patellar resurfacing on knee kinematics is challenging due to individual variations in patient kinematics. The study by Sauer et al. investigates these effects by examining patellar kinematics in an in vitro setup using two different posterior-stabilized implant variants.

The study utilized eight fresh-frozen specimens with minimal varus or valgus deformities. The researchers employed a well-established weight-bearing knee rig to simulate squatting movements while measuring patello-femoral kinematics using an ultrasonic measurement system. The specimens underwent testing both before and after patellar resurfacing, with posterior-stabilized implants placed using a tibia-first technique. The study focused on relative kinematics to isolate the effects of resurfacing from individual specimen differences. A linear regression model was used to analyze the relationship between lateral patellar facet angle and changes in patellar shift post-resurfacing.

The findings revealed that patellar resurfacing significantly influenced patellar shift, resulting in more medial tracking compared to the native state. This shift was associated with the lateral patellar facet angle, explaining a portion of the variance observed. The study suggests that considering native patellar geometry could inform optimal medio-lateral positioning of the patellar implant to minimize deviations from natural kinematics. Future study could explore how these findings can be integrated into clinical workflows to improve surgical outcomes in TKA, particularly for patients with pronounced asymmetry in their patellar facets.

6.4.5 The Effect of Patellar Facet Angle on Patellofemoral Alignment and Arthritis Progression in Posterior-Stabilized Total Knee Arthroplasty Without Patellar Resurfacing [153]

This is a machine-generated summary of:

Kim, Chang-Wan; Lee, Chang-Rack; Huh, Tae-Yung The effect of patellar facet angle on patellofemoral alignment and arthritis progression in posterior-stabilized total knee arthroplasty without patellar resurfacing [153].

Published in: Knee Surgery & Related Research (2020).

Link to original: https://doi.org/10.1186/s43019-020-00045-4

If you want to cite the papers, please refer to the original.

For technical reasons we could not place the page where the original quote is coming from.

6.4.5.1 Research Highlights

Anterior knee pain remains a prevalent issue among patients undergoing total knee arthroplasty (TKA), particularly when the patella is retained. Despite advancements in implant design and surgical techniques aimed at reducing this pain, dissatisfaction persists, suggesting that factors beyond surgery and prosthesis may contribute to the problem. Patient-specific anatomical differences, such as variations in patellar shape, have been proposed as potential contributors to anterior knee pain. The study by Kim et al. investigates the impact of patellar facet angle on pre- and postoperative outcomes in posterior-stabilized (PS) TKA without patellar resurfacing.

The study involved a cohort of patients who underwent PS TKA for varus osteoarthritic knees, excluding those with valgus alignment or other complicating factors. Patients were divided into two groups based on their patellar facet angle: Group A with angles greater than 130° and Group B with angles less than or equal to 130°. The researchers assessed radiologic parameters such as the Kellgren-Lawrence grade, Insall-Salvati ratio, and patellar tilt angle, alongside clinical outcomes like range of motion and patient-reported outcomes (PROs). The study found that while a narrow patellar facet angle was associated with greater preoperative patellar tilt, it did not significantly affect postoperative radiologic or clinical outcomes.

The findings suggest that the patellar shape, as measured by the facet angle, does not have a significant impact on the outcomes of PS TKA when soft tissue balancing and implant placement are appropriately managed. This challenges previous assumptions about the role of patellar shape in postoperative complications. Future study could focus on longer-term follow-up to assess changes in osteosclerosis progression and explore the effects of different implant designs. Additionally, further research could investigate whether these findings hold true across larger and more diverse patient populations to better understand the nuances of patient-specific factors in TKA outcomes.

6.4.6 A Randomized Controlled Trial Comparing Patellar Retention Versus Patellar Resurfacing in Primary Total Knee Arthroplasty: 5–10 Year Follow-Up [154]

This is a machine-generated summary of:

Beaupre, Lauren; Secretan, Charles; Johnston, DWC; Lavoie, Guy A Randomized controlled trial comparing patellar retention versus patellar resurfacing in primary total knee arthroplasty: 5–10 year follow-up [154].

Published in: BMC Research Notes (2012).

Link to original: https://doi.org/10.1186/1756-0500-5-273

If you want to cite the papers, please refer to the original.

For technical reasons we could not place the page where the original quote is coming from.

6.4.6.1 Research Highlights

Total knee arthroplasty (TKA) is a common surgical procedure for treating severe knee arthritis, yet the decision to resurface the patella during the initial surgery remains contentious. Surgeons typically choose between three strategies: never resurfacing, always resurfacing, or selectively resurfacing the patella. Despite numerous studies, no approach has been definitively proven superior. Current evidence is limited by study heterogeneity and short follow-up periods, often less than 5 years. The study by Beaupre et al. investigates long-term outcomes of patellar resurfacing versus retention in TKA patients, focusing on patient-reported pain, stiffness, and function over 10 years.

The study employed a double-blind randomized controlled trial design with 38 subjects undergoing primary TKA for non-inflammatory arthritis. Participants were randomly assigned to either a patellar resurfacing group or a non-resurfacing group using a computer-generated sequence. The Profix™ Total Knee System (Smith and nephew, Memphis, Tenn., USA) was used for all surgeries, ensuring consistency in surgical technique and postoperative care. Subjects were assessed preoperatively and at one, five, and 10 years postoperatively using the Western Ontario McMaster Osteoarthritis Index (WOMAC) and RAND-36 questionnaires. The primary outcomes were knee-specific pain, stiffness, and function as reported by patients. Secondary outcomes included revision rates and general health status.

The study found that both groups reported significant improvements in pain and function over time, with no major differences between them at 10 years postoperatively. However, approximately 8% of subjects who did not undergo patellar resurfacing required reoperation due to persistent anterior knee pain within the first 5 years. The findings suggest that while patient-reported outcomes provide valuable insights into long-term TKA performance, they may not fully capture surgical nuances. Future study should incorporate both patient-reported measures and direct surgical assessments to better understand the impact of different patellar management strategies in TKA.

6.4.7 Impact of Patellar Resurfacing on the Revision Rate in Total Knee Arthroplasty [155]

This is a machine-generated summary of:

Labek, Gerold; Liebensteiner, Michael; Williams, Alexandra; Thaler, Martin; Stöckl, Bernd Impact of patellar resurfacing on the revision rate in total knee arthroplasty [155].

Published in: European Orthopaedics and Traumatology (2010).

Link to original: https://doi.org/10.1007/s12570-010-0027-5

If you want to cite the papers, please refer to the original.

For technical reasons we could not place the page where the original quote is coming from.

6.4.7.1 Research Highlights

The debate over whether to resurface the patella during total knee arthroplasty (TKA) has persisted for years, with no global consensus on the best approach. While many guidelines and expert opinions favor patellar resurfacing, data from Scandinavian Arthroplasty Registers suggest a trend against it in practice. The study by Labek et al. examines the impact of patellar resurfacing on revision rates in TKA, aiming to assess the validity and reproducibility of published data and identify potential bias factors.

Labek et al. conducted a comprehensive literature analysis using the Medline database and manual searches to gather studies that clearly identified whether patellar replacement was performed. They included studies with calculable revision rate data published in English or German peer-reviewed journals. The analysis focused on 21 studies that provided information on re-operation rates for the patellar component. The researchers used a standardized methodology, calculating revisions per observed component years, a method employed by Australian and New Zealand Arthroplasty Registries, to compare data across different follow-up periods. This approach allowed them to adjust for varying risks of revision due to different follow-up durations. They also compared these findings with national arthroplasty register reports from Sweden and Australia to evaluate statistical significance and potential biases.

The study found that clinical studies often report higher revision rates for patients without primary patellar replacement compared to those with resurfacing. However, these results were not replicated in registry-based studies, which showed nearly identical revision rates between groups. The divergence was more pronounced in randomized controlled trials (RCTs) than in case-control or cohort studies. This research study suggests that comprehensive registry data may offer superior quality and reproducibility compared to clinical studies, including RCTs. Future study could focus on implant-specific evaluations using arthroplasty register datasets to better understand complications and revisions related to the patellar component. This could involve analysing combined supra-national datasets to account for specific national factors influencing outcomes.

6.4.8 Do we Need to Restore Patellar Thickness After Total Knee Arthroplasty with Patellar Resurfacing? [156]

This is a machine-generated summary of:

Tammachote, Nattapol; Kraisin, Teeramate; Kanitnate, Supakit Do we need to restore patellar thickness after total knee arthroplasty with patellar resurfacing? [156].

Published in: European Journal of Orthopaedic Surgery & Traumatology (2023).

Link to original: https://doi.org/10.1007/s00590-023-03607-w

If you want to cite the papers, please refer to the original.

For technical reasons we could not place the page where the original quote is coming from.

6.4.8.1 Research Highlights

Patellar resurfacing during total knee arthroplasty (TKA) is a debated practice among surgeons, with some opting for it to reduce reoperation rates and anterior knee pain, while others avoid it due to potential complications such as maltracking and patellar fracture. The restoration of native patellar thickness has been the gold standard, but this can increase fracture risk in patients with thin patellae. The study by Tammachote et al. investigates the effects of increased patellar thickness after subchondral bone resection on postoperative knee flexion and functional outcomes.

The study was conducted as a retrospective, single-center analysis at Thammasat University Hospital, involving patients who underwent primary TKA between October 2015 and February 2018. The researchers compared knees that underwent subchondral patellar bone resection with those that did not undergo resurfacing. All procedures were performed using a standardized surgical technique, including lateral facetectomy and cemented onlay all-polyethylene patellar components. Patellar thickness was measured intraoperatively using a Vernier caliper. The primary outcome was knee flexion angle, while secondary outcomes included the modified Western Ontario and McMaster University Osteoarthritis Index (WOMAC) scores and anterior knee pain assessed via a visual analog scale.

The study found that increasing patellar thickness by an average of 2 mm did not adversely affect post-operative knee flexion or functional outcomes as measured by WOMAC scores. Interestingly, patients in the non-resurfaced group reported more anterior knee pain post-operatively, with some requiring secondary resurfacing. This research suggests that moderate overstuffing of the patella does not compromise knee function or range of motion, potentially offering a viable approach for managing thin patellae during TKA.

6.4.9 Predictors for Secondary Patellar Resurfacing After Primary Total Knee Arthroplasty Using a "Patella-Friendly" Total Knee Arthroplasty System [157]

This is a machine-generated summary of:

Roessler, Philip P.; Moussa, Randa; Jacobs, Cornelius; Schüttler, Karl F.; Stein, Thomas; Schildberg, Frank A.; Wirtz, Dieter C. Predictors for secondary patellar resurfacing after primary total knee arthroplasty using a "patella-friendly" total knee arthroplasty system [157].

Published in: International Orthopaedics (2018).
Link to original: https://doi.org/10.1007/s00264-018-4075-8

If you want to cite the papers, please refer to the original.
For technical reasons we could not place the page where the original quote is coming from.

6.4.9.1 Research Highlights

Patellar resurfacing (PR) during total knee arthroplasty (TKA) remains a contentious issue in orthopedic surgery, with differing practices between the USA and Europe. While complications such as patella fractures and instability are associated with PR, anterior knee pain after TKA without PR is also prevalent. Previous studies have not adequately addressed surgery-related predictors for secondary patellar resurfacing (SPR) following TKA. The study by Roessler et al. aims to identify predictors for SPR after initial TKA, hypothesizing that proper TKA implantation and component positioning, along with maintained patellar geometry, could reduce the risk of SPR.

This is a retrospective case-control analysis involving patients who underwent SPR for persistent anterior knee pain after primary TKA using the Genesis II knee system (Smith and Nephew, Memphis, Tenn., USA). The researchers reviewed records of patients treated with primary TKA over a specified period, identifying 57 patients who required SPR. These patients were matched with controls who retained their primary TKA without revision. The study collected epidemiological and clinical data, and post-operative radiographs were analysed to assess potential predictors such as patella tilt, height, thickness, and delta angle. Statistical analyses, including Kaplan-Meier survival analysis and logistic regression, were employed to evaluate these predictors' significance.

The study identified patella tilt, width, thickness, and delta angle as significant predictors of SPR following primary TKA. These findings suggest that specific radiographic measurements can help predict the need for SPR, providing a rationale for preoperative patient selection to minimize revision rates. While intrinsic factors like body mass index did not prove significant in this model, the study highlights the importance of proper component positioning in reducing SPR risk.

6.4.10 Secondary Patellar Resurfacing Following Total Knee Arthroplasty [158]

This is a machine-generated summary of:

Scheurer, Philip; Reininga, Inge H. F.; van Jonbergen, Hans-Peter W.; van Raay, Jos J. A. M. Secondary patellar resurfacing following total knee arthroplasty [158].

Published in: International Orthopaedics (2015).

Link to original: https://doi.org/10.1007/s00264-015-2684-z

If you want to cite the papers, please refer to the original.

For technical reasons we could not place the page where the original quote is coming from.

6.4.10.1 Research Highlights

Anterior knee pain (AKP) is a common complication following total knee arthroplasty (TKA), with some studies reporting high incidence rates. Secondary patellar resurfacing (SPR) has been proposed as a solution for persistent AKP when the patella is not resurfaced during the initial TKA. However, existing literature on SPR is limited, with small and heterogeneous patient cohorts and varying prosthetic designs. A "hot" bone scan has been suggested as an indicator for SPR, potentially leading to favorable outcomes. The study by Scheurer et al. evaluates the mid-term clinical outcomes of SPR for persistent AKP, aiming to correlate these outcomes with clinical and radiological parameters, including bone scintigraphy.

The study involved patients who experienced persistent AKP after primary TKA with a PCL-retaining AGC knee prosthesis. The primary indication for TKA was osteoarthritis, and SPR was considered when AKP persisted without infection or malposition of components. Patients underwent SPR using a medial parapatellar arthrotomy, where the patella was resected and an AGC polyethylene patella button (Zimmer-Biomet, Warsaw, Indiana, USA) was cemented in place. Outcomes were assessed using the Knee injury and Osteoarthritis Outcome Score (KOOS) and Baldini score, alongside patient satisfaction surveys. The study found that satisfied patients had a longer interval between TKA and SPR compared to dissatisfied ones. A "cold" bone scan was associated with higher satisfaction rates following SPR.

The study highlights that SPR can lead to significant reductions in AKP, with most patients reporting satisfaction post-procedure. However, patellar tilt was more common among dissatisfied patients, suggesting its role in poor outcomes. The findings challenge the utility of a "hot" bone scan as an indicator for SPR success. Future study could explore the timing of SPR after TKA and its impact on outcomes further. Additionally, understanding the role of patellar tilt in patient dissatisfaction could guide surgical techniques to improve results. The study underscores the need for standardized protocols in evaluating candidates for SPR to enhance patient satisfaction and clinical outcomes.

6.4.11 The Efficacy of Patellar Decompression for Improving Anterior Knee Pain Following Total Knee Arthroplasty without Patellar Resurfacing [159]

This is a machine-generated summary of:

Lee, Gun Woo; Lee, Sun-Mi; Jang, Soo-Jin; Son, Jung-Hwan The efficacy of patellar decompression for improving anterior knee pain following total knee arthroplasty without patellar resurfacing [159].

Published in: Archives of Orthopaedic and Trauma Surgery (2013).

Link to original: https://doi.org/10.1007/s00402-013-1702-0

If you want to cite the papers, please refer to the original.

For technical reasons we could not place the page where the original quote is coming from.

6.4.11.1 Research Highlights

Total knee arthroplasty (TKA) is a widely used procedure for treating advanced knee joint arthritis, known for its durability and effectiveness. However, a significant number of patients experience persistent anterior knee pain post-surgery, often linked to issues with the patellofemoral joint. This has led to debates over whether to resurface or retain the patella during TKA. Anterior knee pain remains a poorly understood complication, with recent research shifting focus from structural causes to pathophysiologic factors like intraosseous hypertension. The study by Lee et al. explores an alternative treatment method aimed at reducing anterior knee pain following TKA without patellar resurfacing.

The study involved a clinical trial where patients undergoing primary total knee replacement were divided into two groups: one receiving standard TKA without patellar resurfacing and the other undergoing additional patellar decompression via drilling. All surgeries were performed by a single senior surgeon using consistent protocols. The decompression technique involved drilling the patella to alleviate intraosseous pressure, hypothesized to be a cause of anterior knee pain. Patients were evaluated using the Knee Society rating system and patient satisfaction scores, with follow-ups conducted over several years to assess outcomes such as pain levels and functional recovery.

The findings suggest that patellar decompression via drilling can effectively reduce anterior knee pain after TKA without resurfacing the patella. Patients in the decompression group reported lower rates of significant pain and higher satisfaction scores compared to those who did not receive this treatment. The study highlights the potential of this minimally invasive technique as a viable alternative to more traditional methods like patellar resurfacing, which can have complications. Future study could focus on further understanding the mechanisms behind intraosseous hypertension and refining decompression techniques to enhance patient outcomes in TKA procedures.

6.4.12 Does the Grading of Chondromalacia Patellae Influence Anterior Knee Pain Following Total Knee Arthroplasty without Patellar Resurfacing? [160]

This is a machine-generated summary of:

Zha, Guo-Chun; Feng, Shuo; Chen, Xiang-Yang; Guo, Kai-Jin Does the grading of chondromalacia patellae influence anterior knee pain following total knee arthroplasty without patellar resurfacing? [160].

Published in: International Orthopaedics (2017).

Link to original: https://doi.org/10.1007/s00264-017-3658-0

If you want to cite the papers, please refer to the original.

For technical reasons we could not place the page where the original quote is coming from.

6.4.12.1 Research Highlights

Total knee arthroplasty (TKA) is a common procedure for treating degenerative osteoarthritis, but there is no consensus on whether to resurface the patella during surgery. Some studies suggest that patellar resurfacing reduces anterior knee pain (AKP) and revision rates, while others associate it with higher postoperative complications. The role of chondromalacia patellae (CMP) grading in influencing AKP after TKA remains unclear, with conflicting evidence on whether CMP severity correlates with AKP incidence. The study by Zha et al. investigates the impact of different CMP gradings on AKP incidence following TKA without patellar resurfacing.

The study involved a retrospective analysis of patients with primary degenerative osteoarthritis who underwent TKA without patellar resurfacing. Patients were selected based on specific inclusion and exclusion criteria to ensure a homogeneous study group. The surgical procedure was standardized, involving a midline skin incision and medial parapatellar approach, with careful alignment of the femoral and tibial components. Intraoperative CMP grading was performed using the Outerbridge classification, and clinical outcomes were assessed using the Knee Society clinical scoring system. Postoperative evaluations included radiographic assessments and patient satisfaction surveys at a 12-month follow-up. Statistical analyses were conducted to compare outcomes across different CMP grades.

The study found no significant association between CMP grading and the incidence of postoperative AKP or patient satisfaction after TKA without patellar resurfacing. These findings suggest that factors other than CMP grading, such as prosthesis design, may play a more critical role in influencing AKP outcomes. Future study could explore the impact of prosthesis design on patellofemoral kinematics and its relationship with AKP. The authors note limitations such as the short follow-up period and the use of a single prosthesis type, which may affect the generalizability of the results. Further research could address these limitations by including longer follow-up periods and diverse prosthesis designs to validate these findings.

6.4.13 Is the Patient Aware of the Difference Between Resurfaced and Nonresurfaced Patella After Bilateral Total Knee Arthroplasty? A Systematic Review of Simultaneous Bilateral Randomized Trials [161]

This is a machine-generated summary of:

Choi, Keun Young; In, Yong; Kim, Man Soo; Sohn, Sueen; Koh, In Jun Is the patient aware of the difference between resurfaced and nonresurfaced patella after bilateral total knee arthroplasty? A systematic review of simultaneous bilateral randomized trials [161].

Published in: Knee Surgery & Related Research (2022).

Link to original: https://doi.org/10.1186/s43019-022-00133-7

6.4.13.1 Research Highlights

Total knee arthroplasty (TKA) is a common procedure for alleviating knee pain and improving function in patients with severe arthritis. However, the optimal management of the patella during TKA remains controversial, with three main approaches: patellar resurfacing (PR), non-resurfacing (NPR), and selective resurfacing. While some studies suggest that PR reduces anterior knee pain (AKP), others find no significant difference between PR and NPR, leading to ongoing debate among surgeons. The study by Choi et al. aims to address this uncertainty by comparing patella related patient-reported outcome measures (PROMs), clinical outcomes, and reoperation rates between PR and NPR in patients undergoing bilateral TKA.

The study conducted a comprehensive review of prospective randomized controlled trials (RCTs) that compared PR and NPR in single patients undergoing simultaneous bilateral TKA. The authors searched databases such as PubMed, MEDLINE, and EMBASE for English-language studies that reported on clinical and functional outcomes, radiologic findings, and complication rates related to patellar management. After applying strict inclusion criteria, six studies were selected for analysis. The review found that most studies reported no significant differences in AKP, global knee pain, side preference, or patient satisfaction between PR and NPR. Additionally, objective clinical outcomes such as range of motion (ROM), Knee Society Score (KSS), and Feller score showed no significant differences between the two approaches.

The findings suggest that patients undergoing bilateral TKA with different patellar management strategies are generally unaware of any differences between PR and NPR knees. Objective clinical outcomes were also similar across both groups. The study highlights the need for caution when interpreting higher reoperation rates in NPR groups, as these may be influenced by the option of secondary resurfacing for persistent AKP. Future study could focus on addressing heterogeneities in surgical techniques and implant designs to provide more definitive conclusions. Despite limitations such as small sample sizes and short follow-up periods in the included studies, this review provides valuable insights into the ongoing debate over patellar resurfacing in TKA.

6.4.14 The Predictive Factors of Secondary Patellar Resurfacing in Computer-Assisted Total Knee Arthroplasty. A Prospective Cohort Study [162]

This is a machine-generated summary of:

Franck, Florent; Ouanezar, Hervé; Jacquel, Alexandre; Pibarot, Vincent; Wegrzyn, Julien The predictive factors of secondary patellar resurfacing in computer-assisted total knee arthroplasty. A prospective cohort study [162].

Published in: International Orthopaedics (2017).

Link to original: https://doi.org/10.1007/s00264-017-3630-z

If you want to cite the papers, please refer to the original.

For technical reasons we could not place the page where the original quote is coming from.

6.4.14.1 Research Highlights

The decision to resurface the patella during total knee arthroplasty (TKA) is a topic of ongoing debate among orthopedic surgeons. While some advocate for routine resurfacing to reduce post-operative anterior knee pain (AKP) and avoid secondary procedures, others prefer selective resurfacing, citing potential complications such as patellar fracture and instability. Despite numerous studies, including registry analyses and meta-analyses, the benefits of routine resurfacing in terms of patient satisfaction and TKA outcomes remain inconclusive. The study by Franck et al. investigates the outcomes of computer-assisted surgery (CAS) TKA without patellar resurfacing in patients with primary knee osteoarthritis (OA), aiming to identify pre-operative factors that predict the need for secondary patellar resurfacing (SPR).

The study involved a prospective cohort of patients undergoing CAS TKA using a cementless ultra-congruent mobile-bearing system without patellar resurfacing. The researchers focused on evaluating the survivorship of the native patella and identifying predictive factors for SPR. They utilized a passive imageless navigation system to ensure precise alignment and balance during surgery. Pre-operative and post-operative evaluations included physical examinations, radiographic assessments, and specific scoring systems like the International Knee Society scores. The study found that certain pre-operative radiographic parameters—such as Wiberg stage patellar dysplasia, Iwano stage ≥2 PF OA, femoral sulcus angle >145°, and patellar lateralization >3 mm—were significantly associated with an increased risk of SPR.

The findings suggest that careful pre-operative assessment of patellofemoral (PF) parameters can guide decisions on whether to resurface the patella during TKA. Future study could focus on refining these predictive criteria to enhance surgical decision-making and improve patient outcomes. Additionally, while CAS techniques show promise in optimizing component alignment and PF balance, further research is needed to validate these findings across different TKA designs and surgical practices. The study underscores the importance of individualized treatment plans based on specific anatomical and pathological considerations rather than a one-size-fits-all approach to patellar resurfacing in TKA.

6.4.15 Clinical and Radiological Results of Cruciate-Retaining Total Knee Arthroplasty with the NexGen®-CR System: Comparison of Patellar Resurfacing Versus Retention with More Than 14 Years of Follow-Up [163]

This is a machine-generated summary of:

Chun, Keun Churl; Lee, Sung Hyun; Baik, Jong Seok; Kook, Seng Hwan; Han, Joung Kyue; Chun, Churl Hong Clinical and radiological results of cruciate-retaining total knee arthroplasty with the NexGen®-CR system: comparison of patellar resurfacing versus retention with more than 14 years of follow-up [163].

Published in: Journal of Orthopaedic Surgery and Research (2017).

Link to original: https://doi.org/10.1186/s13018-017-0646-4

If you want to cite the papers, please refer to the original.

For technical reasons we could not place the page where the original quote is coming from.

6.4.15.1 Research Highlights

Total knee arthroplasty (TKA) is a common surgical procedure aimed at alleviating pain and improving joint function in patients with severe knee problems. The decision to retain or resect the posterior cruciate ligament (PCL) during TKA has been debated, as retaining the PCL can enhance knee stability and proprioception. Similarly, whether to resurface the patella during TKA remains controversial, with differing opinions on its impact on pain relief and patient satisfaction. The study by Chun et al. investigates the long-term clinical and radiological outcomes of patellar resurfacing versus retention in patients undergoing cruciate-retaining TKA using the NexGen®-CR system (Zimmer Biomet, Warsaw, Indiana, USA).

The study involved 92 patients who underwent cruciate-retaining TKA with the NexGen®-CR system, followed for an average of 10 years and 8 months. Patellar resurfacing was performed based on preoperative pain levels and intraoperative cartilage damage assessment. A single surgeon conducted all procedures using a standardized surgical approach, including medial parapatellar incision and measured resection techniques. Clinical evaluations included patella scores, functional scores, and range of motion (ROM), while radiological assessments focused on implant alignment and radiolucent lines. Statistical analyses compared preoperative and postoperative outcomes between the patellar resurfacing and retention groups.

The study found significant improvements in clinical scores and ROM for both groups post-operatively, with no significant differences between them. Radiological evaluations showed well-maintained implant alignment without significant loosening or dislocation. The findings suggest that both patellar resurfacing and retention yield satisfactory long-term outcomes in cruciate-retaining TKA using the NexGen®-CR system. Future study could explore more objective criteria for deciding between patellar resurfacing and retention to enhance surgical decision-making.

6.4.16 When to Do Selective Patellar Resurfacing in Total Knee Arthroplasty: A Decision-Making Algorithm Based on Pre-operative and Intra-operative Findings [164]

This is a machine-generated summary of:

Palanisamy, Yuvarajan; Naidu, Surya Prakash; Prasad, Arjun R.; Natarajan, Sugumar; Rajan, David V. When to Do Selective Patellar Resurfacing in Total Knee Arthroplasty: A Decision-Making Algorithm Based on Pre-operative and Intra-operative Findings [164].

Published in: Indian Journal of Orthopaedics (2023).

Link to original: https://doi.org/10.1007/s43465-023-01039-6

If you want to cite the papers, please refer to the original.

For technical reasons we could not place the page where the original quote is coming from.

6.4.16.1 Research Highlights

Persisting anterior knee pain after total knee arthroplasty (TKA) is a significant source of patient dissatisfaction, with uncertainty surrounding the optimal management of osteoarthritis in the patellofemoral joint. Current evidence does not definitively support or oppose routine patellar resurfacing, leaving a gap in effective treatment strategies. Widely used scoring systems fail to adequately address symptoms specific to the patellofemoral joint, potentially contributing to inconsistent outcomes. The study by Palanisamy et al. explores the development of a predictive algorithm using the Hospital for Special Surgery Patella-femoral Assessment (HSS PFA) score and intraoperative findings to guide selective patellar resurfacing decisions in TKA.

The study was conducted as a prospective analysis involving patients undergoing unilateral primary TKA for Kellgren Lawrence Grade IV osteoarthritis. Participants were assessed preoperatively using the HSS PFA score and weight-bearing Baldini X-ray views to evaluate patellar alignment and function. Intraoperative assessments included cartilage wear classification and patellar thickness measurements. The decision to resurface the patella was based on these evaluations, with an algorithm developed to predict the necessity of resurfacing. The study's methodology aimed to refine decision-making by correlating preoperative scores with intraoperative findings, ultimately testing the algorithm's efficiency through follow-up assessments using the HSS PFA score.

The study advances understanding of selective patellar resurfacing in TKA by demonstrating that preoperative HSS PFA scores, combined with intraoperative cartilage wear assessments, can effectively guide surgical decisions. The algorithm developed offers a structured approach to determining when patellar resurfacing is necessary, potentially improving patient outcomes by reducing anterior knee pain. Future study could focus on validating this algorithm across larger cohorts and diverse populations to enhance its applicability and accuracy. Additionally, ongoing research into patellofemoral biomechanics may further refine predictive tools for optimizing TKA outcomes.

6.4.17 Patella Is Rarely Resurfaced During Primary Total Knee Arthroplasty in Clinical Trials Conducted in Greece: A Systematic Review [165]

This is a machine-generated summary of:

Vasiliadis, Angelo V.; Fermín, Theodorakys Marín; Giovanoulis, Vasileios; Al-Dolaymi, Ayyoub A.; Batailler, Cécile; Lustig, Sébastien Patella is rarely resurfaced during primary total knee arthroplasty in clinical trials conducted in Greece: a systematic review [165].

Published in: Archives of Orthopaedic and Trauma Surgery (2024).

Link to original: https://doi.org/10.1007/s00402-024-05485-1

If you want to cite the papers, please refer to the original.

For technical reasons we could not place the page where the original quote is coming from.

6.4.17.1 Research Highlights

Total knee arthroplasty (TKA) is a critical procedure for managing end-stage knee osteoarthritis, yet the approach to patellar management during TKA remains contentious. Options include resurfacing or not resurfacing the patella, with varying practices observed globally. While some studies suggest benefits to both approaches, recent research has not shown significant advantages of resurfacing over non-resurfacing. The study by Vasiliadis et al. examines the practices of Greek surgeons regarding patellar management in TKA and evaluates the outcomes and revision rates associated with these practices.

The study conducted a systematic review following (Preferred Reporting Items for Systematic Reviews and Meta-Analyses) (PRISMA) guidelines, focusing on clinical studies from Greece that evaluated primary TKA outcomes with a minimum follow-up of 2 years. The researchers searched databases such as PubMed and Scopus using specific keywords related to TKA and Greece. They included studies that met predefined criteria, excluding abstracts, surveys, and editorials. Data extraction was performed by two independent investigators who assessed study design, functional outcomes, and complications. The methodological quality was evaluated using the Modified Coleman Methodology Score (mCMS), and publication bias was assessed with the ROBIS (Cochrane, Chicago, Il., USA) tool. The review included six studies from the Evros region, revealing that only 7% of TKAs involved patellar resurfacing. Despite this low rate, patients generally experienced good functional outcomes and low revision rates.

The study highlights significant variability in patellar management practices across different regions and underscores the influence of surgeon preference over geographical factors. While Greek surgeons predominantly opt for non-resurfacing, achieving favorable outcomes, the study suggests that future research could explore trends over different decades or include broader indications for TKA beyond idiopathic osteoarthritis. Establishing consensus-based guidelines for patellar management during TKA could help standardize practices and improve patient outcomes globally. Additionally, implementing a Greek National Registry could enhance the quality of future research in this area by providing comprehensive data on TKA procedures and outcomes in Greece.

6.4.18 Patellar Resurfacing in Posterior Cruciate Ligament Retaining Total Knee Arthroplasty (PATRES): Design of a Randomized Controlled Clinical Trial [166]

This is a machine-generated summary of:

Bischoff, Maria JFJ; van Raaij, Tom M; Reininga, Inge HF; van Raay, Jos JAM Patellar resurfacing in posterior cruciate ligament retaining total knee arthroplasty (PATRES): design of a randomized controlled clinical trial [166].

Published in: BMC Musculoskeletal Disorders (2014).

Link to original: https://doi.org/10.1186/1471-2474-15-358

If you want to cite the papers, please refer to the original.

For technical reasons we could not place the page where the original quote is coming from.

6.4.18.1 Research Highlights

Total knee arthroplasty (TKA) is a widely accepted surgical intervention for alleviating pain and enhancing function in patients with knee osteoarthritis. Despite the high success rate of modern TKA procedures, a significant number of patients continue to experience patellofemoral pain post-surgery. Patellar resurfacing has been suggested as a method to reduce anterior knee pain, but it is not without potential complications such as patellar fracture and instability. The current literature lacks conclusive evidence on the symptomatic impact of unresurfaced patellae after TKA. The study by Bischoff et al. aims to address this gap by evaluating the effectiveness of patellar resurfacing in a selective cohort using the Baldini scoring system.

The study is designed as a randomized controlled trial conducted at Martini Hospital Groningen, Netherlands. Patients with clinical and radiological signs of femorotibial and patellofemoral osteoarthritis are randomly assigned to undergo TKA with or without patellar resurfacing. The trial employs the Baldini tool, a validated scoring system specifically for assessing the patellofemoral joint, to measure outcomes. The surgical procedure involves using a medial parapatellar approach with all patients receiving a posterior cruciate ligament-retaining cemented total knee prosthesis. Postoperative assessments are conducted at multiple intervals up to 24 months, focusing on primary outcomes measured by the Baldini score and secondary outcomes using the Knee Society clinical rating system and the Knee injury and Osteoarthritis Outcome Score (KOOS).

The study's innovative approach lies in its selective patient cohort and use of a specific scoring system for patellofemoral evaluation, which may provide more accurate insights into the benefits of patellar resurfacing. Future study directions could explore different knee systems or alternative designs that might affect patellar kinematics differently. By focusing on patients with both femorotibial and patellofemoral osteoarthritis, this research could refine decision-making processes regarding patellar resurfacing in primary TKA, potentially leading to improved patient outcomes and satisfaction.

6.4.19 Circumferential Patellar Denervation Does Not Reduce Anterior Knee Pain in Total Knee Arthroplasty Wthout Patellar Resurfacing; a Prospective Comparison [167]

This is a machine-generated summary of:

Dogruoz, Fırat; Yapar, Aliekber; Buyukarslan, Volkan; Egerci, Omer Faruk; Etli, Ibrahim; Kose, Ozkan Circumferential patellar denervation does not reduce anterior knee pain in total knee arthroplasty without patellar resurfacing; a prospective comparison [167].

Published in: Journal of Orthopaedic Surgery and Research (2024).

Link to original: https://doi.org/10.1186/s13018-024-05161-5

6.4.19.1 Research Highlights

Total knee arthroplasty (TKA) is a widely used surgical procedure to alleviate pain and improve function in patients with end-stage knee osteoarthritis. Despite its success, a significant number of patients experience postoperative anterior knee pain (AKP), which can hinder recovery and satisfaction. AKP remains a challenging complication, with various strategies like patellar resurfacing and denervation being explored to mitigate it. However, the effectiveness of patellar denervation (PD) in reducing AKP and enhancing knee function is still debated. The study by Dogruoz et al. aims to provide a comprehensive evaluation of PD versus non-denervation on postoperative outcomes in TKA without patellar resurfacing.

The study was conducted as a prospective, non-randomized observational trial at a single institution, involving patients who underwent primary TKA between August 2023 and January 2024. Patients were divided into two groups: those who received PD and those who did not. The decision to perform PD was left to the discretion of the operating surgeon. The primary outcome measured was anterior knee pain, assessed using the Kujala anterior knee pain score. Secondary outcomes included functional assessments using the Western Ontario and McMaster Universities Osteoarthritis Index (WOMAC) and range of motion evaluations. The study ensured ethical compliance through informed consent and adherence to the Declaration of Helsinki. Statistical analyses were performed to compare outcomes between the two groups over time.

The findings suggest that both PD and non-denervation groups showed significant improvements in pain and functional scores over time; however, there were no significant differences between the groups regarding pain reduction or functional improvement at any assessment point. This indicates that circumferential PD does not provide additional benefits compared to non-denervation approaches in TKA without patellar resurfacing. Future study could explore patient-specific factors that may predict better outcomes with PD, potentially tailoring surgical interventions to individual needs.

6.4.20 Bilateral Simultaneous Total Knee Arthroplasty with and Wthout Patellar Resurfacing. A Prospective Single Surgeon Series with a Minimum Follow-Up of 7 Years [168]

This is a machine-generated summary of:

Alamino, Leonel Perez; Garabano, German; Pesciallo, Cesar Ángel; Del Sel, Hernán Bilateral simultaneous total knee arthroplasty with and without patellar resurfacing. A prospective single surgeon series with a minimum follow-up of 7 years [168].

Published in: Knee Surgery & Related Research (2024).

Link to original: https://doi.org/10.1186/s43019-024-00225-6

If you want to cite the papers, please refer to the original.
For technical reasons we could not place the page where the original quote is coming from.

6.4.20.1 Research Highlights

Total knee arthroplasty (TKA) is a widely accepted treatment for end-stage knee osteoarthritis, yet patient satisfaction can vary, often due to anterior knee pain (AKP). The causes of AKP are multifaceted, involving potential issues with the patellofemoral joint, synovial plicae, tendonitis, and other factors. Historically, the decision to resurface the patella during TKA has been debated, with previous implant designs not accounting for patellar tracking. The study by Alamino et al. investigates whether patellar resurfacing impacts clinical outcomes, postoperative AKP, and revision rates in patients undergoing simultaneous bilateral TKA.

The study was conducted at a high-volume TKA center and involved a prospective randomized data registry of patients with severe osteoarthritis undergoing simultaneous bilateral TKA. Each patient had one knee with a resurfaced patella and the other with a patelloplasty. The study excluded patients with prior knee surgeries or rheumatoid arthritis. Surgical procedures were standardized across cases, including spinal anesthesia and specific rehabilitation protocols. Clinical outcomes were assessed using the Knee Society Score (KSS) and Visual Analogue Scale (VAS) for pain. Radiographic evaluations were performed preoperatively and at regular intervals post-surgery to monitor complications such as infection or mechanical loosening.

After an average follow-up of 7 years, the study found no significant differences in clinical or functional outcomes between knees with resurfaced versus non-resurfaced patellae. Both groups showed significant improvement in KSS and VAS scores post-surgery. The findings suggest that patellar resurfacing does not offer clear advantages over non-resurfacing in terms of AKP or revision rates.

Bibliography

1. Insall JN, Ranawat CS, Aglietti P, Shine J (1976) A comparison of four models of total kneereplacement prostheses. J Bone Joint Surg Am 58:754–765
2. Murray DG, Webster DA (1981) The variable-axis knee prosthesis. Two-year follow-up study. J Bone Joint Surg Am 63:687–694
3. Jones EC, Insall JN, Inglis AE, Ranawat CS (1979) GUEPAR knee arthroplasty results and late complications. Clin Orthop Relat Res 140:145–152
4. Ranawat CS (1986) The patellofemoral joint in total condylar knee arthroplasty. Pros and cons based on five-to ten-year follow-up observations. Clin Orthop 205:93–99
5. Insall J, Scott WN, Ranawat CS (1979) The total condylar knee prosthesis. A report of two hundred and twenty cases. J Bone Joint Surg Am 61:173–180
6. Kaufer H, Matthews LS (1981) Spherocentric arthroplasty of the knee. Clinical experience with an average four-year follow-up. J Bone Joint Surg Am 63:545–559
7. Scott RD (1979) Prosthetic replacement of the patellofemoral joint. Orthop Clin N Am 10:129–137
8. Boyd AD Jr, Ewald FC, Thomas WH, Poss R, Sledge CB (1993) Long-term complications after total knee arthroplasty with or without resurfacing of the patella. J Bone Joint Surg Am 75:674–681
9. Muoneke HE, Khan AM, Giannikas KA, Hagglund E, Dunningham TH (2003) Secondary resurfacing of the patella for persistent anterior knee pain after primary knee arthroplasty. J Bone Joint Surg Br 85-B:675–678
10. Patel K, Raut V (2011) Patella in total knee arthroplasty: to resurface or not to—a cohort study of staged bilateral total knee arthroplasty. Int Orthop (SICOT) 35:349–353
11. Pilling RW, Moulder E, Allgar V, Messner J, Sun Z, Mohsen A (2012) Patellar resurfacing in primary total knee replacement: a meta-analysis. J Bone Joint Surg Am 94(24):2270–2278
12. Chen K, Li G, Fu D, Yuan C, Zhang Q, Cai Z (2013) Patellar resurfacing versus nonresurfacing in total knee arthroplasty: a meta-analysis of randomised controlled trials. Int Orthop 37(6):1075–1083
13. Barrack RL, Bertot AJ, Wolfe MW, Waldman DA, Milicic M, Myers L (2001) Patellar resurfacing in total knee arthroplasty. A prospective, randomized, double-blind study with five to seven years of follow-up. J Bone Joint Surg Am 83-A(9):1376–1381
14. Calvisi V, Camillieri G, Lupparelli S (2009) Resurfacing versus nonresurfacing the patella in total knee arthroplasty: a critical appraisal of the available evidence. Arch Orthop Traumatol Surg 129(9):1261–1270
15. Ogon M, Hartig F, Bach C, Nogler M, Steingruber I, Biedermann R (2002) Patella resurfacing: no benefit for the long-term outcome of total knee arthroplasty. A 10- to 16.3-year follow-up. Arch Orthop Trauma Surg 122:229–234

16. Ostermeier S, Buhrmester O, Hurschler C, Stukenborg-Colsman C (2005) Dynamic in vitro measurement of patellar movement after total knee arthroplasty: an in vitro study. BMC Musculoskelet Disord 6:30
17. Burke WV, Ammeen DJ, Engh GA (2005) Isolated revision of failed metal-backed patellar components: outcome with minimum 4-year follow-up. J Arthroplasty 20:998–1001
18. Leopold SS, Silverton CD, Barden RM, Rosenberg AG (2003) Isolated revision of the patellar component in total knee arthroplasty. J Bone Joint Surg Am 85-A(1):41–47
19. Muoneke HE, Khan AM, Giannikas KA, Hägglund E, Dunningham TH (2003) Secondary resurfacing of the patella for persistent anterior knee pain after primary knee arthroplasty. J Bone Joint Surg Br 85:675–678
20. Karnezis IA, Vossinakis IC, Rex C, Fragkiadakis EG, Newman JH (2003) Secondary patellar resurfacing in total knee arthroplasty: results of multivariate analysis in two case-matched groups. J Arthroplasty 18:993–998
21. Spencer SJ, Young D, Blyth MJ (2010) Secondary resurfacing of the patella in total knee arthroplasty. Knee 17:187–190
22. Forster MC (2004) Patellar resurfacing in total knee arthroplasty for osteoarthritis: a systematic review. Knee 11(6):427–430
23. Helmy N, Anglin C, Greidanus NV, Masri BA (2008) To resurface or not to resurface the patella in total knee arthroplasty. Clin Orthop Relat Res 466:2775–2783
24. Nizard RS, Biau D, Porcher R, Ravaud P, Bizot P, Hannouche D, Sedel L (2005) A meta-analysis of patellar replacement in total knee arthroplasty. Clin Orthop Relat Res 432:196–203
25. Parvizi J, Rapuri VR, Saleh KJ, Kuskowski MA, Sharkey PF, Mont MA (2005) Failure to resurface the patella during total knee arthroplasty may result in more knee pain and secondary surgery. Clin Orthop Relat Res 438:191–196
26. Goodfellow JW, O'Connor J. The mechanics of the knee and prosthesis design. J Bone Joint Surg (Br). 1978;60B(3):358–68.
27. Buechel FF, Pappas MJ. The New Jersey low contact stress knee replacement system: biomechanical rationale and review of the first 123 cemented cases. Arch Orthop and Traumatic Surg. 1986;105:197–204.
28. Gandhi R, Tsvetkov D, Davey JR, Mahomed NN. Survival and clinical function of cemented and uncemented prostheses in total knee replacement: a meta-analysis. J Bone Joint Surg Br. 2009;91(7):889–95.
29. Drexler M, Dwyer T, Marmor M, Abolghasemian M, Sternheim A, Cameron HU. Cementless fixation in total knee arthroplasty: down the boulevard of broken dreams - opposes. J Bone Joint Surg Br. 2012;94(11 Suppl A):85–9.
30. Yang JH, Yoon JR, Oh CH, Kim TS. Hybrid component fixation in total knee arthroplasty: minimum of 10-year follow-up study. J Arthroplast. 2012;27(6):1111–8.
31. Nakama GY, Peccin MS, Almeida GJ, Lira Neto Ode A, Queiroz AA, Navarro RD. Cemented, cementless or hybrid fixation options in total knee arthro-

plasty for osteoarthritis and other non-traumatic diseases. Cochrane Database Syst Rev. 2012;10:CD006193.
32. Matsuda S, Ishinishi T, Whiteside LA. Contact stresses with an unresurfaced patella in total knee arthroplasty. The effect of femoral component design. Orthopedics. 2000;23:213–8.
33. Chew JT, Stewart NJ, Hanssen AD, Luo ZP, Rand JA, An KN. Differences in patellar tracking and knee kinematics among three different total knee designs. Clin Orthop Relat Res. 1997;345:87–98.
34. Benjamin JB, Szivek JA, Hammond AS, Kubchandhani Z, Matthews AI Jr, Anderson P. Contact areas and pressures between native patellas and prosthetic femoral components. J Arthroplast. 1998;13:693–8.
35. Arthroplasty Care Practitioners. Available at: http://www.acpa-uk.net. Accessed 27 Apr 2016.
36. Ewald FC. The knee society total knee arthroplasty roentgenographic evaluation and scoring system. Clin Orthop Relat Res. 1989;248:9–12.
37. No authors listed. National Joint Registry for England and Wales: 12th Annual report, 2014. http://www.njrcentre.org.uk.
38. Hailer NP, Garellick G, Kärrholm J. Uncemented and cemented primary total hip arthroplasty in the Swedish hip arthroplasty register. Acta Orthop. 2010;81(1):34–41.
39. Park JW, Kim YH. Simultaneous cemented and cementless total knee replacement in the same patients: a prospective comparison of long-term outcomes using an identical design of NexGen prosthesis. J Bone Joint Surg [Br]. 2011;93-B:1479–86.
40. Baker PN, Khaw FM, Kirk LM, Esler CN, Gregg PJ. A randomised controlled trial of cemented versus cementless press-fit condylar total knee replacement: 15-year survival analysis. J Bone Joint Surg [Br]. 2007;89-B:1608–14.
41. Kono, K. *et al.* Patellar resurfacing has minimal impact on in vitro tibiofemoral kinematics during deep knee flexion in total knee arthroplasty. *Knee 30*, 163–169 (2021).
42. Belvedere, C. *et al.* Does navigated patellar resurfacing in total knee arthroplasty result in proper bone cut, motion and clinical outcomes?. *Clin. Biomech. (Bristol, Avon) 69*, 168–177 (2019).
43. Smith, A. J., Lloyd, D. G. and Wood, D. J. A kinematic and kinetic analysis of walking after total knee arthroplasty with and without patellar resurfacing. *Clin. Biomech. (Bristol, Avon) 21*, 379–386 (2006).
44. Xu, Y., Bai, Y., Zhou, J., Li, Q. and Liang, J. Gait analysis in primary total knee arthroplasty with and without patellar resurfacing: A randomized control study. *J. Shanghai Jiaotong Univ. (Sci.) 15*, 632–636 (2010).
45. Berti, L., Benedetti, M. G., Ensini, A., Catani, F. and Giannini, S. Clinical and biomechanical assessment of patella resurfacing in total knee arthroplasty. *Clin. Biomech. (Bristol, Avon) 21*, 610–616 (2006).
46. Bull, A. M. J., Katchburian, M. V., Shih, Y.-F. and Amis, A. A. Standardisation of the description of patellofemoral motion and comparison between different techniques. *Knee Surg. Sports Traumatol. Arthrosc. 10*, 184–193 (2002).

47. Sauer, A., Kebbach, M., Maas, A., Mihalko, W. M. and Grupp, T. M. The influence of mathematical definitions on patellar kinematics representations. *Materials (Basel, Switzerland) 14*, 7644 (2021).
48. Anglin, C. *et al.* Biomechanical consequences of patellar component medialization in total knee arthroplasty. *J. Arthroplasty 25*, 793–802 (2010).
49. Kawano, T. *et al.* Factors affecting patellar tracking after total knee arthroplasty. *J. Arthroplasty 17*, 942–947 (2002).
50. Longo UG, Ciuffreda M, Mannering N, D'Andrea V, Cimmino M, Denaro V (2018) Patellar resurfacing in total knee arthroplasty: systematic review and meta-analysis. J Arthroplast 33(2):620–632
51. Conrad DN, Dennis DA (2014) Patellofemoral crepitus after total knee arthroplasty: etiology and preventive measures. Clin Orthop Surg 6(1):9–19
52. Putman S, Boureau F, Girard J, Migaud H, Pasquier G (2019) Patellar complications after total knee arthroplasty. Orthop Traumatol Surg Res 105(1S):S43–S51
53. Inoue A, Arai Y, Nakagawa S, Inoue H, Yoshihara Y, Yamazoe S, Kubo T (2017) Differences in patellofemoral alignment as a result of patellar shape in cruciate-retaining total knee arthroplasty without patellar resurfacing at a minimum three-year follow-up. Knee 24(6):1448–1453
54. Panni AS, Cerciello S, Maffulli N, Di Cesare M, Servien E, Neyret P (2011) Patellar shape can be a predisposing factor in patellar instability. Knee Surg Sports Traumatol Arthrosc 19(4):663–670
55. Kellgren JH, Lawrence JS (1957) Radiological assessment of osteo-arthrosis. Ann Rheum Dis 16(4):494–502
56. Burnett RS, Haydon CM, Rorabeck CH, Bourne RB (2004) Patella resurfacing versus nonresurfacing in total knee arthroplasty: results of a randomized controlled clinical trial at a minimum of 10 years' followup. Clin Orthop Relat Res 428:12–25
57. Mayman D, Bourne RB, Rorabeck CH, Vaz M, Kramer J: Resurfacing versus not resurfacing the patella in total knee arthroplasty: 8- to 10-year results. J Arthroplasty. 2003, 18 (5): 541-545. 10.1016/S0883-5403(03)00150-5.
58. Campbell DG, Duncan WW, Ashworth M, Mintz A, Stirling J, Wakefield L, Stevenson TM (2006) Patellar resurfacing in total knee replacement: a ten-year randomised prospective trial. J Bone Joint Surg 88-B(6):734–739
59. Li S, Chen Y, Su W, Zhao J, He S, Luo X (2011) Systematic review of patellar resurfacing in total knee arthroplasty. Int Orthop 35(3):305–316
60. Lygre SH, Espehaug B, Havelin LI, Vollset SE, Furnes O (2010) Does patella resurfacing really matter? Pain and function in 972 patients after primary total knee arthroplasty. Acta Orthop 81(1):99–107
61. Cameron HU, Fedorkow DM (1982) The patella in total knee arthroplasty. Clin Orthop Relat Res 165:197–199
62. Burnett RS, Boone JL, McCarthy KP, Rosenzweig S, Barrack RL (2007) A prospective randomized clinical trial of patellar resurfacing and nonresurfacing in bilateral TKA. Clin Orthop Relat Res 464:65–72

63. Ranawat CS, Rose HA, Bryan WJ (1984) Replacement of the patello-femoral joint with the total condylar knee arthroplasty. Int Orthop 8(1):61–65
64. Gildone A, Manfredini M, Biscione R, Faccini R (2005) Patella resurfacing in posterior stabilised total knee arthroplasty: a follow-up study in 56 patients. Acta Orthop Belg 71(4):445–451
65. Ranawat CS (2002) History of total knee replacement. J South Orthop Assoc 11(4):218–226
66. Pierson JL, Ritter MA, Keating EM, Faris PM, Meding JB, Berend ME, Davis KE (2007) The effect of stuffing the patellofemoral compartment on the outcome of total knee arthroplasty. J Bone Joint Surg Am 89(10):2195–2203. https://doi.org/10.2106/jbjs.E.01223
67. Kuptniratsaikul V, Rattanachaiyanont M (2007) Validation of a modified Thai version of the Western Ontario and McMaster (WOMAC) osteoarthritis index for knee osteoarthritis. Clin Rheumatol 26(10):1641–1645. https://doi.org/10.1007/s10067-007-0560-y
68. Aitken RC (1969) Measurement of feelings using visual analogue scales. Proc R Soc Med 62(10):989–993
69. Koh JS, Yeo SJ, Lee BP, Lo NN, Seow KH, Tan SK (2002) Influence of patellar thickness on results of total knee arthroplasty: does a residual bony patellar thickness of <or = 12 mm lead to poorer clinical outcome and increased complication rates? J Arthroplasty 17(1):56–61
70. Waters TS, Bentley G. Patellar resurfacing in total knee arthroplasty: a prospective randomized study. J Bone Joint Surg Am. 2003;85(2):212–7.
71. Popovic N, Lemaire R (2003) Anterior knee pain with a posterior-stabilized mobile-bearing knee prosthesis: the effect of femoral component design. J Arthroplast 18:396–400
72. Pavlou G, Meyer C, Leonidou A et al (2011) Patellar resurfacing in total knee arthroplasty: does design matter? A meta-analysis of 7075 cases. J Bone Joint Surg Am 93:1301–1309. https://doi.org/10.2106/JBJS.J.00594
73. Pakos EE, Ntzani EE, Trikalinos TA: Patellar resurfacing in total knee arthroplasty. A meta-analysis. J Bone Joint Surg Volume. 2005, 87 (A(7)): 1438-1445.
74. van Hemert, W. L. W. *et al.* Patella retention versus replacement in total knee arthroplasty; functional and clinimetric aspects. *Arch. Orthop. Trauma Surg. 129*, 259–265 (2009).
75. Daniilidis K, Vogt B, Gosheger G et al (2012) Patellar resurfacing as a second stage procedure for persistent anterior knee pain after primary total knee arthroplasty. Int Orthop 36:1181–1183. https://doi.org/10.1007/s00264-011-1463-8
76. Parvizi J, Mortazavi SM, Devulapalli C, Hozack WJ, Sharkey PF, Rothman RH (2012) Secondary resurfacing of the patella after primary total knee arthroplasty: does the anterior knee pain resolve? J Arthroplasty 27:21–26. https://doi.org/10.1016/j.arth.2011.04.027
77. Muñoz-Mahamud E, Popescu D, Nuñez E et al (2011) Secondary patellar resurfacing in the treatment of patellofemoral pain after total knee arthro-

plasty. Knee Surg Sports Traumatol Arthrosc 19:1467–1472. https://doi.org/10.1007/s00167-011-1402-7
78. Ahmad R, Kumar GS, Katam K, Dunlop D, Pozo JL (2009) Significance of a "hot patella" in total knee replacement without primary patellar resurfacing. Knee 16:337–340. https://doi.org/10.1016/j.knee.2009.02.001
79. Insall JN, Dorr LD, Scott RD, Scott WN (1989) Rationale of the knee society clinical rating system. Clin Orthop 248:13–14
80. Aichroth P, Freeman MAR, Smillie IS, Souter WA (1978) A knee function assessment chart. J Bone Joint Surg Br 60:308–309
81. Schneider U, Graf J, Thomsen M et al (1997) Patellares Hypertensions syndrome—Nomenklatur, Diagnostik und Therpaie. Z Orhop Ijre Grenzgeb 135:70–75
82. Kajino A, Yoshino S, Kameyama S, Kohda M, Nagashima S (1997) Comparison of the results of bilateral total knee arthroplasty with and without patellar replacement for rheumatoid arthritis. A follow-up note. J Bone Joint Surg Am 79(4):570–574
83. Boyd AD Jr, Ewald FC, Thomas WH, Poss R, Sledge CB (1993) Long-term complications after total knee arthroplasty with or without resurfacing of the patella. J Bone Joint Surg Am 75(5):674–681
84. Enis JE, Gardner R, Robledo MA, Latta L, Smith R (1990) Comparison of patellar resurfacing versus nonresurfacing in bilateral total knee arthroplasty. Clin Orthop Relat Res 260:38–42
85. Kim BS, Reitman RD, Schai PA, Scott RD (1999) Selective patellar nonresurfacing in total knee arthroplasty. 10 year results. Clin Orthop Relat Res 367:81–88
86. Maradit-Kremers H, Haque OJ, Kremers WK, Berry DJ, Lewallen DG, Trousdale RT, Sierra RJ (2017) Is selectively not resurfacing the patella an acceptable practice in primary total knee arthroplasty? J Arthroplast 32(4):1143–1147
87. Picetti GD 3rd, McGann WA, Welch RB (1990) The patellofemoral joint after total knee arthroplasty without patellar resurfacing. J Bone Joint Surg Am 72(9):1379–1382
88. Rodríguez-Merchán EC, Gómez-Cardero P (2010) The outerbridge classification predicts the need for patellar resurfacing in TKA. Clin Orthop Relat Res 468(5):1254–1257
89. Outerbridge RE (1961) The etiology of chondromalacia patellae. J Bone Joint Surg Br 43:752–757
90. Ewald FC (1989) The Knee Society total knee arthroplasty roentgenographic evaluation and scoring system. Clin Orthop Relat Res 248:9–12
91. Altay MA, Ertürk C, Altay N, Akmeşe R, Işıkan UE (2012) Patellar denervation in total knee arthroplasty without patellar resurfacing: a prospective, randomized controlled study. Orthop Traumatol Surg Res 98(4):421–425
92. Whiteside LA, Nakamura T (2003) Effect of femoral component design on unresurfaced patellas in knee arthroplasty. Clin Orthop Relat Res 410:189–198

93. Pakos EE, Ntzani EE, Trikalinos TA (2005) Patellar resurfacing in total knee arthroplasty. A meta-analysis. J Bone Jt Surg Am 87:1438–45
94. He JY, Jiang LS, Dai LY. Is patellar resurfacing superior than nonresurfacing in total knee arthroplasty? A meta-analysis of randomized trials. Knee. 2011;18(3):137–44.
95. Enis JE, Gardner R, Robledo MA et al (1990) Comparison of patellar resurfacing versus nonresurfacing in bilateral total knee arthroplasty. Clin Orthop Relat Res 260:38–42
96. Koh IJ, Kim MS, Sohn S, Song KY, Choi NY, In Y (2019) Patients undergoing total knee arthroplasty using a contemporary patella-friendly implant are unaware of any differences due to patellar resurfacing. Knee Surg Sports Traumatol Arthrosc 27:1156–1164
97. Burnett RS, Boone JL, McCarthy KP, Rosenzweig S, Barrack RL (2007) A prospective randomized clinical trial of patellar resurfacing and nonresurfacing in bilateral TKA. Clin Orthop Relat Res 464:65–72
98. Smith AJ, Wood DJ, Li MG. Total knee replacement with and without patellar resurfacing: a prospective randomised trial using the Profix total knee system. J Bone Joint Surg (Br). 2008;90(1):43–9.
99. Ha C, Wang B, Li W, Sun K, Wang D, Li Q (2019) Resurfacing versus not-resurfacing the patella in one-stage bilateral total knee arthroplasty: a prospective randomized clinical trial. Int Orthop 43:2519–2527
100. Dong Y, Li T, Zheng Z, Xiang S, Weng X (2018) Adding patella resurfacing after circumpatellar electrocautery did not improve the clinical outcome in bilateral total knee arthroplasty in Chinese population: a prospective randomized study. J Arthroplasty 33:1057–1061
101. Schindler OS (2012) The controversy of patellar resurfacing in total knee arthroplasty: Ibisne in medio tutissimus? Knee Surg Sports Traumatol Arthrosc 20(7):1227–1244
102. Swan JD, Stoney JD, Lim K, Dowsey MM, Choong PF (2010) The need for patellar resurfacing in total knee arthroplasty: a literature review. ANZ J Surg 80(4):223–233
103. Johnson TC, Tatman PJ, Mehle S, Gioe TJ (2012) Revision surgery for patellofemoral problems: should we always resurface? Clin Orthop Relat Res 470:211–219. https://doi.org/10.1007/s11999-011-2036-2
104. Barrack RL, Bertot AJ, Wolfe MW, Waldman DA, Milicic M, Myers L (2001) Patellar resurfacing in total knee arthroplasty. A prospective, randomized, double-blind study with five to seven years of follow-up. J Bone Joint Surg Am 83(9):1376–1381
105. Bourne RB, Burnett RS: The consequences of not resurfacing the patella. Clin Orthop Relat Res. 2004, 428: 166-169.
106. Burnett RS, Boone JL, McCarthy KP, Rosenzweig S, Barrack RL (2007) A prospective randomized clinical trial of patellar resurfacing and nonresurfacing in bilateral TKA. Clin Orthop Relat Res 464:65–72

107. Wood DJ, Smith AJ, Collopy D, White B, Brankov B, Bulsara MK. Patellar resurfacing in total knee arthroplasty: a prospective randomized study. J Bone Joint Surg Am. 2002;84(2):187–93.
108. Abdel MP, Parratte S, Budhiparama NC (2014) The patella in total knee arthroplasty: to resurface or not is the question. Curr Rev Musculoskelet Med 7:117–124
109. Roberts DW, Hayes TD, Tate CT, Lesko JP (2015) Selective patellar resurfacing in total knee arthroplasty: a prospective, randomized, double-blind study. J Arthroplast 30:216–222. https://doi.org/10.1016/j.arth.2014.09.012
110. Ouanezar H, Franck F, Jacquel A, Pibarot V, Wegrzyn J (2016) Does computer-assisted surgery influence survivorship of cementless total knee arthroplasty in patients with primary osteoarthritis? A 10-year follow-up study. Knee Surg Sports Traumatol Arthrosc 24:3448–3456. https://doi.org/10.1007/s00167-016-4112-3
111. Piriou P, Peronne E, Ouanezar H (2013) Rotational alignment of the femoral component using trochlear navigation during total knee arthroplasty: a dual-center study of 145 cases. J Arthroplast 28:1107–1111. https://doi.org/10.1016/j.arth.2013.04.032
112. Nedopil AJ, Howell SM, Hull ML. What clinical characteristics and radiographic parameters are associated with patellofemoral instability after kinematically aligned total knee arthroplasty? Int Orthop. 2017;41:283–91.
113. Assi C, Kheir N, Samaha C et al (2017) Optimizing patellar positioning during total knee arthroplasty: an anatomical and clinical study. Int Orthop 41:2509–2515. https://doi.org/10.1007/s00264-017-3557-4
114. Grelsamer RP, Bazos AN, Proctor CS (1993) Radiographic analysis of patellar tilt. J Bone Joint Surg (Br) 75:822–824
115. Bhattee G, Moonot P, Govindaswamy R, Pope A, Fiddian N, Harvey A (2014) Does malrotation of components correlate with patient dissatisfaction following secondary patellar resurfacing? Knee 21:247–251. https://doi.org/10.1016/j.knee.2012.12.006
116. Freeman MA, Insall JN, Besser W, Walker PS, Hallel T. Excision of the cruciate ligaments in a total knee replacement. Clin Orthop Relat Res. 1977;126:209–12.
117. David CP, Deborah JA, Gerard AE. Synovial entrapment: a complication of posterior stabilized total knee arthroplasty. J Bone Joint Surg. 2002;84-A:2174–8.
118. Ewald FC. The Knee Society total knee arthroplasty roentgenographic evaluation and scoring system. Clin Orthop. 1989;248:9–12.
119. Dorr LD, Boiardo RA. Technical considerations in total knee arthroplasty. Clin Orthop Relat Res. 1986;205:5–11.
120. Freeman MA, Railton GT. Should the posterior cruciate ligament be retained or resected in condylar nonmeniscal knee arthroplasty? The case for resection. J Arthroplast. 1988;3(Suppl):S3–12.
121. Patel, V. V., Hall, K., Ries, M., Lindsey, C., Ozhinsky, E., Lu, Y., and Majumdar, S. (2003). Magnetic resonance imaging of patellofemoral kinematics with

weight-bearing. *The Journal of Bone and Joint Surgery - Series A, 85*, 2419–2424.

122. Baldini A, Anderson JA, Zampetti P, Pavlov H, Sculco TP (2006) A new patellofemoral scoring system for total knee arthroplasty. Clin Orthop Relat Res 452:150–154. https://doi.org/10.1097/01.blo.0000238847.34047.90
123. Matharu, G. S., Blom, A. W., Venkatesh, R., Metcalfe, A. J., and Whitehouse, M. R. (2021). Patellar resurfacing practices in primary total knee replacement: A survey of BASK members. *Knee*, *28*, A3–A5.
124. Benazzo F, Perticarini L, Jannelli E, Ivone A, Ghiara M, Paolo Rossi SM (2020) Controversy: supporting patellar resurfacing in total knee arthroplasty – do it. EFORT Open Rev 5:785–792. https://doi.org/10.1302/2058-5241.5.190075
125. Sato D, Inoue M, Sasaki T, Uchida J, Onodera T, Kondo E, Iwasaki N (2021) No patella resurfacing total knee arthroplasty leads to reduction in the thickness of patellar cartilage to less than half within 5 years: a quantitative longitudinal evaluation using MRI. J Exp Orthop 8:107. https://doi.org/10.1186/s40634-021-00425-z
126. Robben BJ, De Vries AJ, Spekenbrink-Spooren A, Nelissen RGHH, Brouwer RW (2022) Rare primary patellar resurfacing does not lead to more secondary patellar resurfacing: analysis of 70,014 primary total knee arthroplasties in the Dutch Arthroplasty Register (LROI). Acta Orthop 93:334–340. https://doi.org/10.2340/17453674.2022.2078
127. Whiting P, Savović J, Higgins JP, Caldwell DM, Reeves BC, Shea B, Davies P, Kleijnen J, Churchill R, ROBIS group (2016) ROBIS: a new tool to assess risk of bias in systematic reviews was developed. J Clin Epidemiol 69:225–234. https://doi.org/10.1016/j.jclinepi.2015.06.005
128. Touzopoulos P, Ververidis A, Mpogiatzis C, Chatzigiannakis A, Drosos GI (2019) The use of tourniquet may influence the cement mantle thickness under the tibial implant during total knee arthroplasty. Eur J Orthop Surg Traumatol 29:869–875. https://doi.org/10.1007/s00590-019-02369-8
129. Karachalios T, Komnos G, Hantes M, Varitimidis S (2021) Evaluating the patella-friendly' concept in total knee arthroplasty: a minimum 15-year follow-up outcome study comparing constant radius, multiradius cruciate-retaining and nonanatomical cruciate-retaining implants. J Arthroplasty 36:2771–2778. https://doi.org/10.1016/j.arth.2021.03.007
130. Papasoulis E, Karachalios T (2019) A 13- to 16-year clinical and radiological outcome study of the genesis II cruciate retaining total knee arthroplasty with an oxidized zirconium femoral component. Knee 26:492–499. https://doi.org/10.1016/j.knee.2019.01.013
131. Bouras T, Bitas V, Fennema P, Korovessis P (2017) Good long-term results following cementless TKA with a titanium plasma coating. Knee Surg Sports Traumatol Arthrosc 25:2801–2808. https://doi.org/10.1007/s00167-015-3769-3
132. Iosifidis M, Iliopoulos E, Neofytou D, Sakorafas N, Andreou D, Alvanos D, Kyriakidis A (2014) The rotaglide mobile-bearing total knee arthroplasty: no

difference between cemented and hybrid implantation. Knee Surg Sports Traumatol Arthrosc 22:1843–1848. https://doi.org/10.1007/s00167-013-2829-9

133. Georgaklis VA, Karachalios T, Makridis KG, Badras SL, Palaiochorlidis IS, Malizos KN, Badras LS (2019) Genesis 1 posterior cruciate-retaining total knee arthroplasty with asymmetric tibial tray: an 18-to-26-year long-term clinical outcome study. Knee 26:838–846. https://doi.org/10.1016/j.knee.2019.04.014
134. Coory JA, Tan KG, Whitehouse SL, Hatton A, Graves SE, Crawford RW (2020) The outcome of total knee arthroplasty with and without patellar resurfacing up to 17 years: a report from the australian orthopaedic association national joint replacement registry. J Arthroplasty 35(1):132–138. https://doi.org/10.1016/j.arth.2019.08.007
135. Maney AJ, Frampton CM, Young SW (2020) Age and prosthetic design as risk factors for secondary patella resurfacing. J Arthroplasty 35:1563–1568. https://doi.org/10.1016/j.arth.2020.01.018
136. Waters TS, Bentley G: Patellar resurfacing in total knee arthroplasty - A prospective, randomized study. J Bone Joint Surg Am. 2003, 85A (2): 212-217.
137. Wood DJ, Smith AJ, Collopy D, White B, Brankov B, Bulsara MK: Patellar resurfacing in total knee arthroplasty - A prospective, randomized trial. J Bone Joint Surg Am. 2002, 84A (2): 187-193.
138. Barrack RL, Bertot AJ, Wolfe MW, Waldman DA, Milicic M, Myers L: Patellar resurfacing in total knee arthroplasty - A prospective, randomized, double-blind study with five to seven years of follow-up. J Bone Joint Surg Am. 2001, 83A (9): 1376-1381.
139. Breeman S, Campbell M, Dakin H, Fiddian N, Fitzpatrick R et al (2011) Patellar resurfacing in total knee replacement: five-year clinical and economic results of a large randomized controlled trial. J Bone Joint Surg Am 93:1473–1481. https://doi.org/10.2106/JBJS.J.00725
140. Feller JA, Bartlett RJ, Lang DM: Patellar resurfacing versus retention in total knee arthroplasty. J Bone Joint Surg Br. 1996, 78B: 226-228.
141. Insall JN, Dorr LD, Scott RD, Scott WN: Rationale of the knee-society clinical rating system. Clin Orthop. 1989, 248: 13-14.
142. Roos EM, Roos HP, Lohmander LS, Ekdahl C, Beynnon BD: Knee Injury and Osteoarthritis Outcome Score (KOOS)–development of a self-administered outcome measure. J Orthop Sports Phys Ther. 1998, 28 (2): 88-96. 10.2519/jospt.1998.28.2.88.
143. Baldini A, Anderson JA, Cerulli-Mariani P, Kalyvas J, Pavlov H, Sculco TP (2007) Patellofemoral evaluation after total knee arthroplasty. Validation of a new weight-bearing axial radiographic view. J Bone Joint Surg Am 89:1810–1817. https://doi.org/10.2106/JBJS.E.00432
144. Duan G, Liu C, Lin W, Shao J, Fu K, Niu Y, et al. Different factors conduct anterior knee pain following primary total knee arthroplasty: a systematic review and meta-analysis. J Arthroplasty. 2018;33:1962–71. e1963.

145. Budhiparama NC, Hidayat H, Novito K, Utomo DN, Lumban-Gaol I, Nelissen RGHH. Does circumferential patellar denervation result in decreased knee pain and improved patient-reported outcomes in patients undergoing nonresurfaced, simultaneous bilateral TKA? Clin Orthop Relat Res. 2020;478(9):2020–33.
146. Insall J, Scott WN (2008) Desarrollo histórico, clasificación y características de las prótesis de rodilla. En Insall J et al., Rodilla. Vol 2. Ed Marbán Libros S.L., Madrid, España. P1516–1552
147. Burnett RSJ, Boone JL, Rosenzweig SD, Steger-May K, Barrack RL (2009) Patellar resurfacing compared with nonresurfacing in total knee arthroplasty. A concise follow-up of a randomised trial. J Bone Joint Surg 91-A:2562–2567
148. Caton J, Deschamps G, Chambat P, Lerat JL, Dejour H (1982) Patella infera. A propos of 128 cases. Rev Chir Orthop Reparatrice Appar Mot 68(5):317–325
149. Schiavone Panni, Alfredo; Cerciello, Simone; Del Regno, Chiara; Felici, Alessandro; Vasso, Michele Patellar resurfacing complications in total knee arthroplasty. International Orthopaedics (2013). 10.1007/s00264-013-2244-3
150. Daniilidis, Kiriakos; Vogt, Bjoern; Gosheger, Georg; Henrichs, Marcel; Dieckmann, Ralf; Schulz, Dino; Hoell, Steffen Patellar resurfacing as a second stage procedure for persistent anterior knee pain after primary total knee arthroplasty. International Orthopaedics (2012). https://doi.org/10.1007/s00264-011-1463-8
151. Napier, Richard J.; O'Neill, Christopher; O'Brien, Seamus; Doran, Emer; Mockford, Brian; Boldt, Jens; Beverland, David E. A prospective evaluation of a largely cementless total knee arthroplasty cohort Without patellar resurfacing: 10-year outcomes and survivorship. BMC Musculoskeletal Disorders (2018). https://doi.org/10.1186/s12891-018-2128-1
152. Sauer, Adrian; Thorwaechter, Christoph; Dupraz, Ingrid; Maas, Allan; Steinbrueck, Arnd; Grupp, Thomas M.; Woiczinski, Matthias Isolated effects of patellar resurfacing in total knee arthroplasty and their relation to native patellar geometry. Scientific Reports (2022). https://doi.org/10.1038/s41598-022-16810-2
153. Kim, Chang-Wan; Lee, Chang-Rack; Huh, Tae-Yung The effect of patellar facet angle on patellofemoral alignment and arthritis progression in posterior-stabilized total knee arthroplasty without patellar resurfacing. Knee Surgery & Related Research (2020). https://doi.org/10.1186/s43019-020-00045-4
154. Beaupre, Lauren; Secretan, Charles; Johnston, DWC; Lavoie, Guy A Randomized controlled trial comparing patellar retention versus patellar resurfacing in primary total knee arthroplasty: 5–10 year follow-up. BMC Research Notes (2012). https://doi.org/10.1186/1756-0500-5-273
155. Labek, Gerold; Liebensteiner, Michael; Williams, Alexandra; Thaler, Martin; Stöckl, Bernd Impact of patellar resurfacing on the revision rate in total knee arthroplasty. European Orthopaedics and Traumatology (2010). https://doi.org/10.1007/s12570-010-0027-5

156. Tammachote, Nattapol; Kraisin, Teeramate; Kanitnate, Supakit Do we need to restore patellar thickness after total knee arthroplasty with patellar resurfacing?. European Journal of Orthopaedic Surgery & Traumatology (2023). https://doi.org/10.1007/s00590-023-03607-w
157. Roessler, Philip P.; Moussa, Randa; Jacobs, Cornelius; Schüttler, Karl F.; Stein, Thomas; Schildberg, Frank A.; Wirtz, Dieter C. Predictors for secondary patellar resurfacing after primary total knee arthroplasty using a "patella-friendly" total knee arthroplasty system. International Orthopaedics (2018). https://doi.org/10.1007/s00264-018-4075-8
158. Scheurer, Philip; Reininga, Inge H. F.; van Jonbergen, Hans-Peter W.; van Raay, Jos J. A. M. Secondary patellar resurfacing following total knee arthroplasty. International Orthopaedics (2015). https://doi.org/10.1007/s00264-015-2684-z
159. Lee, Gun Woo; Lee, Sun-Mi; Jang, Soo-Jin; Son, Jung-Hwan The efficacy of patellar decompression for improving anterior knee pain following total knee arthroplasty without patellar resurfacing. Archives of Orthopaedic and Trauma Surgery (2013). https://doi.org/10.1007/s00402-013-1702-0
160. Zha, Guo-Chun; Feng, Shuo; Chen, Xiang-Yang; Guo, Kai-Jin Does the grading of chondromalacia patellae influence anterior knee pain following total knee arthroplasty without patellar resurfacing?. International Orthopaedics (2017). https://doi.org/10.1007/s00264-017-3658-0
161. Choi, Keun Young; In, Yong; Kim, Man Soo; Sohn, Sueen; Koh, In Jun Is the patient aware of the difference between resurfaced and nonresurfaced patella after bilateral total knee arthroplasty? A systematic review of simultaneous bilateral randomized trials. Knee Surgery & Related Research (2022). https://doi.org/10.1186/s43019-022-00133-7
162. Franck, Florent; Ouanezar, Hervé; Jacquel, Alexandre; Pibarot, Vincent; Wegrzyn, Julien The predictive factors of secondary patellar resurfacing in computer-assisted total knee arthroplasty. A prospective cohort study. International Orthopaedics (2017). https://doi.org/10.1007/s00264-017-3630-z
163. Chun, Keun Churl; Lee, Sung Hyun; Baik, Jong Seok; Kook, Seng Hwan; Han, Joung Kyue; Chun, Churl Hong Clinical and radiological results of cruciate-retaining total knee arthroplasty with the NexGen®-CR system: comparison of patellar resurfacing versus retention with more than 14 years of follow-up. Journal of Orthopaedic Surgery and Research (2017). https://doi.org/10.1186/s13018-017-0646-4
164. Palanisamy, Yuvarajan; Naidu, Surya Prakash; Prasad, Arjun R.; Natarajan, Sugumar; Rajan, David V. When to Do Selective Patellar Resurfacing in Total Knee Arthroplasty: A Decision-Making Algorithm Based on Pre-operative and Intra-operative Findings. Indian Journal of Orthopaedics (2023). https://doi.org/10.1007/s43465-023-01039-6
165. Vasiliadis, Angelo V.; Fermín, Theodorakys Marín; Giovanoulis, Vasileios; Al-Dolaymi, Ayyoub A.; Batailler, Cécile; Lustig, Sébastien Patella is rarely resurfaced during primary total knee arthroplasty in clinical trials conducted

in Greece: a systematic review. Archives of Orthopaedic and Trauma Surgery (2024). https://doi.org/10.1007/s00402-024-05485-1
166. Bischoff, Maria JFJ; van Raaij, Tom M; Reininga, Inge HF; van Raay, Jos JAM Patellar resurfacing in posterior cruciate ligament retaining total knee arthroplasty (PATRES): design of a randomized controlled clinical trial. BMC Musculoskeletal Disorders (2014). https://doi.org/10.1186/1471-2474-15-358
167. Dogruoz, Fırat; Yapar, Aliekber; Buyukarslan, Volkan; Egerci, Omer Faruk; Etli, Ibrahim; Kose, Ozkan Circumferential patellar denervation does not reduce anterior knee pain in total knee arthroplasty without patellar resurfacing; a prospective comparison. Journal of Orthopaedic Surgery and Research (2024). https://doi.org/10.1186/s13018-024-05161-5
168. Alamino, Leonel Perez; Garabano, German; Pesciallo, Cesar Ángel; Del Sel, Hernán Bilateral simultaneous total knee arthroplasty with and without patellar resurfacing. A prospective single surgeon series with a minimum follow-up of 7 years. Knee Surgery & Related Research (2024). https://doi.org/10.1186/s43019-024-00225-6

Chapter 7
Innovative Technology for Total Knee Arthroplasty

Alfred J. Tria Jr. and Giles R. Scuderi

Introduction by the Editors

Total knee arthroplasty (TKA) has been shown to improve the quality of daily activities for those with disabling knee arthritis. The positive impact this procedure has on the patient's life is significantly influenced by the accuracy of component alignment and restoration of alignment. Precise execution of the surgical technique, with accurate soft tissue balancing and limb alignment is important. Conventional TKA with manual instrumentation is an accepted, safe and cost-effective procedure. Yet in search of improving patient satisfaction, technological advancements have resulted in the invention of more advanced joint navigation and robotic systems.

Initially navigation systems whether image based or imageless and based upon intraoperative bone landmarking were designed to increase the accuracy of the bone resection along a predetermined surgical plan. Over time this improved to take into consideration soft tissue balancing. Robotic surgery has taken this innovation one step further and integrates the computer based surgical plan with the cutting tools. Advocates of robotic surgery emphasize the ability of these systems to improve implant position, alignment and create balanced gaps. The short-term clinical results have been promising, but we will need to see whether the increased investment in this technology will influence the long-term outcomes. Recently artificial intelligence and augmented reality have been introduced as newer interactive technologies to guide the surgical plan. While in its infancy, this may be the future. Understanding that innovative technology has greatly influenced TKA, the references in this chapter will highlight some of these developments.

A. J. Tria Jr. (✉)
Department of Orthopedics, Rutgers-Robert Wood Johnson Medical School, New Brunswick, NJ, USA

G. R. Scuderi
Department of Orthopedic Surgery, Northwell Health, Garden City, NY, USA

A. J. Tria Jr., G. R. Scuderi (eds.), *Total Knee Arthroplasty*,
https://doi.org/10.1007/978-3-032-00175-7_7

One of the simplest navigation systems that has been utilized and brings refined accuracy to familiar manual instruments has been handheld navigation with built in accelerometers and gyroscopes. There are six articles that discuss the accuracy of navigation. Liow et al., Tran et al., Zheng et al., Gao et al., Loh et al., Thiengwittayaporn et al. Each article does support the improved accuracy of the procedure. Further defining the accuracy, Fikert el al. evaluated the flexion-extension gaps using a handheld navigation system and showed that 90% of the knees achieved coronal alignment within 3 degrees of the desired results. Realizing that navigation systems continue to evolve, Inui et al. looked at navigation system updates and showed that the newer design did lead to a decrease in the surgical time with no change in accuracy. When compared to robotic system, Macino et al. showed some early benefits with the robotic system but longer operative times.

Robotics systems continue to grow in popularity. While there are numerous reports of improved accuracy and reproducibility, it does come at a cost. Ezeokoli et al. showed that the robotic system did increase overall cost. Haslhofer et al. looked at surgical time with robotics versus computer assisted and found no differences: however, the procedures were performed by surgeons who were very familiar with the system. Several articles review the results from specific systems and the interaction of those systems in the operating room setting. Tsai et al. were able to include a gap balancing technique with robotics in a small patient population. Further application to a larger population will be necessary to validate these results. Not without complications, Wever et al. outlines the specific complications from a single system.

With ever evolving technology, artifical intelligence and augmented reality are making a breakthrough into TKA. Shaheen et al. did a systematic review and metanalysis of virtual reality rehabilitation showing some early benefits but only 15 randomized controlled trials were included and there was significant heterogeneity among the included studies. Fucentese et al. introduce a novel artificial intelligence system, which is of some interest but very early in its development. Buchlak et al. used natural language processing to facilitate the systematic review process with automated article screening. This is very similar to the approach of this very text.

7.1 Handheld Navigation

Machine Generated Summaries

Disclaimer: The summaries in this chapter were generated from Springer Nature publications using abstractive AI auto-summarization: An abstraction-based summarizer creates new text based on deep learning. New phrases are created to summarize the content. As the constituted sentences are machine selected, they may not fully reflect the body of the work, so we strongly advise that the original content is read and cited. The auto-generated summaries were curated by the editor to meet Springer Nature publication standards.

7.1.1 Computer-Assisted Stereotaxic Navigation Improves the Accuracy of Mechanical Alignment and Component Positioning in Total Knee Arthroplasty [64]

This is a machine-generated summary of:

Liow, Ming Han Lincoln; Goh, Graham Seow-Hng; Pang, Hee-Nee; Tay, Darren Keng Jin; Lo, Ngai Nung; Yeo, Seng Jin Computer-assisted stereotaxic navigation improves the accuracy of mechanical alignment and component positioning in total knee arthroplasty [64].

Published in: Archives of Orthopaedic and Trauma Surgery (2016).

Link to original: https://doi.org/10.1007/s00402-016-2483-z

If you want to cite the papers, please refer to the original.

For technical reasons we could not place the page where the original quote is coming from.

7.1.1.1 Research Highlights

Total knee arthroplasty (TKA) is a widely accepted treatment for advanced knee arthritis, yet the optimal mechanical alignment and component positioning remain subjects of debate due to their potential impact on implant longevity. Traditional TKA techniques often lack precision in achieving ideal mechanical alignment, prompting interest in technologies like computer-assisted surgery (CAS) that promise enhanced accuracy without compromising surgical efficiency. The study by Liow et al. explores the efficacy of the iASSIST knee computer-assisted stereotaxic navigation system (Zimmer-Biomet, Warsaw, IN., USA) in improving mechanical alignment and component positioning in TKA.

The study involved patients with tricompartmental osteoarthritis undergoing TKA using either conventional methods or the iASSIST system at a single institution. Two senior surgeons performed the surgeries, with one using the conventional technique and the other employing the CAS method. The iASSIST system utilizes disposable electronic stereotaxic pods for alignment feedback, eliminating the need for large consoles or navigation arrays. The study assessed post-operative outcomes through radiological evaluations and clinical assessments at six months. Results indicated that while both groups showed significant improvements in clinical scores, the CAS group achieved superior mechanical alignment and component positioning compared to the conventional group. However, surgeries using CASN were longer, and no significant differences in clinical outcomes were observed between the two groups.

The findings suggest that while CAS systems like iASSIST offer improved alignment accuracy, they do not necessarily translate into better short-term clinical outcomes compared to conventional TKA methods. Future study could focus on long-term outcomes to determine if improved alignment leads to enhanced implant survivorship or patient satisfaction over time. Additionally, considerations regarding cost-effectiveness and surgical duration remain critical as these factors influence the broader adoption of CAS technologies in orthopedic practice. The study highlights the need for further research to establish definitive clinical benefits before widespread implementation of new navigation systems in TKA procedures.

7.1.2 Handheld Imageless Robotic Total Knee Arthroplasty Improves Accuracy and Early Clinical Outcomes when Compared with Navigation [65]

This is a machine-generated summary of:

Tran, Joshua Yeuk-Shun; Tang, Abbie Yan-Tung; Wong, Cham-Kit; Lam, Gloria Yan-Ting; Choi, Tsz-Lung; Mak, Rex Wang-Fung; Ng, Jonathan Patrick; Ho, Kevin Ki-Wai; Ong, Michael Tim-Yun; Yung, Patrick Shu-Hang Handheld imageless robotic total knee arthroplasty improves accuracy and early clinical outcomes when compared with navigation [65].

Published in: Arthroplasty (2025).

Link to original: https://doi.org/10.1186/s42836-025-00303-4

If you want to cite the papers, please refer to the original.

For technical reasons we could not place the page where the original quote is coming from.

7.1.2.1 Research Highlights

Total knee arthroplasty (TKA) is a common surgical procedure aimed at alleviating pain and restoring function in patients with degenerative joint disease. Despite advancements in surgical techniques, achieving optimal alignment remains a challenge, as misalignment can lead to complications such as polyethylene wear and prosthetic loosening. This issue is particularly significant given the projected global increase in TKA demand. The study by Tran et al. investigates the effectiveness of semi-active imageless robot-assisted TKA (RATKA) compared to passive imageless accelerometer-based navigation (ABN) systems in improving early functional outcomes and surgical accuracy.

The study conducted a retrospective analysis of data from patients who underwent primary TKA using either RATKA or ABN systems. The research included male and female patients over 18 years old with end-stage osteoarthritis, excluding those with previous surgeries or complicating conditions. Surgeries were performed by experienced orthopedic surgeons using standardized techniques, with the choice of system based on availability. Preoperative and postoperative radiographic analyses were conducted to assess alignment accuracy, while functional outcomes were measured using the Knee Society Knee Score (KSFS). Statistical analyses, including ANCOVA (Analysis of covariance) were used to compare outcomes between the two groups while accounting for preoperative differences.

The study found that RATKA systems provided significantly better alignment accuracy and early postoperative functional outcomes compared to ABN systems. The enhanced precision of RATKA in bone resection and prosthesis positioning likely contributed to these results. While both systems offer advantages over conventional TKA, RATKA's semi-active nature allows for greater control and feedback during surgery. Future study could focus on multi-center trials with larger sample sizes and longer follow-up periods to validate these findings further. Additionally, exploring cost-effectiveness and long-term benefits could help guide clinical decision-making regarding the use of RATKA versus ABN in different healthcare settings.

7.1.3 Precision of Ci-Navigated Extension and Flexion Gap Balancing in Total Knee Arthroplasty and Analysis of Potential Predictive Variables [66]

This is a machine-generated summary of:

Fickert, S.; Jawhar, A.; Sunil, P.; Scharf, H.-P Precision of Ci-navigated extension and flexion gap balancing in total knee arthroplasty and analysis of potential predictive variables [66].

Published in: Archives of Orthopaedic and Trauma Surgery (2011).

Link to original: https://doi.org/10.1007/s00402-011-1419-x

If you want to cite the papers, please refer to the original.
For technical reasons we could not place the page where the original quote is coming from.

7.1.3.1 Research Highlights

Total knee arthroplasty (TKA) success hinges on precise joint line creation, limb alignment, and soft tissue balancing. Malalignment and improper ligamentous balancing can lead to postoperative pain, instability, and long-term complications such as loosening and failure. While computer-assisted navigation in TKA has shown improvements in component positioning and limb alignment, the accuracy of ligament balancing remains underexplored. The study by Fickert et al. evaluates the accuracy of limb alignment and gap balancing in computer-navigated TKA using intraoperative measurements.

The study involved 225 patients with primary osteoarthritis undergoing computer-navigated TKA using the Ci system(Confidential Informant", DePuy Orthopaedics, Raynham, Mass., USA). Excluding other arthritis causes and previous surgeries, the research focused on achieving accurate limb alignment and medial-lateral gap balancing. The Ci Navigation system, a nonimage-based optical wireless system (Hospital for Special Surgery, New York, New York, USA), facilitated precise bone morphing and ligament balancing through data acquisition and tracking. The surgical process included tibial resection followed by femoral adjustments to achieve optimal extension and flexion gaps. Statistical analysis was conducted on various alignment parameters to assess the accuracy of the navigation system.

The study demonstrated that computer-assisted navigation significantly improves gap balancing accuracy in TKA. Over 90% of knees achieved coronal alignment within ±3°, with minimal variance in extension and flexion gaps. The findings suggest that factors such as age, sex, preoperative deformity, and osteoarthritis grade do not influence gap balancing accuracy. Future study could explore the impact of femoral rotation and component flexion on flexion gaps further. This research underscores the potential of navigation systems to enhance surgical precision in TKA while highlighting areas for continued investigation into optimizing ligament balancing techniques.

7.1.4 Influence of Navigation System Updates on Total Knee Arthroplasty [67]

This is a machine-generated summary of:

Inui, Hiroshi; Taketomi, Shuji; Nakamura, Kensuke; Takei, Seira; Takeda, Hideki; Tanaka, Sakae; Nakagawa, Takumi Influence of navigation system updates on total knee arthroplasty [67].

Published in: BMC Sports Science, Medicine and Rehabilitation (2013).
Link to original: https://doi.org/10.1186/2052-1847-5-10

If you want to cite the papers, please refer to the original.

For technical reasons we could not place the page where the original quote is coming from.

7.1.4.1 Research Highlights

Total knee arthroplasty (TKA) is a widely successful procedure in orthopedic surgery, with its success hinging on factors such as surgical techniques and the design and material of the components. Accurate implant positioning, particularly in terms of rotational alignment, is crucial for optimal outcomes. Computer-assisted navigation systems have been developed to enhance the precision of these procedures, yet their effectiveness in consistently improving rotational alignment remains uncertain. The study by Inui et al. investigates whether the latest version of the Stryker image-free navigation system (Stryker Orthopedics, Kalamazoo, Mi., USA) enhances alignment accuracy and reduces operating time in TKA.

In this study, the authors compared two versions of the Stryker navigation system: version 4.0 and version 4.1. They conducted a retrospective analysis of 63 knees operated on with version 4.0 and 33 knees with version 4.1 at their institute. The procedures were performed using an image-free system with infrared cameras and light-emitting diodes to guide implant positioning. The researchers assessed various outcomes, including overall mechanical alignment, individual component positioning, knee scores, range of motion, and operating time. Postoperative alignment was evaluated using radiographs and computerized tomography (CT) scans to measure both frontal and rotational component angles. Statistical analyses were performed to determine any significant differences between the two groups.

The study found that while the updated navigation system reduced operating time by approximately 10 minutes, it did not result in statistically significant improvements in component positioning or clinical outcomes compared to its predecessor. The authors noted that although there was a tendency towards improved alignment with the newer system, further refinements in navigation technology and more precise registration techniques are necessary to achieve better rotational accuracy consistently. Future study could focus on enhancing CT-free navigation systems to improve rotational alignment without incurring additional costs or radiation exposure associated with CT-based methods.

7.1.5 Restoration of Constitutional Alignment Optimizes Outcomes of Computer Navigated Total Knee Arthroplasty: A Prospective Randomized Controlled Trial [68]

This is a machine-generated summary of:

Zheng, Kai; Wang, Yijun; Wang, Tianhao; Zhu, Feng; Zhang, Lianfang; Li, Rongqun; Zhou, Jun; Geng, Dechun; Xu, Yaozeng Restoration of constitutional alignment optimizes outcomes of computer navigated total knee arthroplasty: a prospective randomized controlled trial [68].

Published in: International Orthopaedics (2024).

Link to original: https://doi.org/10.1007/s00264-024-06093-9

If you want to cite the papers, please refer to the original.

For technical reasons we could not place the page where the original quote is coming from.

7.1.5.1 Research Highlights

Computer-navigated total knee arthroplasty (TKA) has been utilized for years to assist surgeons in the precise placement of cutting guides and implants. While proponents argue that navigation systems enhance alignment accuracy and bone resection, some studies have found no significant differences in overall alignment accuracy and patient function between navigated and conventional TKA. Additionally, navigation surgery often involves longer operative times, increased costs, and potential complications. Previous comparisons have been limited by surgical imprecision and radiographic accuracy, with all cases targeting mechanical alignment. The study by Zheng et al. revisits the value of navigated TKA with an updated alignment philosophy, focusing on constitutional alignment and its impact on outcomes.

The study was a prospective, randomized trial involving 41 patients undergoing one-stage bilateral TKA procedures. Each patient's knees were randomly assigned to either constitutional or mechanical alignment using computer navigation for the former. The researchers employed the OrthoPilot (Aesculap AG, Tuttlingen,

Germany) navigation system for constitutional alignment, ensuring precise component positioning based on individual knee phenotypes defined by coronal plane alignment classification. Clinical outcomes were assessed using patient-reported measures and radiographic evaluations preoperatively and postoperatively. The study aimed to determine the efficacy of navigated TKA in achieving accurate component positioning, particularly in knees with moderate to severe deformities.

The findings suggest that computer-navigated TKA allows for restoration of constitutional alignment with minimal soft tissue release, potentially leading to superior early outcomes compared to mechanical alignment. The study highlights the importance of maintaining native knee movements and joint line obliquity, especially in patients with constitutional varus knees. Future study could focus on larger sample sizes and longer follow-up periods to evaluate the long-term survivorship of these techniques. Additionally, multi-center trials may be necessary to generalize these findings across different populations and surgical settings. Despite some limitations, this research underscores the potential benefits of computer navigation in enhancing surgical precision and patient outcomes in TKA.

7.1.6 Comparison of the Accelerometer-Based Navigation System with Conventional Instruments for Total Knee Arthroplasty: A Propensity Score-Matched Analysis [69]

This is a machine-generated summary of:

Gao, Xiang; Sun, Yu; Chen, Zhao-He; Dou, Tian-Xu; Liang, Qing-Wei; Li, Xu Comparison of the accelerometer-based navigation system with conventional instruments for total knee arthroplasty: a propensity score-matched analysis [69].

Published in: Journal of Orthopaedic Surgery and Research (2019).

Link to original: https://doi.org/10.1186/s13018-019-1258-y

7.1.6.1 Research Highlights

Total knee arthroplasty (TKA) is a widely used procedure to alleviate pain and restore function in patients with advanced knee osteoarthritis. Achieving ideal mechanical alignment is crucial for the long-term success of TKA, yet the optimal range remains debated. Traditional methods often struggle with precision, especially in patients with severe deformities or high body mass index (BMI). Computer-assisted systems (CAS) have been introduced to enhance alignment accuracy, but they come with drawbacks such as high costs and a steep learning curve. The study by Gao et al. explores the efficacy of an accelerometer-based navigation (ABN) system as an alternative to conventional instruments in TKA.

The study was conducted as a retrospective case-control analysis at The First Hospital of China Medical University, involving patients who underwent TKA using either conventional instruments or the ABN system. Patients were selected based on specific criteria, including primary tricompartmental osteoarthritis and unilateral TKA history. Propensity score matching was employed to minimize confounding factors between the two groups. The ABN system, which uses positioning sensors and surgical instruments to guide bone resections, was compared against traditional methods in terms of mechanical alignment accuracy and short-term clinical outcomes. Radiographic assessments were performed postoperatively to evaluate alignment deviations, while clinical outcomes were measured using the Knee Society Score (KSS) and Western Ontario and McMaster Universities Osteoarthritis Index (WOMAC).

The findings indicate that the ABN system significantly improved mechanical alignment accuracy compared to conventional instruments, particularly in achieving desired hip-knee-ankle angles and component positioning. Short-term clinical outcomes showed better pain and stiffness scores in the ABN group, although no significant differences were observed in overall KSS or WOMAC scores between the groups. The study also noted reduced blood loss in the ABN group, attributed to less invasive procedures without intramedullary positioning. Future study could focus on long-term outcomes and revision rates to further validate the benefits of ABN systems in TKA. Despite its advantages, further research is needed to establish whether these improvements translate into enhanced quality of life and prosthesis longevity over time.

7.1.7 The Accuracy of a Hand-Held Navigation System in Total Knee Arthroplasty [70]

This is a machine-generated summary of:

Loh, Bryan; Chen, Jerry Yongqiang; Yew, Andy Khye Soon; Pang, Hee Nee; Tay, Darren Keng Jin; Chia, Shi-Lu; Lo, Ngai Nung; Yeo, Seng Jin The accuracy of a hand-held navigation system in total knee arthroplasty [70].

Published in: Archives of Orthopaedic and Trauma Surgery (2017).
Link to original: https://doi.org/10.1007/s00402-016-2612-8

If you want to cite the papers, please refer to the original.
For technical reasons we could not place the page where the original quote is coming from.

7.1.7.1 Research Highlights

Total knee arthroplasty (TKA) is a widely successful procedure for alleviating pain and restoring function in patients with knee issues. The success of TKA is influenced by several factors, including the proper positioning of implants and overall limb alignment. Malalignment can lead to increased stress on the prosthesis, accelerating wear and potentially leading to implant failure. While computer navigation has been shown to improve accuracy in implant positioning compared to conventional techniques, it often results in longer operative times and increased costs. The study by Loh et al. evaluates the effectiveness of a hand-held navigation system, Dash®, which aims to improve surgical workflow without the drawbacks associated with traditional computer-assisted systems.

The study involved a retrospective analysis of patients who underwent primary TKA using either the Dash® hand-held navigation system or conventional techniques. The Dash® system (Brainlab, Munich, Germany) utilizes a sterile draped iPod touch® equipped with software that guides surgeons through the procedure by displaying real-time alignment data. This system eliminates the need for anchoring pins, reducing the risk of complications such as fractures or infections at pin sites. The study included 100 patients using the Dash® system and compared their outcomes with those of patients who underwent conventional TKA. Measurements of limb alignment were taken post-operatively using digital radiographs, ensuring high reliability in assessing implant positioning.

The findings indicate that the Dash® system significantly reduces outliers in femoral component placement compared to conventional methods, while also decreasing surgical duration by an average of 10 minutes. This suggests that Dash® offers an efficient alternative to traditional navigation systems without compromising accuracy. Future studies could focus on randomized controlled trials to further validate these findings and explore functional outcomes associated with this technology. Additionally, while Dash® presents an upfront cost increase, its use in high-volume centers may offset expenses through improved surgical efficiency and reduced complication rates.

7.1.8 The Accelerometer-Based Navigation System Demonstrated Superior Radiological Outcomes in Restoring Mechanical Alignment and Component Sagittal Positioning in Total Knee Arthroplasty [71]

This is a machine-generated summary of:

Gao, Jiaxiang; Hou, Yunfei; Li, Rujun; Ke, Yan; Li, Zhichang; Lin, Jianhao The accelerometer-based navigation system demonstrated superior radiological outcomes in restoring mechanical alignment and component sagittal positioning in total knee arthroplasty [71].

Published in: BMC Musculoskeletal Disorders (2021).

Link to original: https://doi.org/10.1186/s12891-021-04213-9

7.1.8.1 Research Highlights

Total knee arthroplasty (TKA) outcomes are significantly influenced by the precise positioning of components, as malalignment can lead to increased polyethylene wear and higher revision rates. Conventional techniques for bone resection may be limited in cases with extra-articular deformities or excessive anterior femoral bowing, resulting in high outlier ratios. Computer-assisted surgery (CAS) has been developed to improve accuracy in limb alignment and component positioning, with handheld accelerometer-based navigation (ABN) systems emerging as a cost-effective alternative to large-console CAS. The study by Gao et al. investigates the postoperative radiological and clinical outcomes of TKA using the ABN system compared to conventional techniques.

The study conducted a retrospective review of patients who underwent primary TKA using either the ABN system or conventional methods at Peking University People's Hospital. The researchers collected preoperative demographic data and assessed clinical outcomes using Knee Society scores and range of motion (ROM). Radiological evaluations were performed using standardized postoperative radiographs, analysed by independent observers. Propensity score matching was employed to minimize confounding factors, ensuring comparable groups for analysis. The study found that the ABN group had significantly higher proportions of TKAs within a ± 3° deviation in most radiological variables, indicating improved accuracy in component positioning compared to the conventional group.

The findings suggest that while both ABN and conventional techniques resulted in significant clinical improvements postoperatively, the ABN system provided superior radiological outcomes, particularly in sagittal alignment. Future study could explore long-term effects on prosthesis survivorship and functional outcomes. The study highlights potential advantages of ABN in cases with complex anatomical challenges and suggests strategies to minimize technical errors during navigation TKA. Despite some limitations, such as its retrospective nature and short follow-up period, this research underscores the value of ABN systems in enhancing surgical precision in TKA.

7.1.9 Hand-Held Navigation May Improve Accuracy in Minimally Invasive Total Knee Arthroplasty: A Prospective Randomized Controlled Trial [72]

This is a machine-generated summary of:

Thiengwittayaporn, Satit; Fusakul, Yupadee; Kangkano, Nunnapat; Jarupongprapa, Chanintorn; Charoenphandhu, Narattaphol Hand-held navigation may improve accuracy in minimally invasive total knee arthroplasty: a prospective randomized controlled trial [72].

Published in: International Orthopaedics (2015).

Link to original: https://doi.org/10.1007/s00264-015-2848-x

If you want to cite the papers, please refer to the original.

For technical reasons we could not place the page where the original quote is coming from.

7.1.9.1 Research Highlights

Total knee arthroplasty (TKA) requires precise mechanical alignment to ensure long-term success, with a postoperative mechanical axis within ±3° of varus or valgus being crucial. Traditional computer-assisted surgery (CAS) systems have improved alignment but are often complex, time-consuming, and carry risks such as fractures from guidance pins. A new hand-held navigation system called iAssist (Zimmer-Biomet, Warsaw, In., USA) was developed to aid surgeons in positioning prosthetic components during surgery. The study by Thiengwittayaporn et al. investigates the accuracy of knee alignment and component positioning using the iAssist system compared to traditional methods in minimally invasive TKA (MIS-TKA).

The study was a prospective, randomized controlled trial involving patients with knee osteoarthritis undergoing MIS-TKA. Participants were randomly assigned to two groups: one using the iAssist navigation system and the other using standard techniques without navigation. The surgeries were performed by an experienced surgeon, ensuring consistency across procedures. The iAssist system utilized position sensors and surgical instruments to determine alignment axes relative to anatomical landmarks, guiding bone cuts in both coronal and sagittal planes. Postoperative outcomes were assessed through radiographic evaluations at six weeks, focusing on angles such as the hip-knee-ankle angle and coronal femoral angle. Statistical analyses compared deviations from target angles between the two groups.

The study found that the iAssist navigation system resulted in fewer alignment outliers compared to standard techniques, particularly in frontal alignment and tibial slope accuracy. While bone cutting time was slightly longer with iAssist, it was not significantly different from the non-navigation group. Blood loss was also reduced but not significantly so. The findings suggest that the iAssist system offers improved accuracy without increasing surgical complexity or time significantly. Future studies could explore long-term outcomes and further refine this technology to enhance its clinical utility in TKA procedures.

7.1.10 A New Robotically Assisted Technique Can Improve Outcomes of Total Knee Arthroplasty Comparing to an Imageless Navigation System [73]

This is a machine-generated summary of:

Mancino, Fabio; Rossi, Stefano Marco Paolo; Sangaletti, Rudy; Lucenti, Ludovico; Terragnoli, Flavio; Benazzo, Francesco A new robotically assisted technique can improve outcomes of total knee arthroplasty comparing to an imageless navigation system [73].

Published in: Archives of Orthopaedic and Trauma Surgery (2022).

Link to original: https://doi.org/10.1007/s00402-022-04560-9

If you want to cite the papers, please refer to the original.

For technical reasons we could not place the page where the original quote is coming from.

7.1.10.1 Research Highlights

Total Knee Arthroplasty (TKA) is the preferred treatment for end-stage knee osteoarthritis, with limb alignment and implant positioning being critical for long-term success and patient satisfaction. Recent advancements in computer navigation and robotic-assisted surgery aim to enhance the precision of TKA procedures. Robotic technologies, particularly imageless systems, offer potential benefits by improving component positioning accuracy without the need for preoperative computerized tomography (CT) scans, thus reducing patient radiation exposure. However, there is limited evidence comparing robotic TKA (RTKA) with navigated TKA (NTKA). The study by Mancino et al. investigates the clinical outcomes of imageless RTKA versus imageless NTKA over a one-year follow-up period.

The study involved patients who underwent primary TKA for knee osteoarthritis between February and September2020 at a high-volume institution. After excluding certain cases to account for a learning curve, 50 RTKA patients with mild-to-moderate varus deformity were included in the final analysis. A matched cohort of NTKA patients served as a comparison group. Both groups followed standardized postoperative rehabilitation protocols. The study collected demographic data, intraoperative details, and postoperative outcomes, including complications and reoperations. Clinical evaluations were conducted at multiple intervals post-surgery using various scoring systems such as the Knee Society Score (KSS) and Knee injury and Osteoarthritis Outcome Score (KOOS). Radiographic analyses assessed alignment deviations from target angles.

The study found that RTKA resulted in better improvements in range of motion (ROM) and KOOS pain scores compared to NTKA at one-year follow-up, suggesting favorable short-term functional outcomes. Despite longer operative times for RTKA, no significant differences were observed in overall alignment or complication rates between the two groups. The findings indicate that imageless RTKA may offer enhanced ROM and pain relief benefits over NTKA. Future studies should focus on larger cohorts and longer follow-up periods to confirm these preliminary results and explore the potential advantages of personalized component positioning offered by robotic systems.

7.1.11 Handheld Computer-Navigated Constrained Total Knee Arthroplasty for Complex Extra-Articular Deformities [74]

This is a machine-generated summary of:

Pietsch, M.; Hochegger, M.; Djahani, O.; Mlaker, G.; Eder-Halbedl, M.; Hofstädter, Th. Handheld computer-navigated constrained total knee arthroplasty for complex extra-articular deformities [74].

Published in: Archives of Orthopaedic and Trauma Surgery (2021).

Link to original: https://doi.org/10.1007/s00402-021-04053-1

If you want to cite the papers, please refer to the original.

For technical reasons we could not place the page where the original quote is coming from.

7.1.11.1 Research Highlights

Proper alignment is a critical goal in total knee arthroplasty (TKA), particularly in patients with arthritic knees and extra-articular deformities (EADs), where controlling the axis during implantation can be challenging. Computer-assisted surgery (CAS) offers potential benefits by avoiding intramedullary access, yet its application in complex EAD cases requiring constrained TKA with stem extensions remains underexplored. The study by Pietsch et al. investigates the impact of preoperative templating combined with an accelerometer-based handheld navigation system on postoperative alignment and clinical outcomes in patients with complex EADs undergoing constrained TKA.

The study enrolled ten consecutive patients with knee osteoarthritis and ipsilateral EADs, who underwent primary constrained TKA using a standardized surgical technique. Preoperative templating was performed on long-leg films to plan the positions of components and possible stem extensions. The alignment was determined using a Bluetooth accelerometer-based handheld CAS system, which did not require pins or trackers. Postoperative care included standardized physiotherapy, and clinical outcomes were assessed using the Knee Society score and range of motion measurements. Statistical analysis confirmed significant improvements in limb alignment and function post-surgery, with no intra- or postoperative complications reported.

This study advances the understanding of managing complex EADs during TKA by demonstrating that preoperative templating combined with handheld CAS can effectively restore limb alignment and improve function. The findings suggest that templating is crucial for identifying appropriate stem lengths, preventing anatomical conflicts, and ensuring successful outcomes. Future study could explore larger patient cohorts or compare different navigation systems to further validate these results. Additionally, the potential for robotic-assisted TKA in similar contexts may offer another avenue for enhancing surgical precision and patient outcomes.

Bibliography

1. Mason JB, Fehring TK, Estok R, Banel D, Fahrbach K (2007) Meta-analysis of alignment outcomes in computer-assisted total knee arthroplasty surgery. J Arthroplasty 22(8):1097–1106. https://doi.org/10.1016/j.arth.2007.08.001
2. Anderson KC, Buehler KC, Markel DC (2005) Computer assisted navigation in total knee arthroplasty: comparison with conventional methods. J Arthroplasty 20(7 Suppl 3):132–138. https://doi.org/10.1016/j.arth.2005.05.009
3. Ensini A, Catani F, Leardini A, Romagnoli M, Giannini S (2007) Alignments and clinical results in conventional and navigated total knee arthroplasty. Clin Orthop Relat Res 457:156–162. https://doi.org/10.1097/BLO.0b013e3180316c92
4. Lutzner J, Dexel J, Kirschner S (2013) No difference between computer-assisted and conventional total knee arthroplasty: five-year results of a prospective randomised study. Knee Surg Sports Traumatol Arthrosc 21(10):2241–2247. https://doi.org/10.1007/s00167-013-2608-7
5. Kazarian GS, Lawrie CM, Barrack TN, et al. the impact of surgeon volume and training status on implant alignment in total knee arthroplasty. J Bone Joint Surg Am. 2019;101(19):1713–23. https://doi.org/10.2106/JBJS.18.01205.
6. Antonios JK, Korber S, Sivasundaram L, et al. Trends in computer navigation and robotic assistance for total knee arthroplasty in the United States: an analysis of patient and hospital factors. Arthroplast Today. 2019;5(1):88–95. https://doi.org/10.1016/j.artd.2019.01.002. Published 2019 Mar 12.
7. Schrednitzki D, Horn CE, Lampe UA, Halder AM. Imageless robotic-assisted total knee arthroplasty is accurate in vivo: a retrospective study to measure the postoperative bone resection and alignment. Arch Orthop Trauma Surg. 2023;143(6):3471–9. https://doi.org/10.1007/s00402-022-04648-2.
8. Agarwal N, To K, McDonnell S, Khan W. Clinical and Radiological Outcomes in Robotic-Assisted Total Knee Arthroplasty: A Systematic Review and Meta-Analysis. J Arthroplasty. 2020;35(11):3393–409.e2. https://doi.org/10.1016/j.arth.2020.03.005.
9. Kayani B, Konan S, Tahmassebi J, Pietrzak JRT, Haddad FS. Robotic-arm assisted total knee arthroplasty is associated with improved early functional recovery and reduced time to hospital discharge compared with conventional jig-based total knee arthroplasty: a prospective cohort study. Bone Joint J. 2018;100-B(7):930–7. https://doi.org/10.1302/0301-620X.100B7.BJJ-2017-1449.R1.
10. Wainwright TW, Gill M, McDonald DA, et al. Consensus statement for perioperative care in total hip replacement and total knee replacement surgery:

Enhanced Recovery After Surgery (ERAS®) Society recommendations. Acta Orthop. 2020;91(1):3–19. https://doi.org/10.1080/17453674.2019.1683790.

11. Christen B, Tanner L, Ettinger M, Bonnin MP, Koch PP, Calliess T. Comparative cost analysis of four different computer-assisted technologies to implant a total knee arthroplasty over conventional instrumentation. J Personal Med. 2022;12(2):184. https://doi.org/10.3390/jpm12020184.
12. Bottros J, Gad B, Krebs V, Barsoum WK (2006) Gap balancing in total knee arthroplasty. J Arthroplasty 21(4 Suppl 1):11–15. https://doi.org/10.1016/j.arth.2006.02.084
13. Bolognesi M, Hofmann A (2005) Computer navigation versus standard instrumentation for TKA: a single-surgeon experience. Clin Orthop Relat Res 440:162–169 (pii:00003086-200511000-00029)
14. Matziolis G, Krocker D, Weiss U, Tohtz S, Perka C (2007) A prospective, randomized study of computer-assisted and conventional total knee arthroplasty. Three-dimensional evaluation of implant alignment and rotation. J Bone Joint Surg Am 89(2):236–243. https://doi.org/10.2106/JBJS.F.00386
15. Lee DH, Padhy D, Park JH, Jeong WK, Han SB The impact of a rectangular or trapezoidal flexion gap on the femoral component rotation in TKA. Knee Surg Sports Traumatol Arthrosc 19(7):1141–1147. https://doi.org/10.1007/s00167-011-1422-3
16. Longstaff LM, Sloan K, Stamp N, Scaddan M, Beaver R (2009) Good alignment after total knee arthroplasty leads to faster rehabilitation and better function. J Arthroplasty 24(4):570–578. https://doi.org/10.1016/j.arth.2008.03.002
17. Mizu-uchi H, Matsuda S, Miura H, Okazaki K, Akasaki Y, Iwamoto Y: The evaluation of post-operative alignment in total knee replacement using a CT-based navigation system. J Bone Joint Surg Br. 2008, 90: 1025-1031. https://doi.org/10.1302/0301-620X.90B8.20265 .
18. Stockl B, Noquler M, Rosiek R, Fischer M, Krismer M, Kessler O: Navigation improves accuracy of rotational alignment in total knee arthroplasty. Clin Orthop Relat Res. 2004, 426: 180-186.
19. Molli RG, Anderson KC, Buehler KC, Markel DC: Computer-assisted navigation software advancements improve the accuracy of total knee arthroplasty. J Arthroplasty. 2011, 26: 432-438. https://doi.org/10.1016/j.arth.2010.01.002 .
20. Chauhan SK, Clark GW, Lloyd S, Scott RG, Breidahl W, Sikorski JM: Computer-assisted total knee replacement. A controlled cadaver study using a multi-parameter quantitative CT assessment of alignment (the Perth CT protocol). J Bone Joint Surg Br. 2004, 86: 818-823. https://doi.org/10.1302/0301-620X.86B6.15456.
21. Allen CL, Hooper GJ, Oram BJ, Wells JE (2014) Does computer-assisted total knee arthroplasty improve the overall component position and patient function? Int Orthop 38:251–257. https://doi.org/10.1007/s00264-013-1996-0
22. Kim YH, Park JW, Kim JS (2017) The clinical outcome of computer-navigated compared with conventional knee arthroplasty in the same patients: a prospective, randomized, double-blind, long-term study. J Bone Joint Surg Am 99:989–996. https://doi.org/10.2106/JBJS.16.00791

23. Kim YH, Park JW, Kim JS (2012) Computer-navigated versus conventional total knee arthroplasty a prospective randomized trial. J Bone Joint Surg Am 94:2017–2024. https://doi.org/10.2106/JBJS.L.00142
24. Bauwens K, Matthes G, Wich M, Gebhard F, Hanson B, Ekkernkamp A, Stengel D (2007) Navigated total knee replacement. A meta-analysis. J Bone Joint Surg Am 89(2):261–269. https://doi.org/10.2106/JBJS.F.00601
25. Zheng K, Zhu F, Zhang W, Sun H, Zhou J, Li R, Xu Y (2022) Total knee arthroplasty using adjusted restricted kinematic alignment for the treatment of severe varus deformity: technical note. Orthop Surg 14:1892–1901. https://doi.org/10.1111/os.13354
26. Bellemans J, Colyn W, Vandenneucker H, Victor J (2012) The Chitranjan Ranawat award: is neutral mechanical alignment normal for all patients? The concept of constitutional varus. Clin Orthop Relat Res 470(1):45–53. https://doi.org/10.1007/s11999-011-1936-5
27. Huang TW, Hsu WH, Peng KT, Hsu RW, Weng YJ, Shen WJ (2011) Total knee arthroplasty with use of computer-assisted navigation compared with conventional guiding systems in the same patient: radiographic results in Asian patients. J Bone Joint Surg Am 93:1197–1202. https://doi.org/10.2106/JBJS.J.00325
28. Inacio MC, Chen Y, Paxton EW, Namba RS, Kurtz SM, Cafri G. Statistics in brief: an introduction to the use of propensity scores. Clin Orthop Relat Res. 2015;473:2722–6.
29. Bonner TJ, Eardley WG, Patterson P, Gregg PJ (2011) The effect of post-operative mechanical axis alignment on the survival of primary total knee replacements after a follow-up of 15 years. J Bone Joint Surg Br 93(9):1217–1222. https://doi.org/10.1302/0301-620X.93B9.26573
30. Goh GS, Liow MHL, Tay DK, Lo NN, Yeo SJ, Tan MH. Accelerometer-based and computer-assisted navigation in total knee arthroplasty: a reduction in mechanical axis outliers does not lead to improvement in functional outcomes or quality of life when compared to conventional total knee arthroplasty. J Arthroplast. 2018;33:379–85.
31. Matassi F, Cozzi Lepri A, Innocenti M, Zanna L, Civinini R, Innocenti M. Total knee arthroplasty in patients with extra-articular deformity: restoration of mechanical alignment using accelerometer-based navigation system. J Arthroplast. 2019;34:676–81.
32. Bugbee WD, Kermanshahi AY, Munro MM, McCauley JC, Copp SN (2014) Accuracy of a hand-held surgical navigation system for tibial resection in total knee arthroplasty. Knee 21(6):1225–1228. https://doi.org/10.1016/j.knee.2014.09.006
33. Chen JY, Chin PL, Tay DK, Chia SL, Lo NN, Yeo SJ (2014) Less outliers in pinless navigation compared with conventional surgery in total knee arthroplasty. Knee Surg Sports Traumatol Arthrosc 22(8):1827–1832. https://doi.org/10.1007/s00167-013-2456-5

34. Schnurr C, Eysel P, Konig DP (2011) Displays mounted on cutting blocks reduce the learning curve in navigated total knee arthroplasty. Comput Aided Surg 16(5):249–256. https://doi.org/10.3109/10929088.2011.603750
35. Zhu M, Chen JY, Chong HC, Yew AK, Foo LS, Chia SL, Lo NN, Yeo SJ (2015) Outcomes following total knee arthroplasty with CT-based patient-specific instrumentation. Knee Surg Sports Traumatol Arthrosc. https://doi.org/10.1007/s00167-015-3803-5
36. Chauhan SK, Scott RG, Breidahl W, Beaver RJ (2004) Computer-assisted knee arthroplasty versus a conventional jig-based technique. A randomised, prospective trial. J Bone Joint Surg Br. 86(3):372–377. http://www.ncbi.nlm.nih.gov/pubmed/15125124. Accessed 26 March 2015
37. Nam D, Jerabek SA, Haughom B, Cross MB, Reinhardt KR, Mayman DJ (2011) Radiographic analysis of a hand-held surgical navigation system for tibial resection in total knee arthroplasty. J Arthroplasty 26(8):1527–1533. https://doi.org/10.1016/j.arth.2011.01.012
38. Tingart M, Luring C, Bathis H, Beckmann J, Grifka J, Perlick L: Computer-assisted total knee arthroplasty versus the conventional technique: how precise is navigation in clinical routine?. Knee Surg Sports Traumatol Arthrosc. 2008, 16: 44-50. https://doi.org/10.1007/s00167-007-0399-4 .
39. Laskin RS, Beksaç B. Computer-assisted navigation in TKA: where we are and where we are going. Clin Orthop Relat Res. 2006;1:452127–31. https://doi.org/10.1097/01.blo.0000238823.78895.dc.
40. Gao X, Sun Y, Chen ZH, Dou TX, Liang QW, Li X. Comparison of the accelerometer-based navigation system with conventional instruments for total knee arthroplasty: a propensity score-matched analysis. J Orthop Surg Res. 2019;14(1):223. https://doi.org/10.1186/s13018-019-1258-y.
41. Kinney MC, Cidambi KR, Severns DL, Gonzales FB. Comparison of the iAssist handheld guidance system to conventional instruments for mechanical Axis restoration in Total knee arthroplasty. J Arthroplast. 2018;33(1):61–6. https://doi.org/10.1016/j.arth.2017.06.004.
42. Liow MH, Goh GS, Pang HN, Tay DK, Lo NN, Yeo SJ (2016) Computer-assisted stereotaxic navigation improves the accuracy of mechanical alignment and component positioning in total knee arthroplasty. Arch Orthop Trauma Surg 136(8):1173–1180. https://doi.org/10.1007/s00402-016-2483-z
43. Moo IH, Chen JYQ, Chau DHH, Tan SW, Lau ACK, Teo YS. Similar radiological results with accelerometer-based navigation versus conventional technique in total knee arthroplasty. J Orthop Surg (Hong Kong). 2018;26(2):2309499018772374. https://doi.org/10.1177/2309499018772374.
44. Nam D, Cody EA, Nguyen JT, Figgie MP, Mayman DJ (2014) Extramedullary guides versus portable, accelerometer-based navigation for tibial alignment in total knee arthroplasty: a randomized, controlled trial: winner of the 2013 HAP PAUL award. J Arthroplasty 29(2):288–294. https://doi.org/10.1016/j.arth.2013.06.006

45. Kim YH, Park JW, Kim JS, Park SD. The relationship between the survival of total knee arthroplasty and postoperative coronal, sagittal and rotational alignment of knee prosthesis. Int Orthop. 2014;38:379–85.
46. Brin YS, Nikolaou VS, Joseph L, Zukor DJ, Antoniou J (2011) Imageless computer assisted versus conventional total knee replacement. A Bayesian meta-analysis of 23 comparative studies. Int Orthop 35(3):331–339. https://doi.org/10.1007/s00264-010-1008-6
47. Jung KA, Lee SC, Ahn NK, Song MB, Nam CH, Shon OJ (2011) Delayed femoral fracture through a tracker pin site after navigated total knee arthroplasty. J Arthroplasty 26:505 e59-505 e511. https://doi.org/10.1016/j.arth.2010.01.006
48. Scuderi GR, Fallaha M, Masse V, Lavigne P, Amiot LP, Berthiaume MJ (2014) Total knee arthroplasty with a novel navigation system within the surgical field. Orthop Clin North Am 45(2):167–173. https://doi.org/10.1016/j.ocl.2013.11.002
49. Bourne RB, Chesworth BM, Davis AM, Mahomed NN, Charron KD. Patient satisfaction after total knee arthroplasty: who is satisfied and who is not? Clin Orthop Relat Res. 2010;468:57–63.
50. Gunaratne R, Pratt DN, Banda J, Fick DP, Khan RJK, Robertson BW (2017) Patient dissatisfaction following total knee arthroplasty: a systematic review of the literature. J Arthroplasty 32:3854–3860. https://doi.org/10.1016/j.arth.2017.07.021
51. Noble PC, Conditt MA, Cook KF, Mathis KB (2006) The John Insall Award: Patient expectations affect satisfaction with total knee arthroplasty. Clin Orthop Relat Res 2006:35–43. https://doi.org/10.1097/01.blo.0000238825.63648.1e
52. Hampp EL, Chughtai M, Scholl LY, Sodhi N, Bhowmik-Stoker M, Jacofsky DJ et al (2019) Robotic-arm assisted total knee arthroplasty demonstrated greater accuracy and precision to plan compared with manual techniques. J Knee Surg 32(3):239–250. https://doi.org/10.1055/s-0038-1641729
53. Parratte S, Price AJ, Jeys LM, Jackson WF, Clarke HD (2019) Accuracy of a new robotically assisted technique for total knee arthroplasty: a cadaveric study. J Arthroplasty 34(11):2799–2803. https://doi.org/10.1016/j.arth.2019.06.040
54. Savov P, Tuecking LR, Windhagen H, et al. Imageless robotic handpiece-assisted total knee arthroplasty: a learning curve analysis of surgical time and alignment accuracy. Arch Orthop Trauma Surg. 2021;141:2119–28. https://doi.org/10.1007/s00402-021-04036-2.
55. Thiengwittayaporn S, Uthaitas P, Senwiruch C, Hongku N, Tunyasuwanakul R (2021) Imageless robotic-assisted total knee arthroplasty accurately restores the radiological alignment with a short learning curve: a randomized controlled trial. Int Orthop 45(11):2851–2858. https://doi.org/10.1007/s00264-021-05179-y
56. Collins K, Agius PA, Fraval A, Petterwood J (2021) Initial experience with the NAVIO robotic-assisted total knee replacement-coronal alignment accuracy and the learning curve [published online ahead of print, 2021 Jan 28]. J Knee Surg. https://doi.org/10.1055/s-0040-1722693

57. King CA, Jordan M, Bradley AT, Wlodarski C, Tauchen A, Puri L (2022) Transitioning a practice to robotic total knee arthroplasty is correlated with favorable short-term clinical outcomes-a single surgeon experience. J Knee Surg 35(1):78–82. https://doi.org/10.1055/s-0040-1712984
58. Batailler C, Fernandez A, Swan J, Servien E, Haddad FS, Catani F et al (2020) MAKO CT-based robotic arm-assisted system is a reliable procedure for total knee arthroplasty: a systematic review. Knee Surg Sports Traumatol Arthrosc. https://doi.org/10.1007/s00167-020-06283-z
59. Wang JW, Wang CJ (2002) Total knee arthroplasty for arthritis of the knee with extra-articular deformity. J Bone Jt Surg Am 84:1769–1774. https://doi.org/10.2106/00004623-200210000-00005
60. Mabry TM, Vessely MB, Schleck CD, Harmsen WS, Berry DJ (2007) Revision total knee arthroplasty with modular cemented stems: long-term follow-up. J Arthroplasty 22:100–105. https://doi.org/10.1016/j.arth.2007.03.025
61. Lachiewicz PF, Soileau ES (2015) A 30-mm cemented stem extension provides adequate fixation of the tibial component in revision knee arthroplasty. Clin Orthop Relat Res 473:185–189. https://doi.org/10.1007/s11999-014-3529-6
62. Rhee SJ, Seo CH, Suh JT (2013) Navigation-assisted total knee arthroplasty for patients with extra-articular deformity. Knee Surg Relat Res 25:194–201. https://doi.org/10.5792/ksrr.2013.25.4.194
63. Catani F, Digennaro V, Ensini A, Leardini A, Giannini S (2012) Navigation-assisted total knee arthroplasty in knees with osteoarthritis due to extra-articular deformity. Knee Surg Sports Traumatol Arthrosc 20:546–551. https://doi.org/10.1007/s00167-011-1602-1
64. Liow, Ming Han Lincoln; Goh, Graham Seow-Hng; Pang, Hee-Nee; Tay, Darren Keng Jin; Lo, Ngai Nung; Yeo, Seng Jin Computer-assisted stereotaxic navigation improves the accuracy of mechanical alignment and component positioning in total knee arthroplasty. Archives of Orthopaedic and Trauma Surgery (2016). https://doi.org/10.1007/s00402-016-2483-z
65. Tran, Joshua Yeuk-Shun; Tang, Abbie Yan-Tung; Wong, Cham-Kit; Lam, Gloria Yan-Ting; Choi, Tsz-Lung; Mak, Rex Wang-Fung; Ng, Jonathan Patrick; Ho, Kevin Ki-Wai; Ong, Michael Tim-Yun; Yung, Patrick Shu-Hang Handheld imageless robotic total knee arthroplasty improves accuracy and early clinical outcomes when compared with navigation. Arthroplasty (2025). https://doi.org/10.1186/s42836-025-00303-4
66. Fickert, S.; Jawhar, A.; Sunil, P.; Scharf, H.-P Precision of Ci-navigated extension and flexion gap balancing in total knee arthroplasty and analysis of potential predictive variables. Archives of Orthopaedic and Trauma Surgery (2011). https://doi.org/10.1007/s00402-011-1419-x
67. Inui, Hiroshi; Taketomi, Shuji; Nakamura, Kensuke; Takei, Seira; Takeda, Hideki; Tanaka, Sakae; Nakagawa, Takumi Influence of navigation system updates on total knee arthroplasty. BMC Sports Science, Medicine and Rehabilitation (2013). https://doi.org/10.1186/2052-1847-5-10
68. Zheng, Kai; Wang, Yijun; Wang, Tianhao; Zhu, Feng; Zhang, Lianfang; Li, Rongqun; Zhou, Jun; Geng, Dechun; Xu, Yaozeng Restoration of constitutional

alignment optimizes outcomes of computer navigated total knee arthroplasty: a prospective randomized controlled trial. International Orthopaedics (2024). 10.1007/s00264-024-06093-9

69. Gao, Xiang; Sun, Yu; Chen, Zhao-He; Dou, Tian-Xu; Liang, Qing-Wei; Li, Xu Comparison of the accelerometer-based navigation system with conventional instruments for total knee arthroplasty: a propensity score-matched analysis. Journal of Orthopaedic Surgery and Research (2019). https://doi.org/10.1186/s13018-019-1258-y
70. Loh, Bryan; Chen, Jerry Yongqiang; Yew, Andy Khye Soon; Pang, Hee Nee; Tay, Darren Keng Jin; Chia, Shi-Lu; Lo, Ngai Nung; Yeo, Seng Jin The accuracy of a hand-held navigation system in total knee arthroplasty. Archives of Orthopaedic and Trauma Surgery (2017). https://doi.org/10.1007/s00402-016-2612-8
71. Gao, Jiaxiang; Hou, Yunfei; Li, Rujun; Ke, Yan; Li, Zhichang; Lin, Jianhao The accelerometer-based navigation system demonstrated superior radiological outcomes in restoring mechanical alignment and component sagittal positioning in total knee arthroplasty. BMC Musculoskeletal Disorders (2021). https://doi.org/10.1186/s12891-021-04213-9
72. Thiengwittayaporn, Satit; Fusakul, Yupadee; Kangkano, Nunnapat; Jarupongprapa, Chanintorn; Charoenphandhu, Narattaphol Hand-held navigation may improve accuracy in minimally invasive total knee arthroplasty: a prospective randomized controlled trial. International Orthopaedics (2015). https://doi.org/10.1007/s00264-015-2848-x
73. Mancino, Fabio; Rossi, Stefano Marco Paolo; Sangaletti, Rudy; Lucenti, Ludovico; Terragnoli, Flavio; Benazzo, Francesco A new robotically assisted technique can improve outcomes of total knee arthroplasty comparing to an imageless navigation system. Archives of Orthopaedic and Trauma Surgery (2022). https://doi.org/10.1007/s00402-022-04560-9
74. Pietsch, M.; Hochegger, M.; Djahani, O.; Mlaker, G.; Eder-Halbedl, M.; Hofstädter, Th. Handheld computer-navigated constrained total knee arthroplasty for complex extra-articular deformities. Archives of Orthopaedic and Trauma Surgery (2021). https://doi.org/10.1007/s00402-021-04053-1

7.2 Robotic

Machine Generated Summaries

Disclaimer: The summaries in this chapter were generated from Springer Nature publications using abstractive AI auto-summarization: An abstraction-based summarizer creates new text based on deep learning. New phrases are created to summarize the content. As the constituted sentences are machine selected, they may not fully reflect the body of the work, so we strongly advise that the original content is read and cited. The auto-generated summaries were curated by the editor to meet Springer Nature publication standards.

7.2.1 Complications and Learning Curve Associated with an Imageless Burr-Based (CORI) Robotic-Assisted Total Knee Arthroplasty System: Results from First 500 Cases [109]

This is a machine-generated summary of:

Weaver, Douglas J.; Deshmukh, Shobit; Bashyal, Ravi; Bagaria, Vaibhav Complications and Learning Curve Associated with an Imageless Burr-Based (CORI) Robotic-Assisted Total Knee Arthroplasty System: Results from First 500 Cases [109].

Published in: Indian Journal of Orthopaedics (2024).

Link to original: https://doi.org/10.1007/s43465-024-01200-9

If you want to cite the papers, please refer to the original.

For technical reasons we could not place the page where the original quote is coming from.

7.2.1.1 Research Highlights

Total knee arthroplasty (TKA) is a prevalent orthopedic procedure, with its demand expected to rise significantly. Robotic-assisted total knee arthroplasty (RA-TKA) has emerged as a promising approach to enhance precision and implant positioning accuracy. Despite the introduction of various robotic systems with differing haptic feedback and imaging technologies, there remains a lack of comprehensive data on their long-term outcomes and specific complications. The study by Weaver et al. investigates the learning curve and complications associated with a novel burr-based, imageless RA-TKA system, providing valuable insights into its integration into surgical practice.

The study was conducted at an urban tertiary referral center, involving patients undergoing primary TKA using the CORI Surgical System (Smith and Nephew, Memphis Tenn., USA). The research focused on calculating the learning curve for this new robotic system by comparing operative times with conventional TKA performed by the same surgeon. The study also assessed intraoperative and postoperative complications specific to this burr-based system. A standard medial parapatellar approach was used, with pins inserted for registration and intraoperative mapping to create a geometric model for the robotic system. The LEGION Total Knee Implant

System (Smith and Nephew, Memphis Tenn., USA) was utilized in all cases, with bone cuts executed by a handheld burr-based device. Cumulative summation analysis revealed that the learning curve for this system was six cases, after which operative times decreased significantly.

The study highlights several key advances in understanding RA-TKA systems. It establishes a learning curve for integrating the CORI imageless RA-TKA system into surgical workflows, comparable to other robotic platforms. The research identifies specific intraoperative and postoperative complications associated with this system, such as burr over-resection and pin site issues, emphasizing the need for surgeons to be prepared for potential challenges. Future study could focus on optimizing software algorithms to minimize errors and exploring patient-reported outcomes to further evaluate the benefits of RA-TKA systems. This study provides a foundation for evaluating future generations of robotic-assisted knee arthroplasty technologies.

7.2.2 Comparison of the Efficacy and Safety of MAKO Robot-Assisted Total Knee Arthroplasty Versus Conventional Manual Total Knee Arthroplasty in Uncomplicated Unilateral Total Knee Arthroplasty a Single-Centre Retrospective Analysis [110]

This is a machine-generated summary of:

Ma, Nanshan; Sun, Pengfei; Xin, Pengfei; Zhong, Sheng; Xie, Jun; Xiao, Lianbo Comparison of the efficacy and safety of MAKO robot-assisted total knee arthroplasty versus conventional manual total knee arthroplasty in uncomplicated unilateral total knee arthroplasty a single-centre retrospective analysis [110].

Published in: International Orthopaedics (2024).

Link to original: https://doi.org/10.1007/s00264-024-06234-0

If you want to cite the papers, please refer to the original.

For technical reasons we could not place the page where the original quote is coming from.

7.2.2.1 Research Highlights

Total knee arthroplasty (TKA) is a widely performed surgical procedure for patients with severe knee osteoarthritis, offering pain relief and improved joint function. However, traditional TKA relies heavily on the surgeon's experience for precise osteotomy and soft tissue balancing, which are crucial for optimal prosthetic positioning and alignment. Inaccuracies in these areas can lead to increased prosthetic wear and the need for revision surgeries. The study by Ma et al. explores the efficacy of MAKO robot-assisted TKA (Stryker Orthopedics, Kalamazoo, Mi., USA) compared to conventional manual TKA in achieving better surgical outcomes.

The study conducted a retrospective analysis of patients who underwent TKA between April and July,2023, comparing those who received MAKO robot-assisted surgery with those who underwent conventional manual procedures. The MAKO system utilizes preoperative CT scans to create a 3D model of the knee, guiding precise osteotomies during surgery. Both groups followed similar postoperative protocols, including pain management and rehabilitation exercises. The researchers evaluated radiographic outcomes using angles such as the medial proximal tibial angle (MPTA) and hip-knee-ankle angle (HKA), alongside clinical outcomes measured by Visual Analog Scale (VAS) scores and American Knee Society Scores (AKSS).

The findings indicate that MAKO robot-assisted TKA offers superior short-term clinical efficacy compared to traditional methods. Patients in the MAKO group exhibited better alignment with lower HKA angles postoperatively, reduced pain levels, and higher functional scores at one- and three-months post-surgery. The study highlights the potential of robotic assistance in enhancing surgical precision, reducing soft tissue damage, and improving patient satisfaction. However, challenges such as high costs and a learning curve for surgeons remain barriers to widespread adoption. Future studies with larger sample sizes and longer follow-up periods are needed to validate these findings further and explore long-term benefits.

7.2.3 Mako Versus ROSA: Comparing Surgical Accuracy in Robotic Total Knee Arthroplasty [111]

This is a machine-generated summary of:

Rajgor, Harshadkumar D.; Mayne, Alistair; Munasinghe, Chathura; Pagkalos, Joseph; Agrawal, Yuvraj; Davis, Edward T.; Sharma, Akash D. Mako versus ROSA: comparing surgical accuracy in robotic total knee arthroplasty [111].

Published in: Journal of Robotic Surgery (2024).
Link to original: https://doi.org/10.1007/s11701-023-01786-6

If you want to cite the papers, please refer to the original.

For technical reasons we could not place the page where the original quote is coming from.

7.2.3.1 Research Highlights

Primary total knee arthroplasty (TKA) is a widely successful procedure that significantly enhances patients' quality of life. However, despite its success, approximately 20% of patients report dissatisfaction post-surgery, often due to factors like residual pain and implant malalignment. Robotic-assisted surgery has emerged as a promising approach to improve outcomes by enhancing the precision of implant positioning. The study by Rajgor et al. compares the accuracy of two robotic systems, the ROSA Knee (Zimmer-Biomet, Warsaw, In., USA) and MAKO (Stryker Orthopedics, Kalamazoo, Mi., USA) robotic arm-assisted surgery, in component positioning for TKA.

The study was conducted at a single tertiary orthopedic hospital using a retrospective analysis of a prospectively collated database. Two senior fellowship-trained orthopedic surgeons performed the surgeries using either the ROSA or MAKO systems. The MAKO system utilized pre-operative computerized tomography (CT) scans for precise implant positioning, while the ROSA system offered both image-dependent and imageless options for intra-operative guidance. The procedures involved standard surgical approaches with specific registration techniques to ensure accurate component placement. Radiological parameters such as joint line height, patella height, tibial slope, and posterior condylar offset were assessed pre- and post-operatively to evaluate the accuracy of component positioning.

The study found no significant differences between the two robotic systems in terms of accuracy for joint line height, patella height, tibial slope, and posterior condylar offset. Both systems demonstrated high precision in restoring these parameters compared to conventional TKA methods. The findings suggest that both ROSA and MAKO systems are effective in achieving accurate implant positioning with low complication rates. Future study could focus on evaluating patient-reported outcome measures (PROMs) following robotic TKA to further understand the benefits of these technologies in clinical practice. Additionally, considerations regarding cost-effectiveness and compatibility with various implants remain areas for further exploration.

7.2.4 *Imageless Robotic Total Knee Arthroplasty Determines Similar Coronal Plane Alignment of the Knee (CPAK) Parameters to Long Leg Radiographs [112]*

This is a machine-generated summary of:

Edelstein, Adam I.; Orsi, Alexander D.; Plaskos, Christopher; Coffey, Simon; Suleiman, Linda I. Imageless robotic total knee arthroplasty determines similar coronal plane alignment of the knee (CPAK) parameters to long leg radiographs [112].

Published in: Arthroplasty (2024).

Link to original: https://doi.org/10.1186/s42836-024-00231-9

If you want to cite the papers, please refer to the original.

For technical reasons we could not place the page where the original quote is coming from.

7.2.4.1 Research Highlights

The persistence of suboptimal satisfaction outcomes among patients following total knee arthroplasty (TKA) has led to the development of innovative surgical techniques. Personalized alignment strategies, such as kinematic alignment, aim to recreate native knee morphology by precisely replacing the amount of bone and cartilage removed with the implant, thereby restoring natural kinematics and joint laxities. These approaches have shown improved balance and outcomes compared to traditional mechanical alignment. However, a knowledge gap exists regarding the accuracy of imageless intraoperative robotic data in defining coronal plane alignment of the knee (CPAK) parameters, which are crucial for personalized TKA. The study by Edelstein et al. investigates whether imageless robotic data can accurately describe CPAK parameters and determine optimal cartilage wear assumptions for use in imageless navigation systems.

The study retrospectively reviewed 62 robotic TKA procedures performed using the imageless OMNIBotics system (Corin Orthopedics, Cirencester, UK). Patients included had end-stage osteoarthritis and underwent preoperative long leg radiographs (LLR). The researchers compared CPAK parameters derived from LLR with those obtained from intraoperative robotic navigation data using two sets of cartilage wear assumptions: a literature-based nominal wear correction and an optimized wear assumption tailored to the patient cohort. Measurements such as mechanical axis angles were taken from preoperative radiographs, while intraoperative landmarks were acquired using robotic navigation to calculate key angles like MPTA and LDFA. Statistical analyses assessed agreement between LLR-derived and navigated CPAK parameters, evaluating mean differences, standard deviations, and error margins.

The study found that imageless intraoperative robotic navigation data could determine CPAK parameters with mean differences within clinically acceptable limits when compared to LLR-derived values. The optimized wear assumptions led to minor improvements in accuracy over literature-based assumptions. These findings support the use of imageless navigation systems for identifying native knee phenotypes in TKA procedures. Future study could focus on directly comparing CT-based assessments with imageless navigation-based assessments of CPAK parameters to further validate these findings. Additionally, incorporating CPAK planning into computer-assisted TKA workflows may enhance personalized alignment strategies, potentially improving patient satisfaction outcomes in knee arthroplasty.

7.2.5 A New Gap Balancing Technique with Functional Alignment in Total Knee Arthroplasty Using the MAKO Robotic Arm System: A Preliminary Study [113]

This is a machine-generated summary of:

Tsai, Hung-Kang; Bao, Zhengyuan; Wu, Dengxian; Han, Jing; Jiang, Qing; Xu, Zhihong A new gap balancing technique with functional alignment in total knee arthroplasty using the MAKO robotic arm system: a preliminary study [113].

Published in: BMC Surgery (2024).

Link to original: https://doi.org/10.1186/s12893-024-02524-x

If you want to cite the papers, please refer to the original.

For technical reasons we could not place the page where the original quote is coming from.

7.2.5.1 Research Highlights

Traditional mechanical alignment in total knee arthroplasty (TKA) aims for neutral alignment by adjusting bone resections perpendicular to the femoral and tibial mechanical axes, which has shown good implant survivorship but lower patient satisfaction due to soft tissue release. Kinematic alignment (KA) and functional alignment (FA) are newer techniques that aim to improve outcomes by preserving individual anatomical structures and minimizing soft tissue impact, respectively. However, concerns about KA include potential risks of aseptic loosening due to unrestricted alignment. The study by Tsai et al. describes a spacer-based gap balancing technique with FA using the MAKO robotic arm system (Stryker Orthopedics, Kalamazoo, MI.,USA), aiming to enhance precision in TKA procedures.

The study involved 22 patients undergoing primary TKA with the MAKO robotic arm system, performed by a single experienced orthopedic surgeon. The researchers utilized a patented modified spacer-based gap tool under the supervision of a MAKO product specialist. Pre-operative assessments included measuring the hip-knee-ankle angle and recording knee function scores. During surgery, osteophytes were removed to improve gap measurement accuracy, and tibial resections were adjusted to achieve balanced extension-flexion gaps. The modified gap plate instrument was used for ligament tension assessment, allowing fine-tuning of medial and lateral gaps. Post-operative management included routine analgesia and rehabilitation guidance. Clinical outcomes were evaluated at six months and one-year following surgery using various scoring systems.

The study demonstrated that the new technique achieved controlled limb alignment and satisfied clinical outcomes without requiring soft tissue release in most cases. The mean post-operative hip-knee-ankle angle indicated more neutral alignment compared to traditional methods. Future study could focus on larger populations and longer follow-ups to verify the technique's effectiveness and reliability further. Additionally, developing quantifiable gap tension assessments could enhance the tool's utility for beginners in TKA procedures. Overall, this spacer-based gap balancing technique with FA using the MAKO robotic arm system shows promise in improving patient satisfaction and functional outcomes after TKA.

7.2.6 Operating Room Efficiency After the Implementation of MAKO Robotic-Assisted Total Knee Arthroplasty [114]

This is a machine-generated summary of:

Loomans, Laura; Leirs, Geert; Vandenneucker, Hilde Operating room efficiency after the implementation of MAKO robotic-assisted total knee arthroplasty [114].

Published in: Archives of Orthopaedic and Trauma Surgery (2023).

Link to original: https://doi.org/10.1007/s00402-023-04834-w

If you want to cite the papers, please refer to the original.

For technical reasons we could not place the page where the original quote is coming from.

7.2.6.1 Research Highlights

Robotic-assisted surgery for joint arthroplasties has seen rapid advancements over the past decades, particularly in total knee replacements, where robotic-assisted total knee arthroplasty (RATKA) is believed to offer improved clinical outcomes. Despite these advancements, the efficiency and cost-effectiveness of RATKA procedures have not been thoroughly investigated. The study by Loomans et al. examines the efficiency of MAKO (Stryker Orthopedics, Kalamazoo, Mi., USA) robotic-assisted total knee arthroplasty, comparing it to navigation-assisted procedures. The study highlights significant findings such as reduced operating room time, thinner insert thickness, and shorter hospital stays for RATKA.

The study retrospectively analyzed 432 consecutive patients undergoing primary total knee arthroplasty (TKA), with 198 receiving navigation-assisted procedures and 234 undergoing robotic-assisted procedures. Exclusion criteria included previous knee surgeries with implants. The surgeries were performed by an experienced surgeon familiar with both techniques. The RATKA group involved additional steps such as draping the robotic arm and setting up the robot, with a MAKO product specialist present to assist. Both groups followed similar preoperative protocols, except for a computerized tomography (CT) scan required for the RATKA group. Postoperative care was consistent across both groups, focusing on immediate mobilization and continuous passive motion. Statistical analysis revealed that RATKA resulted in a significantly shorter operating room time and length of stay, although surgical time did not differ significantly between the groups.

The study's findings suggest that RATKA offers several advantages over navigation-assisted procedures, including reduced instrumentation needs and improved predictability of implant sizes. These factors contribute to potential cost savings through decreased inventory and sterilization costs. However, the financial benefits must be weighed against the initial costs associated with robotic surgery equipment and maintenance. Future study could focus on long-term follow-up to assess cost-effectiveness more comprehensively, considering factors like implant survivorship and overall health costs. Despite limitations such as its retrospective design and non-randomized group allocation, this study provides valuable insights into the efficiency of RATKA compared to traditional methods.

7.2.7 Individualized Alignment in Total Knee Arthroplasty Using Image-Based Robotic Assistance [115]

This is a machine-generated summary of:

Calliess, Tilman; Ettinger, Max; Savov, Peter; Karkosch, Roman; Windhagen, Henning Individualized alignment in total knee arthroplasty using image-based robotic assistance [115].

Published in: Die Orthopädie (2018).

Link to original: https://doi.org/10.1007/s00132-018-3637-1

If you want to cite the papers, please refer to the original.

For technical reasons we could not place the page where the original quote is coming from.

7.2.7.1 Research Highlights

Total knee arthroplasty (TKA) traditionally aims for neutral mechanical alignment, but this approach may not suit all patients due to variations in individual anatomy and alignment. Despite advancements like computer-assisted surgery, dissatisfaction rates remain high, prompting exploration of more personalized approaches. Recent discussions have focused on kinematic alignment (KA), which seeks to restore the knee's pre-arthritic anatomy, potentially improving outcomes for patients with varus alignment. However, KA's anatomical focus may overlook individual soft tissue conditions. The study by Calliess et al. explores a hybrid technique using image-based semi-automated robotic-assisted surgery to achieve patient-specific alignment in TKA.

The study utilized the Stryker MAKO® robotic system (Stryker Orthopedics, Kalamazoo, Mi., USA) to perform TKA on cadaveric and clinical cases. Preoperative computerized tomography (CT) scans were used to create 3D models of the knee, guiding the KA-based planning process. The robotic system allowed precise bone cuts while considering soft tissue balance, aiming for symmetrical gap balance without excessive soft tissue release. The tibial and femoral components were aligned based on individual anatomy and soft tissue conditions, with adjustments made to achieve optimal balance. Two clinical cases demonstrated the technique's application, with patients enrolled in a trial comparing robotic-assisted TKA with conventional methods.

The study highlights the potential of robotic-assisted TKA to address limitations of traditional approaches by integrating anatomical and soft tissue considerations into surgical planning. This method allows for individualized component positioning while maintaining alignment within accepted ranges. Future study could focus on long-term outcomes and further refinement of balancing algorithms. While initial results are promising, longer follow-up is needed to fully assess the benefits of this technology in improving patient satisfaction and reducing revision rates in TKA.

7.2.8 Robotic-Assisted Total Knee Arthroplasty with the OMNIBot Platform: A Review of the Principles of Use and Outcomes [116]

This is a machine-generated summary of:

Shatrov, J.; Murphy, G. T.; Duong, J.; Fritsch, B. Robotic-assisted total knee arthroplasty with the OMNIBot platform: a review of the principles of use and outcomes [116].

Published in: Archives of Orthopaedic and Trauma Surgery (2021).

Link to original: https://doi.org/10.1007/s00402-021-04173-8

Copyright of the summarized publication:

Crown 2021.

7.2.8.1 Research Highlights

Total knee arthroplasty (TKA) is a common surgical intervention for end-stage osteoarthritis of the knee, aiming to alleviate pain, restore stability, and improve mobility. Achieving optimal outcomes in TKA depends on various factors, including patient selection and technical precision in implant positioning and ligament balancing. Traditional manual techniques have shown variability in accuracy, leading to the development of computer-assisted and robotic systems that enhance precision. The study by Shatrov et al. explores the OMNIBotics robotic platform (Corin Orthopedics, Cirencester, UK), which has been used in over 10,000 knee replacement surgeries, detailing its history, principles, and outcomes.

The study reviews the OMNIBotics system's components: Bone morphing statistical shape modeling, the OMNIBot robotic cutting guide, and the BalanceBot (Corin Orthopedics, Cirencester, UK), ligament balancing tool. The planning stage involves creating a real-time anatomical model using intraoperative data without preoperative imaging. Surgeons use this model to plan bone resections and implant positioning virtually before making any cuts. The OMNIBot assists with precise femoral resections using a bone-mounted guide that ensures accurate cuts through automated adjustments. The BalanceBot aids in achieving optimal soft tissue balance by measuring ligament tension throughout the knee's range of motion. The study conducted a literature review to assess the system's accuracy compared to traditional methods, finding that it offers improved consistency in implant positioning and alignment.

The study highlights that while evidence on long-term outcomes is still accumulating, early results indicate high accuracy and consistency with the OMNIBotics system. Future study could focus on long-term survivorship and patient-reported outcomes to further validate these findings. The authors note that concerns about workflow disruption or increased surgical time with robotic systems have not been substantiated in their experience or existing literature. The OMNIBotics platform presents a promising advancement in TKA technology with its precise planning capabilities and adaptability to different surgical philosophies, offering potential improvements in patient outcomes compared to conventional techniques.

7.2.9 *No Difference in Surgical Time and Total Theatre Time Between Robotically Assisted and Computer Assisted Total Knee Arthroplasty [117]*

This is a machine-generated summary of:

Haslhofer, David Johannes; Anelli-Monti, Victoria; Hausbrandt, Peter; Kammerlander, Christian; Klasan, Antonio No difference in surgical time and total theatre time between robotically assisted and computer assisted total knee arthroplasty [117].

Published in: Journal of Orthopaedics and Traumatology (2024).

Link to original: https://doi.org/10.1186/s10195-024-00798-8

If you want to cite the papers, please refer to the original.

For technical reasons we could not place the page where the original quote is coming from.

7.2.9.1 Research Highlights

Knee arthroplasty is a vital orthopedic procedure for patients with severe knee joint conditions, and recent technological advancements have introduced robotically assisted surgery (RAS) based on computer-assisted surgery (CAS). These innovations promise more personalized, precise, and accurate procedures, potentially improving patient outcomes. However, the impact of RAS and CAS on surgical and total theatre time remains a critical consideration in preoperative planning. The study by Haslhofer et al. evaluates the surgical and total theatre times of RAS compared to CAS, aiming to determine if RAS prolongs these times.

The study was conducted at a single center with a prospectively collected database of patients undergoing total knee arthroplasty (TKA) using either CAS or RAS between January and September. The researchers excluded initial cases for each surgeon using RAS to account for the learning curve, except for one surgeon experienced in RAS. Data collected included patient demographics, surgical and theatre times, length of stay, and 90-day complication and readmission rates. The procedures involved mechanical alignment for CAS and adjusted mechanical alignment for RAS, with all patients receiving cementless TKA. Statistical analysis was performed using IBM SPSS Statistics to compare the outcomes between the two groups.

The study found no significant difference in surgical or total theatre time between RAS-TKA and CAS-TKA, refuting the hypothesis that RAS would increase these times. This finding suggests that previous experience with CAS may facilitate the transition to RAS without additional time costs. The presence of a technician required by the MAKO (Stryker Orthopedics, Kalamazoo, Mi.,USA) system used in this study may aid workflow continuity. Future study could explore clinical outcomes and cost implications further, as well as investigate other robotic systems beyond MAKO. The results highlight that implementing robotic-assisted surgery does not reduce case volume due to time constraints but offers an efficient alternative to traditional methods without compromising safety or increasing complications.

7.2.10 Outcomes Following Robotic Assisted Total Knee Arthroplasty Compared to Conventional Total Knee Arthroplasty [118]

This is a machine-generated summary of:

Aggarwal, Vikram A; Sun, Joshua; Sambandam, Senthil N Outcomes following robotic assisted total knee arthroplasty compared to conventional total knee arthroplasty [118].

Published in: Archives of Orthopaedic and Trauma Surgery (2024).

Link to original: https://doi.org/10.1007/s00402-024-05231-7

If you want to cite the papers, please refer to the original.

For technical reasons we could not place the page where the original quote is coming from.

7.2.10.1 Research Highlights

Conventional total knee arthroplasty (cTKA) is a widely used and effective surgical treatment for knee osteoarthritis, but it carries risks of complications such as joint stiffness, infection, and nerve injury. Robotic total knee arthroplasty (rTKA) has emerged as a potential solution to reduce these complications by offering more precise surgical outcomes tailored to patient-specific anatomy. However, rTKA is not without its own challenges, including higher costs and a steep learning curve. The study by Aggarwal et al. investigates the complication rates and healthcare costs associated with cTKA and rTKA using data from the National Inpatient Sample (NIS) database.

The study retrospectively analyzed NIS records from 2010 to 2019, identifying patients who underwent either cTKA or rTKA. Excluding complex primary and revision TKAs, the researchers compared age at admission, length of stay (LoS), total costs, and various medical and surgical complications between the two groups. Statistical analyses were conducted using SPSS (Statistical Package for the Social Sciences, IBM, Chicago, IL, USA) to assess differences in these factors before and after propensity matching for variables such as age, sex, race, tobacco use, diabetes, and obesity. The results showed that rTKA patients had a significantly shorter LoS but incurred higher average costs compared to cTKA patients. Additionally, rTKA was associated with lower rates of certain complications like blood loss and pneumonia.

The study highlights that while rTKA offers benefits in terms of reduced complication rates and shorter hospital stays, it also comes with significantly higher costs. This cost increase is primarily due to the initial expenses of acquiring specialized equipment for rTKA. Future study could explore ways to make rTKA more cost-effective, particularly in high-volume hospitals where reduced postoperative complications could offset initial expenses. The findings suggest that rTKA may be particularly beneficial for complex cases where reducing severe complications is crucial. Further research is needed to optimize the integration of rTKA into orthopedic practice while addressing its economic challenges.

7.2.11 Real-World Accuracy of Robotic-Assisted Total Knee Arthroplasty and its Impact on Expedited Recovery [119]

This is a machine-generated summary of:

Wong, Wai Kit; Abu Bakar Sajak, Azliana; Chua, Hwa Sen Real-world accuracy of robotic-assisted total knee arthroplasty and its impact on expedited recovery [119].

Published in: Journal of Robotic Surgery (2024).

Link to original: https://doi.org/10.1007/s11701-024-02059-6

If you want to cite the papers, please refer to the original.

For technical reasons we could not place the page where the original quote is coming from.

7.2.11.1 Research Highlights

Total knee arthroplasty (TKA) is the standard treatment for end-stage knee osteoarthritis, yet a significant number of patients remain dissatisfied post-surgery. This dissatisfaction is often attributed to issues such as component malalignment, which can lead to persistent pain and instability. Accurate implant positioning and soft-tissue preservation are crucial for successful outcomes. Traditional methods rely on anatomical landmarks and the surgeon's judgment, but recent technological advancements have introduced robotic systems to enhance precision. The study by Wong et al. evaluates the precision of robotic-assisted TKA in implant positioning, alignment restoration, gap balancing, and early clinical outcomes.

The study enrolled patients with end-stage tricompartmental knee osteoarthritis who were scheduled for robotic primary TKA using the MAKO Robotic Arm Interactive Orthopedic System (Stryker Orthopedics, Kalamazoo, Mi., USA). Exclusion criteria included revision surgeries and recent knee infections. Pre-operative planning involved computerized tomography (CT) scans, and surgical techniques adhered to Functional Alignment principles. The procedure utilized bone cuts for gap balancing, with minimal soft tissue releases when necessary. Post-operative assessments included range of motion, stability tests, and patient-reported outcome measures at various intervals up to six months. Radiological evaluations were conducted pre- and post-operatively to assess alignment and implant positioning accuracy.

The study demonstrated that robotic-assisted TKA offers precise control over implant positioning and gap balancing, resulting in improved early post-operative outcomes. The restoration of the hip-knee-ankle axis showed minimal deviation from intra-operative plans, aligning with previous studies on robotic systems.

Patient-reported outcomes indicated significant improvements in symptoms and satisfaction within weeks post-surgery. While this preliminary report highlights promising short-term results, future studies with longer follow-up periods are needed to fully understand the long-term benefits of robotic-assisted TKA. The study suggests that enhanced accuracy in implant positioning could lead to better knee kinematics and increased implant survivorship, particularly important as more younger patients undergo TKA procedures.

7.2.12 Index Surgery and Ninety Day Re-operation Cost Comparison of Robotic Assisted Versus Manual Total Knee Arthroplasty [120]

This is a machine-generated summary of:

Ezeokoli, Ekene Uchenna; John, Jithin; Gupta, Rohun; Jawad, Ali; Cavinatto, Leonardo Index surgery and ninety day re-operation cost comparison of robotic-assisted versus manual total knee arthroplasty [120].

Published in: International Orthopaedics (2022).

Link to original: https://doi.org/10.1007/s00264-022-05674-w

If you want to cite the papers, please refer to the original.

For technical reasons we could not place the page where the original quote is coming from.

7.2.12.1 Research Highlights

In the last decade, robotic-assisted procedures have increasingly been integrated into orthopedic surgeries, particularly in total knee arthroplasties (TKAs). These robotic systems promise enhanced precision in bone cuts and improved intra-operative feedback, potentially leading to better implant positioning and patient outcomes. However, the financial implications of robotic-assisted TKAs (rTKAs) compared to manual TKAs (mTKAs) remain underexplored, with existing studies showing mixed results regarding cost-effectiveness. The study by Ezeokoliet al. investigates the early variable direct costs associated with rTKA versus mTKA in a high-volume setting at a single institution.

The study utilized data from the Michigan Arthroplasty Registry Collaborative Quality Initiative (MARCQI) database, analyzing cases from January 2018 to March 2020. The researchers included patients who underwent either rTKA or mTKA, excluding those with additional procedures or incomplete cost data. The analysis focused on variable direct costs (VDC), which encompass expenses directly related to patient care such as supplies and operating room time. The study found that rTKA had higher median total encounter costs and day-of-surgery costs compared to mTKA. Specifically, supply costs for rTKA were significantly higher, contributing to the overall increased expense. Despite these higher costs, rTKA patients experienced a shorter length of stay and reduced opioid requirements post-surgery.

The findings suggest that while rTKA incurs higher initial costs primarily due to supply expenses, it may offer clinical benefits such as reduced opioid use and shorter hospital stays. However, these advantages were not sufficient to offset the increased supply costs in this study. Future studies could explore post-operative costs more comprehensively, including readmissions and overall episode of care expenses. Additionally, evaluating the cost implications for payors alongside hospital VDC could provide a more holistic understanding of the financial viability of adopting robotic systems in orthopedic surgery. As rTKA becomes more prevalent, institutions should carefully consider these financial aspects before widespread implementation.

7.2.13 Learning Curve Analysis of Robotic-Assisted Total Knee Arthroplasty with a Chinese Surgical System [121]

This is a machine-generated summary of:

Zhang, Haoran; Bai, Xizhuang; Wang, Huisheng; Zhu, Zhiyong; Li, Xi Learning curve analysis of robotic-assisted total knee arthroplasty with a Chinese surgical system [121].

Published in: Journal of Orthopaedic Surgery and Research (2023).

Link to original: https://doi.org/10.1186/s13018-023-04382-4

If you want to cite the papers, please refer to the original.

For technical reasons we could not place the page where the original quote is coming from.

7.2.13.1 Research Highlights

Knee osteoarthritis (KOA) is a degenerative joint disease that affects millions of individuals in China, often leading to painful deformities and limited mobility. Total knee arthroplasty (TKA) is the most effective treatment for end-stage KOA, with conventional TKA surgeries increasing significantly over the past decade. Recently, robot-assisted TKA (RA-TKA) has gained popularity due to its ability to enhance surgical precision and outcomes. The study by Zhang et al.; investigates the efficacy of the HURWA knee surgery robot, an image-based, semiautomatic robotic arm system designed for RA-TKA, in improving surgical outcomes compared to conventional TKA.

The study conducted a retrospective analysis of RA-TKA procedures performed by three experienced surgeons using the HURWA system (HURWA robotic technology, Beijing, China). The research included patients aged 60 years or older who underwent robotic-assisted primary total knee arthroplasty for KOA. The study excluded patients with high body mass index (BMI), traumatic knee osteoarthritis, or other complicating factors. Surgeons received comprehensive training on the HURWA system before performing surgeries. The study measured operative time, bone cutting accuracy, and limb alignment using standardized protocols and statistical methods like CUSUM (Cumulative Sum) to assess learning curves. Results indicated that while there was a learning curve for operative time with the HURWA system, bone cutting accuracy and limb alignment were not significantly affected by the surgeon's prior experience with conventional TKA.

The findings suggest that the HURWA system can enhance surgical precision and consistency in RA-TKA procedures, potentially reducing postoperative alignment abnormalities. Surgeons reached proficiency in operative time after 10 to 15 procedures without relying heavily on prior experience with conventional TKA. Future studies could focus on optimizing operating procedures to reduce RA-TKA operative time further and explore additional benefits of individualized' osteotomy concepts beyond the mechanical axis approach. Long-term follow-up is necessary to validate these findings and assess the broader implications of robotic systems like HURWA in joint replacement surgeries.

7.2.14 Fracture through Tracking Pin Sites Following a Robotic-Assisted Total Knee Arthroplasty [122]

This is a machine-generated summary of:

Feroe, Aliya G.; Chakraborty, Amit K.; Rosenthal, Daniel I.; Simeone, F. Joseph Fracture through tracking pin sites following a robotic-assisted total knee arthroplasty [122].

Published in: Skeletal Radiology (2022).

Link to original: https://doi.org/10.1007/s00256-022-04034-4

If you want to cite the papers, please refer to the original.

For technical reasons we could not place the page where the original quote is coming from.

7.2.14.1 Research Highlights

Robotic-assisted total knee arthroplasty (TKA) has become increasingly popular over the past decade, offering an alternative to conventional TKA with the potential for improved implant positioning and limb alignment. Despite its advantages, robotic-assisted TKA is associated with unique complications, particularly those related to the pins used for mounting the robotic tracking system. These pins, temporarily placed in the femur and tibia during surgery, can serve as sites for infection or fracture. The study by Feroe et al. presents a case of a periprosthetic femoral shaft fracture through a robotic-assisted TKA pin site, highlighting this rare complication and its radiologic appearance.

The study details the case of a 65-year-old woman who underwent robotic-assisted TKA and later sustained a displaced fracture of the midshaft of her right femur. Radiographs revealed a transverse fracture through the mid-femoral diaphysis, extending between two bicortical pin sites used during her surgery. The fracture was treated with open reduction and internal fixation using a long intramedullary nail, allowing the patient to return to normal activities. The authors emphasize that such fractures can occur due to stress concentration at bone defects created by temporary hardware insertion. They note that risk factors include multiple pin placement attempts, transcortical pin trajectory, larger pin diameters, and diaphyseal placement.

The study underscores the importance of awareness regarding pin site-related femur fractures in robotic-assisted TKA. Future study could focus on optimizing pin placement techniques to minimize fracture risk, such as favoring metaphyseal or unicortical placements over diaphyseal ones. Additionally, documenting pin tracks on post-operative radiographs may help identify potential complications early. As robotic-assisted TKA continues to rise in prevalence, understanding these rare complications will be crucial for improving patient outcomes and guiding surgical planning and follow-up care.

7.2.15 Comparison of Serum Inflammatory Indicators and Radiographic Results in MAKO Robotic-Assisted Versus Conventional Total Knee Arthroplasty for Knee Osteoarthritis: A Retrospective Study of Chinese Patients [123]

This is a machine-generated summary of:

Xu, Jia-Zheng; Li, Liang-Liang; Fu, Jun; Xu, Chi; Zhang, Guo-Qiang; Chai, Wei; Hao, Li-Bo; Li, Xiang; Chen, Ji-Ying Comparison of serum inflammatory indicators and radiographic results in MAKO robotic-assisted versus conventional total knee arthroplasty for knee osteoarthritis: a retrospective study of Chinese patients [123].

Published in: BMC Musculoskeletal Disorders (2022).

Link to original: https://doi.org/10.1186/s12891-022-05373-y

If you want to cite the papers, please refer to the original.

For technical reasons we could not place the page where the original quote is coming from.

7.2.15.1 Research Highlights

As total knee arthroplasty (TKA) technology advances, robot-assisted TKA (RA-TKA) is increasingly utilized, with the MAKO surgical robot being one of the most prominent systems. While RA-TKA is reported to enhance precision and improve imaging and functional outcomes compared to conventional manual TKA (CM-TKA), its impact on early functional recovery remains debated. Some studies suggest no significant difference in postoperative function and pain scores between RA-TKA and CM-TKA. The study by Xu e al. investigates the early clinical outcomes of MAKO robot-assisted TKA (Stryker Orthopedics, Kalamazoo, MI., USA) in the Chinese population, focusing on inflammatory indicators, muscle damage markers, joint function, pain scores, and imaging outcomes.

The study included patients who underwent unilateral TKA for end-stage knee osteoarthritis between December 2020 and November 2021. Participants were divided into two groups: those receiving MAKO-assisted TKA (MA-TKA) and those undergoing conventional manual TKA (CM-TKA). Both groups received similar postoperative care, including enhanced recovery protocols. The researchers measured serum inflammatory markers preoperatively and postoperatively at specific intervals to assess differences between the two surgical approaches. Radiographic evaluations were conducted to determine prosthesis positioning accuracy. The study found that while there was no significant difference in preoperative inflammatory markers between the groups, postoperative levels of interleukin-6 (IL-6), C-reactive protein (CRP), erythrocyte sedimentation rate (ESR), and creatine kinase (CK) were significantly lower in the MA-TKA group. Additionally, radiographic results indicated more precise prosthesis positioning in the MA-TKA group.

The findings suggest that MAKO-assisted TKA may offer advantages in reducing early postoperative inflammatory responses and achieving more accurate prosthesis placement compared to conventional methods. However, no significant differences were observed in short-term functional or pain scores between the two groups. Future study could focus on long-term outcomes to determine if these early benefits translate into improved clinical results over time. The study highlights the need for further research with larger sample sizes and extended follow-up periods to fully understand the potential advantages of robotic assistance in TKA for diverse populations.

7.2.16 Efficacy of the Newly Designed "SkyWalker" Robot Compared to the MAKO Robotic System in Primary Total Knee Arthroplasty: A One-Year Follow-Up Study [124]

This is a machine-generated summary of:

Ping, Hang-Yu; An, Hao-Ming; Cao, Zheng; Nan, Shao-Kui; Li, Hai-Feng; Chai, Wei Efficacy of the newly designed "SkyWalker" robot compared to the MAKO robotic system in primary total knee arthroplasty: a one-year follow-up study [124].

Published in: International Orthopaedics (2023).
Link to original: https://doi.org/10.1007/s00264-023-06023-1

If you want to cite the papers, please refer to the original.
For technical reasons we could not place the page where the original quote is coming from.

7.2.16.1 Research Highlights

Knee osteoarthritis is a common age-related condition that often leads to pain, stiffness, and impaired knee function. Total knee arthroplasty (TKA) is the standard treatment for advanced cases, requiring precise surgical techniques to ensure successful outcomes. Robotic-assisted systems, such as the MAKO (Stryker Orthopedics, Kalamazoo, Mi., USA) robot, have been developed to enhance surgical precision but are limited by high costs and logistical challenges. Recently, a new semiactive robotic system called "SkyWalker" (MicroPort Orthopedics, Arlington, Tenn., USA) has been introduced by Chinese researchers, promising reduced costs and efficient preoperative planning. However, no direct comparisons between the SkyWalker and MAKO systems have been conducted until now. A new study by Hang-Yu Ping et al. addresses this gap by comparing the accuracy of lower limb alignment and surgical outcomes between these two robotic systems.

The study was a retrospective analysis involving patients who underwent primary TKA using either the SkyWalker or MAKO robots. Data were collected prospectively from surgeries performed by the same team within a specified period to ensure consistency. The inclusion criteria focused on patients with advanced knee osteoarthritis requiring TKA, while various exclusion criteria ensured a homogeneous study population. Preoperative planning for both robotic systems was based on computerized tomography (CT) imaging data, with specific osteotomy angles and alignments calculated for each patient. The surgical procedures were meticulously executed using each system's unique features, followed by postoperative assessments of alignment accuracy and clinical outcomes. Radiological measurements were taken shortly after surgery, and follow-ups were conducted at six months and one year to evaluate knee function and complications.

The study found no significant differences in lower limb alignment accuracy or clinical outcomes between the SkyWalker and MAKO groups at both follow-up intervals. Both systems demonstrated comparable performance in terms of operation time, estimated blood loss, and recovery of knee function. However, higher serum levels of IL-6 were observed in the SkyWalker group on the third postoperative day, suggesting a potentially greater stress response. The authors note that this could be due to the learning curve associated with the new system. Future studies with larger sample sizes and longer follow-up periods are recommended to further validate these findings and explore any long-term differences in revision rates or complications between the two robotic systems.

Bibliography

1. Thomas, T. L., Goh, G. S., Nguyen, M. K., and Lonner, J. H. (2022). Pin-related complications in computer navigated and robotic-assisted knee arthroplasty: a systematic review. *The J Arthroplasty., 37*(11), 2291-2307.e2. https://doi.org/10.1016/j.arth.2022.05.012
2. Lonner, J. H., and Kerr, G. J. (2019). Low rate of iatrogenic complications during unicompartmental knee arthroplasty with two semiautonomous robotic systems. *The Knee, 26*(3), 745–749. https://doi.org/10.1016/j.knee.2019.02.005
3. Feroe, A. G., Chakraborty, A. K., Rosenthal, D. I., and Simeone, F. J. (2022). Fracture through tracking pin sites following a robotic-assisted total knee arthroplasty. *Skeletal Radiology, 51*(11), 2217–2221. https://doi.org/10.1007/s00256-022-04034-4
4. Smith TJ, Siddiqi A, Forte SA, Judice A, Sculco PK, Vigdorchik JM et al (2021) Periprosthetic fractures through tracking pin sites following computer navigated and robotic total and unicompartmental knee arthroplasty: a systematic review. JBJS Rev. 9(1):e2000091. https://doi.org/10.2106/JBJS.RVW.20.00091
5. Kayani, B., Konan, S., Huq, S. S., Tahmassebi, J., and Haddad, F. S. (2019). Robotic-arm assisted total knee arthroplasty has a learning curve of seven cases for integration into the surgical workflow but no learning curve effect for accuracy of implant positioning. *Knee Surgery Sports Traumatology Arthroscopy, 27*(4), 1132–1141. https://doi.org/10.1007/s00167-018-5138-5
6. Khlopas, A., Sodhi, N., Sultan, A. A., Chughtai, M., Molloy, R. M., and Mont, M. A. (2018). Robotic arm-assisted total knee arthroplasty. *The Journal of Arthroplasty, 33*(7), 2002–2006. https://doi.org/10.1016/j.arth.2018.01.060
7. Deckey, D. G., Rosenow, C. S., Verhey, J. T., et al. (2021). Robotic-assisted total knee arthroplasty improves accuracy and precision compared to conventional techniques. *The Bone and Joint Journal*. https://doi.org/10.1302/0301-620x.103b6.bjj-2020-2003.r1
8. Liow, M. H., Xia, Z., Wong, M. K., Tay, K. J., Yeo, S. J., and Chin, P. L. (2014). Robot-assisted total knee arthroplasty accurately restores the joint line and mechanical axis a prospective randomised study. *The Journal of Arthroplasty, 29*(12), 2373–7. https://doi.org/10.1016/j.arth.2013.12.010
9. Kayani, B., Konan, S., Pietrzak, J. R. T., and Haddad, F. S. (2018). Iatrogenic bone and soft tissue trauma in robotic-arm assisted total knee arthroplasty compared with conventional jig-based total knee arthroplasty: a prospective cohort study and validation of a new classification system. *The Journal of Arthroplasty, 33*(8), 2496–2501. https://doi.org/10.1016/j.arth.2018.03.042

10. Hampp, E. L., Sodhi, N., Scholl, L., et al. (2019). Less iatrogenic soft-tissue damage utilizing robotic-assisted total knee arthroplasty when compared with a manual approach:a blinded assessment. *Bone and Joint Research, 8*(10), 495–501. https://doi.org/10.1302/2046-3758.810.bjr-2019-0129.r1
11. Fontalis, A., Kayani, B., Asokan, A., et al. (2022). Inflammatory response in robotic-arm-assisted versus conventional jig-based TKA and the correlation with early functional outcomes: results of a prospective randomized controlled trial. *Journal of Bone and Joint Surg America, 104*(21), 1905–1914. https://doi.org/10.2106/jbjs.22.00167
12. Sultan AA, Piuzzi N, Khlopas A, Chughtai M, Sodhi N, Mont MA (2017) Utilization of robotic-arm assisted total knee arthroplasty for soft tissue protection. Expert Rev Med Devices 14(12):925–927. https://doi.org/10.1080/17434440.2017.1392237
13. Loures FB, Góes RFA, Gusmão CV, Albuquerque RSPE, Labronici PJ (2021) Epidemiological and clinical profile of patients submitted to total knee arthroplasty. Rev Bras Ortop 57(2):223–229. https://doi.org/10.1055/s-0041-1724080
14. Schwechter EM, Fitz W (2012) Design rationale for customized TKA: a new idea or revisiting the past? Curr Rev Musculoskelet Med 5(4):303–308. https://doi.org/10.1007/s12178-012-9143-x
15. Bardou-Jacquet J, Murgier J, Laudet F, Fabre T (2022) Combining load sensor and robotic technologies for ligament balance in total knee arthroplasty. Orthop Traumatol Surg Res:OTSR 108(5):102889. https://doi.org/10.1016/j.otsr.2021.102889
16. Daffara V, Zambianchi F, Bazzan G, Matveitchouk N, Berni A, Piacentini L, Cuoghi Costantini R, Catani F (2023) No difference in clinical outcomes between functionally aligned cruciate-retaining and posterior-stabilized robotic-assisted total knee arthroplasty. Int Orthop 47(3):711–717. https://doi.org/10.1007/s00264-023-05693-1
17. Masilamani S, Mulpur P, Annapareddy A, Hippalgaonkar K, Roche MW, Reddy AVG (2022) Enhanced mid-resection workflow technique for severe varus deformity correction using robotic-arm assisted total knee arthroplasty. Surg Technol Int 41:sti41-1612. https://doi.org/10.52198/22.STI.41.OS1621. (Advance online publication)
18. Steelman K, Carlson K, Ketner A (2021) Utilization of robotic arm assistance for revision of primary total knee arthroplasty: a case report. J Orthop Case Rep 11(8):50–54. https://doi.org/10.13107/jocr.2021.v11.i08.2362
19. Wu XD, Zhou Y, Shao H, Yang D, Guo SJ, Huang W (2023) Robotic-assisted revision total joint arthroplasty: a state-of-the-art scoping review. EFORT Open Reviews 8(1):18–25. https://doi.org/10.1530/EOR-22-0105
20. Ngim HJ, Van Bavel D, De Steiger R, Tang AWW (2023) Robotic-assisted revision total knee arthroplasty: a novel surgical technique. Arthroplasty (London, England) 5(1):5. https://doi.org/10.1186/s42836-022-00160-5
21. Sires JD, Craik JD, Wilson CJ. Accuracy of bone resection in MAKO total knee robotic-assisted surgery. J Knee Surg. 2021;34(7):745–8. https://doi.org/10.1055/s-0039-1700570.

22. MacDessi SJ, Griffiths-Jones W, Harris IA, Bellemans J, Chen DB (2021) Coronal Plane Alignment of the Knee (CPAK) classification. Bone Joint J 103-B:329–337. https://doi.org/10.1302/0301-620X.103B2.BJJ-2020-1050.R1
23. Howell SM. Use the right looking glass when you do Caliper-verified Kinematically Aligned TKA! Arthroplast Today. 2022;15:139–40.
24. de Winnock Grave P, Luyckx T, Claeys K, Tampere T, Kellens J, Muller J, et al. Higher satisfaction after total knee arthroplasty using restricted inverse kinematic alignment compared to adjusted mechanical alignment. Knee Surg Sports Traumatol Arthrosc. 2022;30(2):488–99.
25. Kim KK, Howell SM, Won YY. Kinematically aligned total knee arthroplasty with patient-specific instrument. Yonsei Med J. 2020;61(3):201–9.
26. Calliess T, Bauer K, Stukenborg-Colsman C, Windhagen H, Budde S, Ettinger M. PSI kinematic versus non-PSI mechanical alignment in total knee arthroplasty: a prospective, randomized study. Knee Surg Sports Traumatol Arthrosc. 2017;25(6):1743–8.
27. Stindel E, Briard JL, Merloz P, Plaweski S, Dubrana F, Lefevre C, et al. Bone morphing: 3D morphological data for total knee arthroplasty. Comput Aided Surg. 2002;7(3):156–68.
28. Suero EM, Citak M, Claps C, Pearle AD, Plaskos C. Variations in ankle registration using two different anatomic landmarks: a radiographic study. Knee Surg Sports Traumatol Arthrosc. 2013;21(12):2759–63.
29. Howell SM, Roth JD, Hull ML. Kinematic alignment in total knee arthroplasty definition, history, principle, surgical technique, and results of an alignment option for TKA. Arthropaedia. 2014;1:44–53.
30. Murgier J, Clatworthy M. Variable rotation of the femur does not affect outcome with patient specific alignment navigated balanced TKA. Knee Surg Sports Traumatol Arthrosc. 2022;30(2):517–26.
31. Nam D, Lin KM, Howell SM, Hull ML. Femoral bone and cartilage wear is predictable at 0 degrees and 90 degrees in the osteoarthritic knee treated with total knee arthroplasty. Knee Surg Sports Traumatol Arthrosc. 2014;22(12):2975–81.
32. Tarassoli P, Wood JA, Chen DB, Griffiths-Jones W, Bellemans J, MacDessi SJ. Arithmetic hip-knee-ankle angle and stressed hip-knee-ankle angle: equivalent methods for estimating constitutional lower limb alignment in kinematically aligned total knee arthroplasty. Knee Surg Sports Traumatol Arthrosc. 2022;30(9):2980–90.
33. Insall JN, Binazzi R, Soudry M, Mestriner LA. Total knee arthroplasty. Clin Orthop Relat Res. 1985(192):13–22.
34. Oussedik S, Abdel MP, Victor J, Pagnano MW, Haddad FS. Alignment in total knee arthroplasty. Bone Joint J. 2020;102–b(3):276–9.
35. Clark GW, Esposito CI, Wood D. Individualized functional knee alignment in total knee arthroplasty: a robotic-assisted technique. Techniques Orthop. 2022;37(3):185–91.

36. Shatrov J, Battelier C, Sappey-Marinier E, Gunst S, Servien E, Lustig S. Functional alignment philosophy in total knee arthroplasty - rationale and technique for the varus morphotype using a CT based robotic platform and individualized planning. Sicot j. 2022;8:11.
37. Deckey DG, Rosenow CS, Verhey JT, Brinkman JC, Mayfield CK, Clarke HD et al. Robotic-assisted total knee arthroplasty improves accuracy and precision compared to conventional techniques. Bone Joint J. 2021;103-b(6 Supple A):74–80.
38. Rossi SMP, Benazzo F. Individualized alignment and ligament balancing technique with the ROSA® robotic system for total knee arthroplasty. Int Orthop. 2023;47(3):755–62.
39. Murphy GT, Shatrov J, Duong J, Fritsch BA (2023) How does the use of quantified gap-balancing affect component positioning and limb alignment in robotic total knee arthroplasty using functional alignment philosophy? A comparison of two robotic platforms. Int Orthop 47(5):1221–1232. https://doi.org/10.1007/s00264-022-05681-x
40. Mancino F, Rossi SMP, Sangaletti R, Caredda M, Terragnoli F, Benazzo F. Increased accuracy in component positioning using an image-less robotic arm system in primary total knee arthroplasty: a retrospective study. Arch Orthop Trauma Surg. 2024;144(1):393–404.
41. Bollars P, Meshram P, Al Thani S, Schotanus MGM, Albelooshi A. Achieving functional alignment in total knee arthroplasty: early experience using a second-generation imageless semi-autonomous handheld robotic sculpting system. Int Orthop. 2023;47(2):585–93.
42. Almaawi AM, Hutt JRB, Masse V, Lavigne M, Vendittoli PA. The impact of mechanical and restricted kinematic alignment on knee anatomy in total knee arthroplasty. J Arthroplasty. 2017;32(7):2133–40.
43. Aunan E, Kibsgård TJ, Diep LM, Röhrl SM. Intraoperative ligament laxity influences functional outcome 1 year after total knee arthroplasty. Knee Surg Sports Traumatol Arthrosc. 2015;23(6):1684–92.
44. Jacofsky DJ, Allen M. Robotics in arthroplasty: a comprehensive review. J Arthroplasty. 2016;31(10):2353–63. https://doi.org/10.1016/j.arth.2016.05.026.
45. Lonner JH (2009) Indications for unicompartmental knee arthroplasty and rationale for robotic arm-assisted technology. Am J Orthop (Belle Mead NJ) 38:3–6
46. Lonner JH, Moretti VM (2016) The evolution of image-free robotic assistance in unicompartmental knee arthroplasty. Am J Orthop (Belle Mead NJ) 45:249–254
47. Lonner JH, Fillingham YA (2018) Pros and cons: a balanced view of robotics in knee arthroplasty. J Arthroplasty 33:2007–2013. https://doi.org/10.1016/j.arth.2018.03.056
48. Sodhi N, Khlopas A, Piuzzi NS et al (2018) The learning curve associated with robotic total knee arthroplasty. J Knee Surg 31:17–21. https://doi.org/10.1055/S-0037-1608809/ID/JR17SEP0024SSA-15

49. Marchand KB, Ehiorobo J, Mathew KK et al (2020) Learning curve of robotic-assisted total knee arthroplasty for a high-volume surgeon. J Knee Surg. https://doi.org/10.1055/S-0040-1715126/ID/JR190398OA-25
50. Cotter EJ, Wang J, Illgen RL (2020) Comparative cost analysis of robotic-assisted and jig-based manual primary total knee arthroplasty. J Knee Surg. https://doi.org/10.1055/S-0040-1713895
51. Bellemans J, Colyn W, Vandenneucker H, Victor J (2012) The Chitranjan Ranawat award: is neutral mechanical alignment normal for all patients? The concept of constitutional varus. Clin Orthop Relat Res 470(1):45–53. https://doi.org/10.1007/s11999-011-1936-5
52. Gibon E, Goodman MJ, Goodman SB (2017) Patient satisfaction after total knee arthroplasty: a realistic or imaginary goal? Orthop Clin North Am 48(4):421–431. https://doi.org/10.1016/j.ocl.2017.06.001
53. Plaskos C, Cinquin P, Lavallée S, Hodgson AJ (2005) Praxiteles: a miniature bone-mounted robot for minimal access total knee arthroplasty. Int J Med Robot 1(4):67–79
54. Koenig JA, Shalhoub S, Chen EA, Plaskos C (2019) Accuracy of soft tissue balancing in robotic-assisted measured-resection TKA using a robotic distraction tool. CAOS 2019 EPiC Ser Health Sci 3:210–214
55. Shatrov J, Parker D (2020) Computer and robotic - assisted total knee arthroplasty: a review of outcomes. J Exp Orthop 7(1):70
56. Clement ND, Al-Zibari M, Afzal I, Deehan DJ, Kader D (2020) A systematic review of imageless hand-held robotic-assisted knee arthroplasty: learning curve, accuracy, functional outcome and survivorship. EFORT Open Rev 5(5):319–326
57. Gharaibeh MA, Chen DB, MacDessi SJ (2018) Soft tissue balancing in total knee arthroplasty using sensor-guided assessment: is there a learning curve? ANZ J Surg 88(5):497–501
58. Kayani B, Konan S, Pietrzak JRT, Huq SS, Tahmassebi J, Haddad FS (2018) The learning curve associated with robotic-arm assisted unicompartmental knee arthroplasty: a prospective cohort study. Bone Joint J. 100(8):1033–1042
59. Vermue H, Luyckx T, Winnock de Grave P, Ryckaert A, Cools AS, Himpe N, Victor J (2022) Robot-assisted total knee arthroplasty is associated with a learning curve for surgical time but not for component alignment, limb alignment and gap balancing. Knee Surg, Sports Traumatol, Arthrosc: Off J ESSKA 30(2):593–602. https://doi.org/10.1007/s00167-020-06341-6
60. Kort N, Stirling P, Pilot P, Müller JH (2022) Robot-assisted knee arthroplasty improves component positioning and alignment, but results are inconclusive on whether it improves clinical scores or reduces complications and revisions: a systematic overview of meta-analyses. Knee Surg Sports Traumatol Arthrosc 30(8):2639–2653
61. Onggo JR, Onggo JD, De Steiger R, Hau R (2020) Robotic-assisted total knee arthroplasty is comparable to conventional total knee arthroplasty: a meta-analysis and systematic review. Arch Orthop Trauma Surg 140(10):1533–1549. https://doi.org/10.1007/s00402-020-03512-5

62. Chin BZ, Tan SSH, Chua KCX, Budiono GR, Syn NL, O'Neill GK (2021) Robot-assisted versus conventional total and unicompartmental knee arthroplasty: a meta-analysis of radiological and functional outcomes. J Knee Surg 34(10):1064–1075
63. Siddiqi A, Horan T, Molloy RM, Bloomfield MR, Patel PD, Piuzzi NS (2021) A clinical review of robotic navigation in total knee arthroplasty: historical systems to modern design. EFORT Open Rev 6(4):252–269
64. Plaskos C, Blum C, Lynch B, Ackerman M, Islam S, Lepkowsky E, Koenig J. Conventional vs. robotic/computer assisted total knee arthroplasty: a meta-analysis. J Orthop Exp Innov. 2021(Mar 2020-Jan 2022).
65. Liow MHL, Goh GS, Wong MK, Chin PL, Tay DK, Yeo SJ (2017) Robotic-assisted total knee arthroplasty may lead to improvement in quality-of-life measures: a 2-year follow-up of a prospective randomized trial. Knee Surg Sports Traumatol Arthrosc 25(9):2942–2951. https://doi.org/10.1007/s00167-016-4076-3
66. Nogalo C, Meena A, Abermann E, Fink C (2023) Complications and downsides of the robotic total knee arthroplasty: a systematic review. Knee Surg Sports Traumatol Arthrosc Mar 31(3):736–750. https://doi.org/10.1007/s00167-022-07031-1
67. Kayani B, Konan S, Ayuob A, Onochie E, Al-Jabri T, Haddad FS (2019) Robotic technology in total knee arthroplasty: a systematic review. EFORT Open Rev. 4(10):611–617. https://doi.org/10.1302/2058-5241.4.190022
68. Archer A, Salem HS, Coppolecchia A, Mont MA (2021) Lengths of stay and discharge dispositions after total knee arthroplasty: a comparison of robotic-assisted and manual techniques. J Knee Surg. https://doi.org/10.1055/S-0041-1735280
69. Heinz T, Eidmann A, Anderson P et al (2023) Trends in computer-assisted surgery for total knee arthroplasty in Germany: an analysis based on the operative procedure classification system between 2010 to 2021. J Clin Med 12(2):549 Published 2023 Jan 9. https://doi.org/10.3390/jcm12020549
70. Kahlenberg CA, Nwachukwu BU, McLawhorn AS, Cross MB, Cornell CN, Padgett DE. Patient satisfaction after total knee replacement: a systematic review. HSS Journal®. 2018;14(2):192–201.
71. Bourne RB, Chesworth BM, Davis AM, Mahomed NN, Charron KD. Patient satisfaction after total knee arthroplasty: who is satisfied and who is not? Clin Orthop Relat Res. 2010;468:57–63.
72. Price AJ, Alvand A, Troelsen A, Katz JN, Hooper G, Gray A et al (2018) Knee replacement. Lancet 392(10158):1672–1682
73. Vendittoli P-A, Martinov S, Blakeney WG. Restricted kinematic alignment, the fundamentals, and clinical applications. Front Surg. 2021;8:697020.
74. Blakeney W, Clément J, Desmeules F, Hagemeister N, Rivière C, Vendittoli PA. Kinematic alignment in total knee arthroplasty better reproduces normal gait than mechanical alignment. Knee Surg Sports Traumatol Arthrosc. 2019;27(5):1410–7. https://doi.org/10.1007/s00167-018-5174-1.

75. Gao Zx L, Nj Z, Sy, Yu W, Dai Yx, Xiao C. Comparison of kinematic alignment and mechanical alignment in total knee arthroplasty: a meta-analysis of randomized controlled clinical trials. Orthop Surg. 2020;12(6):1567–78.
76. Clatworthy M. Patient-specific TKA with the Velys™ robotic-assisted solution. Surg Technol Int. 2022;40:315–20.
77. Aflatooni JO, Wininger AE, Park KJ, Incavo SJ. Alignment options and robotics in total knee arthroplasty. Front Surg. 2023;10:1106608.
78. Smith AF, Eccles CJ, Bhimani SJ et al (2021) Improved patient satisfaction following robotic-assisted total knee arthroplasty. J Knee Surg 34(7):730–738. https://doi.org/10.1055/s-0039-1700837
79. Kayani B, Konan S, Tahmassebi J, Pietrzak JRT, Haddad FS. Robotic-arm assisted total knee arthroplasty is associated with improved early functional recovery and reduced time to hospital discharge compared with conventional jig-based total knee arthroplasty: a prospective cohort study. Bone Joint J. 2018;100-B(7):930–7. https://doi.org/10.1302/0301-620X.100B7.BJJ-2017-1449.R1.
80. King CA, Jordan M, Bradley AT, Wlodarski C, Tauchen A, Puri L (2022) Transitioning a practice to robotic total knee arthroplasty is correlated with favorable short-term clinical outcomes-a single surgeon experience. J Knee Surg 35(1):78–82. https://doi.org/10.1055/s-0040-1712984
81. Mason JB, Fehring TK, Estok R, Banel D, Fahrbach K (2007) Meta-analysis of alignment outcomes in computer-assisted total knee arthroplasty surgery. J Arthroplasty 22(8):1097–1106. https://doi.org/10.1016/j.arth.2007.08.001
82. Mannan A, Vun J, Lodge C, Eyre-Brook A, Jones S (2018) Increased precision of coronal plane outcomes in robotic-assisted total knee arthroplasty: a systematic review and meta-analysis. Surgeon 16(4):237–244. https://doi.org/10.1016/j.surge.2017.12.003
83. Marchand RC, Sodhi N, Khlopas A, Sultan AA, Harwin SF, Malkani AL et al (2017) Patient satisfaction outcomes after robotic arm-assisted total knee arthroplasty: a short-term evaluation. J Knee Surg 30(9):849–853. https://doi.org/10.1055/s-0037-1607450
84. Zhang J, Ndou WS, Ng N et al (2021) Robotic-arm assisted total knee arthroplasty is associated with improved accuracy and patient reported outcomes: a systematic review and meta-analysis. Knee Surg Sports Traumatol Arthrosc. https://doi.org/10.1007/S00167-021-06464-4
85. Song EK, Seon JK, Yim JH, Netravali NA, Bargar WL (2013) Robotic-assisted TKA reduces postoperative alignment outliers and improves gap balance compared to conventional TKA [published correction appears in Clin Orthop Relat res. 2012;470(9):2627]. Clin Orthop Relat Res 471(1):118–126. https://doi.org/10.1007/s11999-012-2407-3
86. Choong PF, Dowsey MM, Stoney JD (2009) Does accurate anatomical alignment result in better function and quality of life? Comparing conventional and computer-assisted total knee arthroplasty. J Arthroplasty 24(4):560–569. https://doi.org/10.1016/j.arth.2008.02.018

87. Clark G, Steer R, Wood D. Functional alignment achieves a more balanced total knee arthroplasty than either mechanical alignment or kinematic alignment prior to soft tissue releases. Knee Surg Sports Traumatol Arthrosc. 2023;31(4):1420–6.
88. Rossi SMP, Sangaletti R, Perticarini L, Terragnoli F, Benazzo F (2022) High accuracy of a new robotically assisted technique for total knee arthroplasty: an in vivo study. Knee Surg Sports Traumatol Arthrosc 4:1–9. https://doi.org/10.1007/s00167-021-06800-8
89. Mahoney O, Kinsey T, Sodhi N et al (2022) Improved component placement accuracy with robotic-arm assisted total knee arthroplasty. J Knee Surg 35(3):337–344. https://doi.org/10.1055/s-0040-1715571
90. Bautista M, Manrique J, Hozack WJ (2019) Robotics in total knee arthroplasty. J Knee Surg 32(7):600–606. https://doi.org/10.1055/s-0039-1681053
91. Fang CJ, Mazzocco JC, Sun DC et al (2022) Total knee arthroplasty hospital costs by time-driven activity-based costing: robotic vs conventional. Arthroplast Today 13:43. https://doi.org/10.1016/J.ARTD.2021.11.008
92. St Mart JP, Goh EL. The current state of robotics in total knee arthroplasty. EFORT Open Rev. 6, 270–9 (2021).
93. Hetaimish BM, Khan MM, Simunovic N, Al-Harbi HH, Bhandari M, Zalzal PK (2012) Meta-analysis of navigation vs conventional total knee arthroplasty. J Arthroplasty 27(6):1177–1182. https://doi.org/10.1016/j.arth.2011.12.028
94. Kim YH, Yoon SH, Park JW. Does robotic-assisted TKA result in Better Outcome scores or Long-Term Survivorship Than Conventional TKA? A Randomized, Controlled Trial. Clin Orthop Relat Res. 2020;478(2):266–75.
95. Matziolis G, Krocker D, Weiss U, Tohtz S, Perka C. A prospective, randomized study of computer-assisted and conventional total knee arthroplasty. Three-dimensional evaluation of implant alignment and rotation. J Bone Joint Surg Am. 2007;89:236–243.
96. Yang HY, Seon JK, Shin YJ, Lim HA, Song EK (2017) Robotic total knee arthroplasty with a cruciate-retaining implant: a 10-year follow-up study. Clin Orthop Surg 9(2):169–176. https://doi.org/10.4055/cios.2017.9.2.169
97. Kamara E, Robinson J, Bas MA, Rodriguez JA, Hepinstall MS. Adoption of Robotic vs fluoroscopic guidance in total hip arthroplasty: is acetabular positioning improved in the learning curve? J Arthroplasty. 2017;32:125–30.
98. Marchand KB, Ehiorobo J, Mathew KK, Marchand RC, Mont MA. Learning Curve of robotic-assisted total knee arthroplasty for a high-volume surgeon. J Knee Surg. 2020.
99. Skibicki HE, Ponzio DY, Brustein JA, Post ZD, Ong AC, Orozco FR. A cautionary case: osteoporotic femur fracture after robotic-assisted total knee arthroplasty. Osteoporos Int. 2021;32:2125–9.
100. Smith TJ, Siddiqi A, Forte SA, Judice A, Sculco PK, Vigdorchik JM, Schwarzkopf R, Springer BD. Periprosthetic fractures through tracking pin sites following computer navigated and robotic total and unicompartmental knee arthroplasty: a systematic review. JBJS Rev. 2021;9:e20.00091.

101. Yun AG, Qutami M, Pasko KBD. Do bicortical diaphyseal array pins create the risk of periprosthetic fracture in robotic-assisted knee arthroplasties? Arthroplasty. 2021;3:25.
102. Owens RF Jr, Swank ML (2010) Low incidence of postoperative complications due to pin placement in computer-navigated total knee arthroplasty. J Arthroplasty 25(7):1096–1098. https://doi.org/10.1016/j.arth.2009.07.025
103. Cip J, Obwegeser F, Benesch T, Bach C, Ruckenstuhl P, Martin A. Twelve-year follow-up of navigated computer-assisted versus conventional total knee arthroplasty: a prospective randomized comparative trial. J Arthroplast. 2018;33:1404–11.
104. Hamilton DA, Ononuju U, Nowak C, Chen C, Darwiche H. Differences in immediate postoperative outcomes between robotic-assisted TKA and conventional TKA. Arthroplast Today. 2021;8:57–62.
105. Zak SG, Yeroushalmi D, Tang A, Meftah M, Schnaser E, Schwarzkopf R. The use of navigation or robotic-assisted Technology in Total Knee Arthroplasty Does not Reduce Postoperative Pain. J Knee Surg. 2021.
106. Gross JB. Estimating allowable blood loss: corrected for dilution. 1983;58(3):277–80.
107. Batailler C, Fernandez A, Swan J, Servien E, Haddad FS, Catani F, et al. MAKO CT-based robotic arm-assisted system is a reliable procedure for total knee arthroplasty: a systematic review. Knee Surg Sports Traumatol Arthrosc. 2021;29(11):3585–98.
108. Xia R, Zhai Z, Zhang J, Yu D, Wang L, Mao Y, Zhu Z, Wu H, Dai K, Yan M, Li H (2021) Verification and clinical translation of a newly designed "Skywalker" robot for total knee arthroplasty: a prospective clinical study. J Orthop Transl 29:143–151. https://doi.org/10.1016/j.jot.2021.05.006
109. Weaver, Douglas J.; Deshmukh, Shobit; Bashyal, Ravi; Bagaria, Vaibhav Complications and Learning Curve Associated with an Imageless Burr-Based (CORI) Robotic-Assisted Total Knee Arthroplasty System: Results from First 500 Cases. Indian Journal of Orthopaedics (2024). https://doi.org/10.1007/s43465-024-01200-9
110. Ma, Nanshan; Sun, Pengfei; Xin, Pengfei; Zhong, Sheng; Xie, Jun; Xiao, Lianbo Comparison of the efficacy and safety of MAKO robot-assisted total knee arthroplasty versus conventional manual total knee arthroplasty in uncomplicated unilateral total knee arthroplasty a single-centre retrospective analysis. International Orthopaedics (2024). https://doi.org/10.1007/s00264-024-06234-0
111. Rajgor, Harshadkumar D.; Mayne, Alistair; Munasinghe, Chathura; Pagkalos, Joseph; Agrawal, Yuvraj; Davis, Edward T.; Sharma, Akash D. Mako versus ROSA: comparing surgical accuracy in robotic total knee arthroplasty. Journal of Robotic Surgery (2024). https://doi.org/10.1007/s11701-023-01786-6
112. Edelstein, Adam I.; Orsi, Alexander D.; Plaskos, Christopher; Coffey, Simon; Suleiman, Linda I. Imageless robotic total knee arthroplasty determines similar coronal plane alignment of the knee (CPAK) parameters to long leg radiographs. Arthroplasty (2024). https://doi.org/10.1186/s42836-024-00231-9

113. Tsai, Hung-Kang; Bao, Zhengyuan; Wu, Dengxian; Han, Jing; Jiang, Qing; Xu, Zhihong A new gap balancing technique with functional alignment in total knee arthroplasty using the MAKO robotic arm system: a preliminary study. BMC Surgery (2024). https://doi.org/10.1186/s12893-024-02524-x
114. Loomans, Laura; Leirs, Geert; Vandenneucker, Hilde Operating room efficiency after the implementation of MAKO robotic-assisted total knee arthroplasty. Archives of Orthopaedic and Trauma Surgery (2023). https://doi.org/10.1007/s00402-023-04834-w
115. Calliess, Tilman; Ettinger, Max; Savov, Peter; Karkosch, Roman; Windhagen, Henning Individualized alignment in total knee arthroplasty using image-based robotic assistance. Die Orthopädie (2018). https://doi.org/10.1007/s00132-018-3637-1
116. Shatrov, J.; Murphy, G. T.; Duong, J.; Fritsch, B. Robotic-assisted total knee arthroplasty with the OMNIBot platform: a review of the principles of use and outcomes. Archives of Orthopaedic and Trauma Surgery (2021). https://doi.org/10.1007/s00402-021-04173-8
117. Haslhofer, David Johannes; Anelli-Monti, Victoria; Hausbrandt, Peter; Kammerlander, Christian; Klasan, Antonio No difference in surgical time and total theatre time between robotically assisted and computer assisted total knee arthroplasty. Journal of Orthopaedics and Traumatology (2024). https://doi.org/10.1186/s10195-024-00798-8
118. Aggarwal, Vikram A; Sun, Joshua; Sambandam, Senthil N Outcomes following robotic assisted total knee arthroplasty compared to conventional total knee arthroplasty. Archives of Orthopaedic and Trauma Surgery (2024). https://doi.org/10.1007/s00402-024-05231-7
119. Wong, Wai Kit; Abu Bakar Sajak, Azliana; Chua, Hwa Sen Real-world accuracy of robotic-assisted total knee arthroplasty and its impact on expedited recovery. Journal of Robotic Surgery (2024). https://doi.org/10.1007/s11701-024-02059-6
120. Ezeokoli, Ekene Uchenna; John, Jithin; Gupta, Rohun; Jawad, Ali; Cavinatto, Leonardo Index surgery and ninety day re-operation cost comparison of robotic-assisted versus manual total knee arthroplasty. International Orthopaedics (2022). https://doi.org/10.1007/s00264-022-05674-w
121. Zhang, Haoran; Bai, Xizhuang; Wang, Huisheng; Zhu, Zhiyong; Li, Xi Learning curve analysis of robotic-assisted total knee arthroplasty with a Chinese surgical system. Journal of Orthopaedic Surgery and Research (2023). https://doi.org/10.1186/s13018-023-04382-4
122. Feroe, Aliya G.; Chakraborty, Amit K.; Rosenthal, Daniel I.; Simeone, F. Joseph Fracture through tracking pin sites following a robotic-assisted total knee arthroplasty. Skeletal Radiology (2022). https://doi.org/10.1007/s00256-022-04034-4
123. Xu, Jia-Zheng; Li, Liang-Liang; Fu, Jun; Xu, Chi; Zhang, Guo-Qiang; Chai, Wei; Hao, Li-Bo; Li, Xiang; Chen, Ji-Ying Comparison of serum inflammatory indicators and radiographic results in MAKO robotic-assisted versus conventional total knee arthroplasty for knee osteoarthritis: a retrospective study

of Chinese patients. BMC Musculoskeletal Disorders (2022). https://doi.org/10.1186/s12891-022-05373-y

124. Ping, Hang-Yu; An, Hao-Ming; Cao, Zheng; Nan, Shao-Kui; Li, Hai-Feng; Chai, Wei Efficacy of the newly designed "SkyWalker" robot compared to the MAKO robotic system in primary total knee arthroplasty: a one-year follow-up study. International Orthopaedics (2023). https://doi.org/10.1007/s00264-023-06023-1

7.3 Augmented Reality

Machine Generated Summaries

Disclaimer: The summaries in this chapter were generated from Springer Nature publications using abstractive AI auto-summarization: An abstraction-based summarizer creates new text based on deep learning. New phrases are created to summarize the content. As the constituted sentences are machine selected, they may not fully reflect the body of the work, so we strongly advise that the original content is read and cited. The auto-generated summaries were curated by the editor to meet Springer Nature publication standards.

7.3.1 Efficacy of Virtual Reality-Based Rehabilitation Following Total Knee Replacement: A Systematic Review and Meta-Analysis of Randomized Control Trials [48]

This is a machine-generated summary of:

Shaheen, Afaf A. M.; Algabbani, Maha F.; Alshahrani, Manar M.; Alshahrani, Fatimah A. Z.; Alsobayel, Hana I.; Omar, Mohammed Taher Ahmed; Alsubiheen, Abdulrahman M. Efficacy of virtual reality-based rehabilitation following total knee replacement: a systematic review and meta-analysis of randomized control trials [48].

Published in: Bulletin of Faculty of Physical Therapy (2025).

Link to original: https://doi.org/10.1186/s43161-024-00246-y

If you want to cite the papers, please refer to the original.

For technical reasons we could not place the page where the original quote is coming from.

7.3.1.1 Research Highlights

Total knee replacement (TKR) is a widely successful orthopedic procedure, with increasing demand projected globally over the coming decades. Despite its benefits, TKR patients often experience persistent postural balance impairments, which can lead to an increased risk of falls. Rehabilitation plays a crucial role in optimizing outcomes, and virtual reality-based rehabilitation (VRBR) has emerged as a promising tool for enhancing recovery. However, the effectiveness of VRBR compared to conventional therapy remains uncertain. The study by Shaheen et al. aims to provide a comprehensive analysis of randomized controlled trials (RCTs) to determine whether VRBR significantly reduces knee pain and improves balance, proprioception, joint function, gait speed, and health-related quality of life (HRQOL) following TKR.

The study conducted a systematic review and meta-analysis following Preferred Reporting Items for Systematic Reviews and Meta-Analyses (PRISMA) guidelines, searching multiple databases for RCTs up to September 2023. The authors included studies that compared VRBR with control therapy or usual care in patients aged 65 and older who underwent TKR for knee osteoarthritis. The review assessed various outcomes such as pain, balance, proprioception, joint function using the Western Ontario and McMaster Universities Osteoarthritis Index (WOMAC), gait speed, and HRQOL. The meta-analysis included 15 RCTs with 1200 participants and evaluated both immersive and non-immersive VR devices. The results indicated that VRBR significantly reduced pain and improved dynamic balance and knee function immediately post-intervention but showed no significant advantages over conventional therapy in terms of proprioception, gait speed, or HRQOL.

The study highlights that while VRBR can effectively reduce pain and improve certain functional outcomes immediately after TKR, its long-term benefits remain unclear due to significant heterogeneity among studies. Immersive VR devices were found to be more effective than non-immersive ones in improving knee function. Future study should focus on large-scale multicenter RCTs to explore the potential advantages of different VR tools over conventional therapy in improving balance, proprioception, gait speed, and HRQOL. Additionally, developing standardized protocols for VRBR could enhance its application in clinical practice following TKR.

7.3.2 A Novel Augmented Reality-Based Surgical Guidance System for Total Knee Arthroplasty [49]

This is a machine-generated summary of:

Fucentese, Sandro F.; Koch, Peter P. A novel augmented reality-based surgical guidance system for total knee arthroplasty [49].

Published in: Archives of Orthopaedic and Trauma Surgery (2021).

Link to original: https://doi.org/10.1007/s00402-021-04204-4

If you want to cite the papers, please refer to the original.

For technical reasons we could not place the page where the original quote is coming from.

7.3.2.1 Research Highlights

There is a growing interest in enhancing the outcomes of total knee arthroplasty (TKA) within the orthopaedics community. Despite advancements in surgical safety, a significant percentage of TKA patients remain dissatisfied with their post-operative lifestyle, particularly among younger, more active individuals. Precision in implant alignment and soft tissue balance is crucial for improving patient satisfaction, yet traditional computer-assisted surgery has not consistently demonstrated superior outcomes compared to conventional techniques. The study by Fucentese et al. introduces an augmented reality (AR)-based surgical guidance system designed to improve accuracy and efficiency in TKA procedures.

The study details the development and application of the NextAR TKA system (Medacta International, Castel San Pietro, Switzerland) which utilizes AR technology to provide real-time visual guidance during surgery. The system comprises smart glasses, two small sensors, and a control unit, offering a compact and efficient solution without the need for external cameras. The smart glasses display critical information directly in the surgeon's field of view, enhancing hand-eye coordination and surgical precision. The system tracks the spatial position of sensors attached to the femur and tibia, allowing for accurate measurement of prosthesis alignment and soft tissue balance. A novel feature of this system is its ability to assess ligament strain by tracking their origins and insertions in three dimensions, providing a more comprehensive evaluation than traditional gap measurements.

The introduction of this AR-based system represents a potential advancement in TKA by improving surgical accuracy and soft tissue balance while maintaining cost-effectiveness. Future study will focus on collecting clinical data to validate the system's performance and its impact on patient outcomes. The ongoing clinical investigations aim to establish reliable baselines for ligament assessment and explore the integration of biomechanical models to predict surgical outcomes. Additionally, the technology platform's versatility extends beyond knee surgery, with applications for shoulder and spine procedures already available, suggesting a promising future for AR technology in various orthopaedic specialties.

7.3.3 Clinical Outcomes Associated with Robotic and Computer-Navigated Total Knee Arthroplasty: A Machine Learning-Augmented Systematic Review [50]

This is a machine-generated summary of:

Buchlak, Quinlan D.; Clair, Joe; Esmaili, Nazanin; Barmare, Arshad; Chandrasekaran, Siva Clinical outcomes associated with robotic and computer-navigated total knee arthroplasty: a machine learning-augmented systematic review [50].

Published in: European Journal of Orthopaedic Surgery & Traumatology (2021).

Link to original: https://doi.org/10.1007/s00590-021-03059-0

If you want to cite the papers, please refer to the original.

For technical reasons we could not place the page where the original quote is coming from.

7.3.3.1 Research Highlights

Total knee arthroplasty (TKA) is a widely performed surgical procedure aimed at alleviating pain and disability in patients with knee issues, significantly improving their quality of life. With the rising demand for TKA, advancements in surgical technology, such as computer-navigated TKA (CNTKA) and robotic TKA (RTKA), have been developed to enhance surgical precision and outcomes. These technologies offer real-time intraoperative assessment of alignment, potentially reducing errors associated with manual TKA (mTKA). However, the comparative clinical outcomes of RTKA and CNTKA remain unclear. The study by Buchlak et al. systematically reviews and compares the clinical outcomes associated with RTKA and CNTKA, while also exploring the application of natural language processing (NLP) to facilitate the systematic review process.

The study employed a comprehensive search strategy guided by the Preferred Reporting Items for Systematic Reviews and Meta-Analyses guidelines to identify relevant studies on RTKA and CNTKA. The researchers included randomized controlled trials (RCTs) and cohort studies published in English over the past five years that reported clinical outcomes for these techniques. Data extraction focused on patient-reported outcome measures such as the Hospital for Special Surgery score, Western Ontario and McMaster Universities Osteoarthritis Index score, and others. Quantitative analyses were conducted to compare surgical techniques, while NLP was used to automate article screening through document classification models like BERT (Bidirectional Encoder Representations from Transformers, Google, Mountain View, California) and RoBERTa (Robustly Optimized BERT Approach, Google, Mountain View, California, USA). The study found that both RTKA and CNTKA are associated with satisfactory clinical outcomes, although RTKA may offer advantages such as shorter operative time and reduced length of stay.

The findings suggest that both RTKA and CNTKA have distinct strengths, with RTKA potentially providing more accurate alignment and less blood loss compared to CNTKA. However, each system type has its own limitations, including cost considerations for robotic systems. Future study could focus on directly comparing RTKA with CNTKA through high-quality RCTs to better understand their relative benefits. Additionally, further research into cost-effectiveness analyses could guide investment decisions in healthcare systems. The study also highlights the potential of NLP technologies to streamline literature synthesis processes in systematic reviews, suggesting avenues for improving NLP document classification performance in future research endeavors.

Bibliography

1. Laverdière C, Corban J, Khoury J, Ge SM, Schupbach J, Harvey EJ, Reindl R, Martineau PA (2019) Augmented reality in orthopaedics: a systematic review and a window on future possibilities. Bone Joint J 101-B(12):1479–1488. https://doi.org/10.1302/0301-620X.101B12.BJJ-2019-0315.R1 (*PMID: 31786992*)
2. Keating TC, Jacobs JJ (2021) Augmented reality in orthopedic practice and education. Orthop Clin North Am 52(1):15–26. https://doi.org/10.1016/j.ocl.2020.08.002 (*PMID: 33222981*)
3. Polce EM, Kunze KN, Williams BT, Krivicich LM, Maheshwer B, Beletsky A, Cohn MR, Kogan M, Chahla J (2020) Efficacy and validity of orthopaedic simulators in surgical training: a systematic review and meta-analysis of randomized controlled trials. J Am Acad Orthop Surg 28(24):1027–1040. https://doi.org/10.5435/JAAOS-D-19-00839 (*PMID: 32398408*)

4. Eberlein TJ (2014) A new paradigm in surgical training. J Am Coll Surg 218(4):511–518. https://doi.org/10.1016/j.jamcollsurg.2013.12.045 (*Epub 2014 Jan 24 PMID: 24655837*)
5. Harris JD, Staheli G, LeClere L, Andersone D, McCormick F (2015) What effects have resident work-hour changes had on education, quality of life, and safety? A systematic review. Clin Orthop Relat Res 473(5):1600–1608. https://doi.org/10.1007/s11999-014-3968-0 (*PMID:25269530; PMCID:PMC4385350*)
6. Pokhrel S, Alsadoon A, Prasad PWC et al (2019) A novel augmented reality (AR) scheme for knee replacement surgery by considering cutting error accuracy. Int J Med Robot 15(1):e1958
7. Wang L, Sun Z, Zhang X et al (2019) A HoloLens based augmented reality navigation system for minimally invasive total knee arthroplasty. In: Yu H, Liu J, Liu L et al (eds) Intelligent robotics and applications. Springer, pp 519–530
8. Daniel C, Ramos O (2016) Augmented reality for assistance of total knee replacement. J Electrical Comput Eng 16:1–6. https://doi.org/10.1155/2016/9358369
9. Ogawa H, Kurosaka K, Sato A, Hirasawa N, Matsubara M, Tsukada S (2020) Does an augmented reality-based portable navigation system improve the accuracy of acetabular component orientation during tha? a randomized controlled trial. Clin Orthop Relat Res 478(5):935–943. https://doi.org/10.1097/CORR.0000000000001083 (*PMID:31834164;PMCID:PMC7170692*)
10. Logishetty K, Western L, Morgan R, Iranpour F, Cobb JP, Auvinet E (2019) Can an augmented reality headset improve accuracy of acetabular cup orientation in simulated THA? A randomized trial. Clin Orthop Relat Res 477(5):1190–1199. https://doi.org/10.1097/CORR.0000000000000542 (*PMID:30507832;PMCID:PMC6494316*)
11. Peltola M, Malmivaara A, Paavola M (2013) Learning curve for new technology?: A nationwide register-based study of 46,363 total knee arthroplasties. J Bone Joint Surg Am 95(23):2097–2103. https://doi.org/10.2106/JBJS.L.01296 (*PMID: 24306696*)
12. Harrington CM, Kavanagh DO, Quinlan JF, Ryan D, Dicker P, O'Keeffe D, Traynor O, Tierney S (2018) Development and evaluation of a trauma decision-making simulator in Oculus virtual reality. Am J Surg 215(1):42–47. https://doi.org/10.1016/j.amjsurg.2017.02.011 (*Epub 2017 Feb 10 PMID: 28262203*)
13. Bartlett JD, Lawrence JE, Stewart ME, Nakano N, Khanduja V (2018) Does virtual reality simulation have a role in training trauma and orthopaedic surgeons? Bone Joint J 100B(5):559–565. https://doi.org/10.1302/0301-620X.100B5.BJJ-2017-1439 (*PMID: 29701089*)
14. Cui A, Li H, Wang D, Zhong J, Chen Y, Lu H. Global, regional prevalence, incidence and risk factors of knee osteoarthritis in population-based studies. EClinicalMedicine. 2020;29.
15. Moutzouri M, Gleeson N, Billis E, Panoutsopoulou I, Gliatis J. What is the effect of sensori-motor training on functional outcome and balance perfor-

mance of patients undergoing TKR? A systematic review Physiotherapy. 2016;102:136–44.
16. Blasco J, Igual-Camacho C, Blasco M, Anton-Anton V, Ortiz-Llueca l, Roig-Casasus S. The efficacy of virtual reality tools for total knee replacement rehabilitation: A systematic review. Physiother Theory Pract. 2021;37:682–692.
17. Peng L, Zeng Y, Wu Y, Si H, Shen B. Virtual reality-based rehabilitation in patients following total knee arthroplasty: a systematic review and meta-analysis of randomized controlled trials. Chin Med J. 2022;135:153–63.
18. Maher CG, Sherrington C, Herbert RD, Moseley AM, Elkins M. Reliability of the PEDro scale for rating quality of randomized controlled trials. Phys Ther. 2003;83:713–21.
19. Bettger JP, Green CL, Holmes DN, Chokshi A, Mather RC III, Hoch BT, et al. Effects of virtual exercise rehabilitation in-home therapy compared with traditional care after total knee arthroplasty: VERITAS, a randomized controlled trial. JBJS. 2020;102:101–9.
20. Piqueras M, Marco E, Coll M, Escalada F, Ballester A, Cinca C, et al. Effectiveness of an interactive virtual telerehabilitation system in patients after total knee arthroplasty: a randomized controlled trial. J Rehabil Med. 2013;45:392–6.
21. Jin C, Feng Y, Ni Y, Shan Z. Virtual reality intervention in postoperative rehabilitation after total knee arthroplasty: a prospective and randomized controlled clinical trial. Int J Clin Exp Med. 2018;11:6119–24.
22. Gianola S, Stucovitz E, Castellini G, Mascali M, Vanni F, Tramacere I, et al. Effects of early virtual reality-based rehabilitation in patients with total knee arthroplasty: a randomized controlled trial. Medicine. 2020; 99.
23. Pournajaf, Goffredo M, Pellicciari L, Piscitelli D, Criscuolo S, Le Pera D, et al. Effect of balance training using virtual reality-based serious games in individuals with total knee replacement: A randomized controlled trial. Ann Phys Rehabil Med. 2022;65:101609.
24. Janhunen M, Katajapuu N, Paloneva J, Pamilo K, Oksanen A, Keemu H, et al. Effects of a home-based, exergaming intervention on physical function and pain after total knee replacement in older adults: a randomized controlled trial. BMJ Open Sport Exerc Med. 2023;9: e001416.
25. Fung V, Ho A, Shaffer J, Chung E, Gomez M. Use of Nintendo Wii Fit™ in the rehabilitation of outpatients following total knee replacement: a preliminary randomised controlled trial. Physiotherapy. 2012;98:183–8.
26. Fuchs L, Kluska A, Novak D, Kosashvili Y. The influence of early virtual reality intervention on pain, anxiety, and function following primary total knee arthroplasty. Complement Ther Clin Pract. 2022;49: 101687.
27. Yoon S, Son H. Effects of full immersion virtual reality training on balance and knee function in total knee replacement patients: a randomized controlled study. Journal of Mechanics in Medicine and Biology. 2020;20:2040007.
28. Roig-Casasús S, Blasco JM, López-Bueno L, Blasco-Igual MC. Balance training with a dynamometric platform following total knee replacement: a randomized controlled trial. Journal of geriatric physical therapy. 2018;41:204–9.

29. Eichler S, Salzwedel A, Rabe S, Mueller S, Wochatz FMM, Hadzic M, et al. The effectiveness of telerehabilitation as a supplement to rehabilitation in patients after total knee or hip replacement. JMIR Rehabil Assist Technol. 2019;6(2):e14236.
30. Gür O, Başar S. The effect of virtual reality on pain, kinesiophobia and function in total knee arthroplasty patients: A randomized controlled trial. Knee. 2023;45:187–97.
31. Christiansen CL, Bade MJ, Davidson BS, Dayton MR, Stevens-Lapsley JE. Effects of weight-bearing biofeedback training on functional movement patterns following total knee arthroplasty: a randomized controlled trial. J Orthop Sports Phys Ther. 2015;45:647–655.
32. Choi H-S, Shin W-S. Effects of game-based balance training with constraint-induced movement therapy on lower extremity function and balance confidence levels in women with total knee replacement. Physical Therapy Rehabilitation Science. 2019;8:8–14.
33. Yu J-H, Nekar DM, Kang H-Y, Lee J-W, Oh S-Y. Comparison of Physical Activity Training Using Augmented Reality and Conventional Therapy on Physical Performance following a Total Knee Replacement: A Randomized Controlled Trial. Appl Sci. 2023;13:894.
34. Bini S, Mahajan J. Clinical outcomes of remote asynchronous telerehabilitation are equivalent to traditional therapy following total knee arthroplasty: a randomized control study. J Telemed Telecare. 2017;23:239–47.
35. García-Sánchez M, García-Robles P, Osuna-Pérez MC, Lomas-Vega R, Obrero-Gaitán E, Cortés-Pérez I. Effectiveness of Virtual Reality-Based Early Postoperative Rehabilitation after Total Knee Arthroplasty: A Systematic Review with Meta-Analysis of Randomized Controlled Trials. Appl Sci. 2023;13:4597.
36. Shatrov J, Parker D (2020) Computer and robotic - assisted total knee arthroplasty: a review of outcomes. J Exp Orthop 7(1):70
37. Attard A, Tawy GF, Simons M, Riches P, Rowe P, Biant LC (2019) Health costs and efficiencies of patient-specific and single-use instrumentation in total knee arthroplasty: a randomised controlled trial. BMJ Open Quality. 8(2):e000493
38. Ascani D, Mazzà C, De Lollis A, Bernardoni M, Viceconti M (2015) A procedure to estimate the origins and the insertions of the knee ligaments from computed tomography images. J Biomech 48(2):233–237. https://doi.org/10.1016/j.jbiomech.2014.11.041
39. Gaukel S, Vuille-dit-Bille RN, Schläppi M, Koch PP (2020) CT-based patient-specific instrumentation for total knee arthroplasty in over 700 cases: single-use instruments are as accurate as standard instruments. Knee Surg Sports Traumatol Arthrosc. https://doi.org/10.1007/s00167-020-06150-x
40. Abane L, Zaoui A, Anract P, Lefevre N, Herman S, Hamadouche M (2018) Can a single-use and patient-specific instrumentation be reliably used in primary total knee arthroplasty? A multicenter controlled study. J Arthroplasty 33(7):2111–2118

41. Goldberg TD, Maltry JA, Ahuja M, Inzana JA (2019) Logistical and economic advantages of sterile-packed, single-use instruments for total knee arthroplasty. J Arthroplasty 34(9):1876-1883.e2. https://doi.org/10.1016/j.arth.2019.03.011
42. Viceconti M, Ascani D, Mazzà C (2019) Pre-operative prediction of soft tissue balancing in knee arthoplasty part 1: effect of surgical parameters during level walking. J Orthop Res 37(7):1537–1545. https://doi.org/10.1002/jor.24289
43. Zamora LA, Humphreys KJ, Watt AM, Forel D, Cameron AL (2013) Systematic review of computer-navigated total knee arthroplasty. ANZ J Surg 83:22–30
44. Kayani B, Konan S, Ayuob A, Onochie E, Al-Jabri T, Haddad FS (2019) Robotic technology in total knee arthroplasty: a systematic review. EFORT Open Rev. 4(10):611–617. https://doi.org/10.1302/2058-5241.4.190022
45. Selim AJ, Rogers W, Fleishman JA, Qian SX, Fincke BG, Rothendler JA et al (2009) Updated US population standard for the Veterans RAND 12-item health survey (VR-12). Qual Life Res 18:43–52
46. Clark TC, Schmidt FH (2013) Robot-assisted navigation versus computer-assisted navigation in primary total knee arthroplasty: efficiency and accuracy. ISRN Orthop 2013:794827
47. Jacofsky DJ, Allen M. Robotics in arthroplasty: a comprehensive review. J Arthroplasty. 2016;31(10):2353–63. https://doi.org/10.1016/j.arth.2016.05.026.
48. Shaheen, Afaf A. M.; Algabbani, Maha F.; Alshahrani, Manar M.; Alshahrani, Fatimah A. Z.; Alsobayel, Hana I.; Omar, Mohammed Taher Ahmed; Alsubiheen, Abdulrahman M. Efficacy of virtual reality-based rehabilitation following total knee replacement: a systematic review and meta-analysis of randomized control trials. Bulletin of Faculty of Physical Therapy (2025). https://doi.org/10.1186/s43161-024-00246-y
49. Fucentese, Sandro F.; Koch, Peter P. A novel augmented reality-based surgical guidance system for total knee arthroplasty. Archives of Orthopaedic and Trauma Surgery (2021). https://doi.org/10.1007/s00402-021-04204-4
50. Buchlak, Quinlan D.; Clair, Joe; Esmaili, Nazanin; Barmare, Arshad; Chandrasekaran, Siva Clinical outcomes associated with robotic and computer-navigated total knee arthroplasty: a machine learning-augmented systematic review. European Journal of Orthopaedic Surgery & Traumatology (2021). https://doi.org/10.1007/s00590-021-03059-0

Chapter 8
Fixation Methods for Total Knee Arthroplasty

Alfred J. Tria Jr. and Giles R. Scuderi

Introduction by the Editors

Total knee arthroplasty (TKA) remains one of the most successful and frequently performed orthopedic procedures. With an aging population and expanding indications, the demand for TKA is expected to rise dramatically. This highlights the increasing clinical and economic impact of TKA and the need to optimize implant selection, surgical efficiency, and patient outcomes. While cemented fixation has long been the gold standard in TKA, cementless fixation has gained popularity due to improved implant technology, biologic coatings with enhanced osseointegration. Current porous materials offer improved initial stability and long-term fixation. Over recent years, registry has supported comparable outcomes with cemented and cementless implants.

This chapter reviews references that highlights the fixation in TKA. With our editorial prerogative, we reviewed each of the referenced articles and summarized our own conclusions, as detailed below. As you read each of the computer-generated summaries that follow in this chapter you can draw your own conclusions.

Advocates of cement fixation stress the importance of surgical technique, especially bone preparation and management of bone defects. Several of the papers in this chapter review techniques when using cement. Realizing that tibial bone defects are not uncommon, especially in the varus knee, Harna et al. Review the results of a screw-cement construct for managing the defect and report that it is a viable approach. Kim et al. recommends a modified cementing technique for stem pain,

A. J. Tria Jr. (✉)
Department of Orthopedics, Rutgers-Robert Wood Johnson Medical School, New Brunswick, NJ, USA

G. R. Scuderi
Department of Orthopedic Surgery, Northwell Health, Garden City, NY, USA

A. J. Tria Jr., G. R. Scuderi (eds.), *Total Knee Arthroplasty*,
https://doi.org/10.1007/978-3-032-00175-7_8

while Bosebeck et al. used a "pastry cement" whose properties are not entirely clear from the article. Having a clean and dry bone surface for cementing is important, so Touzopoulos et al. concluded that tourniquet use increased the thickness of the cement mantle. While this may be true, this is a multifactorial issue and other factors may influence the penetration of the cement into the bone, such as bone quality and viscosity of the cement. While controversial and not completely supported by the literature, Schlegel et al. found no difference in 10–12-year survival of surface or full cementing for the tibial component. Zhao et al. showed that the PEEK prostheses had good cement penetration with short term follow-up: however, the need for this implant is minimal.

Cementless fixation continues to grow. Rodriguez et al. show a trend in use of cementless implants. Several articles in this chapter compare cemented and cementless fixation and appear to have comparable short-term and long-term outcomes. Tay et al. in a 5-year follow up study and Kim et al. in a greater than 10-year follow up study showed no differences in outcomes. Liu et al. in a systematic review reported that cementless implants did not lower the revision rate, while Chen et al. in a metanalysis showed no difference in functional outcomes or loosening. Rassir et al. reported similar cost effectiveness with only 1 year of follow up to comment on function. Therbo et al. describes a bioactive coating which may have some application to enhance cementless fixation. Initial stable fixation is important. Yilmaz et al. showed prosthesis settling in the uncemented design during the first 6 months followed by stabilization. This may be a way to monitor this design for loosening. The remainder of the papers review bone density, modified cementing, and single implant results.

There are situations, especially in the revision setting where hybrid fixation is utilized. This means cementing the core implant and cementless press-fit stems. Moya-Angeler et al. present an excellent review of the options. Van Es et al. reviewed all three modes of fixation with similar results at 5 years in a single mobile bearing design. Sheridan et al. performed a systematic review and metanalysis that favored hybrid stems in revision with a good results. In contrast, Thever et al. looked at hybrid versus cemented stems in revision and reported no difference. This observation is similar to Gomez-Vallejo et al. who reported no differences in a 7 year follow-up comparing hybrid versus standard fixation for revision TKA. Schnetz et al. looked at a modular hinge knee with cementless stems. With a short follow-up of only 24–36 months and 92% survivorship.

Conclusions

While cemented TKA appears the more popular mode of fixation in TKA, there is a continued, steady rise in cementless TKA. Factors that appear to influence fixation is patient age, sex and bone quality. There have also been advancements in implant technology and materials supporting biologic fixation. The current comparative studies report comparable short-term and long-term results.

8.1 Cement

Machine Generated Summaries

Disclaimer: The summaries in this chapter were generated from Springer Nature publications using abstractive AI auto-summarization: An abstraction-based summarizer creates new text based on deep learning. New phrases are created to summarize the content. As the constituted sentences are machine selected, they may not fully reflect the body of the work, so we strongly advise that the original content is read and cited. The auto-generated summaries were curated by the editor to meet Springer Nature publication standards.

8.1.1 Long-Term Comparative Study Evaluating the Screw-Cement Construct for Tibial Defects in Total Knee Arthroplasty: Our Experience [58]

This is a machine-generated summary of:

Harna, Bushu; Kapoor, Anil; Arora, Anil; Arya, Shivali Long-term comparative study evaluating the screw-cement construct for tibial defects in total knee arthroplasty: our experience [58].

Published in: International Orthopaedics (2025).

Link to original: https://doi.org/10.1007/s00264-025-06439-x

If you want to cite the papers, please refer to the original.

For technical reasons we could not place the page where the original quote is coming from.

8.1.1.1 Research Highlights

Total knee arthroplasty (TKA) is a widely accepted treatment for end-stage osteoarthritis of the knee, often complicated by tibial plateau bone loss in cases of severe angular deformities. Managing these bone defects effectively is crucial for ensuring a stable and well-aligned implant. Various surgical techniques are available, including the use of screws with cement, which is favored for its quick, economical, and bone-preserving attributes. However, the compressibility of cement can lead to subsidence and loosening of the tibial component over time. The study by Harna et al. investigates the long-term functional outcomes and success rate of the screw-cement construct in patients with significant tibial defects.

The study was conducted as a retrospective analysis involving patients undergoing TKA due to various forms of arthritis. Participants were divided into two groups: Group A received conventional TKA, while Group B was treated with TKA using a screw-cement construct. The groups were matched demographically, and all patients were assessed preoperatively using radiographs and scannograms. The study excluded patients requiring more extensive hardware or those with large tibial defects beyond the scope of screw-cement management. Surgical procedures involved standard mid-patellar approaches with specific attention to defect assessment and management using screws and cement. Postoperative rehabilitation was consistent across both groups, focusing on early mobilization and pain management.

The findings suggest that the screw-cement construct is a viable option for managing large tibial defects up to 10 mm involving two quadrants of the resected tibial plateau surface. The study reported similar implant survival rates between both groups over an 8-year follow-up period. While radiolucency was more frequent in the screw-cement group, it did not correlate with implant loosening or failure.

8.1.2 Cemented Fixed-Bearing PFC Total Knee Arthroplasty: Survival and Failure Analysis at 12–17 Years [59]

This is a machine-generated summary of:

Bistolfi, A.; Massazza, G.; Rosso, F.; Deledda, D.; Gaito, V.; Lagalla, F.; Olivero, C.; Crova, M. Cemented fixed-bearing PFC total knee arthroplasty: survival and failure analysis at 12–17 years [59].

Published in: Journal of Orthopaedics and Traumatology (2011).

Link to original: https://doi.org/10.1007/s10195-011-0142-2

If you want to cite the papers, please refer to the original.

For technical reasons we could not place the page where the original quote is coming from.

8.1.2.1 Research Highlights

Total knee arthroplasty (TKA) is a widely accepted treatment for degenerative knee pathology, with the Press Fit Condylar (PFC) (DePuy-Synthes, Raynham, Mass., USA) total knee prosthesis being one of the prominent options due to its strong interface between prosthesis and bone. Despite advancements in implant technology, cemented models with fixed bearings remain the gold standard, demonstrating good long-term results. However, the primary reasons for TKA failure are not fully understood, with issues such as malalignment, wear, loosening, infections, and persistent pain being observed. Additionally, the decision to resurface the patella during TKA is still debated among surgeons. The study by Bistolfi et al. investigates a series of cemented fixed bearing TKA and selective patellar resurfacing in non-randomized patients operated on by different surgeons within the same orthopedic division.

The study was conducted as a prospective case series involving several surgeons performing TKA using PFC fixed-bearing prostheses on patients with different indications for surgery, including knee arthritis and consequences of tibial plateau fractures. The surgical technique involved a medial parapatellar approach with general or spinal anesthesia, followed by specific steps such as osteophyte removal and ligamentous balance. Selective patellar resurfacing was performed based on cartilage damage severity. Clinical evaluations were conducted pre- and post-operatively using the Hospital for Special Surgery (HSS) knee score questionnaire at specified intervals. Radiographic evaluations were standardized using the Knee Society Roentgenographic Evaluation System to assess implant position and potential signs of failure. Data were analyzed statistically to determine implant survival rates and patient satisfaction.

The study's findings indicate that the PFC prosthesis with fixed bearing and cemented fixation is an effective solution for TKA, showing significant improvements in clinical outcomes such as HSS scores and range of motion. The cumulative average implant survival rate at 10 years was approximately 95%, aligning with existing literature. While no significant differences were found between resurfaced and unresurfaced patella groups in terms of failure rates or patient satisfaction, secondary surgeries were more common in the unresurfaced group.

8.1.3 Modified Hybrid Cementing Technique Reduces Stem Tip Pain and Improves Patient's Satisfaction after Revision Total Knee Arthroplasty [60]

This is a machine-generated summary of:

Kim, Man Soo; Koh, In Jun; Sohn, Sueen; Park, Hyung Chul; In, Yong Modified hybrid cementing technique reduces stem tip pain and improves patient's satisfaction after revision total knee arthroplasty [60].

Published in: Journal of Orthopaedic Surgery and Research (2020).
Link to original: https://doi.org/10.1186/s13018-020-01921-1

If you want to cite the papers, please refer to the original.
For technical reasons we could not place the page where the original quote is coming from.

8.1.3.1 Research Highlights

Revision total knee arthroplasty (TKA) presents significant challenges compared to primary TKA due to severe bone defects and insufficient soft tissue, necessitating the use of stems for effective load transmission and stress distribution. Diaphyseal fixation with a long stem is often preferred for its enhanced joint stability, but it can lead to end-of-stem tip pain, impacting patient satisfaction. Traditional cementing techniques, such as hybrid and total cementation, have their own pros and cons, with hybrid cementing generally favored for its ease of removal. However, the occurrence of end-of-stem tip pain with hybrid cementing has prompted the development of a modified hybrid technique. The study by Kim et al. investigates the impact of this modified hybrid cementing technique on patient-reported outcomes and satisfaction in revision TKAs.

The study retrospectively reviewed clinical and radiological data from patients who underwent revision TKA using either the traditional hybrid or the modified hybrid cementing technique. The modified approach involved additional cementation at the stem tip to potentially reduce end-of-stem tip pain. Patients were excluded if they had septic revisions or were not followed up for at least 2 years post-operation. The study compared variables such as age, comorbidities, prosthesis type, and post-operative outcomes between the two groups. Patient-reported outcomes were assessed using the Western Ontario and McMaster Universities Osteoarthritis Index (WOMAC) score and New Knee Society Score for satisfaction. Statistical analyses were conducted to evaluate differences in outcomes between the groups.

The findings revealed that patients treated with the modified hybrid cementing technique experienced significantly less shin pain and improved WOMAC scores compared to those treated with the traditional hybrid method. Satisfaction rates were higher in the modified group, suggesting that this approach may better address end-of-stem tip pain issues. The study highlights that future studies could focus on larger sample sizes to confirm these results and explore further refinements in cementing techniques to enhance patient outcomes in revision TKA procedures.

8.1.4 Cementing Technique for Total Knee Arthroplasty in Cadavers Using a Pastry Bone Cement [61]

This is a machine-generated summary of:

Bösebeck, Hans; Holl, Anna-Maria; Ochsner, Peter; Groth, Manuel; Stippich, Kevin; Nowakowski, Andrej M.; Egloff, Christian; Hoechel, Sebastian; Göpfert, Beat; Vogt, Sebastian Cementing technique for total knee arthroplasty in cadavers using a pastry bone cement [61].

Published in: Journal of Orthopaedic Surgery and Research (2021).

Link to original: https://doi.org/10.1186/s13018-021-02436-z

If you want to cite the papers, please refer to the original.

For technical reasons we could not place the page where the original quote is coming from.

8.1.4.1 Research Highlights

In the field of joint replacement surgery, cemented and cement-less techniques are employed for implant fixation, with bone cement being the predominant method in total knee arthroplasty (TKA). Despite advancements in cementing techniques, aseptic loosening remains a common cause for TKA revisions. While some studies suggest that cemented TKAs have lower failure rates compared to uncemented ones, others report similar outcomes for both methods. The study by Bösebeck et al. investigates the efficacy of a novel pastry bone cement compared to conventional powder/liquid cement in a pre-clinical TKA setting.

The study was conducted at the Anatomical Institute of the University of Basel using cadaver knees to evaluate the quality of cementation, handling, and mechanical properties of the pastry bone cement. Standardized implantations were performed on bilateral knee cadavers, with one side using conventional powder/liquid cement and the other using pastry bone cement. The researchers used high-viscous polymethylmethacrylate cements with comparable compositions and gentamicin content. The surgical procedures were executed by trained orthopedic surgeons, and various parameters such as temperature, handling characteristics, and mechanical properties were assessed. Pull-out trials were conducted to measure the maximum tractive force of knee implants for each type of cement.

The findings suggest that both cements exhibited similar characteristics during preparation and application, although the pastry cement had a longer curing time. This extended curing time may facilitate better penetration but was not conclusively supported by the results. The study indicates that the pastry bone cement may offer slightly improved properties over conventional powder/liquid cement, potentially reducing preparation-associated errors due to its ready-to-use nature. Future study could involve clinical trials to further verify these findings and assess biological reactions related to polymerization heat and monomer toxicity in vivo.

8.1.5 The Use of Tourniquet May Influence the Cement Mantle Thickness under the Tibial Implant during Total Knee Arthroplasty [62]

This is a machine-generated summary of:

Touzopoulos, Panagiotis; Ververidis, Athanasios; Mpogiatzis, Christos; Chatzigiannakis, Athanasios; Drosos, Georgios I. The use of tourniquet may influence the cement mantle thickness under the tibial implant during total knee arthroplasty [62].

Published in: European Journal of Orthopaedic Surgery & Traumatology (2019).

Link to original: https://doi.org/10.1007/s00590-019-02369-8

Copyright of the summarized publication:

If you want to cite the papers, please refer to the original.

For technical reasons we could not place the page where the original quote is coming from.

8.1.5.1 Research Highlights

Total knee arthroplasty (TKA) is a common surgical procedure aimed at alleviating pain and restoring function in patients with end-stage osteoarthritis. A critical factor for the success of TKA is the long-term mechanical fixation of the implants, which is influenced by the cement mantle thickness between the tibial implant and the trabecular bone. Despite advancements in cementing techniques, aseptic loosening remains a prevalent cause for revision surgeries. The use of a tourniquet during surgery is thought to improve visualization and potentially enhance cement penetration by creating a bloodless field, but its impact on implant stability remains unclear. The study by Touzopoulos et al. investigates whether tourniquet use during TKA affects cement mantle thickness and implant stability over a 3-year follow-up period.

The study was a retrospective comparative clinical analysis using data from patients who underwent primary TKA for osteoarthritis. The researchers compared two groups: one where a tourniquet was used during surgery and another where it was not. Both groups were matched for baseline characteristics such as age, gender, body mass index (BMI), and osteoarthritis stage. The surgical technique involved using a hybrid cruciate-retaining TKA with fixed bearing design, and radiological evaluations were conducted to measure cement mantle thickness and radiolucent lines (RLLs) under the tibial component. The study found that the use of a tourniquet increased the cement mantle thickness slightly but significantly compared to the non-tourniquet group. Radiological assessments at 3 years postoperatively showed that RLLs were more prevalent in the non-tourniquet group.

The findings suggest that using a tourniquet during TKA may enhance cement mantle thickness, potentially reducing the occurrence of progressive RLLs at the bone-cement interface. This could have implications for long-term implant survivorship, although further research is needed to confirm these outcomes over extended follow-up periods. Future study could focus on randomized clinical trials with larger sample sizes to validate these results and explore whether increased cement mantle thickness directly correlates with improved implant longevity. Additionally, investigating alternative methods to achieve optimal cement penetration without tourniquet use could provide valuable insights into enhancing TKA outcomes.

8.1.6 Tibial Stem Extension Versus Standard Configuration in Primary Cemented Total Knee Arthroplasty: Systematic Review and Meta-Analysis [63]

This is a machine-generated summary of:

Heidari, Arash; Ebrahimzadeh, Mohammad H.; Daliri, Mahla; Moradi, Ali; Sahebi, Mahdieh; Sadeghi, Masoumeh Tibial stem extension versus standard configuration in primary cemented total knee arthroplasty: systematic review and meta-analysis [63].

Published in: Journal of Orthopaedic Surgery and Research (2025).

Link to original: https://doi.org/10.1186/s13018-024-05342-2

If you want to cite the papers, please refer to the original.

For technical reasons we could not place the page where the original quote is coming from.

8.1.6.1 Research Highlights

Total Knee Arthroplasty (TKA) relies heavily on the mechanical stability of the implanted components, with aseptic loosening now recognized as a leading cause of failure post-surgery. Intramedullary stems have been developed to enhance stability by redistributing loads and reducing strain at the bone-component interface, particularly in complex cases and revision surgeries. However, the use of longer tibial stems in primary TKA (pTKA) remains controversial due to potential drawbacks like stress shielding and increased costs. The study by Heidari et al. addresses this knowledge gap by conducting a comprehensive systematic review and meta-analysis comparing post-operative outcomes and complications between tibial components with stem extensions (SE) and standard configurations (SC) in cemented pTKA.

The study followed Preferred Reporting Items for Systematic Reviews and Meta-Analyses (PRISMA) guidelines and involved a thorough search of multiple databases up to March 2023, focusing on clinical trials published in English. The researchers applied strict inclusion criteria, excluding studies on joints other than the knee, uncemented arthroplasty, and those with less than 12 months of follow-up. Ultimately, 15 studies were included in the meta-analysis, comprising both randomized controlled trials (RCTs) and non-randomized studies of interventions (NRSIs). Data extraction was performed using a pre-designed Excel form, capturing key characteristics such as study design, population demographics, clinical outcomes, and complication rates. The quality of included studies was assessed using Cochrane tools for bias evaluation. The primary outcome focused on comparing tibial implant loosening revision rates between SE and SC groups. Statistical analyses were conducted using Stata software (Stata Corp, College Station, TX. USA) to calculate pooled estimates and assess heterogeneity.

The findings suggest that tibial SE in pTKA is associated with a reduced risk of revision due to tibial loosening, higher Knee Society Score functional scores, and improved prosthesis survival rates compared to SC. However, the study acknowledges limitations such as low overall incidence of aseptic loosening events and potential heterogeneity due to variations in implant types and surgical expertise. Future study could focus on high-quality research to further explore patient selection criteria and optimize surgical techniques for using tibial stems in pTKA. Additionally, addressing factors like patient BMI and pre-operative deformity could enhance the generalizability of these findings.

8.1.7 Surface or Full Cementation of the Tibial Component in Total Knee Arthroplasty: A Matched-Pair Analysis of Mid- to Long-Term Results [64]

This is a machine-generated summary of:

Schlegel, U. J.; Bruckner, T.; Schneider, M.; Parsch, D.; Geiger, F.; Breusch, S. J. Surface or full cementation of the tibial component in total knee arthroplasty: a matched-pair analysis of mid- to long-term results [64].

Published in: Archives of Orthopaedic and Trauma Surgery (2015).

Link to original: https://doi.org/10.1007/s00402-015-2190-1

If you want to cite the papers, please refer to the original.

For technical reasons we could not place the page where the original quote is coming from.

8.1.7.1 Research Highlights

Total knee arthroplasty (TKA) is widely regarded as the gold standard for treating advanced osteoarthritis of the knee, with demand for the procedure increasing significantly over recent decades. Despite low overall revision rates, the absolute number of revisions is rising, with aseptic loosening of the tibial component being a major concern. This highlights the importance of optimal cementing techniques to ensure stable primary fixation. The debate continues over whether full cementation or surface cementation of the tibial tray provides better long-term outcomes. The study by Schlegel et al. investigates this issue by analyzing long-term clinical outcomes of full versus surface cemented tibial trays in TKA, including cases with rheumatoid arthritis (RA).

The study utilized data from a local arthroplasty registry, focusing on patients who underwent unilateral primary TKA with either surface or full cementation techniques. Patients were matched based on initial diagnosis, gender, and age to ensure comparability between groups. The surgical technique was consistent across all cases, involving a standard medial parapatellar approach and a modular knee system retaining the posterior cruciate ligament. Clinical outcomes were assessed using pre- and postoperative Knee Society Scores and patient satisfaction ratings, while radiographic analysis evaluated signs of loosening or migration. Survival analysis considered aseptic loosening as an endpoint, excluding other causes of revision such as septic loosening or isolated femoral component failure.

The findings revealed no significant difference in long-term implant survival between the two cementing techniques, aligning with previous non-comparative studies suggesting that surface cementation provides adequate fixation strength while potentially reducing stress shielding and preserving bone stock for future revisions. Interestingly, RA did not increase revision risk in the surface cementation group despite concerns about excessive cement penetration in porous bone. However, limitations such as small sample size and lack of pulsed lavage during surgery suggest that further randomized controlled trials with larger populations are needed to conclusively determine the optimal cementing technique for TKA.

8.1.8 Consequences of Using Poly-Ether-Ether-Ketone Versus Traditional Implant on Tibial Cement Penetration and Short-Term Clinical Outcomes during Total Knee Arthroplasty: A Randomized Controlled Trial [65]

This is a machine-generated summary of:

Zhao, Guanghui; Yao, Shuxin; Sun, Xiangxiang; Ma, Jianbing; Wang, Jianpeng Consequences of using poly-ether-ether-ketone versus traditional implant on tibial cement penetration and short-term clinical outcomes during total knee arthroplasty: a randomized controlled trial [65].

Published in: Journal of Orthopaedic Surgery and Research (2023).
Link to original: https://doi.org/10.1186/s13018-023-04064-1

If you want to cite the papers, please refer to the original.

For technical reasons we could not place the page where the original quote is coming from.

8.1.8.1 Research Highlights

Total knee arthroplasty (TKA) is a widely used procedure for treating osteoarthritis, but the aseptic loosening of the tibial component remains a significant issue. The longevity of TKA is largely dependent on the strength of the cement-bone bond, which is influenced by the depth and uniformity of cement penetration into the cancellous bone beneath the tibial component. Previous studies have shown that cement penetration is affected by factors such as cement type, technique, and tourniquet use. The study by Zhao et al. explores the use of poly-ether-ether-ketone (PEEK) as an alternative material for knee prostheses, comparing its effects on cement penetration and short-term clinical outcomes to those of conventional cobalt chromium molybdenum (CoCrMo) prostheses.

The study was conducted as a prospective randomized clinical trial at Honghui Hospital affiliated with Xi'An Jiaotong University. Patients aged 50–80 years scheduled for elective primary TKA were enrolled and randomly assigned to receive either PEEK or CoCrMo knee implants. The surgical procedures were standardized across both groups, including preoperative and postoperative care protocols. Cement penetration depth was measured using radiographs taken on the second day postoperatively, focusing on the tibial plateau zones. Clinical outcomes were assessed using the Knee Society Score and visual analog scale for pain at 1 year post-surgery. Statistical analyses were performed to compare outcomes between the two groups.

The study found no statistically significant difference in cement penetration depth between PEEK and CoCrMo prostheses, with both achieving satisfactory penetration levels. Additionally, both groups showed significant improvements in clinical outcomes and pain reduction at 1 year postoperatively, with no increased risk of complications in the PEEK group. These findings suggest that PEEK is a viable alternative to CoCrMo for knee prostheses in TKA, offering similar short-term safety and efficacy. Future studies could focus on evaluating long-term outcomes and potential benefits of PEEK implants in TKA to further establish their role in orthopedic applications.

Bibliography

1. Aggarwal A, Baburaj V (2021) Managing bone defects in primary total knee arthroplasty: options and current trends. Musculoskelet Surg 105(1):31–38
2. Gurazhev MB, Baitov VS, Gavrilov AA, Pavlov VV, Korytkin AA (2021) Methods of the Tibia Bone Defect Management in primary knee arthroplasty: systematic review. Traumatol Orthop Russia 27(3):173–188
3. Berend ME, Ritter MA, Keating EM, Jackson MD, Davis KE (2014) Use of screws and cement in primary TKA with up to 20 years follow-up. J Arthroplasty 29(6):1207–1210
4. Ritter MA (1986) Screw and cement fixation of large defects in total knee arthroplasty. J Arthroplasty 1(2):125–129
5. Lotke PA, Wong RY, Ecker ML (1991) The use of methylmethacrylate in primary total knee replacements with large tibial defects. Clinc Orthop Relat Res (1976–2007) 270:288–294
6. Marx RG (2003) Knee rating scales. J Arthroplasty 19(10):1103–1108
7. Rodricks DJ, Patil S, Pulido P, Colwell CW (2007) Press-fit condylar design total knee artroplasty. Fourteen to seventeen-year follow-up. J Bone Joint Surg Am 89(A):89–95
8. Khaw FM, Kirk LM, Morris RW, Gregg PJ (2002) A randomised, controlled trial of cemented versus cementless press-fit condylar total knee replacement. Ten-year survival analysis. J Bone Joint Surg Br 84-B:658–666
9. Parratte S, Pagnano MW, Trousdale RT, Berry DJ (2010) Effect of postoperative mechanical axis alignment on the fifteen-year survival of modern, cemented total knee replacements. J Bone Joint Surg Am 192(12):2143–2149
10. Buechel FF Sr (2006) Long-term follow up after mobile-bearing total knee replacement. Clin Orthop Rel Res 404:40–50
11. Vessely MB, Whaley AL, Harmsen WS, Scheleck CD, Berry DJ (2006) Long-term survivorship and failure modes of 1,000 cemented condylar total knee arthroplasties. Clin Orthop Rel Res 452:28–34
12. Kang SG, Park CH, Song SJ. Stem fixation in revision total knee arthroplasty: indications, stem dimensions, and fixation methods. Knee Surg Relat Res. 2018;30:187–92.
13. Bottner F, Laskin R, Windsor RE, Haas SB. Hybrid component fixation in revision total knee arthroplasty. Clin Orthop Relat Res. 2006;446:127–31.

14. Wang C, Pfitzner T, von Roth P, Mayr HO, Sostheim M, Hube R. Fixation of stem in revision of total knee arthroplasty: cemented versus cementless-a meta-analysis. Knee Surg Sports Traumatol Arthrosc. 2016;24:3200–11.
15. Barrack RL, Rorabeck C, Burt M, Sawhney J. Pain at the end of the stem after revision total knee arthroplasty. Clin Orthop Relat Res. 1999:216–25.
16. Cameron HU, Jung YB. Noncemented stem tibial component in total knee replacement: the 2- to 6-year results. Can J Surg. 1993;36:555–9.
17. Scuderi GR, Bourne RB, Noble PC, Benjamin JB, Lonner JH, Scott WN. The new knee society knee scoring system. Clin Orthop Relat Res. 2012;470:3–19.
18. Vaishya R, Chauhan M, Vaish A. Bone cement. J Clin Orthop Trauma. 2013;4(4):157–63. https://doi.org/10.1016/j.jcot.2013.11.005.
19. Köster U, Jaeger R, Bardts M, Wahnes C, Büchner H, Kühn K-D, et al. Creep and fatigue behavior of a novel 2-component paste-like formulation of acrylic bone cements. J Mater Sci Mater Med. 2013;24(6):1395–406. https://doi.org/10.1007/s10856-013-4909-2.
20. Graham J, Ries M, Pruitt L. Effect of bone porosity on the mechanical integrity of the bone-cement interface. J Bone Joint Surg Am. 2003;85-A:1901–8.
21. Krause WR, Krug W, Miller J. Strength of the cement-bone interface. Clin Orthop Relat Res. 1982;163:290–9.
22. Mann KA, Ayers DC, Werner FW, Nicoletta RJ, Fortino MD. Tensile strength of the cement-bone interface depends on the amount of bone interdigitated with PMMA cement. J Biomech. 1997;30(4):339–46. https://doi.org/10.1016/S0021-9290(96)00164-9.
23. Song Y, Zhu F, Lin F, Zhang F, Zhang S. Bone quality, and the combination and penetration of cement-bone interface: A comparative micro-CT study of osteoarthritis and rheumatoid arthritis. Medicine (Baltimore). 2018;97(35):e11987. https://doi.org/10.1097/MD.0000000000011987.
24. Dorr LD, Lindberg JP, Claude-Faugere M et al (1984) Factors influencing the intrusion of methylmethacrylate into human tibiae. Clin Orthop Relat Res 183:147–152
25. Walker PS, Soudry M, Ewald FC, McVickar H (1984) Control of cement penetration in total knee arthroplasty. Clin Orthop Relat Res 185:155–164
26. Ritter MA, Herbst SA, Keating EM, Faris PM (1994) Radiolucency at the bone-cement interface in TKR. J Bone Joint Surg Am 76:60–65
27. Schneider R, Hood RW, Ranawat CS (1982) Radiologic evaluation of knee arthroplasty. Orthop Clin North Am 13:225–244
28. Ecker ML, Lotke PA, Windsor RE, Cella JP (1987) Long-term results after total condylar knee arthroplasty: significance of radiolucent lines. Clin Orthop Relat Res 216:151–158
29. Hofmann AA, Goldberg TD, Tanner AM, Cook TM (2006) Surface cementation of stemmed tibial components in primary total knee arthroplasty: minimum 5-year follow-up. J Arthroplasty 21:353–357
30. Smith S, Naima VS, Freeman MA (1999) The natural history of tibial radiolucent lines in a proximally cemented stemmed total knee arthroplasty. J Arthroplasty 14:3–8

31. Ledin H, Aspenberg P, Good L (2012) Tourniquet use in total knee replacement does not improve fixation, but appears to reduce final range of motion. Acta Orthop 83(5):499–503
32. Molt M, Harsten A, Toksvig-Larsen S (2014) The effect of tourniquet use on fixation quality in cemented total knee arthroplasty a prospective randomized clinical controlled RSA trial. Knee 21(2):396–401
33. Scott C, Biant L. The role of the design of tibial components and stems in knee replacement. J Bone Joint Surg Br. 2012;94(8):1009–15.
34. Rawlinson JJ, Peters LE, Campbell DA, Windsor R, Wright TM, Bartel DL. Cancellous bone strains indicate efficacy of stem augmentation in constrained condylar knees. Clin Orthop Relat Res. 2005;440:107–16.
35. Haas SB, Insall JN, Montgomery W 3rd, Windsor RE. Revision total knee arthroplasty with use of modular components with stems inserted without cement. J Bone Joint Surg Am. 1995;77:1700–7.
36. Jazrawi LM, Bai B, Kummer FJ, Hiebert R, Stuchin SA. The effect of stem modularity and mode of fixation on tibial component stability in revision total knee arthroplasty. J Arthroplasty. 2001;16(6):759–67.
37. Yoshii I, Whiteside LA, Milliano MT, White SE. The effect of central stem and stem length on micromovement of the tibial tray. J Arthroplasty. 1992;7:433–8.
38. Zhou Y, Rele S, Elsewaisy O. Does the use of tibial stem extensions reduce the risk of aseptic loosening in obese patients undergoing primary total knee arthroplasty: a systematic review and meta-analysis. Knee. 2024;48:35–45.
39. Molt M, Toksvig-Larsen S. 2-year follow-up report on micromotion of a short tibia stem: a prospective, randomized RSA study of 59 patients. Acta Orthop. 2015;86(5):594–8.
40. Ries C, Heinichen M, Dietrich F, Jakubowitz E, Sobau C, Heisel C. Short-keeled cemented tibial components show an increased risk for aseptic loosening. Clin Orthop Relat Res. 2013;471:1008–13.
41. Lonner JH, Klotz M, Levitz C et al (2001) Changes in bone density after cemented total knee arthroplasty: influence of stem design. J Arthroplasty 16:107–111
42. Robertsson O, Sundberg M, Sezgin EA, Lidgren L, Annette W. Higher risk of loosening for a four-pegged TKA tibial baseplate than for a stemmed one: a register-based study. Clin Orthop Relat Res. 2020;478(1):58–65.
43. Stern SH, Wills RD, Gilbert JL. The effect of tibial stem design on component micromotion in knee arthroplasty. Clin Orthop Relat Res. 1997;345:44–52.
44. Cawley DT, Kelly N, McGarry JP, Shannon FJ (2013) Cementing techniques for the tibial component in primary total knee replacement. Bone Joint J 95-B:295–300
45. Clarius M, Hauck C, Seeger JB, James A, Murray DW, Aldinger PR (2009) Pulsed lavage reduces the incidence of radiolucent lines under the tibial tray of Oxford unicompartmental knee arthroplasty: pulsed lavage versus syringe lavage. Int Orthop 33:1585–1590

46. Schlegel UJ, Siewe J, Delank KS, Eysel P, Puschel K, Morlock MM, de Uhlenbrock AG (2011) Pulsed lavage improves fixation strength of cemented tibial components. Int Orthop 35:1165–1169
47. Bert JM, McShane M (1998) Is it necessary to cement the tibial stem in cemented total knee arthroplasty? Clin Orthop Relat Res 356:73–78
48. Peters CL, Craig MA, Mohr RA, Bachus KN (2003) Tibial component fixation with cement: full- versus surface-cementation techniques. Clin Orthop Relat Res 409:158–168
49. Sharkey PF, Hozack WJ, Rothman RH, Shastri S, Jacoby SM (2002) Insall Award paper. Why are total knee arthroplasties failing today? Clin Orthop Relat Res 404:7–13
50. Kolisek FR, Mont MA, Seyler TM, Marker DR, Jessup NM, Siddiqui JA, Monesmith E, Ulrich SD (2009) Total knee arthroplasty using cementless keels and cemented tibial trays: 10-year results. Int Orthop 33:117–121
51. Greene JW, Reynolds SM, Stimac JD, Malkani AL, Massini MA (2013) Midterm results of hybrid cement technique in revision total knee arthroplasty. J Arthroplast 28:570–574
52. Pfitzner T, von Roth P, Voerkelius N, Mayr H, Perka C, Hube R (2016) Influence of the tourniquet on tibial cement mantle thickness in primary total knee arthroplasty. Knee Surg Sports Traumatol Arthrosc 24(1):96–101
53. Scholes SC, Unsworth A. Wear studies on the likely performance of CFR-PEEK/CoCrMo for use as artificial joint bearing materials. J Mater Sci Mater Med. 2009;20(1):163–70.
54. Li CS, Vannabouathong C, Sprague S, Bhandari M. The use of carbon-fiber-reinforced (CFR) PEEK material in orthopedic implants: a systematic review. Clin Med Insights Arthritis Musculoskelet Disord. 2015;8:33–45.
55. Najeeb S, Zafar MS, Khurshid Z, Siddiqui F. Applications of polyetheretherketone (PEEK) in oral implantology and prosthodontics. J Prosthodont Res. 2016;60(1):12–9.
56. Nakahara I, Takao M, Bandoh S, Bertollo N, Walsh WR, Sugano N. In vivo implant fixation of carbon fiber-reinforced PEEK hip prostheses in an ovine model. J Orthop Res. 2013;31(3):485–92.
57. Du Z, Zhu Z, Yue B, Li Z, Wang Y. Feasibility and safety of a cemented PEEK-on-PE knee replacement in a goat model: a preliminary study. Artif Organs. 2018;42(8):E204–14.
58. Harna, Bushu; Kapoor, Anil; Arora, Anil; Arya, Shivali Long-term comparative study evaluating the screw-cement construct for tibial defects in total knee arthroplasty: our experience. International Orthopaedics (2025). https://doi.org/10.1007/s00264-025-06439-x
59. Bistolfi, A.; Massazza, G.; Rosso, F.; Deledda, D.; Gaito, V.; Lagalla, F.; Olivero, C.; Crova, M. Cemented fixed-bearing PFC total knee arthroplasty: survival and failure analysis at 12–17 years. Journal of Orthopaedics and Traumatology (2011). https://doi.org/10.1007/s10195-011-0142-2

60. Kim, Man Soo; Koh, In Jun; Sohn, Sueen; Park, Hyung Chul; In, Yong Modified hybrid cementing technique reduces stem tip pain and improves patient's satisfaction after revision total knee arthroplasty. Journal of Orthopaedic Surgery and Research (2020). https://doi.org/10.1186/s13018-020-01921-1
61. Bösebeck, Hans; Holl, Anna-Maria; Ochsner, Peter; Groth, Manuel; Stippich, Kevin; Nowakowski, Andrej M.; Egloff, Christian; Hoechel, Sebastian; Göpfert, Beat; Vogt, Sebastian Cementing technique for total knee arthroplasty in cadavers using a pastry bone cement. Journal of Orthopaedic Surgery and Research (2021). https://doi.org/10.1186/s13018-021-02436-z
62. Touzopoulos, Panagiotis; Ververidis, Athanasios; Mpogiatzis, Christos; Chatzigiannakis, Athanasios; Drosos, Georgios I. The use of tourniquet may influence the cement mantle thickness under the tibial implant during total knee arthroplasty. European Journal of Orthopaedic Surgery & Traumatology (2019). https://doi.org/10.1007/s00590-019-02369-8
63. Heidari, Arash; Ebrahimzadeh, Mohammad H.; Daliri, Mahla; Moradi, Ali; Sahebi, Mahdieh; Sadeghi, Masoumeh Tibial stem extension versus standard configuration in primary cemented total knee arthroplasty: systematic review and meta-analysis. Journal of Orthopaedic Surgery and Research (2025). https://doi.org/10.1186/s13018-024-05342-2
64. Schlegel, U. J.; Bruckner, T.; Schneider, M.; Parsch, D.; Geiger, F.; Breusch, S. J. Surface or full cementation of the tibial component in total knee arthroplasty: a matched-pair analysis of mid- to long-term results. Archives of Orthopaedic and Trauma Surgery (2015). https://doi.org/10.1007/s00402-015-2190-1
65. Zhao, Guanghui; Yao, Shuxin; Sun, Xiangxiang; Ma, Jianbing; Wang, Jianpeng Consequences of using poly-ether-ether-ketone versus traditional implant on tibial cement penetration and short-term clinical outcomes during total knee arthroplasty: a randomized controlled trial. Journal of Orthopaedic Surgery and Research (2023). https://doi.org/10.1186/s13018-023-04064-1

8.2 Non-Cemented implants

Machine Generated Summaries

Disclaimer: The summaries in this chapter were generated from Springer Nature publications using abstractive AI auto-summarization: An abstraction-based summarizer creates new text based on deep learning. New phrases are created to summarize the content. As the constituted sentences are machine selected, they may not fully reflect the body of the work, so we strongly advise that the original content is read and cited. The auto-generated summaries were curated by the editor to meet Springer Nature publication standards.

8.2.1 *The Knee-Fix Study: Study Protocol for a Randomised Controlled Trial Evaluating Cemented and Cementless Components in Total Knee Arthroplasty [73]*

This is a machine-generated summary of:

Tay, Mei Lin; Zeng, Nina; Holland, Sherina; Bayan, Ali; Farrington, Bill J.; van Rooyen, Rupert; Sharp, Rob; Elliott, Robert S. J.; Walker, Matthew L.; Young, Simon W. The Knee-Fix study: study protocol for a randomised controlled trial evaluating cemented and cementless components in total knee arthroplasty [73].

Published in: Trials (2022).

Link to original: https://doi.org/10.1186/s13063-022-06974-7

8.2.1.1 Research Highlights

Total knee arthroplasty (TKA) is a widely used procedure for treating various knee conditions, such as osteoarthritis and rheumatoid arthritis, with a high success rate in improving patient outcomes. However, the longevity of TKA implants is crucial, especially as younger patients with higher functional expectations increasingly undergo this surgery. Aseptic loosening, often due to poor cement mantle quality, is the leading cause of TKA failure. While cementless components have shown promise in total hip arthroplasty by reducing aseptic loosening, their efficacy in TKA remains underexplored. The study by Tay et al. investigates the long-term survival and patient outcomes of fully uncemented versus cemented fixation in TKA.

The Knee-Fix study is a prospective, single-centre, single-blinded, non-inferiority randomized controlled trial conducted at North Shore Hospital in Auckland, New Zealand. Participants eligible for cruciate-retaining knee replacement are randomly assigned to receive either a fully uncemented or fully cemented TKA using the Stryker Triathlon system (Stryker Orthopedics, Mawah, New Jersey, USA). The trial aims to assess whether uncemented TKA can match the clinical reliability and durability of the gold-standard cemented approach. The primary outcome focuses on implant fixation assessed through radiographic evaluation of progressive radiolucencies over 5 years. Secondary outcomes include health status and functional measures using validated questionnaires like the Oxford Knee Score. The study employs rigorous randomization and blinding procedures to ensure unbiased results.

These findings could significantly impact clinical practice by providing evidence on the viability of fully uncemented TKA as an alternative to traditional cemented methods. If successful, this approach may offer benefits such as better bone stock preservation and reduced operating time. Future study directions could involve longer follow-up periods to assess implant longevity further or exploring different patient demographics to generalize findings. The results will be disseminated through peer-reviewed publications and conferences, contributing valuable data to the ongoing debate over optimal fixation methods in TKA.

8.2.2 The Future Is Non-cemented Total Knee Arthroplasty: Volume Trends at the Hospital for Special Surgery [74]

This is a machine-generated summary of:

Rodriguez, Samuel; Ranawat, Amar S. The Future is Non-cemented Total Knee Arthroplasty: Volume Trends at the Hospital for Special Surgery [74].

Published in: Indian Journal of Orthopaedics (2021).

Link to original: https://doi.org/10.1007/s43465-021-00508-0

If you want to cite the papers, please refer to the original.

For technical reasons we could not place the page where the original quote is coming from.

8.2.2.1 Research Highlights

Total knee arthroplasty (TKA) is a widely performed elective surgery, with cemented fixation being the gold standard due to its excellent long-term outcomes. However, aseptic loosening remains a significant cause for revision surgeries, particularly in younger, more active patients. The bone-cement interface's inability to remodel under cyclical loading contributes to this issue. The study by Rodriguez et al. explores the potential of cementless TKA as an alternative, leveraging advancements in implant technology and design to address these challenges.

The study conducted a retrospective review of a prospectively collected database at a single academic institution, focusing on patients aged 65 and older who underwent primary TKA with cementless implants. Researchers analyzed trends in the utilization of cementless TKA prostheses over several years. A consistent surgical approach was used across all procedures, including a midline skin incision and medial parapatellar approach, with standardized preoperative and postoperative protocols. The study evaluated patient demographics, surgical variables, and outcomes such as time to revision and reasons for failure. Statistical analyses revealed an upward trend in the use of cementless TKA implants, with nine aseptic failures identified during the study period.

The findings suggest that modern cementless TKA implants have improved short- and mid-term survivorship rates due to technological advancements like porous titanium surfaces and biologically active coatings. While early designs had flaws leading to failures, current iterations show promise in reducing aseptic loosening. Future study could focus on long-term outcomes and randomized clinical trials to further validate these findings. The increasing interest in cementless TKA parallels the successful transition seen in total hip arthroplasty (THA), indicating potential for broader adoption as technology continues to evolve. However, challenges remain, particularly regarding tibial design changes needed for osteoporotic bone conditions.

8.2.3 A Comprehensive Comparison Between Cementless and Cemented Fixation in the Total Knee Arthroplasty: An Updated Systematic Review and Meta-Analysis [75]

This is a machine-generated summary of:

Liu, Yuan; Zeng, Yi; Wu, Yuangang; Li, Mingyang; Xie, Huiqi; Shen, Bin A comprehensive comparison between cementless and cemented fixation in the total knee arthroplasty: an updated systematic review and meta-analysis [75].

Published in: Journal of Orthopaedic Surgery and Research (2021).

Link to original: https://doi.org/10.1186/s13018-021-02299-4

If you want to cite the papers, please refer to the original.

For technical reasons we could not place the page where the original quote is coming from.

8.2.3.1 Research Highlights

Total knee arthroplasty (TKA) is a common procedure for patients with severe knee arthritis, and cemented fixation has traditionally been the gold standard due to its advantages in handling bone defects, delivering antibiotics, and preventing osteolysis. However, as the demographic of TKA patients shifts towards younger individuals with more active lifestyles, concerns about bone resorption at the bone-cement interface have emerged. Cementless fixation, which offers a biological bone-implant interface, has shown promise in reducing osteolysis and aseptic loosening. The study by Liu et al. compares the outcomes of cemented versus cementless fixation in TKA to address these evolving needs.

The study conducted a systematic review and meta-analysis following Preferred Reporting Items for Systematic Reviews and Meta-Analyses (PRISMA) guidelines, searching databases such as MEDLINE and Cochrane for relevant studies on cementless TKA. The researchers included studies that reported on revision rates, reasons for revision, functional recovery, and complications over a minimum follow-up period of 2 years. A total of 26 studies were analyzed, involving thousands of patients across both fixation groups. The analysis revealed no significant difference in overall revision rates between cemented and cementless groups over the follow-up period. However, the cementless group showed better functional recovery scores and required fewer manipulations under anesthesia compared to the cemented group.

The findings suggest that while cementless fixation does not reduce revision rates compared to cemented fixation in TKA, it may offer superior long-term functional recovery. This could be particularly beneficial for younger or more active patients who place greater stress on the implant interface. Future study could focus on longer follow-up periods to better understand the long-term benefits of cementless fixation.

8.2.4 *Effect of Bioactive Coating of the Tibial Component on Migration Pattern in Uncemented Total Knee Arthroplasty: A Randomized RSA Study of 14 Knees Presented According to New RSA-Guidelines [76]*

This is a machine-generated summary of:

Therbo, M.; Lund, B.; Jensen, K.-E.; Schrøder, H. M. Effect of bioactive coating of the tibial component on migration pattern in uncemented total knee arthroplasty: a randomized RSA study of 14 knees presented according to new RSA-guidelines [76].

Published in: Journal of Orthopaedics and Traumatology (2008).

Link to original: https://doi.org/10.1007/s10195-008-0008-4

If you want to cite the papers, please refer to the original.

For technical reasons we could not place the page where the original quote is coming from.

8.2.4.1 Research Highlights

Early fixation of the tibial component in total knee arthroplasty (TKA) is essential for the long-term success of the implant. In uncemented TKA, bone ingrowth into the implant's porous surface can be hindered by a fibrous membrane, which bioactive coatings like hydroxyapatite (HA) aim to convert into bony anchorage. Despite the potential benefits of HA coatings, predicting long-term outcomes of TKA remains challenging. Traditional methods such as DEXA and X-ray examinations have limitations in assessing implant stability over time. The study by Therbo et al. explores the use of Roentgen stereophotogrammetric analysis (RSA) to evaluate the migration patterns of HA-coated versus non-HA-coated tibial implants in TKA.

The study involved 23 patients with osteoarthritis undergoing uncemented TKA, randomly assigned to receive either HA-coated or non-HA-coated tibial implants. RSA was employed to track implant migration over a 12-month period, using tantalum markers inserted during surgery for precise measurement. The RSA examinations were conducted postoperatively and at several intervals up to 12 months, with meticulous attention to technical parameters such as condition number and rigid body error to ensure data reliability. Statistical analyses were performed to compare migration patterns between the two groups, revealing that HA-coated implants demonstrated less migration and variation compared to non-HA-coated implants.

The findings suggest that bioactive coating with HA may enhance the stability of uncemented TKA implants by reducing migration over time. However, due to the small sample size and short follow-up period, these results should be interpreted cautiously. Future study could benefit from larger patient cohorts and extended follow-up durations to confirm these preliminary findings. Additionally, standardizing RSA protocols across studies would facilitate more consistent comparisons and improve our understanding of implant behavior in TKA. The study underscores the potential of HA coatings in improving implant longevity and highlights the importance of methodological rigor in RSA studies.

8.2.5 Short-Term Results of the Uncemented Triathlon Total Knee Arthroplasty: A Large Cohort Single-Centre Comparative Study [77]

This is a machine-generated summary of:

Sheridan, G. A.; Garbuz, D. S.; Nazaroff, H.; Howard, L. C.; Masri, B. A. Short-term results of the uncemented triathlon total knee arthroplasty: a large cohort single-centre comparative study [77].

Published in: European Journal of Orthopaedic Surgery & Traumatology (2022).

Link to original: https://doi.org/10.1007/s00590-022-03422-9

If you want to cite the papers, please refer to the original.

For technical reasons we could not place the page where the original quote is coming from.

8.2.5.1 Research Highlights

Uncemented total knee arthroplasty (TKA) has faced challenges over the years due to issues such as aseptic loosening and tibial tray subsidence, which were prevalent in early designs. These failures were often attributed to inadequate bone ingrowth and mechanical instability. Recent advancements in uncemented TKA technology, including the introduction of the Triathlon Tritanium TKA (Stryker Orthopedics, Kalamazoo, Mi, US) with enhanced porous designs and bullet cruciform pegs, aim to address these shortcomings by improving initial fixation and promoting better bone integration. The study by Sheridan et al. evaluates the short-term survivorship of this novel uncemented TKA design in a high-volume single-center setting.

The study conducted was a retrospective cohort analysis involving consecutive primary Triathlon TKAs performed at a single center over a specified period. The researchers included both cemented and uncemented TKAs, with cemented patellar components used when resurfacing was necessary. Primary outcomes focused on aseptic and all-cause revision rates, while secondary outcomes assessed radiological indicators such as tibial tray subsidence and radiolucent lines (RLLs). Statistical analyses included chi-squared tests for categorical variables and logistic regression for interval variables, with Kaplan-Meier curves illustrating all-cause revision rates. The study found no significant differences in demographic factors like BMI or ASA grades between cohorts but noted shorter operative times for uncemented procedures.

These findings suggest that the uncemented Triathlon TKA demonstrates excellent short-term survivorship with no aseptic failures reported in the uncemented cohort. The study highlights the potential benefits of reduced operative times and improved mechanical stability due to advanced design features like porous metal integration and cruciform pegs. While these results are promising, future studies should focus on long-term outcomes and include diverse patient populations to validate these findings further. Additionally, larger multicenter trials could provide more comprehensive insights into the performance of uncemented TKAs compared to traditional cemented options.

8.2.6 No Differences in Cost-Effectiveness and Short-Term Functional Outcomes Between Cemented and Uncemented Total Knee Arthroplasty [78]

This is a machine-generated summary of:

Rassir, R.; Nolte, P. A.; van der Lugt, J. C. T.; Nelissen, R. G. H. H.; Sierevelt, I. N.; Verra, W. C. No differences in cost-effectiveness and short-term functional outcomes between cemented and uncemented total knee arthroplasty [78].

Published in: BMC Musculoskeletal Disorders (2020).

Link to original: https://doi.org/10.1186/s12891-020-03477-x

If you want to cite the papers, please refer to the original.

For technical reasons we could not place the page where the original quote is coming from.

8.2.6.1 Research Highlights

Total knee arthroplasty (TKA) is one of the most performed surgeries worldwide, with a significant portion of these procedures utilizing cemented implants. Despite the prevalence of cemented TKA, there is ongoing debate regarding the benefits of uncemented fixation, which features a porous coating to enhance biological ingrowth and potentially offers advantages such as bone stock preservation and ease of revision. However, high-quality evidence comparing the two methods has been limited, particularly in terms of cost-effectiveness. The study by Rassir et al. evaluates the cost-effectiveness and patient-reported outcomes of cemented versus uncemented TKA within the first-year following surgery.

The study conducted a post-hoc prospective multicenter observational cohort analysis involving patients who underwent TKA with either cemented or uncemented Low Contact Stress knee systems (DePuy Orthopedics, Warsaw, IN, USA). Participants were selected from a larger randomized controlled trial cohort and followed a standardized surgical protocol with multimodal analgesia to facilitate fast rehabilitation. Data collection was managed using Castor data management software, and cost-effectiveness was assessed from a societal perspective, considering both direct healthcare costs and indirect costs outside the healthcare system. The primary outcome was cost per quality-adjusted life year (QALY), while secondary outcomes included patient-reported measures of knee function and pain 1 year after surgery. Statistical analyses revealed no significant differences in overall costs or cost-effectiveness between the two groups, with comparable patient-reported outcomes at the 1-year mark.

The findings suggest that both cemented and uncemented TKA offer similar cost-effectiveness within the first-year following surgery, challenging previous assumptions about higher costs associated with uncemented implants. The study highlights that implant prices are becoming more comparable due to market changes, reducing concerns about cost disparities. Future study could focus on long-term outcomes and survivorship to further inform decision-making regarding fixation methods. Additionally, comparative meta-analyses pooling data from modern uncemented implants may provide further insights into optimal fixation strategies for long-term implant survival.

8.2.7 Bone Remodeling and Implant Migration of Uncemented Femoral and Cemented Asymmetrical Tibial Components in Total Knee Arthroplasty - DXA and RSA Evaluation with 2-Year Follow Up [79]

This is a machine-generated summary of:

Yilmaz, Müjgan; Holm, Christina Enciso; Lind, Thomas; Flivik, Gunnar; Odgaard, Anders; Petersen, Michael Mørk Bone remodeling and implant migration of uncemented femoral and cemented asymmetrical tibial components in total knee arthroplasty - DXA and RSA evaluation with 2-year follow up [79].

Published in: Knee Surgery & Related Research (2021).

Link to original: https://doi.org/10.1186/s43019-021-00111-5

If you want to cite the papers, please refer to the original.

For technical reasons we could not place the page where the original quote is coming from.

8.2.7.1 Research Highlights

Total knee arthroplasty (TKA) is a widely successful treatment for patients with symptomatic osteoarthritis, with implant survival rates exceeding 90% over 10 years. However, aseptic loosening remains a significant cause of long-term revision. Radiostereometric analysis (RSA) is a recommended method for detecting micromovements, or migration, of implants, which can indicate the risk of aseptic loosening. Dual-energy X-ray absorptiometry (DXA) can measure changes in bone mineral density (BMD) post-TKA, which may correlate with implant migration.

The study by Yilmaz et al. evaluates implant migration using model-based RSA (MBRSA) and bone remodeling using DXA in patients with cemented asymmetrical tibial and uncemented femoral TKA components over a two-year follow-up period.

The study was conducted as a prospective longitudinal cohort at Gentofte Hospital(Hellerup, Denmark), involving patients aged 55 to 75 who underwent primary hybrid TKA for osteoarthritis. The hybrid Persona® TKA implant (Zimer-Biomet, Warsaw, In., USA) included cemented asymmetrical tibial and uncemented femoral components. RSA was performed at one-week post-surgery as a baseline and followed up at 3, 6, 12, and 24 months. DXA scans were conducted at similar intervals to assess BMD changes in the distal femur and proximal tibia. The study aimed to correlate implant migration with bone remodeling by analyzing MTPM (maximal total point of motion) and BMD changes. The results showed that the greatest increase in MTPM occurred within the first 6 months for both femoral and tibial components, followed by stabilization. A significant decrease in BMD was observed at both the distal femur and proximal tibia over 2 years.

These findings align with previous research on implant migration patterns and BMD changes post-TKA. While no significant correlation between MTPM and BMD was found, the study highlights the importance of monitoring components at risk of aseptic loosening. Future studies could focus on examining migration patterns in patients who undergo revision due to aseptic loosening to identify potential predictive factors. Additionally, further evaluation of components at risk is planned with a 5-year postoperative follow-up to better understand long-term outcomes and improve clinical decision-making regarding TKA implants.

8.2.8 Changes in Bone Mineral Density of the Proximal Tibia after Uncemented Total Knee Arthroplasty. A Prospective Randomized Study [80]

This is a machine-generated summary of:

Winther, Nikolaj; Jensen, Claus; Petersen, Morten; Lind, Thomas; Schrøder, Henrik; Petersen, Michael Changes in bone mineral density of the proximal tibia after uncemented total knee arthroplasty. A prospective randomized study [80].

Published in: International Orthopaedics (2015).

Link to original: https://doi.org/10.1007/s00264-015-2852-1

If you want to cite the papers, please refer to the original.

For technical reasons we could not place the page where the original quote is coming from.

8.2.8.1 Research Highlights

After total knee arthroplasty (TKA), adaptive bone remodeling often leads to a reduction in bone mineral density (BMD) due to stress shielding, surgical trauma, and immobilization. Uncemented implants, which rely on bone ingrowth for fixation, are being developed with porous surfaces to support tissue integration and improve mechanical stability. The study by Winther et al. investigates the effects of a novel porous titanium construct, Regenerex (Zimmer-Biomet, Warsaw, IN USA) on BMD changes in the proximal tibia following TKA compared to a porous plasma-sprayed (PPS) coated implant.

The study employed a prospective, randomized design involving patients undergoing uncemented TKA due to osteoarthritis. Participants were assigned to receive either the Regenerex or PPS tibial component. Dual-energy X-ray absorptiometry (DEXA) was used to measure BMD at various intervals post-surgery. The Regenerex implant features a large pore size and interconnecting structure that mimics trabecular bone, potentially enhancing bone ingrowth and fixation. The study aimed to determine if this novel construct could minimize the typical post-operative decrease in BMD. Despite some logistical exclusions and patient dropouts, the study maintained rigorous follow-up protocols and statistical analyses to ensure reliable results.

The findings revealed that both implants led to significant improvements in knee function scores over 2 years. However, no significant differences in BMD changes were observed between the two groups at any follow-up point. Both implants showed similar patterns of peri-prosthetic bone remodeling, with an early decrease in BMD in the distal tibia that stabilized after 6 months. The Regenerex group exhibited an overall increase in BMD in certain regions, aligning with the hypothesis that its design could mitigate BMD loss. Future study could explore long-term outcomes and further refine implant designs to enhance initial stability and bone integration.

8.2.9 Total Knee Arthroplasty Using Cementless Keels and Cemented Tibial Trays: 10-Year Results [81]

This is a machine-generated summary of:

Kolisek, Frank R.; Mont, Michael A.; Seyler, Thorsten M.; Marker, David R.; Jessup, Nenette M.; Siddiqui, Junaed A.; Monesmith, Eric; Ulrich, Slif D. Total knee arthroplasty using cementless keels and cemented tibial trays: 10-year results [81].

Published in: International Orthopaedics (2008).

Link to original: https://doi.org/10.1007/s00264-007-0502-y

If you want to cite the papers, please refer to the original.

For technical reasons we could not place the page where the original quote is coming from.

8.2.9.1 Research Highlights

Total knee arthroplasty (TKA) is a common procedure aimed at alleviating pain and restoring function in patients with severe knee joint conditions. A critical aspect of TKA is the fixation and mechanical stability of the tibial component, which can be achieved using either cemented or cementless techniques. While most TKAs in the United States utilize cemented tibial components, there is ongoing debate about the efficacy of cementless fixation methods, particularly those involving additional devices like screws or keels. The study by Kolisek et al. explores the clinical outcomes of a hybrid fixation technique using a proximally cemented tibial tray with a cementless keel.

The study involved a review of clinical and radiographic outcomes for patients who underwent TKA with this hybrid technique. The researchers collected data prospectively from patients who had at least 5 years of follow-up. The surgical procedure involved press-fitting the keel into the proximal tibia while cementing the baseplate onto the tibial surface. Post-operative assessments included pain and function evaluations using the Knee Society's objective rating system, along with routine X-rays to monitor for radiolucent lines and mechanical alignment. A Kaplan-Meier survival analysis was conducted to assess prosthetic survival, using aseptic loosening or radiographic evidence of loosening as endpoints.

The study demonstrated excellent 5-year clinical results with significant improvements in Knee Society Scores and functional outcomes. The hybrid fixation technique showed a 98% survival rate at 5 years, with minimal complications reported. The authors noted that this approach is bone-conserving, potentially limiting bone loss during future revisions. However, they caution that these results are specific to the Series 7000 Stryker® TKR design (Stryker Orthopedics, Mahwah, New Jersey) and may not be generalizable to other prosthetic designs. Future studies should focus on comparing different TKA designs with cementless keels and cemented trays to further evaluate their efficacy and long-term survivorship.

8.2.10 Cementless Versus Cemented Total Knee Arthroplasty in Young Patients: A Meta-Analysis of Randomized Controlled Trials [82]

This is a machine-generated summary of:

Chen, Chengyu; Li, Ruodong Cementless versus cemented total knee arthroplasty in young patients: a meta-analysis of randomized controlled trials [82].

Published in: Journal of Orthopaedic Surgery and Research (2019).
Link to original: https://doi.org/10.1186/s13018-019-1293-8

If you want to cite the papers, please refer to the original.
For technical reasons we could not place the page where the original quote is coming from.

8.2.10.1 Research Highlights

Total knee arthroplasty (TKA) is a widely performed surgical procedure for managing knee osteoarthritis, particularly in younger patients whose demographics are shifting according to the Australian Joint Replacement Register. Younger patients undergoing TKA face unique challenges due to longer life expectancy and higher activity levels, which increase the risk of complications such as aseptic loosening and periprosthetic infection. The optimal type of prosthesis for these patients remains controversial, with cemented prostheses offering early fixation benefits but posing revision challenges, while cementless options promise long-term survival but lack widespread acceptance. The study by Chen et al. provides insights into this debate by conducting a meta-analysis of recent randomized controlled trials (RCTs) to evaluate the clinical outcomes of cemented versus cementless TKA in younger patients.

The study employed a comprehensive literature search across multiple databases, including Embase, Medline, the Cochrane Library, and Web of Science, focusing on RCTs that compared cemented and cementless TKA in patients aged 60 years or younger. The researchers extracted data on functional outcomes, radiological evaluations, pain scores, and complications from eligible studies. Quality assessment was conducted using the Cochrane Handbook for systematic reviews, and statistical analyses were performed using Stata software (Stata Corp, College Station, Texas, USA). The meta-analysis included six RCTs with a total of 1000 patients and revealed that while there was no significant difference in functional outcomes or aseptic loosening between the two groups, cementless fixation was associated with improved pain scores and radiological outcomes.

The findings suggest that cementless TKA may offer advantages in terms of pain relief and radiological results for younger patients without compromising functional recovery or increasing the risk of aseptic loosening. However, the study acknowledges limitations such as the small number of included RCTs and potential publication bias due to language restrictions. Future study could focus on larger-scale RCTs with diverse populations to further validate these findings and explore long-term outcomes. High-quality research is essential to guide clinical decision-making for optimizing prosthesis selection in young TKA patients.

8.2.11 Cementless and Cemented Total Knee Arthroplasty in Patients Younger than Fifty Five Years. Which Is Better? [83]

This is a machine-generated summary of:

Kim, Young-Hoo; Park, Jang-Won; Lim, Hyung-Mook; Park, Eun-Soo Cementless and cemented total knee arthroplasty in patients younger than 55 years. Which is better? [83].

Published in: International Orthopaedics (2014).

Link to original: https://doi.org/10.1007/s00264-013-2243-4

If you want to cite the papers, please refer to the original.

For technical reasons we could not place the page where the original quote is coming from.

8.2.11.1 Research Highlights

Cemented total knee arthroplasties (TKAs) have demonstrated low rates of aseptic loosening and favorable clinical outcomes over the long term. However, concerns about osteolysis at the cement-bone interface have raised questions about their durability, especially in younger patients. Cementless TKAs were developed to potentially enhance implant longevity by fostering a more physiological bond between bone and implant. Despite this, signs of osteolysis and early migration have also been observed in cementless TKAs, leading to doubts about their long-term effectiveness compared to cemented TKAs. The study by Kim et al. investigates the long-term clinical outcomes of cemented versus cementless TKAs in younger patients.

The study was a prospective, randomized trial involving patients under 65 years who underwent bilateral, simultaneous, sequential TKAs with either cemented or cementless fixation using the NexGen posterior-cruciate-retaining prosthesis (Zimmer-Biomet, Warsaw, In., USA). Conducted between January 2000 and March

2001, the procedures were performed by a single surgeon under consistent conditions. Patients were followed up for a mean duration of 10.8 years, with assessments including Knee Society scores, Western Ontario and McMaster Universities Osteoarthritis Index scores, radiographic evaluations, and patient satisfaction surveys. The study found no significant differences in clinical outcomes or prosthesis survival rates between the two groups. Both groups showed improved long-term survival rates without notable issues of aseptic loosening necessitating revision.

The findings suggest that both cemented and cementless TKAs offer comparable long-term outcomes in younger patients with osteoarthritis. The study highlights that neither method showed superiority over the other in terms of survival or clinical results at an average follow-up of 10.8 years. Future study could focus on larger sample sizes and diverse patient populations to validate these findings further. Additionally, exploring advancements in prosthesis design and materials may provide insights into enhancing TKA longevity across different patient demographics.

Bibliography

1. Ewald FC (1989) The Knee Society total knee arthroplasty roentgenographic evaluation and scoring system. Clin Orthop Relat Res 248:9–12
2. Kheir MM, Drayer NJ, Chen AF. An update on cementless femoral fixation in total hip arthroplasty. J Bone Jt Surg Am. 2020;102:1646–61.
3. Harwin SF, Degouveia W, Sodhi N, Gold PA, Garbarino LJ, Ehiorobo JO, et al. Outcomes of cementless-backed patellar components. J Knee Surg. 2020;33:856–61.
4. Stryker Orthopaedics. OrthoMap ® Precision Knee Product Guide. 9100-001-756 Rev. None. 2012.
5. Stryker Orthopaedics. Triathlon Knee System Surgical Protocol. TRIATH-SP-3. 2015.
6. New Zealand Orthopaedic Association. The New Zealand Joint Registry twenty-one year report January 1999 to December 2019. 2019. Available from: https://nzoa.org.nz/nzoa-joint-registry.
7. Minoda Y, Kobayashi A, Ikebuchi M, Iwaki H, Inori F, Nakamura H. Porous tantalum tibial component prevents periprosthetic loss of bone mineral density after total knee arthroplasty for five years-a matched cohort study. J Arthroplasty. 2013;28:1760–4.
8. Young SW, Mutu-Grigg J, Frampton CM, Cullen J. Does speed matter? Revision rates and functional outcomes in TKA in relation to duration of surgery. J Arthroplasty. 2014;29:1473–1477.e1. https://doi.org/10.1016/j.arth.2014.03.004.
9. Restrepo S, Smith EB, Hozack WJ. Excellent mid-term follow-up for a new 3D-printed cementless total knee arthroplasty. Bone Joint J. 2021;103-B:32–7.
10. Australian Orthopaedic Association, Australian Orthopaedic Association National Joint Replacement Registry (AOANJRR). Hip, knee and shoulder arthroplasty: 2019 annual report. Adelaide; 2019. Available from: https://aoanjrr.sahmri.com/annual-reports

11. Nugent M, Wyatt MC, Frampton CM, Hooper GJ. Despite improved survivorship of uncemented fixation in total knee arthroplasty for osteoarthritis, cemented fixation remains the gold standard: an analysis of a national joint registry. J Arthroplasty. 2019;34:1626–33. https://doi.org/10.1016/j.arth.2019.03.047.
12. American Joint Replacement Registry (AJRR). (2020). *2020 annual report*. Rosemont, IL: American Academy of Orthopaedic Surgeons AAOS.
13. Vasarhelyi, E. M., and Petis, S. M. (2020). Use of national joint registries to evaluate a new knee arthroplasty design. *Journal of Arthroplasty, 35*, 413–416. https://doi.org/10.1016/j.arth.2019.09.018
14. Quispel, C. R., Duivenvoorden, T., Beekhuizen, S. R., Verburg, H., Spekenbrink-Spooren, A., Van Steenbergen, L. N., et al. (2020). Comparable mid-term revision rates of primary cemented and cementless total knee arthroplasties in 201,211 cases in the Dutch Arthroplasty Register (2007–2017). *Knee Surgery and Sport Traumatology, Arthroscopy*. https://doi.org/10.1007/s00167-020-06183-2
15. Niemeläinen, M. J., Mäkelä, K. T., Robertsson, O., W-Dahl, A., Furnes, O., Fenstad, A. M., et al. (2020). The effect of fixation type on the survivorship of contemporary total knee arthroplasty in patients younger than 65 years of age: a register-based study of 115,177 knees in the Nordic Arthroplasty Register Association (NARA) 2000–2016. *Acta Orthopaedica, 91*, 184–190.
16. Hampton CB, Berliner ZP, Nguyen JT, Mendez L, Smith SS, Joseph AD, et al. Aseptic loosening at the tibia in total knee arthroplasty: a function of cement mantle quality? J Arthroplasty. 2020;35:S190–6.
17. Lawrie, C. M., Schwabe, M., Nunley, R. M., Barrack, R. L., and Pierce, A. (2019). The cost of implanting a cemented versus cementless total knee arthroplasty. *Bone Joint Journal, 101*, 61–63.
18. Kim, Y.-H., Park, J.-W., and Jang, Y.-S. (2021). The 22 to 25-year survival of cemented and cementless total knee arthroplasty in young patients. *Journal of Arthroplasty, 36*, 566–572.
19. Matassi F, Carulli C, Civinini R, Innocenti M. Cemented versus cementless fixation in total knee arthroplasty. Joints. 2013;1(3):121.
20. Hungerford DS, Krackow KA, Kenna RV. Cementless total knee replacement in patients 50 years old and under. Orthop Clin North Am. 1989;20(2):131.
21. Hartling L, Ospina M, Liang Y, et al. Risk of bias versus quality assessment of randomised controlled trials: cross sectional study. BMJ. 2009;339:b4012.
22. Slim K, Nini E, Forestier D, Kwiatkowski F, Panis Y, Chipponi J. Methodological index for non-randomized studies (minors): development and validation of a new instrument. ANZ J Surg. 2003;73(9):712.
23. Bagsby DT, Issa K, Smith LS, Elmallah RK, Mast LE, Harwin SF, Mont MA, Bhimani SJ, Malkani AL. Cemented vs cementless total knee arthroplasty in morbidly obese patients. J Arthroplasty. 2016;31(8):1727.
24. Søballe K, Overgaard S (1996) The current status of hydroxyapatite coating of prostheses. J Bone Joint Surg Br 78:689–691

25. Søballe K, Hansen ES, B-Rasmussen H, Jørgensen PH, Bünger C (1992) Tissue ingrowth into titanium- and hydroxyapatite-coated implants during stable and unstable mechanical conditions. J Orthop Res 10:285–299
26. Ryd L, Albrektsson BEJ, Carlsson L, Dansgård F, Herberts P, Lindstrand A, Regner L, Toksvig-Larsen S (1995) Roentgen stereophotogrammetric analysis as a predictor of mechanical loosening of knee prostheses. J Bone Joint Surg Br 77:377–383
27. Ryd L, Lindstrand A, Stenström A, Selvik G (1990) Porous coated anatomic tricompartmental tibial components. The relationship between prosthetic position and micromotion. Clin Orthop Relat Res 251:189–197
28. Therbo M, Petersen MM, Varmarken JE, Olsen CA, Lund B (2003) Influence of pre-operative bone mineral content of the proximal tibia on revision rate after uncemented knee arthroplasty. J Bone Joint Surg Br 85:975–979
29. Petersen MM, Gehrchen M, Østgaard SE, Nielsen PK, Lund B (2005) Effect of hydroxyapatite-coated tibial components on change in bone mineral density of the proximal tibia after uncemented total knee arthroplasty. J Arthroplasty 20:516–520
30. Østgaard SE, Gottlieb L, Toksvig-Larsen S, Lebech A, Talbot A, Lund B (1997) Roentgen stereophotogrammetric analysis using computer-based image-analysis. J Biomech 30:993–995
31. Valstar ER (2001) Digital roentgen stereophotogrammetry: development, validation and clinical application (Thesis). University of Leiden, Holland pp 1–179
32. Nelissen RG, Valstar ER, Rozing PM (1998) The effect of hydroxyapatite on the micromotion af total knee prostheses. A prospective, randomized, double-blind study. J Bone Joint Surg Am 80:1665–1672
33. van der Linde MJA, Garling EH, Valstar ER, Tonino AJ, Nelissen RGHH (2006) Periapatite may not improve micromotion of knee prostheses in rheumatoid arthritis. Clin Orthop Relat Res 448:122–128
34. Behery OA, Kearns SM, Rabinowitz JM, Levine BR (2017) Cementless vs cemented tibial fixation in primary total knee arthroplasty. J Arthroplasty 32(5):1510–1515
35. Meneghini RM, de Beaubien BC (2013) Early failure of cementless porous tantalum monoblock tibial components. J Arthroplasty 28(9):1505–1508
36. Barrack RL, Nakamura SJ, Hopkins SG, Rosenzweig S (2004) Winner of the 2003 James A. Rand young investigator's award. Early failure of cementless mobile-bearing total knee arthroplasty. J Arthroplasty 19(7 Suppl 2):101–106
37. Nam D, Kopinski JE, Meyer Z, Rames RD, Nunley RM, Barrack RL (2017) Perioperative and early postoperative comparison of a modern cemented and cementless total knee arthroplasty of the same design. J Arthroplasty 32(7):2151–2155
38. Miller AJ, Stimac JD, Smith LS, Feher AW, Yakkanti MR, Malkani AL. Results of cemented vs cementless primary total knee arthroplasty using the same implant design. J Arthroplasty. 2018;33:1089–93. https://doi.org/10.1016/j.arth.2017.11.048.
39. Online LROI annual report 2019 (2019). Stichting LROI,.

40. The NJR Editorial Board. 16th Annual Report, National Joint Registry for England, Wales, Northern Ireland and the Isle of Man. National Joint Registry. 2019. https://reports.njrcentre.org.uk/. Accesed 1 Mar 2020.
41. Australian Orthopaedic Association National Joint Replacement Registry (AOANJRR). Hip, Knee and Shoulder Arthroplasty: 2019 Annual Report. Adelaide: Australian Orthopaedic Association (AOA); 2019.
42. Malchau H (2000) Introducing new technology: a stepwise algorithm. Spine (Phila Pa 1976) 25(3):285
43. Nelissen RG, Pijls BG, Karrholm J, Malchau H, Nieuwenhuijse MJ, Valstar ER. RSA and registries: the quest for phased introduction of new implants. J Bone Joint Surg Am. 2011;93(Suppl 3):62–5. https://doi.org/10.2106/jbjs.K.00907.
44. Ryd L et al (1995) Roentgen stereophotogrammetric analysis as a predictor of mechanical loosening of knee prostheses. J Bone Joint Surg Br 77(3):377–383
45. Henricson A, Wojtowicz R, Nilsson KG, Crnalic S (2019) Uncemented or cemented femoral components work equally well in total knee arthroplasty. Knee Surg Sports Traumatol Arthrosc 27(4):1251–1258. https://doi.org/10.1007/s00167-018-5227-5
46. Selvik G (1989) Roentgen stereophotogrammetry. A Method for the study of the kinematics of the skeletal system. Acta Orthop (Suppl) 60:1–51 (Reprint)
47. Petersen MM, Nielsen PT, Lauritzen JB, Lund B (1995) Changes in bone mineral density of the proximal tibia after uncemented total knee arthroplasty. A 3-year follow-up of 25 knees. Acta Orthop Scand 66(6):513–516. https://doi.org/10.3109/17453679509002305
48. Abu-Rajab RB, Watson WS, Walker B, Roberts J, Gallacher SJ, Meek RM. Periprosthetic bone mineral density after total knee arthroplasty. Cemented versus cementless fixation. J Bone Joint Surg Br. 2006;88(5):606.
49. Andersen MR, Winther NS, Lind T, Schrøder HM, Mørk Petersen M (2018) bone remodeling of the distal femur after uncemented total knee arthroplasty-a 2-year prospective DXA study. J Clin Densitom 21(2):236–243. https://doi.org/10.1016/j.jocd.2017.05.001
50. Minoda Y, Kobayashi A, Iwaki H, Ikebuchi M, Inori F, Takaoka K (2010) Comparison of bone mineral density between porous tantalum and cemented tibial total knee arthroplasty components. J Bone Joint Surg Am 92(3):700–706. https://doi.org/10.2106/JBJS.H.01349
51. Bohr HH, Lund B (1987) Bone mineral density of the proximal tibia following uncemented arthroplasty. J Arthroplasty 2(4):309–312
52. Cameron HU, Pilliar RM, MacNab I (1973) The effect of movement on the bonding of porous metal to bone. J Biomed Mater Res 7(4):301–311
53. Henricson A, Linder L, Nilsson KG (2008) A trabecular metal tibial component in total knee replacement in patients younger than 60 years: a two-year radiostereophotogrammetric analysis. J Bone Joint Surg (Br) 90(12):1585–1593
54. Ryd L (1986) Micromotion in knee arthroplasty. A roentgen stereophotogrammetric analysis of tibial component fixation. Acta Orthop Scand Suppl 220:1–80

55. Fehring TK, Odum S, Griffin WL, Mason JB, Nadaud M (2001) Early failures in total knee arthroplasty. Clin Orthop Relat Res 392:315–318
56. Mikulak SA, Mahoney OM, de la Rosa MA, Schmalzried TP (2001) Loosening and osteolysis with the press-fit condylar posterior-cruciate-substituting total knee replacement. J Bone Joint Surg Am 83(3):398–403
57. Bert JM, McShane M (1998) Is it necessary to cement the tibial stem in cemented total knee arthroplasty? Clin Orthop Relat Res 356:73–78
58. Sekundiak T (2001) Tibial component cement technique for longevity of total knee arthroplasty. Annual Meeting of the American Academy of Orthopaedic Surgeons, San Francisco, CA
59. Labutti RS, Bayers-Thering M, Krackow KA. Enhancing femoral cement fixation in total knee arthroplasty. J Arthroplasty. 2003;18(8):979–83.
60. Badawy M, Espehaug B, Indrekvam K, Engesaeter LB, Havelin LI, Furnes O. Influence of hospital volume on revision rate after total knee arthroplasty with cement. J Bone Joint Surg Am. 2013;95(18):e131.
61. Namba RS, Chen Y, Paxton EW, Slipchenko T, Fithian DC. Outcomes of routine use of antibiotic-loaded cement in primary total knee arthroplasty. J Arthroplasty. 2009;24(6 Suppl):44–7.
62. Lonner JH, Hershman S, Mont M, Lotke PA. Total knee arthroplasty in patients 40 years of age and younger with osteoarthritis. Clin Orthop Relat Res. 2000;380:85–90.
63. Diduch DR, Insall JN, Scott WN, Scuderi GR, Font-Rodriguez D. Total knee replacement in young, active patients. Long-term follow-up and functional outcome. J Bone Joint Surg Am. 1997;79(4):575–82.
64. Naudie DD, Ammeen DJ, Engh GA, Rorabeck CH (2007) Wear and osteolysis around total knee arthroplasty. J Am Acad Orthop Surg 15(1):53–64
65. O̕Rourke MR, Callaghan JJ, Goetz DD, Sullivan PM, Johnston RC (2002) Osteolysis associated with a cemented modular posterior –cruciate-substituting total knee design: five to eight- year follow-up. J Bone Joint Surg Am 84(8):1362–1371
66. Duffy GP, Crowder AR, Trousdale RR, Berry DJ. Cemented total knee arthroplasty using a modern prosthesis in young patients with osteoarthritis - The Journal of Arthroplasty. J Arthroplasty. 2007;22(6):67–70.
67. McCaskie AW, Deehan DJ, Green TP, Lock KR, Rhompson JR, Harper WM, Gregg PJ (1998) Randomised, prospective study comparing cemented and cementless total knee replacement: results of press-fit condylar total knee replacement at five years. J Bone Joint Surg Br 80(6):971–975
68. Duffy GP, Berry DJ, Rand JA. Cement versus cementless fixation in total knee arthroplasty. Clin Orthop Relat Res. 1998;356:66.
69. Park JW, Kim YH. Simultaneous cemented and cementless total knee replacement in the same patients: a prospective comparison of long-term outcomes using an identical design of NexGen prosthesis. J Bone Joint Surg Br. 2011;93(11):1479.
70. Insall JN, Dorr LD, Scott RD, Scott RN (1989) Rationale of the Knee Society clinical rating system. Clin Orthop Relat Res 248:13–14

71. Belllamy N, Buchanan WW, Goldsmith CH, Campbell J, Stitt LW (1988) Validation study of WOMAC: a health status instrument for measuring clinically important patient relevant outcomes to antirheumatic drug therapy in patient with osteoarthritis of the hip or knee. J Rheumatol 15(2):1833–1840
72. Baker PN, Khaw FM, Kirk LM, Esler CN, Gregg PJ. A randomised controlled trial of cemented versus cementless press-fit condylar total knee replacement: 15-year survival analysis. J Bone Joint Surg Br. 2007;89(12):1608.
73. Tay, Mei Lin; Zeng, Nina; Holland, Sherina; Bayan, Ali; Farrington, Bill J.; van Rooyen, Rupert; Sharp, Rob; Elliott, Robert S. J.; Walker, Matthew L.; Young, Simon W. The Knee-Fix study: study protocol for a randomised controlled trial evaluating cemented and cementless components in total knee arthroplasty. Trials (2022). https://doi.org/10.1186/s13063-022-06974-7
74. Rodriguez, Samuel; Ranawat, Amar S. The Future is Non-cemented Total Knee Arthroplasty: Volume Trends at the Hospital for Special Surgery. Indian Journal of Orthopaedics (2021). https://doi.org/10.1007/s43465-021-00508-0
75. Liu, Yuan; Zeng, Yi; Wu, Yuangang; Li, Mingyang; Xie, Huiqi; Shen, Bin A comprehensive comparison between cementless and cemented fixation in the total knee arthroplasty: an updated systematic review and meta-analysis. Journal of Orthopaedic Surgery and Research (2021). https://doi.org/10.1186/s13018-021-02299-4
76. Therbo, M.; Lund, B.; Jensen, K.-E.; Schrøder, H. M. Effect of bioactive coating of the tibial component on migration pattern in uncemented total knee arthroplasty: a randomized RSA study of 14 knees presented according to new RSA-guidelines. Journal of Orthopaedics and Traumatology (2008). https://doi.org/10.1007/s10195-008-0008-4
77. Sheridan, G. A.; Garbuz, D. S.; Nazaroff, H.; Howard, L. C.; Masri, B. A. Short-term results of the uncemented triathlon total knee arthroplasty: a large cohort single-centre comparative study. European Journal of Orthopaedic Surgery & Traumatology (2022). https://doi.org/10.1007/s00590-022-03422-9
78. Rassir, R.; Nolte, P. A.; van der Lugt, J. C. T.; Nelissen, R. G. H. H.; Sierevelt, I. N.; Verra, W. C. No differences in cost-effectiveness and short-term functional outcomes between cemented and uncemented total knee arthroplasty. BMC Musculoskeletal Disorders (2020). https://doi.org/10.1186/s12891-020-03477-x
79. Yilmaz, Müjgan; Holm, Christina Enciso; Lind, Thomas; Flivik, Gunnar; Odgaard, Anders; Petersen, Michael Mørk Bone remodeling and implant migration of uncemented femoral and cemented asymmetrical tibial components in total knee arthroplasty - DXA and RSA evaluation with 2-year follow up. Knee Surgery & Related Research (2021). https://doi.org/10.1186/s43019-021-00111-5
80. Winther, Nikolaj; Jensen, Claus; Petersen, Morten; Lind, Thomas; Schrøder, Henrik; Petersen, Michael Changes in bone mineral density of the proximal tibia after uncemented total knee arthroplasty. A prospective randomized study. International Orthopaedics (2015). https://doi.org/10.1007/s00264-015-2852-1

81. Kolisek, Frank R.; Mont, Michael A.; Seyler, Thorsten M.; Marker, David R.; Jessup, Nenette M.; Siddiqui, Junaed A.; Monesmith, Eric; Ulrich, Slif D. Total knee arthroplasty using cementless keels and cemented tibial trays: 10-year results. International Orthopaedics (2008). https://doi.org/10.1007/s00264-007-0502-y
82. Chen, Chengyu; Li, Ruodong Cementless versus cemented total knee arthroplasty in young patients: a meta-analysis of randomized controlled trials. Journal of Orthopaedic Surgery and Research (2019). https://doi.org/10.1186/s13018-019-1293-8
83. Kim, Young-Hoo; Park, Jang-Won; Lim, Hyung-Mook; Park, Eun-Soo Cementless and cemented total knee arthroplasty in patients younger than fifty five years. Which is better?. International Orthopaedics (2014). https://doi.org/10.1007/s00264-013-2243-4

8.3 Hybrid Total Knee

Machine Generated Summaries

Disclaimer: The summaries in this chapter were generated from Springer Nature publications using abstractive AI auto-summarization: An abstraction-based summarizer creates new text based on deep learning. New phrases are created to summarize the content. As the constituted sentences are machine selected, they may not fully reflect the body of the work, so we strongly advise that the original content is read and cited. The auto-generated summaries were curated by the editor to meet Springer Nature publication standards.

8.3.1 Micromotion in Cemented Rotating Platform Total Knee Arthroplasty: Cemented Tibial Stem Versus Hybrid Fixation [67]

This is a machine-generated summary of:

Luring, C.; Perlick, L.; Trepte, C.; Linhardt, O.; Perlick, C.; Plitz, W.; Grifka, J. Micromotion in cemented rotating platform total knee arthroplasty: cemented tibial stem versus hybrid fixation [67].

Published in: Archives of Orthopaedic and Trauma Surgery (2005).

Link to original: https://doi.org/10.1007/s00402-005-0082-5

If you want to cite the papers, please refer to the original.

For technical reasons we could not place the page where the original quote is coming from.

8.3.1.1 Research Highlights

Total knee arthroplasty (TKA) is a widely accepted surgical procedure, but aseptic loosening due to micromotion remains a significant challenge. The rotating platform design in TKA has garnered attention for its potential to reduce polyethylene wear through axial rotation and greater articular conformity. However, the initial stability of cemented versus hybrid fixation in rotating platform TKA is not well understood. The study by Lüring et al. investigates whether cementing the tibial stem in TKA with a mobile bearing design reduces micromotion of the tibial tray.

The study employed an experimental in vitro approach using the PFC Sigma® total knee prosthesis (DePuy Orthopedics, Warsaw, In., USA) with a rotating platform design. Ten tibial trays were implanted into sawbone models, with five trays having a cement mantle around the stem and five without, all with 2 mm of cement beneath the baseplate. The models were subjected to four loading conditions—anterior, medial, lateral, and posterior—using Zwick's machine (Zwick Roell, *Kennesaw, GA., USA)* to simulate forces equivalent to three times the body weight of a 70-kg patient. Micromotion was measured using inductive pickups at various points on the tibial tray. Statistical analysis using paired Student's t-test revealed significantly increased maximum liftoff for hybrid fixation compared to cemented stems under all test conditions.

The findings suggest that cementing the tibial stem in TKA with a rotating platform design significantly enhances initial fixation by reducing micromotion. This study highlights the importance of deep cement penetration for achieving optimal stability. While current literature on this topic is limited and varied, future studies could explore different tibial tray designs using consistent experimental setups to better understand their impact on initial stability. These insights could inform surgical practices and improve long-term outcomes for patients undergoing TKA with rotating platform designs.

8.3.2 Fixation Options for Total Knee Arthroplasty: A Comprehensive Literature Review [68]

This is a machine-generated summary of:

Moya-Angeler, J.; Akkaya, M.; Innocenti, M.; Bergadano, D.; Martin-Alguacil, J.; León-Muñoz, V. Fixation options for total knee arthroplasty: a comprehensive literature review [68].

Published in: Journal of Orthopaedic Surgery and Research (2024).

Link to original: https://doi.org/10.1186/s13018-024-04966-8

If you want to cite the papers, please refer to the original.

For technical reasons we could not place the page where the original quote is coming from.

8.3.2.1 Research Highlights

Total Knee Arthroplasty (TKA) is a widely performed surgical procedure aimed at alleviating pain and restoring function in patients with end-stage knee osteoarthritis. The choice of fixation method for the prosthetic components—cemented, cementless, or hybrid—significantly impacts postoperative stability, implant longevity, and patient outcomes. Cemented fixation has traditionally been the gold standard due to its high survival rates, while cementless options offer potential benefits such as biological fixation and reduced third-body wear. The study by Moya-Angeler et al. provides an in-depth review of these fixation methods, examining their biomechanical properties, clinical performance, and current usage trends.

The study employs a comprehensive review methodology to evaluate the three primary fixation methods in TKA. Cemented fixation involves using polymethylmethacrylate bone cement to create a robust bond between the implant and bone, ensuring immediate stability. The authors highlight that successful cementation depends on factors such as cement type, application technique, and surface preparation. Cementless fixation relies on biological integration through porous surfaces that promote osseointegration. Recent advancements in implant materials have improved the clinical outcomes of cementless TKA, particularly for younger patients. Hybrid fixation combines cemented tibial components with cementless femoral components to leverage the strengths of both methods. The study synthesizes evidence from various clinical trials and meta-analyses to compare the efficacy and complications associated with each method.

Their conclusions were that the choice of fixation method in TKA is critical to the procedure's success and longevity. Cemented fixation remains reliable for older patients and those with poor bone quality, providing immediate stability and proven long-term results. Cementless fixation offers significant advantages for younger, more active patients, with advancements in materials improving long-term outcomes. Hybrid fixation provides a balanced approach, combining the benefits of both techniques. Future research should focus on optimising these methods and refining patient-specific approaches to improve overall TKA outcomes.

The findings underscore the importance of tailoring TKA procedures based on patient-specific factors such as age, bone quality, and activity level. The study suggests that while cemented fixation remains reliable for older patients with poor bone quality, cementless options are increasingly viable for younger, active individuals due to material advancements enhancing osseointegration. Hybrid fixation offers a balanced approach by combining immediate stability with long-term biological benefits. Future study directions include optimizing these methods through advanced materials and technologies like robotic surgery to improve precision and outcomes further. The authors recommend ongoing evaluation of patient-specific factors to refine surgical techniques and enhance overall patient care in TKA.

8.3.3 The Mid-Term Survival of Cemented, Uncemented, and Hybrid Fixation of the ACS Mobile Bearing Total Knee Arthroplasty [69]

This is a machine-generated summary of:

van Es, Laurian J. M.; Sierevelt, Inger N.; Hoornenborg, Daniël; van Ooij, Bas; Haverkamp, Daniël The mid-term survival of cemented, uncemented, and hybrid fixation of the ACS mobile bearing total knee arthroplasty [69].

Published in: Indian Journal of Orthopaedics (2022).

Link to original: https://doi.org/10.1007/s43465-022-00715-3

If you want to cite the papers, please refer to the original.

For technical reasons we could not place the page where the original quote is coming from.

8.3.3.1 Research Highlights

Cementation of both prosthesis components has long been the standard in Total Knee Arthroplasty (TKA), with cemented fixation being more prevalent than hybrid or uncemented methods. Despite the excellent overall results of TKA, differences between fixation methods are challenging to detect, particularly concerning survival rates and functional outcomes. Recent studies have shown varying long-term survival rates for cemented fixation, with some indicating an increased risk of aseptic loosening compared to uncemented components. The study by Es et al. investigates the mid-term outcomes of cemented, uncemented, and hybrid fixation methods in primary Advanced Coated System® Mobile Bearing Total Knee Arthroplasties (ACS MB TKAs) (ACS Manufacturing, Verona, Wisconsin, USA).

The study is an extended data report from a prospective single-center, single-blinded randomized controlled trial (RCT) conducted between 2010 and 2015. It involved 120 patients with disabling osteoarthritis who were randomized into three groups: cemented femur and tibia components, uncemented femur component with cemented tibia component, and hybrid fixation. The primary outcome was the five-year survival rate without revision surgery, while secondary outcomes included pain, function, and quality of life assessed through patient-reported outcome measures (PROMs). Data were analyzed using Kaplan–Meier survival analysis and ANOVA tests to compare differences between groups. The study found no statistically significant difference in five-year survival rates or functional outcomes among the three fixation methods.

The findings suggest that at mid-term follow-up, there is no significant difference in survival or function between cemented, uncemented, and hybrid fixation methods for ACS MB TKA. This aligns with previous systematic reviews showing comparable outcomes across different fixation types. However, the study highlights limitations such as high loss to follow-up and a smaller sample size than initially calculated. Future study directions include continuing follow-up for up to 10 years to assess long-term outcomes more comprehensively. Additionally, the study underscores the need for further research into specific TKA designs and their impact on fixation success to better inform clinical practice.

8.3.4 Hybrid Stems Are Superior to Cemented Stems in Revision Total Knee Arthroplasty: A Systematic Review and Meta-Analysis of Recent Comparative Studies [70]

This is a machine-generated summary of:

Sheridan, Gerard A.; Garbuz, Donald S.; Masri, Bassam A. Hybrid stems are superior to cemented stems in revision total knee arthroplasty: a systematic review and meta-analysis of recent comparative studies [70].

Published in: European Journal of Orthopaedic Surgery & Traumatology (2020).

Link to original: https://doi.org/10.1007/s00590-020-02752-w

If you want to cite the papers, please refer to the original.

For technical reasons we could not place the page where the original quote is coming from.

8.3.4.1 Research Highlights

The demand for revision total knee arthroplasty (TKA) has been increasing globally, with projections indicating a continued rise in these procedures. In revision TKA, femoral and tibial stems are often used to enhance the stability of primary components, especially in cases of bone loss and instability. Fixation can be achieved in three anatomical zones: the epiphysis, metaphysis, and diaphysis. However, there is ongoing debate regarding the most effective fixation method for these stems—cemented versus hybrid fixation. The study by Sheridan et al. addresses this knowledge gap by conducting a systematic review and meta-analysis of recent comparative studies to determine the optimal fixation method for stems in revision TKA.

The study employed a rigorous methodology adhering to Preferred Reporting Items for Systematic Reviews and Meta-Analyses (PRISMA) guidelines, analyzing comparative studies published within the last decade that directly compared cemented and hybrid stem outcomes in revision TKA. The researchers conducted an extensive search across multiple electronic databases using specific MeSH terms to identify relevant studies. After applying strict inclusion criteria, seven comparative studies were selected for systematic review. Data extraction was performed using an electronic form, and any disagreements were resolved through consensus among the authors. Statistical analyses were conducted using random-effects meta-analysis to account for missing data and potential inter-study heterogeneity. The primary outcome measure was "all-cause failure," which included re-revision for any reason and radiographic failure.

The findings of this study indicate that hybrid stem fixation in revision TKA is associated with a significantly lower overall failure rate compared to cemented stems across all assessed outcome measures. This suggests that hybrid stems may offer advantages such as preservation of bone stock and ease of implant removal if re-revision is necessary. The study highlights the importance of recent advancements in uncemented fixation technology and improved surgical proficiency with hybrid techniques. Future study could focus on further refining these techniques and exploring long-term outcomes to enhance the success rates of revision TKA procedures.

8.3.5 Revision Total Knee Arthroplasty: Hybrid Vs Standard Cemented Fixation [71]

This is a machine-generated summary of:

Gómez-Vallejo, Jesús; Albareda-Albareda, Jorge; Seral-García, Belén; Blanco-Rubio, Nieves; Ezquerra-Herrando, Laura Revision total knee arthroplasty: hybrid vs standard cemented fixation [71].

Published in: Journal of Orthopaedics and Traumatology (2018).

Link to original: https://doi.org/10.1186/s10195-018-0494-y

If you want to cite the papers, please refer to the original.
For technical reasons we could not place the page where the original quote is coming from.

8.3.5.1 Research Highlights

Revision arthroplasty of the knee presents significant challenges in orthopedic surgery due to the increasing number of procedures and the demanding nature of the surgery, which often involves poor bone quality and complex issues such as bone loss and insufficient soft tissue. Modular revision prostheses, which utilize metal wedges and augmentations, have become a standard treatment option to address these challenges. However, a critical question remains: is it necessary to cement central-medullary devices in these procedures? While cemented stems are known for their durability, they also pose drawbacks like stress shielding and difficulty in removal during further revisions. The study by Gómez-Vallejo et al. investigates whether hybrid fixation methods offer better clinical and radiographic outcomes compared to cemented stem methods in total knee arthroplasty revision.

The study was analytical and retrospective, utilizing data from patients who underwent revision total knee arthroplasty at the authors' institution within a specified period. Patients were selected based on specific criteria, including aseptic failure of the primary prosthesis and replacement of at least the tibial and femoral components. The study compared outcomes between patients receiving cemented arthroplasty and those with hybrid fixation, with all surgeries performed by a single surgeon. Postoperative care included standardized physical therapy protocols. The primary outcome measures were assessed using the American Knee Society Score (AKSS), Western Ontario and McMaster Universities Arthritis Index (WOMAC), and SF-36 indices. Radiological stability was evaluated using modified AKSS criteria. Statistical analyses were conducted to compare clinical outcomes, survival rates, and radiographic results between the two groups.

The study concluded that both cemented and hybrid fixation methods achieve similar clinical results and survival times in knee arthroplasty revisions. Although WOMAC scores indicated some differences in function and stiffness favoring hybrid fixation, no significant differences were found in pain scores or overall improvement according to AKSS indices. Radiological assessments showed comparable stability between the two fixation types. Given these findings, both methods are deemed safe and effective; however, due to potential future revision needs and the complexity of cement removal, hybrid stems may be preferred. Future studies could focus on larger sample sizes or randomized trials to further validate these findings.

8.3.6 Midterm Results of Modular Hinge Total Knee Arthroplasty Using Cementless Osseointegrating Stems: Low Fixation Associated Complications and Good Functional Outcome in Primary and Revision Knee Arthroplasty [72]

This is a machine-generated summary of:

Schnetz, M.; Hofmann, L.; Ewald, L.; Klug, A.; Hoffmann, R.; Gramlich, Y. Midterm results of modular hinge total knee arthroplasty using cementless osseointegrating stems: low fixation associated complications and good functional outcome in primary and revision knee arthroplasty [72].

Published in: Archives of Orthopaedic and Trauma Surgery (2023).

Link to original: https://doi.org/10.1007/s00402-023-05148-7

If you want to cite the papers, please refer to the original.

For technical reasons we could not place the page where the original quote is coming from.

8.3.6.1 Research Highlights

Hinged total knee arthroplasty (H-TKA) is often employed in cases of severe bone or soft tissue damage, particularly in revision surgeries where traditional implants fail. The demand for revision total knee arthroplasty (TKA) is expected to rise significantly in the coming years, driven by issues such as aseptic loosening, infection, and implant failure. Despite advancements in implant design and improved survival rates of up to 95% for third-generation hinged TKA, there remains no international consensus on the optimal choice between cemented and cementless fixation techniques. The study by Schnetz et al. investigates the functional outcomes and complication rates associated with a hybrid modular rotating hinge implant using cementless osseointegrating stems.

The study was conducted as a prospective single center trial at a primary academic referral center for arthroplasty. It included patients who underwent H-TKA with the MUTARS® GenuX® MK System (Implantcast GmbH, Dallas, Tx.,USA) between 2015 and 2020. The hybrid implantation approach involved cemented femoral and tibial components with cementless stems and modular components like augments, sleeves, or cones. Surgeries were performed by experienced surgeons using preoperative planning software, and patients were followed up for a minimum of 24 months. The study assessed functional outcomes using the Knee Society Score (KSS) and Western Ontario McMasters Universities Osteoarthritis Index (WOMAC), alongside radiological evaluations to monitor implant survival and complications.

The study found significant improvements in KSS scores postoperatively, indicating enhanced functional outcomes and reduced pain levels. Implant survivorship was reported at 92% after an average follow-up of 36 months, with complications related to cementless stem fixation occurring in only 5% of cases. While the overall complication rate was relatively high due to the complex nature of cases involved, fixation-associated complications were low compared to existing literature. Future study directions could focus on long-term outcomes beyond the midterm results presented here, as well as comparisons between hybrid and fully cemented fixation methods to further refine surgical approaches in complex primary and revision arthroplasty cases.

8.3.7 A Systematic Review and Meta-Analysis of Hybrid Vs. Cemented Stems—Which Method Is More Optimal for Revision Total Knee Arthroplasty? [73]

This is a machine-generated summary of:

Thever, Yogen; James Loh, Sir Young; Raghavan, Raghuraman; Toh, Rong Chuin; Moo, Ing How A systematic review and meta-analysis of hybrid vs. cemented stems—which method is more optimal for revision total knee arthroplasty? [73].

Published in: BMC Musculoskeletal Disorders (2024).

Link to original: https://doi.org/10.1186/s12891-024-07389-y

If you want to cite the papers, please refer to the original.

For technical reasons we could not place the page where the original quote is coming from.

8.3.7.1 Research Highlights

The increasing demand for Total Knee Arthroplasty (TKA) and subsequent revision surgeries poses significant challenges for orthopedic surgeons, particularly due to bone deficiencies and deformities that complicate implant stability. Intramedullary stems, either cemented or hybrid, are commonly used to enhance stability in revision TKA. However, the optimal fixation method remains controversial, with existing studies offering conflicting results. The study by Thever et al. conducted a systematic review and meta-analysis to compare the outcomes of cemented versus hybrid stem fixation in revision TKA.

The study adhered to the Preferred Reporting Items for Systematic Reviews and Meta-Analyses (PRISMA) guidelines, utilizing databases such as PubMed, Cochrane Library, Embase, and Web of Science to identify relevant studies. The authors included studies published in English that directly compared cemented and hybrid stems in revision TKA with a minimum follow-up period of 2 years. After a rigorous selection process, eight studies were included in the analysis. The meta-analysis employed a random-effects model to assess outcomes such as total re-revision rates and radiological failure. The results indicated no significant difference between the two fixation methods in terms of re-revision rates or radiological loosening, although trends slightly favored hybrid stems.

The findings suggest that both cemented and hybrid stem fixations offer similar clinical and radiological outcomes in revision TKA. While hybrid stems may provide better alignment and bone preservation, they can also cause end-of-stem pain. Cemented stems offer initial stability but may complicate future revisions. Future study could explore other fixation techniques like metaphyseal cones for enhanced outcomes. The authors recommend considering surgeon expertise and patient-specific factors when choosing the fixation method, as both techniques have proven effective but require further investigation into functional and patient-reported outcomes post-operatively.

Bibliography

1. McEwen HMJ, Goldsmith AAJ, Auger DD, Hardaker CH, Stone MH, Fisher J (2001) Wear of fixed bearing and rotating platform mobile bearing knees subjected to high levels of internal and external tibial rotation. J Mater Sci Mater Med 12:1049–1052
2. Davies J, Harris W (1994) Tensile bonding strength of the cement–prosthesis interface. Orthopedics 17:171–178
3. Dempsey A, Finlay J, Bourne R, Rorabeck CH, Scott MA, Millman JC (1989) Stability and anchorage considerations for cementless tibial components. J Arthroplasty 4:223–229
4. James S, Schmalzried T, McGarry FJ, Harris W (1991) Corrosity reduction at the femoral prosthesis/cement interface. Trans Soc Biomater 14:50
5. Keller JC, Lautenschlager E, Grayson W, Meyer P (1980) Factors affecting surgical alloy/bone cement interface adhesion. J Biomed Mater Res 14:639–644
6. Miller JE, Burke DO, Krause W, Kelebay LC (1979) An experimental technique for improved fixation of implant components in human TKA. Trans Orthop Res Soc 4:303
7. Strickland A, Chan K, Andriacchi T, Miller J (1998) The initial fixation of porous-coated tibial components evaluated by the study of rigid body motion under static load. Trans Orthop Res Soc 13:476
8. Volz R, Lee R (1988) The effect of the stem and stem length on mechanical stability of tibial components. Trans Orthop Res Soc 13:472
9. Ahmed AM, Raad S, Miller JE (1984) Metal/cement interface strength in cemented stem fixation. J Orthop Res 2:105–111
10. Seki T, Bourgeault C, Chareancholvanich AK (1997) Does a central stem affect bone strain and the stability of cemented tibial tray in primary revision TKA? Trans Orthop Res Soc 22:635
11. Bert JM, McShane M (1998) Is it necessary to cement the tibial stem in cemented total knee arthroplasty? Clin Orthop Relat Res 356:73–78
12. Chon JG, Lombardi AV, Berend KR (2004) Hybrid stem fixation in revision total knee arthroplasty (TKA). Surg Technol Int 12:214–220
13. Peters CL, Craig MA, Mohr RA, Bachus KN (2003) Tibial component fixation with cement: full- versus surface-cementation techniques. Clin Orthop Relat Res 409:158–168
14. Nivbrant NO, Khan RJK, Fick DP, Haebich S, Smith E. Cementless versus cemented tibial fixation in posterior stabilized total knee replacement: a randomized trial. J Bone Joint Surg Am. 2020;102(12):1075–82.
15. Huddleston JI, Wiley JW, Scott RD. Zone 4 femoral radiolucent lines in hybrid versus cemented total knee arthroplasties: are they clinically significant? Clin Orthop Relat Res. 2005;441(NA):334–9.
16. Gandhi R, Tsvetkov D, Davey JR, Mahomed NN. Survival and clinical function of cemented and uncemented prostheses in total knee replacement: a meta-analysis. J Bone Joint Surg Br. 2009;91(7):889.

17. DeFrancesco CJ, Canseco JA, Nelson CL, Israelite CL, Kamath AF. Uncemented tantalum monoblock tibial fixation for total knee arthroplasty in patients less than 60 years of age. J Bone Joint Surg. 2018;100(10):865–70.
18. Nam, D., Lawrie, C. M., Salih, R., Nahhas, C. R., Barrack, R. L., and Nunley, R. M. (2019). Cemented versus cementless total knee arthroplasty of the same modern design. *Journal of Bone Joint Surgery, 101*, 1185–1192.
19. Henricson A, Wojtowicz R, Nilsson KG, Crnalic S (2019) Uncemented or cemented femoral components work equally well in total knee arthroplasty. Knee Surg Sports Traumatol Arthrosc 27(4):1251–1258. https://doi.org/10.1007/s00167-018-5227-5
20. Cameron HU, Pilliar RM, MacNab I (1973) The effect of movement on the bonding of porous metal to bone. J Biomed Mater Res 7(4):301–311
21. Hampton M, Balachandar V, Charalambous CP, Sutton PM. Cementing techniques in knee surgery (CeTIKS): a UK expert consensus study. Bone Jt Open. 2023;4(9):682–8.
22. Mosher ZA, Bolognesi MP, Malkani AL, Meneghini RM, Oni JK, Fricka KB. Cementless total knee arthroplasty: a resurgence—who, when, where, and how? J Arthroplast. 2024. https://doi.org/10.1016/j.arth.2024.02.078
23. Whiteside LA, Viganò R. Young and heavy patients with a cementless TKA do as well as older and lightweight patients. Clin Orthop Relat Res. 2007;464:93–8.
24. Haeberle HS, Salem HS, Ehiorobo JO, Sodhi N, Mont MA. Newer generation of cementless total knee arthroplasty: a systematic review. Surg Technol Int. 2020;36:351–9.
25. Goh GS, Fillingham YA, Sutton RM, Small I, Courtney PM, Hozack WJ. Cemented versus cementless total knee arthroplasty in obese patients with body mass index ≥35 kg/m^2: a contemporary analysis of 812 patients. J Arthroplast. 2022;37(4):688-693.e1.
26. Nakama GY, Peccin MS, Almeida GJM, Lira Neto OA, Queiroz AAB, Navarro RD. Cemented cementless or hybrid fixation options in total knee arthroplasty for osteoarthritis and other non-traumatic diseases. Cochrane Database Syst Rev. 2012;10:CD006193.
27. Faris PM, Keating EM, Farris A, Meding JB, Ritter MA. Hybrid total knee arthroplasty: 13-year survivorship of AGC total knee systems with average 7 years followup. Clin Orthop Relat Res. 2008;466(5):1204–9.
28. van Ooij B et al (2021) What is the role of cemented fixation in total knee arthroplasty? The two-year results of a randomized RSA controlled trial. Bone Joint J 103-b(1):98–104
29. Kim YH, Park JW, Lim HM, Park ES. Cementless and cemented total knee arthroplasty in patients younger than fifty five years. Which is better? Int Orthop. 2014;38(2):297.
30. Nugent M, Wyatt MC, Frampton CM, Hooper GJ. Despite improved survivorship of uncemented fixation in total knee arthroplasty for osteoarthritis, cemented fixation remains the gold standard: an analysis of a national joint registry. J Arthroplasty. 2019;34:1626–33. https://doi.org/10.1016/j.arth.2019.03.047.

31. Lizaur-Utrilla, A., Miralles-Muoz, F. A., Ruiz-Lozano, M., Gonzlez-Parreo, S., Alonso-Montero, C., and Lopez-Prats, F. A. (2020). Better clinical outcomes and overall higher survival with hybrid versus cemented primary total knee arthroplasty: a minimum 15 years follow-up. *Knee surgery, sports traumatology, arthroscopy : official journal of the ESSKA.* https://doi.org/10.1007/s00167-020-06028-y PubMed PMID: Lizaur-Utrilla2020.
32. Irmola, T., Ponkilainen, V., and Mkel. (2020). Association between fixation type and revision risk in total knee arthroplasty patients aged 65 years and older: a cohort study of 265,877 patients from the Nordic arthroplasty register association 2000-2016. *Acta orthopaedica.* https://doi.org/10.1080/17453674.2020.1837422 PubMed PMID: Irmola2020.
33. Batailler C, Malemo Y, Demey G, Kenney R, Lustig S, Servien E (2020) Cemented vs uncemented femoral components: a randomized, controlled trial at 10 years minimum follow-up. J Arthroplasty 35(8):2090–2096
34. Breugem, S. J. M., Linnartz, J., Sierevelt, I., Bruijn, J. D., and Driessen, M. J. M. (2017). Evaluation of 1031 primary titanium nitride coated mobile bearing total knee arthroplasties in an orthopedic clinic. *World journal of orthopedics., 8*(12), 922–928. https://doi.org/10.5312/wjo.v8.i12.922. PubMed PMID: 29312851; PubMed Central PMCID: PMCPMC5745435.
35. de Groot, I. B., Favejee, M. M., Reijman, M., Verhaar, J. A., and Terwee, C. B. (2008). The Dutch version of the knee injury and osteoarthritis outcome score: a validation study. *Health and quality of life outcomes., 6*, 16. https://doi.org/10.1186/1477-7525-6-16 PubMed PMID: 18302729; PubMed Central PMCID: PMCPMC2289810.
36. Prudhon J-L, Verdier R. Cemented or cementless total knee arthroplasty? Comparative results of 200 cases at a minimum follow-up of 11 years. SICOT J. 2017;3:70. https://doi.org/10.1051/sicotj/2017046.
37. Kim, Y.-H., Park, J.-W., and Jang, Y.-S. (2021). The 22 to 25-year survival of cemented and cementless total knee arthroplasty in young patients. *Journal of Arthroplasty, 36*, 566–572.
38. Stempin, R., Stempin, K., Kaczmarek, W., and Dutka, J. (2018). Midterm results of cementless total knee arthroplasty: a retrospective case series. *The open orthopaedics journal., 2018*(12), 196–202. https://doi.org/10.2174/1874325001812010196 PubMedPMID:Stempin.
39. Bottner F, Laskin R, Windsor RE, Haas SB. Hybrid component fixation in revision total knee arthroplasty. Clin Orthop Relat Res. 2006;446:127–31.
40. Egger M, Davey Smith G, Schneider M, Minder C (1997) Bias in meta-analysis detected by a simple, graphical test. BMJ 315(7109):629–634
41. Edwards PK, Fehring TK, Hamilton WG, Perricelli B, Beaver WB, Odum SM (2014) Are cementless stems more durable than cemented stems in two-stage revisions of infected total knee arthroplasties? Clin Orthopaedics Related Res 472(1):206–211
42. Lachiewicz PF, O'Dell JA (2020) Is there a difference between cemented and uncemented femoral stem extensions in revision knee arthroplasty? J Knee Surg 33(1):84–88. https://doi.org/10.1055/s-0038-1676567

43. Wood GC, Naudie DD, MacDonald SJ, McCalden RW, Bourne RB. Results of press-fit stems in revision knee arthroplasties. Clin Orthop Relat Res. 2009;467:810–7.
44. Bertin KC, Freeman MAR, Samuelson KM et al (1985) Stemmed revision arthroplasty for aseptic loosening of total knee arthroplasty. J Bone Jt Surg (Br) 67:242–248
45. Mullaji A, Shetty GM (2014) Cemented stems: a requisite in revision total knee replacement. Bone Jt J 96-B(11 Suppl A):115–117
46. Baggio L, Gil-González S, Barra-González X et al (2016) Cemented stems in revision total knee arthroplasty on patients older than 75 y/o. Clinical and radiological analysis. Acta Ortop Mex 30(2):85–90
47. Fehring TK, Odum S, Olekson C, Griffin WL, Mason JB, McCoy TH (2003) Stem fixation in revision total knee arthroplasty: a comparative analysis. Clin Orthopaedics Relat Res 416:217–224
48. Tarazi JM, Chen Z, Scuderi GR, Mont MA (2021) The epidemiology of revision total knee arthroplasty. J Knee Surg 34(13):1396–1401
49. Sadoghi P, Liebensteiner M, Agreiter M, Leithner A, Böhler N, Labek G (2013) Revision surgery after total joint arthroplasty: a complication-based analysis using worldwide arthroplasty registers. J Arthroplasty 28(8):1329–1332
50. Wignadasan W, Chang JS, Kayani B, Kontoghiorghe C, Haddad FS (2021) Long-term results of revision total knee arthroplasty using a rotating hinge implant. Knee 28:72–80
51. Kang SG, Park CH, Song SJ. Stem fixation in revision total knee arthroplasty: indications, stem dimensions, and fixation methods. Knee Surg Relat Res. 2018;30:187–92.
52. Lizaur-Utrilla A, Gonzalez-Parreño S, Martinez-Mendez D, Miralles-Muñoz FA, Lopez-Prats FA (2020) Minimal clinically important differences and substantial clinical benefits for Knee Society Scores. Knee Surg Sports Traumatol Arthrosc 28(5):1473–1478
53. Bingham JS, Bukowski BR, Wyles CC, Pareek A, Berry DJ, Abdel MP (2019) Rotating-hinge revision total knee arthroplasty for treatment of severe arthrofibrosis. J Arthroplasty 34(7s):S271-s276
54. Houfani F, Mainard D, Rubens-Duval B, Papin PE, Pasquier G, Ehlinger M (2021) Rotating-hinge prosthesis for aseptic revision knee arthroplasty: a multicentre retrospective study of 127 cases with a mean follow-up of five years. Orthop Traumatol Surg Res 107(3):102855
55. Theil C, Schmidt-Braekling T, Gosheger G et al (2020) Acceptable mid- to long-term survival rates and functional outcomes following a single design rotating hinge total knee arthroplasty. Knee Surg Sports Traumatol Arthrosc 28(6):1868–1875
56. Mabry TM, Vessely MB, Schleck CD, Harmsen WS, Berry DJ. Revision total knee arthroplasty with modular cemented stems: long-term follow-up. J Arthroplast. 2007;22:100–5.
57. Murray PB, Rand JA, Hanssen AD. Cemented long-stem revision total knee arthroplasty. Clin Orthop 1994:116–23.

58. Peters CL, Erickson J, Kloepper RG, Mohr RA. Revision total knee arthroplasty with modular components inserted with metaphyseal cement and stems without cement. J Arthroplasty. 2005;20(3):302–8.
59. Peters CL, Erickson JA, Gililland JM. Clinical and radiographic results of 184 consecutive revision total knee arthroplasties placed with modular Cementless stems. J Arthroplasty. 2009;24:48–53. https://doi.org/10.1016/j.arth.2009.04.033.
60. Shannon BD, Klassen JF, Rand JA, Berry DJ, Trousdale RT (2003) Revision total knee arthroplasty with cemented components and uncemented intramedullary stems. J Arthroplasty 18(7 Suppl 1):27–32
61. Sheridan GA, Garbuz DS, Masri BA (2021) Hybrid stems are superior to cemented stems in revision total knee arthroplasty: a systematic review and meta-analysis of recent comparative studies. Eur J Orthop Surgery Traumatol 31(1):131–141
62. Gomez-Vallejo J, Albareda-Albareda J, Seral-Garcia B, Blanco-Rubio N, Ezquerra-Herrando L (2018) Revision total knee arthroplasty: hybrid vs standard cemented fixation. J Orthop Traumatol 19(1):9
63. Gililland JM, Gaffney CJ, Odum SM, Fehring TK, Peters CL, Beaver WB (2014) Clinical and radiographic outcomes of cemented vs. diaphyseal engaging cementless stems in aseptic revision TKA. J Arthroplasty 29(9 Suppl):224–228.
64. Fleischman AN, Azboy I, Fuery M, Restrepo C, Shao H, Parvizi J (2017) Effect of stem size and fixation method on mechanical failure after revision total knee arthroplasty. J Arthroplasty 32(9S):S202-S208.e1.
65. Mills K, Wymenga AB, van Hellemondt GG, Heesterbeek PJC. No difference in long-term micromotion between fully cemented and hybrid fixation in revision total knee arthroplasty: a randomized controlled trial. Bone Jt J. 2022;104-B:875–83. https://doi.org/10.1302/0301-620X.104B7.BJJ-2021-1600.R1.
66. Jacquet C, Ros F, Guy S, Parratte S, Ollivier M, Argenson J-N. Trabecular metal cones combined with short cemented stem allow favorable outcomes in aseptic revision total knee arthroplasty. J Arthroplasty. 2021;36:657–63. https://doi.org/10.1016/j.arth.2020.08.058.
67. Luring, C.; Perlick, L.; Trepte, C.; Linhardt, O.; Perlick, C.; Plitz, W.; Grifka, J. Micromotion in cemented rotating platform total knee arthroplasty: cemented tibial stem versus hybrid fixation. Archives of Orthopaedic and Trauma Surgery (2005). https://doi.org/10.1007/s00402-005-0082-5
68. Moya-Angeler, J.; Akkaya, M.; Innocenti, M.; Bergadano, D.; Martin-Alguacil, J.; León-Muñoz, V. Fixation options for total knee arthroplasty: a comprehensive literature review. Journal of Orthopaedic Surgery and Research (2024). https://doi.org/10.1186/s13018-024-04966-8
69. van Es, Laurian J. M.; Sierevelt, Inger N.; Hoornenborg, Daniël; van Ooij, Bas; Haverkamp, Daniël The mid-term survival of cemented, uncemented, and hybrid fixation of the ACS mobile bearing total knee arthroplasty. Indian Journal of Orthopaedics (2022). https://doi.org/10.1007/s43465-022-00715-3

70. Sheridan, Gerard A.; Garbuz, Donald S.; Masri, Bassam A. Hybrid stems are superior to cemented stems in revision total knee arthroplasty: a systematic review and meta-analysis of recent comparative studies. European Journal of Orthopaedic Surgery & Traumatology (2020). https://doi.org/10.1007/s00590-020-02752-w
71. Gómez-Vallejo, Jesús; Albareda-Albareda, Jorge; Seral-García, Belén; Blanco-Rubio, Nieves; Ezquerra-Herrando, Laura Revision total knee arthroplasty: hybrid vs standard cemented fixation. Journal of Orthopaedics and Traumatology (2018). https://doi.org/10.1186/s10195-018-0494-y
72. Schnetz, M.; Hofmann, L.; Ewald, L.; Klug, A.; Hoffmann, R.; Gramlich, Y. Midterm results of modular hinge total knee arthroplasty using cementless osseointegrating stems: low fixation associated complications and good functional outcome in primary and revision knee arthroplasty. Archives of Orthopaedic and Trauma Surgery (2023). https://doi.org/10.1007/s00402-023-05148-7
73. Thever, Yogen; James Loh, Sir Young; Raghavan, Raghuraman; Toh, Rong Chuin; Moo, Ing How A systematic review and meta-analysis of hybrid vs. cemented stems – which method is more optimal for revision total knee arthroplasty?. BMC Musculoskeletal Disorders (2024). https://doi.org/10.1186/s12891-024-07389-y

Chapter 9
Revision Total Knee Arthroplasty

Alfred J. Tria Jr. and Giles R. Scuderi

Introduction by the Editors

Total knee arthroplasty (TKA) is one of the most successful orthopedic procedures. As the incidence of primary TKA continues to increase without any signs of slowing, it is expected that revision TKA will follow suit. While improvements in TKA design and instrumentation have greatly reduced the number of revisions required for polyethylene wear and osteolysis, patients still commonly undergo revision TKA for septic and aseptic issues such as loosening and instability.

The success of revision TKA necessitates a well-planned surgical with thoughtful assessment of the potential problems that may be encountered, such as exposure and component removal. Adequate exposure is necessary for removal of the components, soft tissue balancing, management of the bone loss, and ultimately accurate placement of the final components. Revision TKA involves a wide variation in complexity, from the relatively straightforward revision with little or no bone loss to those with severely compromised bone stock and supporting soft tissue structures. These complex cases often necessitate a constrained condylar prosthesis or rotating hinge for stability or a megaprosthesis for severe bone loss.

While there is a significant improvement in patient reported outcome measures following revision TKA, patient satisfaction remains low. This is because the outcome of revision TKA is difficult to quantify, since the results are dependent upon the mode of failure. Revisions for periprosthetic joint infection have worse patient outcomes than aseptic revisions. The comparison is further complicated when considering a simple tibial polyethylene exchange versus a complex revision with a megaprosthesis.

A. J. Tria Jr. (✉)
Department of Orthopedics, Rutgers-Robert Wood Johnson Medical School, New Brunswick, NJ, USA

G. R. Scuderi
Department of Orthopedic Surgery, Northwell Health, Garden City, NY, USA

A. J. Tria Jr., G. R. Scuderi (eds.), *Total Knee Arthroplasty*,
https://doi.org/10.1007/978-3-032-00175-7_9

This chapter will focus on multiple elements of revision TKA. With our editorial prerogative, we reviewed each of the referenced articles and summarized our conclusions, as detailed below. As you read each of the computer-generated summaries that follow in this chapter you can draw your own conclusions.

One of the elements of a successful revision TKA is integrity of the collateral ligaments that afford stability to the final construct. It is not uncommon that the supporting soft tissue envelope is compromised with loss of collateral ligament integrity. In these cases, a higher level of varus-valgus constraint may be needed. In this chapter there are several reports on the use of varus-valgus constrained implants in revision TKA. Colyn et al. showed good results at 1-year in high grade varus deformity, while Algatub et al. showed significant improvement but with 36 months of follow up. A varus-valgus constrained implant does not guarantee absolute stability. Rai et al. reported 93.8% survival with 3 years of follow up but with 18% complications showing that the severe deformities are challenging even with a constrained device. Li et al. reported on high dislocation rate in the valgus knee. However, this is probably related more to the releases that were performed rather than the prosthesis. Ren et al. also looked at the valgus knee and concluded that less constraint was required if the lateral soft tissues were selectively released.

There are situations with incompetent collateral ligaments when a varus-valgus constrained implant does not provide appropriate stability. In these cases a hinged implant is necessary. Several articles in this chapter, while heterogenetic in their case distribution, do provide insight into the short-term outcomes. While there is concern about the durability of hinged implants, survivorship analysis in multiple studies have demonstrated similar results: Sanguineti e al. reported 93.5% survivorship at 5 years; Von Hintz et al. reported 81% at 6.2 years; and Gudnason et al. reported 78.6% at 10 years. This does give the impression that with longer follow up, survivorship may be declining, however a more detailed analysis is needed to determine the etiology of this observation.

Adequate surgical exposure is an absolute pre-requisite in the setting of revision TKA. If the standard medial parapatellar arthrotomy, is not sufficient for exposure in the revision TKA setting, there are several options to enhance surgical exposure. Langen et al. compared the tibial tubercle osteotomy to the medial parapatellar arthrotomy and observed that the clinical results were si milar, but the former is more difficult. Sun et al. compared the quadriceps snip to the tubercle osteotomy and found no clinical differences; however, there were more patellar tendon partial avulsions in the quadriceps snip cohort perhaps due to difficulty with the exposure. When preforming the tibial tubercle osteotomy, surgical technique is important. Wishart et al. reported higher complications when the tibial osteotomy was <55.4 mm long or < 14 mm wide; or when the fixation screws were placed too far medially. These parameters are valuable when performing this extensile exposure. As an alternative to screw fixation Zonnenberg et al. describes an absorbable suture for fixation but there is concern that fixation may be questionable. Divano et al. reviewed the literature to deterimine "is it worth it" to perform a tibial tubercle osteotomy and concluded that it does have good functional results but has more complications with a longer surgical time. The V-Y quadriceps turndown is uncommonly utilized due to the possibility of a postoperative extensor lag, but Miralles-Munoz et al. describe a helpful technique to use the V-Y quadriceps turndown for augmentation of acute quadriceps tendon ruptures.

Like primary TKA, the principles of revision TKA focuses on balancing the flexion and extension gaps. This can be achieved by manual instrumentation or more recently with innovative technology. Yu t al. observed that there was no difference with manual and robotic ligament balancing but the robotic technique required fewer soft tissue releases. There are other techniques described in this chapter including Aunan et al. who introduced a manual technique with spatulas for ligament balancing; Ghijselings et al. who recommend a patella in place balancing technique; Rossi et al. who used the ROSA robotic system;, and Cho et al. used VERASENCE. Universal utility of these techniques needs further investigation.

In contrast to most primary TKAs, epiphyseal bone alone may not be sufficient for component fixation in the revision TKA. This has led to the concept of zonal fixation in revision TKA with fixation extending into the metaphysis, the diaphysis, or both. There are several options for metaphyseal bone fixation and Ponzio et al. present a good review of the options for metaphyseal bone loss. Dzidzishvili et al. used metaphyseal cones with and without impaction grafting. Russo et al. evaluated femoral and tibial metaphyseal cone fixation and favored both femoral and tibial cones when feasible. Spinello et al. reported results with tantalum cones and diaphyseal engaging tibial stems with hybrid fixation. At 36 month follow up there was 95% survivorship with favorable clinical outcomes. As another alternative, Gattsche et al. evaluated metaphyseal sleeves without a stem, however this is a small study with limited follow up.

Diaphyseal fixation in revision TKA is achieved with either cemented or uncemented press-fit stems. Cemented stems are preferred in the presence of poor diaphyseal bone, in large canals, or in cases where reliable uncemented press-fit stems cannot be obtained. Cemented stems are usually shorter than uncemented press-fit stems. Uncemented press-fit stems are indicated when there is good diaphyseal bone and the canal geometry allows secure fixation. Sheridan et al. performed a systematic review and concluded that the hybrid fixation with cementing of the metaphysis and uncemented press-fit stems is associated with lower failure rates. Thever et al. used the same analysis approach and showed that trends favored the hybrid over the fully cemented stem. Stem design does influence fixation. Maslaris et al. studied stem profiles and found in a subgroup of cemented stems that the cylindrical stems had a greater loosening rate than the conical stems. As mentioned earlier, metaphyseal and diaphyseal fixation is important for a durable construct in revision TKA. Piovan et al. reported that patient specific cones provide better stress distribution. The results will need to be validated in a clinical setting and the implants certainly add significant cost to the surgical procedure.

Revision TKA can present various case scenarios: but, for each case, an organized step-wise approach including exposure, implant removal, reconstruction, and closure is a requirement for success.. Using a systematic approach to each of these steps allows the surgeon to perform revision TKA in a safe, predictable, and reproducible fashion. The following articles may provide further insights.

9.1 Knee Designs

Machine Generated Summaries

Disclaimer: The summaries in this chapter were generated from Springer Nature publications using abstractive AI auto-summarization: An abstraction-based summarizer creates new text based on deep learning. New phrases are created to summarize the content. As the constituted sentences are machine selected, they may not fully reflect the body of the work, so we strongly advise that the original content is read and cited. The auto-generated summaries were curated by the editor to meet Springer Nature publication standards.

9.1.1 Varus/Valgus Constraint

9.1.1.1 Primary Constrained-Condylar-Knee Designs Outperform Posterior-Stabilized and Cruciate-Retaining Designs in High-Grade Varus Osteoarthritic Knees During Short-Term Follow-Up: A Pilot Study [119]

This is a machine-generated summary of:

Colyn, William; Neirynck, J.; Vanlommel, E.; Bruckers, L.; Bellemans, J. Primary constrained-condylar-knee designs outperform posterior-stabilized and cruciate-retaining designs in high-grade varus osteoarthritic knees during short-term follow-up: a pilot study [119].

Published in: Archives of Orthopaedic and Trauma Surgery (2022).

Link to original: https://doi.org/10.1007/s00402-022-04447-9

If you want to cite the papers, please refer to the original.

For technical reasons we could not place the page where the original quote is coming from.

Research Highlights

Varus osteoarthritis (OA) is characterized by increased loading of the medial compartment, leading to cartilage degeneration, varus deformity, and lateral ligamentous insufficiency. This progression often results in dynamic varus thrust during the stance phase. Total knee arthroplasty (TKA) for varus deformities typically requires extensive medial release to achieve balance, which can lead to instability if not properly managed. Constrained Condylar Knee (CCK) implants have been developed to address these challenges, offering improved stability in cases of significant coronal deformity. The study by Colyn et al. investigates the outcomes of CCK implants in high-grade varus knees with lateral laxity, hypothesizing that these designs provide better clinical stability and functionality compared to conventional primary designs.

The study utilized a joint database from two centers to retrospectively review data from patients undergoing primary TKA between 2016 and 2019. Inclusion criteria required patients to be over 60 years old with a minimum follow-up of 1 year and a preoperative varus alignment greater than 10 degrees. Patients with prior fractures or infections were excluded. The study included 100 primary patients divided into groups based on implant design: CCK, Posterior-Stabilized (PS), and Cruciate-Retaining (CR). Surgeries were performed by senior arthroplasty surgeons using a measured resection technique without soft tissue releases for CCK knees. Outcome measures included Range of Motion (ROM), clinical stability, and various patient-reported outcome measures (PROMs). Radiographic analyses assessed alignment and potential loosening.

The findings indicate that CCK implants significantly improve clinical stability and functional outcomes compared to less constrained designs in high-grade varus OA knees with lateral laxity. The study reported no revisions or implant failures during short-term follow-up, suggesting that CCK designs may offer a viable solution for managing complex varus deformities without the need for extensive medial release. Future studies could focus on prospective randomized trials with larger populations and longer follow-up periods to confirm these results and assess long-term effects such as aseptic loosening. Despite limitations like small cohort size and lack of preoperative PROMs, this pilot study provides valuable insights into the benefits of CCK implants in challenging TKA cases.

9.1.1.2 Primary Constrained Condylar Knee Arthroplasty in Severe Varus Deformity: A Prospective 5-Year Functional Follow-Up Study in Iraqi Patients [120]

This is a machine-generated summary of:

Alqatub, Ahmed; Hasan, Ghazwan A.; Wahab, Mahmood Shihab; Katran, Mustafa Hayder; Wais, Yasameen Bani; Masaoodi, Abbas F.; Shetty, Gautam M. Primary constrained condylar knee arthroplasty in severe varus deformity: a prospective 5-year functional follow-up study in Iraqi patients [120].

Published in: European Journal of Orthopaedic Surgery & Traumatology (2023).

Link to original: https://doi.org/10.1007/s00590-022-03470-1

If you want to cite the papers, please refer to the original.

For technical reasons we could not place the page where the original quote is coming from.

Research Highlights

Total knee arthroplasty (TKA) is a common procedure for treating arthritic knees, often using a posterior stabilized (PS) design. However, in cases of severe deformities with significant ligament attenuation and bone loss, a more constrained implant design, such as the constrained condylar knee (CCK) implant, may be necessary. While CCK implants have shown high clinical success rates in high-income countries (HICs), their outcomes in low- and middle-income countries (LMICs) like Iraq remain unclear due to differences in demographics and healthcare settings. The study by Alqatub et al. investigates the mid-term clinical outcomes of primary CCK TKA in Iraqi patients with severe varus deformities.

The study was conducted prospectively at a tertiary care hospital in Iraq, focusing on patients who underwent primary TKA using the CCK implant design. The inclusion criteria targeted patients with severe knee arthritis and instability, confirmed through physical examination and radiographic findings. Exclusion criteria included traumatic arthritis or known ligament ruptures. The surgical procedure involved standard techniques with specific attention to achieving mediolateral stability through soft-tissue releases. Postoperative care included antibiotics, anticoagulants, and physiotherapy. Clinical outcomes were assessed using the Knee Society Score (KSS), comparing pre- and post-operative scores to evaluate improvements in knee function and deformity correction.

The study found significant improvements in both knee and functional scores at a mean follow-up of 36 months, with most patients achieving excellent outcomes. These results align with similar studies conducted in HICs, suggesting that CCK implants can provide effective solutions for severe varus deformities even in LMIC settings. However, some patients experienced fair to poor function due to issues like contralateral knee pain. Future study directions could include long-term follow-up to assess implant survival and function over time. Additionally, addressing limitations such as the lack of a control group or multicentric data could enhance understanding of CCK TKA outcomes across diverse populations.

9.1.1.3 Primary Total Knee Arthroplasty Using Constrained Condylar Knee Design for Severe Deformity and Stiffness of Knee Secondary to Post-Traumatic Arthritis [121]

This is a machine-generated summary of:

Rai, Saroj; Liu, Xianzhe; Feng, Xiaobo; Rai, Bimal; Tamang, Nira; Wang, Jing; Ye, Shunan; Yang, Shuhua Primary total knee arthroplasty using constrained condylar knee design for severe deformity and stiffness of knee secondary to post-traumatic arthritis [121].

Published in: Journal of Orthopaedic Surgery and Research (2018).

Link to original: https://doi.org/10.1186/s13018-018-0761-x

If you want to cite the papers, please refer to the original.

For technical reasons we could not place the page where the original quote is coming from.

Research Highlights

Intra-articular or peri-articular injuries are prevalent among young and active individuals, often resulting in post-traumatic arthritis of the affected joint. This condition is particularly common in the knee, where it can lead to severe bone loss, ligamentous injuries, instability, stiffness, and deformity. Total knee arthroplasty (TKA) aims to achieve optimal alignment, balance, and deformity correction. While posterior stabilized designs are typically effective for primary TKA, severe cases with significant bony defects or ligament insufficiency may require constrained condylar knee (CCK) prostheses. However, CCK prostheses have drawbacks such as potential mechanical loosening and complications during revision surgeries. Previous studies have assessed CCK prostheses' effectiveness in various conditions but not specifically in primary TKAs following post-traumatic arthritis. The study by Rai et al. evaluates the clinical outcomes and mid-term prosthesis survival of patients undergoing primary CCK TKA for severe knee deformity due to post-traumatic arthritis.

The study was conducted retrospectively on patients who received cemented primary Zimmer® NexGen® Legacy® Constrained Condylar Knee prostheses (Zimmer-Biomet Orthopedics, Warsaw, In, USA) between February 2007 and November 2013. Out of the initial cohort, several patients were excluded due to death, loss to follow-up, or complications requiring implant removal or revision surgery. Ultimately, 32 patients were included in the final analysis with an average follow-up of 5.6 years. The surgical procedure involved a standard medial parapatellar approach with specific techniques for tibial and femoral preparation. Decisions regarding the use of CCK prostheses were made pre-operatively based on severe deformity or intra-operatively when adequate balance could not be achieved through soft tissue release alone. Post-operative care included antibiotics, analgesics, prophylactic anticoagulants, and a structured rehabilitation program starting with passive mobilization followed by active rehabilitation.

The study found that primary CCK TKA effectively corrected severe knee deformities associated with post-traumatic arthritis, achieving a prosthesis survival rate of 93.8% at mid-term follow-up. Patients experienced significant improvements in clinical scores such as the Knee Society Score (KSS) and Hospital for Special Surgery (HSS) score, as well as range of motion (ROM). Despite these positive outcomes, the complication rate was notable at 18%, including issues like infection and mechanical loosening. The study highlights that while CCK TKA is a viable option for treating post-traumatic arthritis with severe deformities, it is not without risks. Future studies could focus on long-term outcomes and strategies to minimize complications further. The authors acknowledge limitations such as retrospective design and potential selection bias but conclude that CCK TKA offers satisfactory mid-term results for this challenging patient population.

9.1.1.4 Abnormally High Dislocation Rate Following Constrained Condylar Knee Arthroplasty for Valgus Knee: A Case-Control Study [122]

This is a machine-generated summary of:

Li, Feng; Liu, Ning; Li, Zijian; Wood, Kirkham B.; Tian, Hua Abnormally high dislocation rate following constrained condylar knee arthroplasty for valgus knee: a case-control study [122].

Published in: Journal of Orthopaedic Surgery and Research (2019).

Link to original: https://doi.org/10.1186/s13018-019-1325-4

If you want to cite the papers, please refer to the original.

For technical reasons we could not place the page where the original quote is coming from.

Research Highlights

Achieving soft-tissue balance is crucial in total knee arthroplasty (TKA) for patients with valgus deformity, where the lateral structures, such as the lateral collateral ligament (LCL) and posterolateral capsule (PLC), are often contracted. This necessitates careful release of these structures, as both excessive and insufficient release can lead to postoperative knee instability. Despite advancements in stabilizing prostheses like the constrained condylar knee (CCK), adequate lateral release remains a key determinant of surgical outcomes. However, there is ongoing debate about whether the LCL and/or popliteus tendon (PT) should be released first during surgery. The study by Li et al. investigates the association between releasing both the LCL and PT together and the risk of dislocation following CCK TKA in patients with valgus deformity.

The study employed a retrospective case-control design involving 43 patients who underwent primary CCK TKA for valgus knee deformity at a single institution. Patients were divided into two groups: those with postoperative dislocation and those without. The researchers compared clinical characteristics, radiological parameters, and the extent of intraoperative soft tissue release between these groups. All surgeries were performed using a standard anterior midline incision and medial parapatellar approach, with lateral structure releases tailored to intraoperative findings. The study found that patients who experienced dislocation were more likely to have had both the LCL and PT released during surgery, suggesting an association between this release strategy and increased dislocation risk.

The findings indicate that releasing both the LCL and PT together may increase the risk of dislocation in CCK TKA for valgus deformity, highlighting the need for caution when employing this approach. Future study could explore alternative strategies such as releasing the iliotibial band (ITB) and PLC first or using more constrained prostheses in cases requiring extensive lateral release. Additionally, postoperative management should include advising patients to avoid certain postures that may predispose them to dislocation. While limited by its retrospective design and small sample size, this study underscores the importance of surgical technique in achieving optimal outcomes in TKA for valgus deformity.

9.1.1.5 Satisfactory Mid-Term Outcomes of Condylar-Constrained Knee Implants in Primary Total Knee Arthroplasty: Clinical and Radiological Follow-Up [123]

This is a machine-generated summary of:

Mancino, Fabio; De Martino, Ivan; Burrofato, Aaron; De Ieso, Carmine; Saccomanno, Maristella F.; Maccauro, Giulio; De Santis, Vincenzo Satisfactory mid-term outcomes of condylar-constrained knee implants in primary total knee arthroplasty: clinical and radiological follow-up [123].

Published in: Journal of Orthopaedics and Traumatology (2020).

Link to original: https://doi.org/10.1186/s10195-020-00561-9

If you want to cite the papers, please refer to the original.
For technical reasons we could not place the page where the original quote is coming from.

Research Highlights

Total knee arthroplasty (TKA) is a common orthopaedic procedure, with over 600,000 surgeries performed annually in the United States. Despite high success rates, aseptic loosening and instability remain significant causes of TKA failure, necessitating revision surgeries. In cases of severe coronal deformities or when standard implants fail to achieve stability, condylar-constrained knee (CCK) prostheses are often used. These implants provide enhanced stability but have been associated with complications such as aseptic loosening and patellar issues. The study by Mancino et al. evaluates the outcomes of second-generation CCK implants in primary TKA for patients with severe coronal deformity and/or medial-lateral instability.

The study retrospectively analyzed records from patients who underwent primary TKA using a second-generation CCK implant at a single institution between 2010 and 2015. The cohort included 97 patients with severe coronal deformities or ligamentous instability where standard implants were inadequate. The surgical technique involved experienced knee surgeons using a standardized approach, including the use of stem extensions for enhanced fixation. Patients were followed clinically and radiographically for an average of 5 years, with assessments based on the Knee Society scoring system. Statistical analyses compared preoperative and postoperative outcomes to evaluate improvements in knee function and implant survivorship.

The study found that CCK implants provided high survivorship rates at midterm follow-up, comparable to less constrained implants. The mean Knee Society scores improved significantly postoperatively, indicating better knee function. While infection was the most common complication leading to reoperation, no cases of aseptic loosening were reported at follow-up. Future study could explore the long-term outcomes of CCK implants in younger, more active patients and compare them with newer mid-level constrained designs. These findings suggest that while CCK implants are effective for severe deformities, careful patient selection is crucial to optimize outcomes and minimize complications.

9.1.1.6 Revision TKA with a Condylar Constrained Prosthesis Using Metaphyseal and Surface Cementation: A Minimum 6-Year Follow-Up Analysis [124]

This is a machine-generated summary of:

Sanz-Ruiz, Pablo; Villanueva-Martínez, Manuel; Matas-Diez, Jose Antonio; Vaquero-Martín, Javier Revision TKA with a condylar constrained prosthesis using metaphyseal and surface cementation: a minimum 6-year follow-up analysis [124].

Published in: BMC Musculoskeletal Disorders (2015).

Link to original: https://doi.org/10.1186/s12891-015-0485-6

If you want to cite the papers, please refer to the original.

For technical reasons we could not place the page where the original quote is coming from.

Research Highlights

The increasing number of patients undergoing primary total knee arthroplasty has led to a rise in revision knee arthroplasty procedures, which are costly and complex. The goal of revision knee arthroplasty is to restore joint anatomy and function, but challenges such as bone loss and soft tissue instability complicate the process. The constrained condylar knee (CCK) prosthesis was developed to address these issues by resisting coronal plane stresses. However, previous studies on CCK prostheses have been difficult to compare due to variations in prosthesis types and short follow-up periods. The study by Sanz-Ruiz et al. provides a comprehensive clinical and radiographic evaluation of CCK arthroplasty procedures using a consistent prosthesis type for patients with instability or severe bone loss.

The study was conducted at a single institution where consecutive revision total knee arthroplasties were performed using the NexGen Legacy Constrained Condylar Knee prosthesis (Zimmer-Biomet, Warsaw, In., USA). The researchers included both aseptic and septic cases, excluding those with posterior stabilized liners or rotating hinge knee prostheses. Data from the procedures were entered into a computerized registry, and follow-up evaluations were conducted at regular intervals. The surgical technique involved removing failed components while preserving bone stock, extensive debridement, and meticulous preparation of osseous surfaces. Two cementing techniques were compared: surface cementation and metaphyseal cementation. Clinical outcomes were assessed using the Knee Society Score, while radiographic outcomes focused on alignment, component positioning, and radiolucent lines.

The study found that the Knee Society clinical score improved significantly after revision surgery, with excellent or good results at the end of follow-up. Radiolucent lines were more frequent with surface cementation than metaphyseal cementation, although this did not translate into significant clinical differences. The projected survival rate of the prostheses at 5 years was 85%. Despite some limitations such as retrospective data analysis and lack of a control group, the study's strengths include its homogeneity in approach and consistent use of a single knee revision system. Future studies could further explore the long-term significance of radiolucent lines and compare different stem types and fixation methods in revision TKA.

9.1.1.7 Improved Surgical Procedure of Primary Constrained Total Knee Arthroplasty Which Enables Use of the Femoral Diaphyseal Straight Extension Stem [125]

This is a machine-generated summary of:

Kawahara, Shinya; Mawatari, Taro; Matsui, Gen; Hamai, Satoshi; Akasaki, Yukio; Tsushima, Hidetoshi; Nakashima, Yasuharu Improved surgical procedure of primary constrained total knee arthroplasty which enables use of the femoral diaphyseal straight extension stem [125].

Published in: BMC Musculoskeletal Disorders (2022).

Link to original: https://doi.org/10.1186/s12891-022-05367-w

If you want to cite the papers, please refer to the original.

For technical reasons we could not place the page where the original quote is coming from.

Research Highlights

Ongoing ligament instability is a significant cause of early revision in total knee arthroplasty (TKA), particularly when severe instability in the coronal plane is present. Constrained condylar knee (CCK) implants, typically used in revision TKA, are sometimes employed in primary TKA to enhance stability for patients with severe varus/valgus deformities or ligament instability. These implants often include modular extension stems to reduce mechanical loosening risks. However, the optimal surgical approach for positioning these stems remains challenging. The study by Kawahara et al. investigates whether three-dimensional templating during primary CCK TKA can ensure the appropriate positioning and diameter of the femoral straight extension stem using a component-first procedure.

The study recruited patients with varus osteoarthritis or prior high tibial osteotomy osteoarthritis undergoing primary TKA with a CCK implant. Preoperative CT scans were used to create three-dimensional templates of the femoral component and straight extension stem. The component-first procedure involved resecting the distal femur with reference to an intramedullary rod and adjusting the mediolateral position of the femoral component to minimize overhang or underhang. The suitability of inserting a straight extension stem was assessed through computer simulations and actual surgeries, comparing templated and actual stem diameters using statistical analyses. The study found that the component-first procedure effectively compensated for appropriate anteroposterior and mediolateral positions without anterior notching, with high concordance between simulations and surgeries.

The study's findings suggest that using a straight extension stem in primary CCK TKA is feasible with the component-first procedure, potentially simplifying surgery for cases with coronal imbalance. Future study should focus on mid- and long-term outcomes of this approach, as well as its applicability across different populations given anatomical variations. Additionally, further research could explore comparisons between cementless diaphyseal stems and cemented metaphyseal stems to determine optimal fixation strategies in constrained TKA procedures.

9.1.1.8 Total Knee Arthroplasty with the least-Constrained Implant Possible for Type II Valgus Knee >20°: A 3–14 Years' Follow-Up [126]

This is a machine-generated summary of:

Ren, Jiangdong; Zhang, Xiaogang; Wulamu, Wuhuzi; Yushan, Nuerailijiang; Aaimaiti, Abudousaimi; Cao, Li Total knee arthroplasty with the least-constrained implant possible for type II valgus knee >20°: a 3–14 years' follow-up [126].

Published in: Arthroplasty (2020).

Link to original: https://doi.org/10.1186/s42836-020-00036-6

If you want to cite the papers, please refer to the original.

For technical reasons we could not place the page where the original quote is coming from.

Research Highlights

Approximately 10% of patients requiring total knee arthroplasty (TKA) present with valgus deformity, which can arise from conditions such as osteoarthritis, rheumatoid arthritis, or post-traumatic arthritis. Correcting severe valgus deformities, particularly types II and III, poses significant surgical challenges due to the complex interplay of osseous deficiencies and soft tissue contractures. Despite advancements in surgical techniques and instrumentation, achieving optimal alignment and soft tissue balance without resorting to constrained implants remains difficult. The study by Ren et al. explores a novel approach to TKA for severe valgus knees using a medial parapatellar approach with selective lateral soft tissue release and minimal constraint prostheses.

The study involved a retrospective analysis of patients with severe type II valgus knee deformities who underwent TKA. The surgical procedure was standardized across cases, utilizing a medial parapatellar approach for osteotomy and selective release of lateral soft tissues. The least-constrained total knee prosthesis possible was used to avoid late-onset instability. Intraoperative techniques included the use of extramedullary tibial guides for bone resection and step-by-step release of tight lateral structures such as the iliotibial band (ITB) and lateral collateral ligament (LCL). Postoperative assessments were conducted using the Knee Society Knee and Functional Scoring System, with radiographic evaluations confirming improvements in femorotibial alignment. The study reported good or excellent clinical outcomes in most cases, with significant improvements in range of motion and joint stability.

The findings suggest that selective lateral soft tissue release combined with the use of non-constrained prostheses can effectively address severe valgus deformities without compromising long-term stability. This approach minimizes the need for high-constraint implants, which are associated with higher risks of loosening and technical difficulties during revision surgeries. Future study could focus on refining these techniques further or exploring their applicability to other complex knee deformities. The results underscore the importance of individualized surgical strategies that consider both osseous and soft tissue components to achieve successful TKA outcomes in patients with severe valgus knees.

9.1.1.9 Clinical Outcome and Survival Rate of Condylar Constrained Knee Prosthesis in Revision Total Knee Arthroplasty: An Average Nine Point Six Year Follow-Up [127]

This is a machine-generated summary of:

Yu, Muyang; Xu, Yiming; Weng, Xisheng; Feng, Bin Clinical outcome and survival rate of condylar constrained knee prosthesis in revision total knee arthroplasty: an average nine point 6 year follow-up [127].

Published in: International Orthopaedics (2024).

Link to original: https://doi.org/10.1007/s00264-024-06096-6

If you want to cite the papers, please refer to the original.

For technical reasons we could not place the page where the original quote is coming from.

Research Highlights

Total knee arthroplasty (TKA) is widely regarded as the most effective treatment for end-stage knee arthritis. However, with an aging population and more younger patients undergoing TKA, there has been a notable increase in revision total knee arthroplasty (rTKA). In China, rTKA accounts for a significant percentage of all knee replacements, with infection and aseptic loosening being the primary causes of failure. The complexity of rTKA, especially in cases with severe deformities and ligament damage, necessitates the use of more restrictive prostheses like the condylar constrained knee (CCK). The study by Yu et al. explores the application of CCK in rTKA, providing insights into its long-term clinical and radiographic outcomes.

The study conducted a retrospective analysis of patients who underwent rTKA using CCK prostheses at their center from January 2010 to January 2020. Data were collected from a joint arthroplasty registry, focusing on patients with more than 1 year of follow-up. The surgical procedures involved one-stage surgeries for non-infected knees and two-stage surgeries for infected knees. The study employed hybrid fixation techniques using press-fit stems with cement fixation in proximal components. Clinical outcomes were assessed using various scoring systems such as the Hospital for Special Surgery score and the Western Ontario and McMaster University Osteoarthritis Index. Radiographic evaluations were performed to assess limb alignment and prosthesis stability. Statistical analyses included paired t-tests and Kaplan-Meier survival analysis to evaluate prosthesis survival rates.

The study demonstrated that CCK prostheses in rTKA significantly improved knee function over an average follow-up period of 5.8 years. The findings suggest that CCK prostheses offer reliable implant survival while maintaining surgical safety. However, infection remains a major postoperative complication and cause of failure in rTKA. Future studies could focus on larger sample sizes and randomized clinical trials to further explore risk factors for re-revision and compare different prosthetic options. Additionally, investigating optimal fixation techniques could enhance outcomes in revision TKA procedures.

9.1.1.10 Comparison of Early Curative Effects of Lateral Unicompartmental Knee Arthroplasty with Total Knee Arthroplasty and the Legacy Constrained Condylar Knee Arthroplasty in the Treatment of Isolated Lateral Osteoarthritis: A Single-Center Retrospective Study [128]

This is a machine-generated summary of:

Yu, Hui; Meng, Jiahong; Xu, Yibo; Xu, Kai; Lin, Changjian; Bao, Jiapeng Comparison of early curative effects of lateral unicompartmental knee arthroplasty with total knee arthroplasty and the legacy constrained condylar knee arthroplasty in the treatment of isolated lateral osteoarthritis: a single-center retrospective study [128].

Published in: Journal of Orthopaedic Surgery and Research (2024).

Link to original: https://doi.org/10.1186/s13018-024-05076-1

If you want to cite the papers, please refer to the original.
For technical reasons we could not place the page where the original quote is coming from.

Research Highlights

Knee osteoarthritis (KOA) is a prevalent joint disease among the elderly, with symptomatic cases increasing with age, particularly in women. Surgical interventions are often recommended for patients unresponsive to conservative treatments, with options including total knee arthroplasty (TKA) and unicompartmental knee arthroplasty (UKA). Lateral unicompartmental knee arthroplasty (LUKA) has historically been less effective than medial UKA, but recent advancements in surgical techniques and prosthesis design have shown promising results. The study by Yu et al. retrospectively analyzes the outcomes of LUKA compared to TKA and lateral condylar constrained knee (LCCK) arthroplasty in patients with lateral compartment knee osteoarthritis (LCKOA).

The study involved a retrospective analysis of 74 patients treated for LCKOA using LUKA, TKA, or LCCK arthroplasty. Propensity score matching was employed to minimize confounding biases, ensuring comparability between groups. Surgical procedures were performed by the same experienced surgeon, and postoperative protocols were standardized across all groups. The study assessed various outcomes, including operation time, blood loss, range of motion (ROM), and pain scores. Results indicated that LUKA had shorter operation times, less blood loss, and lower postoperative pain scores compared to TKA and LCCK. Additionally, improvements in ROM and valgus angle correction were significant across all groups.

The findings suggest that LUKA offers comparable clinical outcomes to TKA while providing benefits such as reduced trauma and quicker recovery. However, patient selection remains crucial; LUKA is recommended for those with specific indications like isolated lateral compartment degeneration and stable collateral ligaments. Future study could focus on long-term efficacy through larger sample sizes and multicenter randomized controlled trials to further validate these findings. The study highlights the potential of LUKA as a viable alternative for treating LCKOA but emphasizes the need for careful evaluation of surgical indications and contraindications.

9.1.2 Rotating Hinge

9.1.2.1 Outcomes of the Rotating Hinge Knee in Revision Total Knee Arthroplasty with a Median Follow-Up of 6.2 Years [129]

This is a machine-generated summary of:

von Hintze, Jake; Niemeläinen, Mika; Sintonen, Harri; Nieminen, Jyrki; Eskelinen, Antti Outcomes of the rotating hinge knee in revision total knee arthroplasty with a median follow-up of 6.2 years [129].

Published in: BMC Musculoskeletal Disorders (2021).

Link to original: https://doi.org/10.1186/s12891-021-04205-9

If you want to cite the papers, please refer to the original.

For technical reasons we could not place the page where the original quote is coming from.

Research Highlights

In recent years, the incidence of total knee arthroplasty (TKA) has increased globally, with projections indicating a further rise in procedures and subsequent revision burdens. Instability, aseptic loosening, and infections are frequent causes of knee revision and re-revision, necessitating the use of implants with varying levels of constraint to ensure stability. The study by Hintze et al. investigates the mid-term clinical, radiographic, and health-related quality of life outcomes in patients who underwent revision TKA using the NexGen® Rotating Hinge Knee (RHK) (Zimmer-Biomet, Warsaw, In, USA) implant at their institution.

The study was conducted at an academic high-volume tertiary referral center and involved three phases: a prospective follow-up of surviving patients, a retrospective analysis of outcome data from an electronic joint replacement database, and cross-checking revision surgeries from the Finnish Arthroplasty Register. All RHK revision knee arthroplasties were performed using a medial parapatellar approach under spinal anesthesia with immediate full weight-bearing postoperatively. The study included detailed perioperative care documentation and utilized patient-reported outcome measures (PROMs) such as the Oxford Knee Score (OKS), Knee Injury and Osteoarthritis Outcome Score (KOOS), and Forgotten Joint Score (FJS). Radiographic evaluations were conducted pre- and post-operatively to assess osteolytic defects and component stability.

The study found that the NexGen® RHK implant provided fair mid-term clinical outcomes with acceptable implant survivorship in complex revision TKA cases. A slight majority of patients reported good or excellent OKS scores at final follow-up, although health-related quality of life was lower compared to the general population. The 10-year Kaplan-Meier survival rate was 84.3% for revisions due to any reason. While mechanical hinge failures were rare, infections remained a significant complication. Future study could focus on improving patient selection criteria and exploring strategies to reduce infection rates in this challenging patient group.

9.1.2.2 Risk Factors for Aseptic Loosening in Complex Revision Total Knee Arthroplasty Using Rotating Hinge Implants [130]

This is a machine-generated summary of:

Levent, Ali; Suero, Eduardo M.; Gehrke, Thorsten; Bakhtiari, Iman Godarzi; Citak, Mustafa Risk factors for aseptic loosening in complex revision total knee arthroplasty using rotating hinge implants [130].

Published in: International Orthopaedics (2020).

Link to original: https://doi.org/10.1007/s00264-020-04878-2

If you want to cite the papers, please refer to the original.

For technical reasons we could not place the page where the original quote is coming from.

Research Highlights

Total knee arthroplasty (TKA) is a widely performed surgery aimed at alleviating pain and dysfunction caused by advanced knee arthritis. Despite generally favorable outcomes, complications such as infection, instability, and aseptic loosening (AL) can necessitate revision surgeries. AL, characterized by the loss of prosthesis attachment to the bone, poses significant challenges in revision TKA due to associated bone defects. Various grafting techniques, including tantalum cones and impaction bone grafting, are employed to address these defects. The study by Levent et al. investigates the risk factors for AL development following re-revision surgeries in patients with rotating hinge prostheses.

The study was conducted at a high-volume arthroplasty center and involved a retrospective review of patients who underwent revision rotating hinge prosthesis between January 2012, and December 2017. Patients included in the study had undergone at least two revision operations after primary TKA and developed AL. The control group consisted of patients who had similar surgical histories but did not develop AL. The researchers evaluated bone defects using pre-operative radiographs and intra-operative assessments, with most cases classified as type II defects. Surgical techniques included synovectomy, removal of loose implants, and treatment of bone defects using impaction grafting or tantalum cones based on surgeon preference. Statistical analyses were performed to identify risk factors for AL, revealing that smoking, right-sided TKA, and large femoral canal diameter increased AL risk while tibial tantalum cone application decreased it.

The study highlights several factors influencing AL development in re-revision TKA with rotating hinge prostheses. Smoking and right-sided prosthesis were associated with increased AL risk, while impaction grafting and tantalum cone application reduced it. The findings suggest that careful consideration of these factors could improve surgical outcomes. Future studies could benefit from larger sample sizes and multi-center collaborations to further elucidate variables affecting AL development in this specific patient group.

9.1.2.3 Implant Survival and Outcome after Rotating-Hinge Total Knee Revision Arthroplasty: A Minimum 6-Year Follow-Up [131]

This is a machine-generated summary of:

Gudnason, Asgeir; Milbrink, Jan; Hailer, Nils P. Implant survival and outcome after rotating-hinge total knee revision arthroplasty: a minimum 6-year follow-up [131].

Published in: Archives of Orthopaedic and Trauma Surgery (2011).

Link to original: https://doi.org/10.1007/s00402-011-1330-5

If you want to cite the papers, please refer to the original.

For technical reasons we could not place the page where the original quote is coming from.

Research Highlights

Historically, hinged knee prostheses were the first generation of implants used in total knee arthroplasty (TKA), but their restricted biomechanics led to issues such as early loosening and excessive wear. This prompted the development of rotating hinge designs, which are now primarily used in complex revision surgeries or cases with severe deformities. Despite their use, the literature on the clinical and radiological outcomes of rotating hinge TKA is inconsistent, with studies often including a wide range of indications and short follow-up periods. The study by Gudnason et al. evaluates the long-term survival and outcomes of the Endo-model rotating hinge prosthesis (Waldemar Link, Barkhausenweg, Hamburg, Germany) specifically in cases of aseptic loosening.

The study was a retrospective analysis focusing on patients who underwent revision TKA due to aseptic loosening using the Endo-model rotating hinge prosthesis. The researchers included patients operated on between 2000 and 2010, ensuring a minimum follow-up period of 10 years. Data collection involved demographic information, medical histories, and radiographic evaluations before and after surgery. The study utilized standard revision TKA procedures with cemented components and peri-operative antibiotic prophylaxis. Clinical outcomes were assessed using the Hospital for Special Surgery score, while implant survival was analyzed using the Kaplan-Meier method. The study found that with revision due to aseptic loosening as the endpoint, 10-year implant survival was 85.7%, while survival for any reason was 78.6%.

The findings suggest that the Endo-model rotating hinge prosthesis can achieve satisfactory long-term results in elderly patients with significant comorbidities' undergoing revision TKA for aseptic loosening. While knee function was generally good to satisfactory among surviving patients, global function scores were lower due to age-related comorbidities. Radiographic evaluations showed no signs of impending revisions. The study highlights the potential benefits of using rotating hinge devices in complex cases but also underscores the need for further research comparing these devices with unconstrained designs in revision TKA settings. Future studies could provide more definitive evidence on optimal prosthetic choices for specific patient populations in revision knee arthroplasty.

9.1.2.4 Total Knee Arthroplasty with Rotating-Hinge Endo-Model Prosthesis: Clinical Results in Complex Primary and Revision Surgery [132]

This is a machine-generated summary of:

Sanguineti, F.; Mangano, T.; Formica, M.; Franchin, F. Total knee arthroplasty with rotating-hinge Endo-Model prosthesis: clinical results in complex primary and revision surgery [132].

Published in: Archives of Orthopaedic and Trauma Surgery (2014).
Link to original: https://doi.org/10.1007/s00402-014-2061-1

If you want to cite the papers, please refer to the original.

For technical reasons we could not place the page where the original quote is coming from.

Research Highlights

Total knee arthroplasty (TKA) is a common procedure for patients with severe knee damage, where the choice of implant constraint is crucial for successful outcomes. In cases of significant bone and ligament damage, high-constrained devices like rotating-hinge designs are often used to restore joint stability. These implants offer rotational freedom and stability, reducing patellofemoral instability and stress at the prosthesis interface. However, concerns about mechanical failure and infection persist, with outcomes varying widely. The study by Sanguineti et al. evaluates the clinical, functional, and radiographic outcomes of the Endo-Model® rotating-hinge prosthesis (Waldemar Link, Barkhausenweg, Hamburg, Germany) in complex primary and revision knee surgeries.

The study retrospectively analyzed patients who received the Endo-Model prosthesis at their institution. The researchers performed total knee arthroplasties using a standardized surgical approach with cemented long-stemmed implants. Antibiotic-loaded cement was used in revision surgeries to mitigate infection risks. Post-operative care included continuous passive motion therapy and a structured rehabilitation program. The study evaluated 100 knees using clinical assessments like the Knee Society score and radiographic analysis for signs of implant loosening or malalignment. Statistical analyses were conducted to compare outcomes between primary and revision surgeries.

The findings suggest that the Endo-Model prosthesis provides satisfactory clinical outcomes with a high survival rate over an average follow-up of 60 months. Despite some limitations due to its non-modular design, the implant demonstrated good adaptability to various anatomical conditions without significant complications like loosening or instability. While pain was reported in some patients, it did not significantly impact daily activities. Future studies could focus on implant-specific revisions and further refine surgical techniques to enhance outcomes. The Endo-Model device remains a viable option for complex knee surgeries, offering stability and functionality in challenging cases.

9.1.2.5 Implant Survivorship, Functional Outcomes and Complications with the Use of Rotating Hinge Knee Implants: A Systematic Review [133]

This is a machine-generated summary of:

Xu, Joshua; von Fritsch, Lennart; Sabah, Shiraz A.; Price, Andrew J.; Alvand, Abtin Implant survivorship, functional outcomes and complications with the use of rotating hinge knee implants: a systematic review [133].

Published in: Knee Surgery & Related Research (2022).

Link to original: https://doi.org/10.1186/s43019-022-00138-2

Research Highlights

Total knee arthroplasty (TKA) is a widely used surgical procedure for managing knee osteoarthritis, with increasing demand among younger, more active patients and those with complex conditions. The need for more constrained knee replacements has grown, particularly in complex primary and revision TKA cases, to ensure optimal reconstruction. However, selecting the appropriate implant involves balancing the need for stability with minimizing stress at the bone-cement-implant interface to prevent aseptic loosening. The study by Xu et al. systematically reviews the evidence on patient-relevant outcomes following modern rotating-hinge TKA, focusing on implant survivorship, joint function, health-related quality of life, and complications.

The study followed the Preferred Reporting Items for Systematic Reviews and Meta-Analyses guidelines and conducted comprehensive electronic database searches. Eligible studies included patients undergoing primary or revision TKA with rotating hinge implants, reporting post-operative knee function. The review excluded studies with mixed cohorts or non-English publications. Data extraction involved two independent reviewers who resolved discrepancies through discussion. The primary outcome was implant survivorship at various time points, while secondary outcomes included knee range of motion and surgical complications. Due to clinical diversity and incomplete reporting in the included studies, a systematic review without meta-analysis was performed to present medians and ranges for each outcome measure.

The systematic review highlights several areas for improvement in future research on hinged knee replacements. The quality of evidence was generally poor due to heterogeneity in study design and reporting practices. Future studies should aim to provide Kaplan-Meier survivorship estimates with uncertainty measures and use patient-completed instruments like the Oxford Knee Score to assess joint function from the patient's perspective. Additionally, consensus on categorizing indications for surgery could enhance consistency across studies. Despite these limitations, the review offers valuable insights into shared decision-making with patients considering hinged knee arthroplasty, emphasizing the need for further research to refine surgical approaches and improve patient outcomes.

9.1.2.6 Failure Rate of a Rotating Hinge Knee Design Due to Yoke Fracture of the Hinged Tibial Insert: A Retrospective Data Analysis and Review of the Literature [134]

This is a machine-generated summary of:

Friesenbichler, Joerg; Schwarzkopf, Ran; Sadoghi, Patrick; Marwin, Scott E.; Glehr, Mathias; Maurer-Ertl, Werner; Leithner, Andreas Failure rate of a rotating hinge knee design due to yoke fracture of the hinged tibial insert: a retrospective data analysis and review of the literature [134].

Published in: International Orthopaedics (2011).

Link to original: https://doi.org/10.1007/s00264-011-1462-9

If you want to cite the papers, please refer to the original.

For technical reasons we could not place the page where the original quote is coming from.

Research Highlights

The third generation of hinged knee prostheses, featuring a rotating hinge articulation with a metal-on-polyethylene bearing surface, has been developed to address the failure modes of earlier designs. These prostheses allow motion in three planes and are designed to distribute weight-bearing forces through the femoral condyles, producing good short- and mid-term results. However, dislocation of rotating hinge knee prostheses remains a rare but serious complication, often associated with mechanical failures such as yoke fractures. The study by riesenbichler et al. investigates yoke fractures in the Limb Preservation System™ (LPS™) hinged tibial insert (DePuy—Syntheses, Warsaw, In,USA) aiming to identify this mechanical complication and describe patient management.

The study was a retrospective analysis of patients who underwent total knee arthroplasties using the LPS™ knee system at two centers. The cohort included patients treated for tumor indications and revision surgeries. The researchers focused on identifying occurrences of yoke fractures and managing these events. Out of the group, four yoke fractures were observed in four patients within months post-surgery. The study utilized Kaplan-Meier curves to calculate implant survival rates for specific mechanical failures and other revision causes. The findings revealed that yoke fractures occurred at the transition zone from the conical to cylindrical part of the insert, possibly due to high axial loads during flexion combined with distraction and anterior load.

The study highlights that despite modifications by the manufacturer to address these issues, such as changing the production method from casting to forging and altering internal geometry, users should remain vigilant about potential mechanical failures. Future study could focus on further improving implant design to prevent reoccurrence of yoke fractures.

9.1.2.7 Increased Constraint of Rotating Hinge Knee Prosthesis Is Associated with poorer Clinical Outcomes as Compared to Constrained Condylar Knee Prosthesis in Total Knee Arthroplasty [135]

This is a machine-generated summary of:

Lim, Jason Beng Teck; Pang, Hee Nee; Tay, Keng Jin Darren; Chia, Shi-lu; Lo, Ngai Nung; Yeo, Seng Jin Increased constraint of rotating hinge knee prosthesis is associated with poorer clinical outcomes as compared to constrained condylar knee prosthesis in total knee arthroplasty [135].

Published in: European Journal of Orthopaedic Surgery & Traumatology (2019).

Link to original: https://doi.org/10.1007/s00590-019-02598-x

If you want to cite the papers, please refer to the original.

For technical reasons we could not place the page where the original quote is coming from.

Research Highlights

Total knee arthroplasty (TKA) stability relies on the prosthesis, bone, and soft tissue structures to resist deforming forces across the knee joint. Condylar constrained knee (CCK) and rotating hinge knee (RHK) prostheses are used to address varying degrees of ligamentous laxity and bone loss. While CCK prostheses are semi-constrained and used for intermediate instability, RHK prostheses are fully constrained and employed in cases of global instability. There is limited research comparing the outcomes of these two types of implants. The study by Lim et al. evaluates the indications, post-operative patient-reported outcomes, and complications associated with CCK and RHK prostheses.

The study retrospectively reviewed data from a tertiary hospital arthroplasty registry, identifying patients who underwent CCK and RHK TKA with a minimum follow-up of several years. Thirty-nine patients with RHK prostheses were matched with a control group of CCK patients based on demographics and pre-operative clinical scores. All surgeries were performed by fellowship-trained arthroplasty surgeons using standardized post-operative pathways. Patient-reported outcome measures (PROMs) such as the Knee Society Score (KSS), Oxford Knee Score (OKS), and Short Form-36 (SF-36) were evaluated at 6 months and 2 years post-operatively. Statistical analyses revealed that while both groups had similar pre-operative scores, CCK patients reported better functional outcomes at midterm follow-up.

The study found that at 2-year follow-up, patients with CCK prostheses had significantly better clinical outcomes compared to those with RHK prostheses in terms of KSS functional scores and SF-36 physical functioning subdomains. Although both groups experienced complications, the RHK group had higher rates of issues such as deep infection requiring revision surgery. The authors suggest that future studies should explore the biomechanical relationship between component constraint, knee kinematics, and clinical outcomes to better understand these differences. The findings highlight the need for careful consideration when selecting implant types for complex knee conditions.

9.1.2.8 Revision Knee Arthroplasty with Rotating Hinge Systems in Patients with Gross Ligament Instability [136]

This is a machine-generated summary of:

Boelch, Sebastian P.; Arnholdt, Joerg; Holzapfel, Boris M.; Jakuscheit, Axel; Rudert, Maximilian; Hoberg, Maik Revision knee arthroplasty with rotating hinge systems in patients with gross ligament instability [136].

Published in: International Orthopaedics (2018).

Link to original: https://doi.org/10.1007/s00264-018-3982-z

Research Highlights

Primary total knee arthroplasty (TKA) is a widely used treatment for end-stage osteoarthritis, with patient satisfaction and implant survivorship improving over recent decades. However, as the population ages and the number of TKAs increases, the absolute number of TKA revisions is also rising, with instability being a major cause. Addressing this issue, hinged knee prostheses have been developed to manage instability after TKA, but fixed hinged designs have shown high failure rates due to increased rotational forces. The study by Boelch et al. compares two rotating hinge knee (RHK) designs—the Link Endo-Model SL™™(WaldemarLink, Barkhausenweg,Hamburg, Germany) and the EnduRo RHK (Aesculap, Center Valley, PA, USA) in a randomized prospective study to evaluate their effectiveness in revision TKA for instability.

The study included patients undergoing TKA revision for gross ligament insufficiency, excluding those with other indications such as infection or implant failure. Patients were randomized into two groups to receive either the EnduRo or Endo-Model RHK. Surgical procedures involved standard medial arthrotomy and cemented stem extensions where necessary. Postoperative care included partial weight-bearing mobilization and unrestricted range of motion. Clinical scores, patient function, and radiographic evaluations were conducted preoperatively and at several postoperative intervals up to 1 year. Statistical analyses revealed no significant differences in patient demographics or surgical outcomes between the two groups. Both RHK designs showed significant improvements in function and patient-reported outcomes, with no intraoperative complications or postoperative implant failures reported.

The study concludes that both RHK designs are reliable options for TKA revision due to instability, providing good clinical results in terms of knee function and pain reduction. However, despite improvements in overall status, revision remains a salvage procedure with potential for persistent impairment in daily activities and unsatisfactory physical health perception. The authors note that infection remains a significant threat post-revision. Future studies should focus on mid- and long-term outcomes to better understand the clinical relevance of observed radiolucency lines and further explore differences between RHK designs in larger patient cohorts.

9.1.3 *Mega Prosthesis*

9.1.3.1 Comparison of Continuous Epidural Analgesia and Intravenous Patient-Controlled Analgesia with Opioids in Terms of Postoperative Pain and Their Complications in Mega-Prosthesis Total Knee Arthroplasty for Bone Cancers [137]

This is a machine-generated summary of:

Solanki, Sohan Lal; Katwale, Bhushan; Jain, Anuja A.; Chatterjee, Aparna; Gehdoo, Raghuveersingh P. Comparison of Continuous Epidural Analgesia and Intravenous Patient-Controlled Analgesia with Opioids in Terms of Postoperative Pain and Their Complications in Mega-Prosthesis Total Knee Arthroplasty for Bone Cancers [137].

Published in: Indian Journal of Surgical Oncology (2019).

Link to original: https://doi.org/10.1007/s13193-019-00940-7

If you want to cite the papers, please refer to the original.

For technical reasons we could not place the page where the original quote is coming from.

Research Highlights

Patients undergoing bone cancer surgeries, such as total knee arthroplasty (TKA), often experience significant postoperative pain and are at risk for nerve complications, including peroneal nerve palsy. This condition can lead to motor weakness and sensory impairments, complicating recovery. Effective pain management is crucial to mitigate these issues. However, the choice between epidural analgesia (EA) and intravenous patient-controlled analgesia (IV PCA) remains debated due to potential complications associated with each method. The study by Solanki et al. investigates the incidence of motor weakness in patients receiving EA compared to those using IV PCA for postoperative pain relief in TKA with megaprosthesis.

The study conducted a retrospective analysis of data from patients who underwent TKA at their institute, comparing outcomes between those who received EA and those who used IV PCA. Patients were divided into two groups based on their analgesia method, and data were collected on demographics, comorbidities, pain scores, motor weakness, and sedation levels. The primary outcome was the incidence of motor weakness, while secondary outcomes included pain and sedation scores. The analysis revealed that none of the patients in the IV PCA group experienced motor weakness, whereas some patients in the EA group did. The study also examined the concentration of bupivacaine used in EA and its correlation with motor weakness, finding that higher concentrations were associated with increased motor block but not statistically significant.

The findings suggest that while EA can lead to neurological complications like motor weakness, these can be managed by an attentive acute pain service team using lower concentrations of local anesthetics. The study highlights the importance of careful monitoring and individualized analgesia plans to optimize patient outcomes post-TKA. Future study could focus on larger sample sizes and explore alternative analgesic strategies to further reduce the risk of neurological deficits while ensuring effective pain management.

Bibliography

1. Bellemans J, Vandenneucker H, Vanlauwe J, Victor J (2010) The influence of coronal plane deformity on mediolateral ligament status: an observational study in varus knees. Knee Surg Sports Traumatol Arthrosc 18(2):152–156.
2. Benjamin J (2006) Component alignment in total knee arthroplasty. Instr Course Lect 55:405–412.
3. Bellemans J, Colyn W, Vandenneucker H, Victor J (2012) The Chitranjan Ranawat award: is neutral mechanical alignment normal for all patients? The concept of constitutional varus. Clin Orthop Relat Res 470(1):45–53.
4. Fang DM, Ritter MA, Davis KE (2009) Coronal alignment in total knee arthroplasty: just how important is it? J Arthroplasty 24(6 Suppl):39–43.
5. Feng XB, Yang C, Fu DH, Ye SN, Liu XZ, Chen Z, Rai S, Yang SH (2016) Mid-term outcomes of primary constrained condylar knee arthroplasty for severe knee deformity. J Huazhong Univ Sci Technolog Med Sci 36:231–236. https://doi.org/10.1007/s11596-016-1572-0
6. Mancino F, De Martino I, Burrofato A, De Ieso C, Saccomanno MF, Maccauro G, De Santis V (2020) Satisfactory mid-term outcomes of condylar-constrained knee implants in primary total knee arthroplasty: clinical and radiological follow-up. J Orthop Traumatol 21:22. https://doi.org/10.1186/s10195-020-00561-9
7. Sculco TP. The role of constraint in total knee arthoplasty. J Arthroplast. 2006;21(4 Suppl 1):54–6.
8. Insall JN, Ranawat CS, Aglietti P, Shine J. A comparison of four models of total knee-replacement prostheses. J Bone Joint Surg Am. 1976;58(6):754–65.
9. Donaldson WF 3rd, Sculco TP, Insall JN, Ranawat CS. Total condylar III knee prosthesis. Long-term follow-up study. Clin Orthop Relat Res. 1988;226:21–8.
10. Easley ME, Insall JN, Scuderi GR, Bullek DD. Primary constrained condylar knee arthroplasty for the arthritic valgus knee. Clin Orthop Relat Res. 2000;380:58–64.
11. Anderson JA, Baldini A, MacDonald JH, Pellicci PM, Sculco TP. Primary constrained condylar knee arthroplasty without stem extensions for the valgus knee. Clin Orthop Relat Res. 2006;442:199–203.
12. Cholewinski P, Putman S, Vasseur L et al. (2015) Long-term outcomes of primary constrained condylar knee arthroplasty. Orthop Traumatol Surg Res 101(4):449–454.

13. Hartford JM, Goodman SB, Schurman DJ, Knoblick G. Complex primary and revision total knee arthroplasty using the condylar constrained prosthesis: an average 5-year follow-up. J Arthroplast. 1998;13(4):380–7.
14. Lachiewicz PF, Soileau ES (2011) Results of a second-generation constrained condylar prosthesis in primary total knee arthroplasty. J Arthroplasty 26(8):1228–1231.
15. Weiss NG, Parvizi J, Hanssen AD, Trousdale RT, Lewallen DG. Total knee arthroplasty in post-traumatic arthrosis of the knee. J Arthroplast. 2003;18(3 Suppl 1):23–6.
16. Bala A, Penrose CT, Seyler TM, Mather RC 3rd, Wellman SS, Bolognesi MP. Outcomes after total knee arthroplasty for post-traumatic arthritis. Knee. 2015;22(6):630–9.
17. Weiss NG, Parvizi J, Trousdale RT, Bryce RD, Lewallen DG. Total knee arthroplasty in patients with a prior fracture of the tibial plateau. J Bone Joint Surg Am. 2003;85-A(2):218–21.
18. Lunebourg A, Parratte S, Gay A, Ollivier M, Garcia-Parra K, Argenson JN. Lower function, quality of life, and survival rate after total knee arthroplasty for posttraumatic arthritis than for primary arthritis. Acta Orthop. 2015;86(2):189–94.
19. Parratte S, Boyer P, Piriou P, Argenson JN, Deschamps G, Massin P, Sfhg. Total knee replacement following intra-articular malunion. Orthop Traumatol Surg Res. 2011;97(6 Suppl):S118–23.
20. Ye CY, Xue DT, Jiang S, He RX (2016) Results of a second-generation constrained condylar prosthesis in complex primary and revision total knee arthroplasty: A mean 5.5-year follow-up. Chin Med J (Engl) 129(11):1334–1339.
21. Peters CL, Mohr RA, Bachus KN. Primary total knee arthroplasty in the valgus knee: Creating a balanced soft tissue envelope. J Arthroplasty. 2001;16(6):721–9. https://doi.org/10.1054/arth.2001.25504.
22. Ranawat AS, Ranawat CS, Elkus M, Rasquinha VJ, Rossi R, Babhulkar S. Total knee arthroplasty for severe valgus deformity. J Bone Joint Surg Am. 2005;87(1_suppl_2):271–84. https://doi.org/10.2106/JBJS.E.00308.
23. Lachiewicz PF, Soileau ES (2006) Ten-year survival and clinical results of constrained components in primary total knee arthroplasty. J Arthroplasty 21:803–808. https://doi.org/10.1016/j.arth.2005.09.008
24. Insall JN. Surgical techniques and instrumentation in total knee arthroplasty. In: Insall JN, editor. Surgery of the knee. 2nd ed. New York: Churchill Livingstone; 1993. p. 781–7.
25. Whiteside LA. Selective ligament release in total knee arthroplasty of the knee in valgus. Clin Orthop Relat Res. 1999;367:130–40. https://doi.org/10.1097/00003086-199910000-00016.
26. Clayton ML, Thompson TR, Mack RP. Correction of alignment deformities during total knee arthroplasties: staged soft-tissue releases. Clin Orthop Relat Res. 1986;202:117–24.

27. Favorito PJ, Mihalko WM, Krackow KA. Total knee arthroplasty in the valgus knee. J Am Acad Orthop Surg. 2002;10(1):16–24.
28. Mansour E, Whiteside LA. Ligament balancing in the valgus knee. Semin Arthroplast. 2018;29(1):27–35. https://doi.org/10.1053/j.sart.2018.04.004.
29. Luque R, Rizo B, Urda A, Garcia-Crespo R, Moro E, López-Durán L. Primary modular total knee replacement in severe and unstable osteoarthritis. Predictive factors for failure. Int Orthop. 2015;39(11):2125–33. https://doi.org/10.1007/s00264-015-2807-6.
30. Avino RJ, King CA, Landy DC, Martell JM (2020) Varus-valgus constraint in primary total knee arthroplasty: a short-term solution but will it last? J Arthroplasty 35(3):741–746.e2. https://doi.org/10.1016/j.arth.2019.09.048
31. Li F, Liu N, Li Z, Wood KB, Tian H (2019) Abnormally high dislocation rate following constrained condylar knee arthroplasty for valgus knee: A case-control study. J Orthop Surg Res 14(1):268. https://doi.org/10.1186/s13018-019-1325-4
32. Sabatini L, Risitano S, Rissolio L, Bonani A, Atzori F, Massè A (2017) Condylar constrained system in primary total knee replacement: our experience and literature review. Ann Transl Med 5(6):135.
33. Callaghan JJ, O'Rourke MR, Liu SS (2005) The role of implant constraint in revision total knee arthroplasty: not too little, not too much. J Arthroplasty 20(4):41–43. https://doi.org/10.1016/j.arth.2005.03.008
34. Maynard LM, Sauber TJ, Kostopoulos VK, Lavigne GS, Sewecke JJ, Sotereanos NG. Survival of primary condylar-constrained total knee arthroplasty at a minimum of 7 years. J Arthroplast. 2014;29(6):1197–201.
35. Garrido-Gomez J, Arrabal-Polo MA, Giron-Prieto MS, Cabello-Salas J, Torres-Barroso J, Parra-Ruiz J. Descriptive analysis of the economic costs of periprosthetic joint infection of the knee for the public health system of Andalusia. J Arthroplasty. 2013;28:1057–60.
36. Kurtz SM, Ong KL, Schmier J, Mowat F, Saleh K, Dybvik E, et al. Future clinical and economic impact of revision total hip and knee arthroplasty. J Bone Joint Surg Am. 2007;89 Suppl 3:144–51.
37. Insall JN, Dorr LD, Scott RD, Scott WN. Rationale of the Knee Society clinical rating system. Clin Orthop Relat Res. 1989;248:13–4.
38. Hossain F, Patel S, Haddad FS (2010) Midterm assessment of causes and results of revision total knee arthroplasty. Clin Orthop Relat Res 468(5):1221–1228. https://doi.org/10.1007/s11999-009-1204-0
39. Kim YH, Kim JS. Revision total knee arthroplasty with use of a constrained condylar knee prosthesis. J Bone Joint Surg Am. 2009;91:1440–7.
40. Jacobs MA, Hungerford DS, Krackow KA, Lennox DW. Revision total knee arthroplasty for aseptic failure. Clin Orthop Relat Res. 1988;226:78–85.
41. Insall JN, Dethmers DA. Revision of total knee arthroplasty. Clin Orthop Relat Res. 1982;170:123–30.
42. Rosenberg AG, Verner JJ, Galante JO. Clinical results of total knee revision using the Total Condylar III prosthesis. Clin Orthop Relat Res. 1991;273:83–90.

43. Mow CS, Wiedel JD. Revision total knee arthroplasty using the porous-coated anatomic revision prosthesis: six- to twelve-year results. J Arthroplasty. 1998;13:681–6.
44. Takahashi Y, Gustilo RB. Nonconstrained implants in revision total knee arthroplasty. Clin Orthop Relat Res. 1994;309:156–62.
45. Morgan H, Battista V, Leopold SS. Constraint in primary total knee arthroplasty. J Am Acad Orthop Surg. 2005;13(8):515–24.
46. Matsuda S, Kawahara S, Okazaki K, Tashiro Y, Iwamoto Y. Postoperative alignment and ROM affect patient satisfaction after TKA. Clin Orthop Relat Res. 2013;471(1):127–33.
47. Ranawat AS, Ranawat CS, Elkus M, Rasquinha VJ, Rossi R, Babhulkar S. Total knee arthroplasty for severe valgus deformity. J Bone Joint Surg Am. 2005;87 Suppl 1(Pt 2):271–84.
48. Ritter MA, Faris GW, Faris PM, Davis KE. Total knee arthroplasty in patients with angular varus or valgus deformities of > or = 20 degrees. J Arthroplast. 2004;19(7):862–6.
49. Girard J, Amzallag M, Pasquier G, Mulliez A, Brosset T, Gougeon F, Duhamel A, Migaud H. Total knee arthroplasty in valgus knees: predictive preoperative parameters influencing a constrained design selection. Orthop Traumatol Surg Res. 2009;95(4):260–6.
50. Luring C, Oczipka F, Grifka J, Perlick L. The computer-assisted sequential lateral soft-tissue release in total knee arthroplasty for valgus knees. Int Orthop. 2008;32(2):229–35.
51. Sasanuma H, Sekiya H, Takatoku K, Takada H, Sugimoto N. Evaluation of soft-tissue balance during total knee arthroplasty. J Orthop Surg (Hong Kong). 2010;18(1):26–30.
52. Sappey-Marinier E, Fratini S, Kremer H, Shatrov J, Batailler C, Servien E, Lustig S (2022) Similar outcomes to primary total knee arthroplasty achievable for aseptic revision using the same primary posterior-stabilised prosthesis at a mean follow-up of 49 months. Knee Surg Sports Traumatol Arthrosc 30:2854–2861. https://doi.org/10.1007/s00167-021-06716-3
53. Digennaro V, Brunello M, Di Martino A, Panciera A, Bordini B, Bulzacki Bogucki BD, Ferri R, Cecchin D, Faldini C (2023) Constraint degree in revision total knee replacement: a registry study on 1432 patients. Musculoskelet Surg. https://doi.org/10.1007/s12306-023-00790-1
54. Mei F, Li JJ, Lin J, Zhou D, Xing D (2023) Constrained condylar prostheses for the treatment of charcot arthropathy: a case report and literature review. Orthop Surg 15:1423–1430. https://doi.org/10.1111/os.13686
55. Limberg AK, Tibbo ME, Pagnano MW, Perry KI, Hanssen AD, Abdel MP (2020) Varus-valgus constraint in 416 revision total knee arthroplasties with cemented stems provides a reliable reconstruction with a low subsequent revision rate at early to mid-term review. Bone Joint J 102:458–462. https://doi.org/10.1302/0301-620x.102b4.Bjj-2019-0719.R2
56. Wilke BK, Wagner ER, Trousdale RT. Long-term survival of semi-constrained total knee arthroplasty for revision surgery. J Arthroplasty. 2014;29(5):1005–8.

57. Rand JA, Bryan RS (1988) Results of revision total knee arthroplasties using condylar prostheses. A review of fifty knees. J Bone Joint Surg Am 70:738–745.
58. Laudren A, Delacroix R, Huten D (2023) Is hybrid fixation in revision TKA using LCCK prostheses reliable? Orthop Traumatol Surg Res 109:747–753. https://doi.org/10.1016/j.otsr.2023.103583
59. Plancher KD, Briggs KK, Chinnakkannu K, Dotterweich KA, Commaroto SA, Wang KH, Petterson SC. Isolated lateral Tibiofemoral Compartment Osteoarthritis: Survivorship and Patient Acceptable Symptom State after lateral fixed-bearing unicompartmental knee arthroplasty at Mean 10-Year follow-up. J Bone Joint Surg Am. 2022;104(18):1621–8.
60. Jansen K, Beckert M, Deckard ER, Ziemba-Davis M, Meneghini RM. Satisfaction and functional outcomes in Unicompartmental Compared with total knee arthroplasty: Radiographically Matched Cohort Analysis. JB JS Open Access. 2020;5(3):e2000051.
61. Fabre-Aubrespy M, Ollivier M, Pesenti S, Parratte S, Argenson JN. Unicompartmental Knee Arthroplasty in patients older Than 75 results in Better Clinical outcomes and similar survivorship compared to total knee arthroplasty. A matched controlled study. J Arthroplasty. 2016;31 (12):2668–71.
62. Edmiston TA, Manista GC, Courtney PM, Sporer SM, Della Valle CJ, Levine BR. Clinical outcomes and survivorship of lateral unicompartmental knee arthroplasty: does Surgical Approach Matter? J Arthroplasty. 2018;33(2):362–5.
63. Hussain SM, Neilly DW, Baliga S, Patil S, Meek R. Knee osteoarthritis: a review of management options. Scott Med J. 2016;61(1):7–16.
64. Böhler C, Kolbitsch P, Schuh R, Lass R, Kubista B, Giurea A. Midterm results of a new rotating hinge knee implant: a 5-year follow-up. Biomed Res Int. 2017;2017:7532745 [cited 2018 Jun 8]. Available from: http://www.ncbi.nlm.nih.gov/pubmed/29376075.
65. Helito CP, Giglio PN, Cavalheiro CM, Gobbi RG, Demange MK, Camanho GL. Knee arthroplasty with rotating-hinge implant: an option for complex primary cases and revisions. Rev. Bras Ortop (English Ed). 2018;53(2):151–7. Available from:. https://doi.org/10.1016/j.rboe.2017.01.010.
66. Röhner E, Benad K, Zippelius T, Kloss N, Jacob B, Kirschberg J, et al. Good clinical and radiological results of total knee arthroplasty using varus valgus constrained or rotating hinge implants in ligamentous laxity. Knee Surg Sport Traumatol Arthrosc. 2019;27(5):1665–70. Available from:. https://doi.org/10.1007/s00167-018-5307-6.
67. Lotke PA, Carolan GF, Puri N (2006) Impaction grafting for bone defects in revision total knee arthroplasty. Clin Orthop Relat Res 446:99–103.
68. Lachiewicz PF, Watters TS (2014) Porous metal metaphyseal cones for severe bone loss: when only metal will do. Bone Joint J 96-B(11 Supple A):118–121.
69. Pasquier G, Ehlinger M, Mainard D (2019) The role of rotating hinge implants in revision total knee arthroplasty. EFORT Open Rev. 4(6):269–278.

70. Klasan A, Magill P, Frampton C, Zhu M, Young SW (2020) Factors predicting repeat revision and outcome after aseptic revision total knee arthroplasty: results from the New Zealand Joint Registry. Knee Surg Sports Traumatol Arthrosc. https://doi.org/10.1007/s00167-020-05985-8 (Online ahead of print).
71. Lachiewicz PF, Bolognesi MP, Henderson RA, Soileau ES, Vail TP (2012) Can tantalum cones provide fixation in complex revision knee arthroplasty? Clin Orthop Relat Res 470(1):199–204.
72. Schiffner E, Latz D, Thelen S, Grassmann JP, Karbowski A, Windolf J, Jungbluth P, Schneppendahl J (2019) Aseptic loosening after THA and TKA - do gender, tobacco use and BMI have an impact on implant survival time? J Orthop 16(3):269–272.
73. Springer BD, Hanssen AD, Sim FH, Lewallen DG (2001) The kinematic rotating hinge prosthesis for complex knee arthroplasty. Clin Orthop Relat Res 392:283–291.
74. Bae DK, Song SJ, Yoon KH, Noh JH (2009) Long-term outcome of total knee arthroplasty in charcot joint. J Arthroplast 24(8):1152–1156.
75. Hwang SC, Kong JY, Nam DC, Kim DH, Park HB, Jeong ST, Cho SH (2010) Revision total knee arthroplasty with a cemented posterior stabilized, condylar constrained or fully constrained prosthesis: a minimum 2-year follow-up analysis. Clinics Orthop Surg 2(2):112–120.
76. Joshi N, Navarro-Quilis A. Is there a place for rotating-hinge arthroplasty in knee revision surgery for aseptic loosening? J Arthroplasty. 2008;23(8):1204–11. Available from: http://www.sciencedirect.com/science/article/pii/S0883540307006110. https://doi.org/10.1016/j.arth.2007.10.016.
77. Insall JN, Ranawat CS, Aglietti P, Shine J (1976) A comparison of four models of total knee-replacement prostheses. J Bone Joint Surg Am 58(6):754–765.
78. Insall JN, Dorr LD, Scott RD, Scott WN (1989) Rationale of the knee society clinical rating system. Clin Orthop Relat Res 248:13–14.
79. Barrack RL, Lyons TR, Ingraham RQ, Johnson JC (2000) The use of a modular rotating hinge component in salvage revision total knee arthroplasty. J Arthroplast 15(7):858–866.
80. Pradhan NR, Bale L, Kay P, Porter ML (2004) Salvage revision total knee replacement using the endo-model rotating hinge prosthesis. Knee 11(6):469–473.
81. Petrou G, Petrou H, Tilkeridis C, Stavrakis T, Kapetsis T, Kremmidas N, Gavras M (2004) Medium-term results with a primary cemented rotating-hinge total knee replacement. A 7- to 15-year follow-up. J Bone Joint Surg Br 86(6):813–817.
82. Morgan H, Battista V, Leopold SS (2005) Constraint in primary total knee arthroplasty. J Am Acad Orthop Surg 13:515–524.
83. Barrack RL (2001) Evolution of rotating hinge for complex total knee arthroplasty. Clin Orthop Relat Res 392:292–299.

84. Engelbrecht E, Nieder E, Strickle E, Keller A (1981) Intracondylare Kniegelenksendo-prosthese mit Rotationsmöglichkeit Endo-Modell. Chirurg 52:368–375.
85. Wylde V, Beswick AD, Dennis J, Gooberman-Hill R (2017) Post-operative patient-related risk factors for chronic pain after total knee replacement: a systematic review. BMJ Open 7:e018105.
86. NJR. National Joint Registry for England Wales Northern Ireland and the Isle of Man; 2020.
87. Gehrke T, Kendoff D, Haasper C. The role of hinges in primary total knee replacement. Bone Joint J. 2014;96(11):93–5.
88. Rodriguez-Merchan EC (2019) Total knee arthroplasty using hinge joints: Indications and results. EFORT Open Rev. 4:121–132.
89. Pasquier G, Ehlinger M, Mainard D. The role of rotating hinge implants in revision total knee arthroplasty. EFORT Open Rev. 2019;4(6):269–78. https://doi.org/10.1302/2058-5241.4.180070.
90. Cuckler JM (1995) Revision total knee arthroplasty: how much constraint is necessary? Orthopedics 18(932–3):6.
91. Makaram N, Clement ND, Hoo T, Nutton R, Burnett R (2018) Survival of the low contact stress rotating platform total knee replacement is influenced by age: 1058 implants with a minimum follow-up of 10 years. Knee 25:1283–1291.
92. Campbell M, McKenzie JE, Sowden A et al. (2020) Synthesis without meta-analysis (SWiM) in systematic reviews: reporting guideline. BMJ 368:6890.
93. Bistolfi A, Lustig S, Rosso F, Dalmasso P, Crova M, Massazza G (2013) Results with 98 endo-modell rotating hinge prostheses for primary knee arthroplasty. Orthopedics 36:e746–e752.
94. Lozano LM, Lopez V, Rios J et al. (2012) Better outcomes in severe and morbid obese patients (BMI > 35 kg/m^2) in primary Endo-Model rotating-hinge total knee arthroplasty. Scientific World J 2012:249391.
95. Yang JH, Yoon JR, Oh CH, Kim TS (2012) Primary total knee arthroplasty using rotating-hinge prosthesis in severely affected knees. Knee Surg Sports Traumatol Arthrosc 20(3):517–523.
96. Ward WG, Haight D, Ritchie P, Gordon S, Eckardt JJ (2003) Dislocation of rotating hinge total knee prostheses. A biomechanical analysis. J Bone Joint Surg Am 85-A(3):448–453.
97. Bickels J, Wittig JC, Kollender Y, Henshaw RM, Kellar-Graney KL, Meller I, Malawer MM (2002) Distal femur resection with endoprosthetic reconstruction: a long-term followup study. Clin Orthop Relat Res 400:225–235.
98. Westrich GH, Mollano AV, Sculco TP, Buly RL, Laskins RS, Windsor S (2000) Rotating hinge total knee arthroplasty in severely affected knees. Clin Orthop Relat Res 379:195–208.
99. Kawai A, Healey JH, Boland PJ, Athanasian EA, Jeon DG (1999) A rotating-hinge knee replacement for malignant tumors of the femur and tibia. J Arthroplasty 14(2):187–196.
100. Rand JA, Chao EY, Stauffer RN (1987) Kinematic rotating-hinge total knee arthroplasty. J Bone Joint Surg Am 69(4):489–497.

101. Schwarzkopf R, Chaudhry S, Kummer FJ, Marwin SE (2011) Failure of the tibial insert in a rotating hinge total knee arthroplasty. J Arthroplasty 26(6):977, e5–8
102. David HG, Bishay M, James ET (1998) Problems with the rotaflex: a 10 year review of a rotating hinge prosthesis. J Arthroplast 13(4):402–408
103. Pacha-Vicente D, Malik A, Castellet-Feliu E, Nardi-Vilardaga J (2008) Dislocation of rotating-hinge knee prostheses with antidislocation mechanism. J Arthroplast 23(2):299–303
104. Wang CJ, Wang HE (2000) Early catastrophic failure of rotating hinge total knee prosthesis. J Arthroplast 15(3):387–391
105. Ward WG, Haight D, Ritchie P, Gordon S, Eckardt JJ (2005) Dislocation of rotating hinge knee prostheses. A report of four cases. J Bone Joint Surg Am 87(5):1108–1112
106. Zeegen EN, Aponte-Tinao LA, Hornicek FJ, Gebhardt MC, Mankin HJ (2004) Survivorship analysis of 141 modular metallic endoprostheses at early followup. Clin Orthop Relat Res 420:239–250
107. Malcolm TL, Bederman SS, Schwarzkopf R (2016) Outcomes of varus valgus constrained versus rotating-hinge implants in total knee arthroplasty. Orthopedics 39(1):e140–e148. https://doi.org/10.3928/01477447-20151228-07
108. Vasso M, Beaufils P, Schiavone Panni A (2013) Constraint choice in revision knee arthroplasty. Int Orthop 37:1279–1284. https://doi.org/10.1007/s00264-013-1929-y
109. Shen C, Lichstein PM, Austin MS, Sharkey PF, Parvizi J. Revision knee Arthroplasty for bone loss: choosing the right degree of constraint. J Arthroplasty. 2014;29(1):127–31. Available from: http://www.sciencedirect.com/science/article/pii/S088354031300346X. https://doi.org/10.1016/j.arth.2013.04.042.
110. Bistolfi A, Massazza G, Rosso F, Crova M (2012) Rotating-hinge total knee for revision total knee arthroplasty. Orthopedics 35:e325–e330
111. Guenoun B, Latargez L, Freslon M, Defossez G, Salas N, Gayet LE. Complications following rotating hinge Endo-Modell (Link®) knee arthroplasty. Orthop Traumatol Surg Res. 2009;95(7):529–36 Nov [cited 2018 Jun 20]Available from: http://linkinghub.elsevier.com/retrieve/pii/S1877056809001479.
112. Whittaker JP, Dharmarajan R, Toms AD (2008) The management of bone loss in revision total knee replacement. J Bone Joint Surg (Br) 90(8):981–987. https://doi.org/10.1302/0301-620X.90B8.19948
113. Ochs BG, Schreiner AJ, de Zwart PM, Stockle U, Gonser CE (2016) Computer-assisted navigation is beneficial both in primary and revision surgery with modular rotating-hinge knee arthroplasty. Knee Surg Sports Traumatol Arthrosc 24(1):64–73. https://doi.org/10.1007/s00167-014-3316-7
114. Efe T, Roessler PP, Heyse TJ, Hauk C, Pahrmann C, Getgood A, et al. Mid-term results after implantation of rotating-hinge knee prostheses: primary versus revision. Orthop Rev. (Pavia). 2012;4(4):35 2 [cited 2018

May 5] Available from: http://www.pagepress.org/journals/index.php/or/article/view/or.2012.e35.
115. Soffin EM, YaDeau JT (2016) Enhanced recovery after surgery for primary hip and knee arthroplasty: a review of evidence. Br J Anaesth 117(suppl 3):iii62–iii72
116. Anderson MR, Jeng CL, Witting JC, Rosenblatt MA (2010) Anesthesia for patients undergoing orthopedic oncologic surgeries. J Clin Anesth 22:565–572
117. Guerra ML, Sigh PJ, Taylor NF (2015) Early mobilization of patients who have had a hip or knee replacement reduces length of stay in hospital: a systematic review. Clin Rehab 29:844–854
118. Ahmed A, Baig T (2016) Incidence of lower limb motor weakness in patients receiving postoperative epidural analgesia and factors associated with it: an observational study. Saudi J Anaesth 10:149–153
119. Colyn, William; Neirynck, J.; Vanlommel, E.; Bruckers, L.; Bellemans, J. Primary constrained-condylar-knee designs outperform posterior-stabilized and cruciate-retaining designs in high-grade varus osteoarthritic knees during short-term follow-up: a pilot study. Archives of Orthopaedic and Trauma Surgery (2022). https://doi.org/10.1007/s00402-022-04447-9
120. Alqatub, Ahmed; Hasan, Ghazwan A.; Wahab, Mahmood Shihab; Katran, Mustafa Hayder; Wais, Yasameen Bani; Masaoodi, Abbas F.; Shetty, Gautam M. Primary constrained condylar knee arthroplasty in severe varus deformity: a prospective 5-year functional follow-up study in Iraqi patients. European Journal of Orthopaedic Surgery & Traumatology (2023). https://doi.org/10.1007/s00590-022-03470-1
121. Rai, Saroj; Liu, Xianzhe; Feng, Xiaobo; Rai, Bimal; Tamang, Nira; Wang, Jing; Ye, Shunan; Yang, Shuhua Primary total knee arthroplasty using constrained condylar knee design for severe deformity and stiffness of knee secondary to post-traumatic arthritis. Journal of Orthopaedic Surgery and Research (2018). https://doi.org/10.1186/s13018-018-0761-x
122. Li, Feng; Liu, Ning; Li, Zijian; Wood, Kirkham B.; Tian, Hua Abnormally high dislocation rate following constrained condylar knee arthroplasty for valgus knee: a case-control study. Journal of Orthopaedic Surgery and Research (2019). https://doi.org/10.1186/s13018-019-1325-4
123. Mancino, Fabio; De Martino, Ivan; Burrofato, Aaron; De Ieso, Carmine; Saccomanno, Maristella F.; Maccauro, Giulio; De Santis, Vincenzo Satisfactory mid-term outcomes of condylar-constrained knee implants in primary total knee arthroplasty: clinical and radiological follow-up. Journal of Orthopaedics and Traumatology (2020). https://doi.org/10.1186/s10195-020-00561-9
124. Sanz-Ruiz, Pablo; Villanueva-Martínez, Manuel; Matas-Diez, Jose Antonio; Vaquero-Martín, Javier Revision TKA with a condylar constrained prosthesis using metaphyseal and surface cementation: a minimum 6-year follow-up analysis. BMC Musculoskeletal Disorders (2015). https://doi.org/10.1186/s12891-015-0485-6

125. Kawahara, Shinya; Mawatari, Taro; Matsui, Gen; Hamai, Satoshi; Akasaki, Yukio; Tsushima, Hidetoshi; Nakashima, Yasuharu Improved surgical procedure of primary constrained total knee arthroplasty which enables use of the femoral diaphyseal straight extension stem. BMC Musculoskeletal Disorders (2022). https://doi.org/10.1186/s12891-022-05367-w
126. Ren, Jiangdong; Zhang, Xiaogang; Wulamu, Wuhuzi; Yushan, Nuerailijiang; Aaimaiti, Abudousaimi; Cao, Li Total knee arthroplasty with the least-constrained implant possible for type II valgus knee >20°: a 3–14 years' follow-up. Arthroplasty (2020). https://doi.org/10.1186/s42836-020-00036-6
127. Yu, Muyang; Xu, Yiming; Weng, Xisheng; Feng, Bin Clinical outcome and survival rate of condylar constrained knee prosthesis in revision total knee arthroplasty: an average nine point six year follow-up. International Orthopaedics (2024). https://doi.org/10.1007/s00264-024-06096-6
128. Yu, Hui; Meng, Jiahong; Xu, Yibo; Xu, Kai; Lin, Changjian; Bao, Jiapeng Comparison of early curative effects of lateral unicompartmental knee arthroplasty with total knee arthroplasty and the legacy constrained condylar knee arthroplasty in the treatment of isolated lateral osteoarthritis: a single-center retrospective study. Journal of Orthopaedic Surgery and Research (2024). https://doi.org/10.1186/s13018-024-05076-1
129. von Hintze, Jake; Niemeläinen, Mika; Sintonen, Harri; Nieminen, Jyrki; Eskelinen, Antti Outcomes of the rotating hinge knee in revision total knee arthroplasty with a median follow-up of 6.2 years. BMC Musculoskeletal Disorders (2021). https://doi.org/10.1186/s12891-021-04205-9
130. Levent, Ali; Suero, Eduardo M.; Gehrke, Thorsten; Bakhtiari, Iman Godarzi; Citak, Mustafa Risk factors for aseptic loosening in complex revision total knee arthroplasty using rotating hinge implants. International Orthopaedics (2020). https://doi.org/10.1007/s00264-020-04878-2
131. Gudnason, Asgeir; Milbrink, Jan; Hailer, Nils P. Implant survival and outcome after rotating-hinge total knee revision arthroplasty: a minimum 6-year follow-up. Archives of Orthopaedic and Trauma Surgery (2011). https://doi.org/10.1007/s00402-011-1330-5
132. Sanguineti, F.; Mangano, T.; Formica, M.; Franchin, F. Total knee arthroplasty with rotating-hinge Endo-Model prosthesis: clinical results in complex primary and revision surgery. Archives of Orthopaedic and Trauma Surgery (2014). https://doi.org/10.1007/s00402-014-2061-1
133. Xu, Joshua; von Fritsch, Lennart; Sabah, Shiraz A.; Price, Andrew J.; Alvand, Abtin Implant survivorship, functional outcomes and complications with the use of rotating hinge knee implants: a systematic review. Knee Surgery & Related Research (2022). https://doi.org/10.1186/s43019-022-00138-2
134. Friesenbichler, Joerg; Schwarzkopf, Ran; Sadoghi, Patrick; Marwin, Scott E.; Glehr, Mathias; Maurer-Ertl, Werner; Leithner, Andreas Failure rate of a rotating hinge knee design due to yoke fracture of the hinged tibial insert: a retrospective data analysis and review of the literature. International Orthopaedics (2011). https://doi.org/10.1007/s00264-011-1462-9

135. Lim, Jason Beng Teck; Pang, Hee Nee; Tay, Keng Jin Darren; Chia, Shi-lu; Lo, Ngai Nung; Yeo, Seng Jin Increased constraint of rotating hinge knee prosthesis is associated with poorer clinical outcomes as compared to constrained condylar knee prosthesis in total knee arthroplasty. European Journal of Orthopaedic Surgery & Traumatology (2019). https://doi.org/10.1007/s00590-019-02598-x
136. Boelch, Sebastian P.; Arnholdt, Joerg; Holzapfel, Boris M.; Jakuscheit, Axel; Rudert, Maximilian; Hoberg, Maik Revision knee arthroplasty with rotating hinge systems in patients with gross ligament instability. International Orthopaedics (2018). https://doi.org/10.1007/s00264-018-3982-z
137. Solanki, Sohan Lal; Katwale, Bhushan; Jain, Anuja A.; Chatterjee, Aparna; Gehdoo, Raghuveersingh P. Comparison of Continuous Epidural Analgesia and Intravenous Patient-Controlled Analgesia with Opioids in Terms of Postoperative Pain and Their Complications in Mega-Prosthesis Total Knee Arthroplasty for Bone Cancers. Indian Journal of Surgical Oncology (2019). https://doi.org/10.1007/s13193-019-00940-7

9.2 Surgical Techniques

Machine Generated Summaries

Disclaimer: The summaries in this chapter were generated from Springer Nature publications using abstractive AI auto-summarization: An abstraction-based summarizer creates new text based on deep learning. New phrases are created to summarize the content. As the constituted sentences are machine selected, they may not fully reflect the body of the work, so we strongly advise that the original content is read and cited. The auto-generated summaries were curated by the editor to meet Springer Nature publication standards.

9.2.1 Exposure

9.2.1.1 Quad Snip

Comparison of Quadriceps Snip and Tibial Tubercle Osteotomy in Revision for Infected Total Knee Arthroplasty [243]

This is a machine-generated summary of:

Sun, Zhenhui; Patil, Abhishek; Song, Eun-Kyoo; Kim, Hyun-Tae; Seon, Jong-Keun Comparison of quadriceps snip and tibial tubercle osteotomy in revision for infected total knee arthroplasty [243].

Published in: International Orthopaedics (2014).
Link to original: https://doi.org/10.1007/s00264-014-2546-0

If you want to cite the papers, please refer to the original.
For technical reasons we could not place the page where the original quote is coming from.

Research Highlights

Infection following total knee arthroplasty (TKA) is a significant concern, with a notable percentage of revision surgeries attributed to prosthetic knee infections, particularly within the first 5 years post-operation. The choice of surgical approach during revision TKA is crucial, especially in cases complicated by infection, scarring, and joint stiffness. Despite various available methods for surgical exposure, such as the medial parapatellar and quadriceps snip (QS) approaches, there is no consensus on the optimal technique. The study by Sun et al. evaluates the clinical and radiological outcomes of second-stage revision for infected primary TKA using the tibial tubercle osteotomy (TTO) approach compared to the QS approach.

The study involved a retrospective review of patients who underwent second-stage revision TKA for infected primary TKA at their institution. Patients were divided into two groups based on the surgical approach used: QS or TTO. All surgeries were performed by the same senior surgeon following a two-stage revision procedure. The first stage involved implant removal and insertion of an antibiotic-impregnated cement spacer, followed by 6 weeks of intravenous antibiotics. Once infection eradication was confirmed, the second stage was performed using either QS or TTO for surgical exposure. Clinical assessments were conducted preoperatively and at regular intervals postoperatively using standardized scoring systems. Radiographic evaluations were also performed to assess limb alignment and component positioning.

The study found no significant differences in clinical scores, range of motion (ROM), or radiological parameters between the QS and TTO groups at final follow-up. However, patellar tendon partial avulsion was more frequent in the QS group, suggesting that TTO might better protect against this complication. The study highlights that both approaches can achieve satisfactory outcomes in revision TKA for infected cases but emphasizes caution to minimize complications such as patellar tendon avulsion or issues related to tubercle osteotomy. Future studies with longer follow-up periods are recommended to provide more definitive conclusions regarding these surgical techniques' long-term efficacy and safety.

9.2.1.2 Tibial Tubercle Osteotomy

Utility of Tibial Tubercle Osteotomy in the Setting of Periprosthetic Infection After Total Knee Arthroplasty [244]

This is a machine-generated summary of:

Choi, Ho-Rim; Burke, Dennis; Malchau, Henrik; Kwon, Young-Min Utility of tibial tubercle osteotomy in the setting of periprosthetic infection after total knee arthroplasty [244].

Published in: International Orthopaedics (2012).

Link to original: https://doi.org/10.1007/s00264-012-1541-6

If you want to cite the papers, please refer to the original.

For technical reasons we could not place the page where the original quote is coming from.

Research Highlights

Adequate surgical exposure is essential for the successful performance of total knee arthroplasty (TKA), particularly in complex cases such as revision surgeries or those involving severe deformities. Traditional approaches like the medial parapatellar arthrotomy often suffice, but in challenging scenarios, such as infections or poor bone quality, extensile approaches are necessary to prevent complications. Despite the known benefits of tibial tubercle osteotomy (TTO) for improving exposure, there is limited data on its outcomes in infected TKA cases. The study by Choi et al. evaluates the radiographic and functional outcomes of TTO in revision arthroplasty for infected TKA.

The study retrospectively analyzed patients who underwent staged revision procedures with TTO at their institution. The decision to perform TTO was based on the need for adequate surgical exposure without compromising the patellar tendon attachment. The procedure involved a midline skin incision extended below the tibial tubercle, followed by a carefully executed osteotomy to allow access to the knee joint. After implant removal and debridement, antibiotic-loaded cement spacers were used before reattachment of the osteotomy with stainless steel wires. Patients received postoperative antibiotics and were allowed partial weight-bearing. The second stage reimplantation followed a similar protocol, with radiographic evaluations confirming implant position and bony union over time.

The study found that despite occurrences of proximal migration and avulsion fractures of the osteotomy segment, satisfactory radiographic and functional outcomes were achieved. The mean range of motion improved significantly from preoperative levels, and Knee Society scores showed marked enhancement at follow-up. While some patients experienced complications like proximal migration or avulsion fractures, these did not adversely affect long-term functionality. The findings suggest that TTO can be effectively used in revision arthroplasty for infected TKA without impeding bony union or functional recovery. Future studies could explore comparative investigations with different fixation methods to further validate these results.

Anterolateral Approach Using Tibial Tubercle Osteotomy for Total Knee Arthroplasty: Can we Predict Failure? [245]

This is a machine-generated summary of:

Wishart, Marc; Arnold, Markus P.; Huegli, Rolf W.; Amsler, Felix; Friederich, Niklaus F.; Hirschmann, Michael T. Anterolateral approach using tibial tubercle osteotomy for total knee arthroplasty: can we predict failure? [245].

Published in: International Orthopaedics (2012).

Link to original: https://doi.org/10.1007/s00264-012-1693-4

If you want to cite the papers, please refer to the original.

For technical reasons we could not place the page where the original quote is coming from.

Research Highlights

Tibial tubercle osteotomy (TTO) is a valuable surgical technique used in orthopaedics, particularly for revision surgeries, due to its benefits in improving exposure and preserving the medial blood supply to the patella. Despite its advantages, TTO is considered technically demanding and is associated with several complications, such as skin necrosis, haematoma, and insufficient consolidation. Surgeons have identified key factors to mitigate these complications, including the size and depth of the TTO and the type of refixation material used. However, there is a lack of clinical studies investigating these factors as predictors for complications. The study by Wishart et al. examines the predictive factors for complications in patients undergoing primary total knee arthroplasty (TKA) with TTO.

The study involved a retrospective review of patients who underwent primary TKA with an anterolateral approach combined with TTO. The researchers focused on patients who had two fixation screws for consistency in statistical analysis. They collected data on age, sex, comorbidities, and any complications related to TTO from surgical reports and radiological data. Standardized radiographs were used to measure the length and depth of the TTO, the size of the proximal abutment, and the orientation of screws. Statistical analyses were conducted to identify correlations between these variables and complication rates. The study found that shorter TTO lengths (<30 mm), narrower proximal abutments (<10 mm), and certain screw placements significantly correlated with higher complication rates.

The findings suggest that specific surgical techniques can reduce complication rates associated with TTO in primary TKA. The study highlights the importance of maintaining adequate TTO length and proximal abutment width to prevent complications such as proximal displacement of the osteotomized bone. Future studies could explore these predictive factors in larger patient cohorts or different surgical settings to validate these findings further. Additionally, refining surgical techniques based on these insights may enhance patient outcomes in orthopaedic surgeries involving TTO.

Tibial Tubercle Osteotomy with Absorbable Suture Fixation in Revision Total Knee Arthroplasty: A Report of 23 Cases [246]

This is a machine-generated summary of:

Zonnenberg, Christian B. L.; van den Bekerom, Michel P. J.; de Jong, Tjitte; Nolte, Peter A. Tibial tubercle osteotomy with absorbable suture fixation in revision total knee arthroplasty: a report of 23 cases [246].

Published in: Archives of Orthopaedic and Trauma Surgery (2014).

Link to original: https://doi.org/10.1007/s00402-014-1950-7

If you want to cite the papers, please refer to the original.

For technical reasons we could not place the page where the original quote is coming from.

Research Highlights

Total knee arthroplasty (TKA) is a common procedure, but achieving adequate exposure during revision surgeries can be challenging due to factors like peripatellar contracture and capsular inflammation. These issues often result in adhesion formation near the quadriceps mechanism, complicating patellar eversion or lateral translation and potentially leading to patellar tendon avulsion. Various techniques have been developed to improve exposure, such as V-Y quadriceps-plasty and tibial tubercle osteotomy (TTO), each with its own set of complications. The study by Zonnenberg et al. explores the use of absorbable suture fixation for TTO in revision TKA, aiming to provide adequate stability without the need for hardware removal.

The study involved 27 patients who underwent TTO as part of their revision TKA procedure, with three exclusions due to preoperative infections or alternative fixation methods. The surgical approach included a medial parapatellar incision and a medial TTO performed with an osteotome, preserving blood supply by leaving the laterally attached periosteum intact. The tibial tubercle was fixated using absorbable Vicryl® sutures (Ethicon, Raritan, New Jersey, USA) without drill holes, allowing immediate full weight-bearing postoperatively with a knee extension splint for support. Patients were followed up at regular intervals to assess clinical outcomes and radiographic healing, with Knee Society Scores (KSS) and SF-36 scores assigned at the latest follow-up.

The study found that absorbable suture fixation provided satisfactory functional outcomes comparable to other fixation techniques, with no cases of anterior knee pain or patellar tendon avulsion reported. Although some limitations exist, such as the small sample size and lack of a control group, the results suggest that this method is a reliable and cost-effective alternative for enhancing surgical exposure in difficult revision TKA cases. Future studies could focus on multicenter trials to gather more evidence-based data on this technique and compare it with other exposure methods at different levels of the extensor mechanism.

Tibial Tubercle Osteotomy in Septic Revision Total Knee Arthroplasty [247]

This is a machine-generated summary of:

Segur, Josep M.; Vilchez-Cavazos, Felix; Martinez-Pastor, Juan Carlos; Macule, Francisco; Suso, Santiago; Acosta-Olivo, Carlos Tibial tubercle osteotomy in septic revision total knee arthroplasty [247].

Published in: Archives of Orthopaedic and Trauma Surgery (2014).

Link to original: https://doi.org/10.1007/s00402-014-2064-y

If you want to cite the papers, please refer to the original.

For technical reasons we could not place the page where the original quote is coming from.

Research Highlights

The incidence of revision knee arthroplasty due to infection is on the rise, presenting significant challenges for surgeons. Limited knee mobility, quadriceps contracture, or patella baja can complicate surgical approaches, risking damage to the extensor mechanism. Traditional extensile approaches like rectus snip and tibial tubercle osteotomy (TTO) have been employed to improve exposure without harming the extensor mechanism. Previous studies have shown promising results with TTO, particularly in two-stage revisions for infected total knee arthroplasty. The study by Segur et al. explores the efficacy of TTO in patients undergoing the second stage of revision for prosthesis infection, providing insights into functional outcomes and complications.

The study involved a retrospective analysis of patients who underwent TTO during the second stage of revision knee arthroplasty for infection. The average patient age and body mass index were both recorded. All patients received an antibiotic-loaded dynamic cement spacer between stages, with surgery proceeding after C-reactive protein normalization. The surgical technique involved a medial parapatellar arthrotomy and intraoperative decision-making regarding TTO use based on patellar retraction feasibility. Postoperative rehabilitation followed standard protocols for primary total knee arthroplasty, including early mobilization and home rehabilitation support. Functional outcomes were assessed using KSS and WOMAC scales, with follow-ups extending up to several years post-surgery.

The study found that TTO provided effective surgical exposure without compromising the extensor mechanism or postoperative rehabilitation outcomes. Most patients experienced improved knee flexion postoperatively, with minor complications reported in a few cases. The osteotomy healed well in most patients by follow-up visits, aligning with previous findings by Whiteside and Mendes et al. Future study could focus on optimizing osteotomy fixation techniques to further minimize complications and enhance functional recovery in revision knee arthroplasty for infection. This research underscores the importance of careful surgical planning and execution in achieving favorable outcomes in complex revision procedures.

Anterolateral Approach with Tibial Tubercle Osteotomy Versus Standard Medial Approach for Primary Total Knee Arthroplasty: Does it Matter? [248]

This is a machine-generated summary of:

Hirschmann, Michael T; Hoffmann, Mathias; Krause, Robert; Jenabzadeh, Reza-Amir; Arnold, Markus P; Friederich, Niklaus F Anterolateral approach with tibial tubercle osteotomy versus standard medial approach for primary total knee arthroplasty: does it matter? [248].

Published in: BMC Musculoskeletal Disorders (2010).

Link to original: https://doi.org/10.1186/1471-2474-11-167

Research Highlights

Total knee arthroplasty (TKA) is a common surgical procedure for patients with severe osteoarthritis, typically performed using a medial parapatellar approach. However, this approach can lead to complications such as painful scarring and reduced extensor strength. An alternative is the lateral parapatellar subvastus approach with tibial tubercle osteotomy, which preserves the quadriceps muscle and patellar blood supply but is considered technically challenging and potentially riskier. The study by Hirschmann et al. investigates whether the choice of surgical approach affects early clinical and radiological outcomes in ligament balancing primary TKA.

The study was a prospective multicenter trial involving patients undergoing primary, ligament balancing, posterior cruciate-retaining TKA for tri-compartmental osteoarthritis. Patients were divided into two groups based on the surgical approach: medial parapatellar (MPA) or lateral parapatellar subvastus with tibial tubercle osteotomy (TubOT). Experienced surgeons performed the procedures across three centers, with standardized postoperative care and follow-up at 6 and 12 months. Clinical outcomes were assessed using pain scores, range of motion, and functional evaluations like the American Knee Society Score. Radiological assessments included implant positioning and mechanical alignment. Statistical analyses compared outcomes between the two groups.

The study found that patients treated with the lateral TubOT approach experienced better functional outcomes, less pain, and higher satisfaction at 2 years post-surgery compared to those who underwent the MPA approach. However, the TubOT group also had a higher early revision rate due to complications like tibial tubercle migration. Despite these complications, no significant differences in prosthetic alignment or radiolucencies were observed between groups. Future studies should focus on long-term outcomes to determine if the benefits of the TubOT approach outweigh its risks and whether it impacts prosthesis longevity compared to traditional methods.

Lateral Subvastus Approach with Tibial Tubercle Osteotomy for Primary Total Knee Arthroplasty: Clinical Outcome and Complications Compared to Medial Parapatellar Approach [249]

This is a machine-generated summary of:

Langen, Susanne; Gaber, Sonja; Zdravkovic, Vilijam; Giesinger, Karlmeinrad; Jost, Bernhard; Behrend, Henrik Lateral subvastus approach with tibial tubercle osteotomy for primary total knee arthroplasty: clinical outcome and complications compared to medial parapatellar approach [249].

Published in: European Journal of Orthopaedic Surgery & Traumatology (2015).

Link to original: https://doi.org/10.1007/s00590-015-1718-y

If you want to cite the papers, please refer to the original.

For technical reasons we could not place the page where the original quote is coming from.

Research Highlights

Total knee arthroplasty (TKA) is a common surgical procedure with generally positive outcomes and high patient satisfaction. Key factors influencing long-term success include anatomical leg alignment, ligament balancing, and precise prosthetic component positioning. The surgical approach also significantly impacts outcomes, with the medial parapatellar arthrotomy being the most common. However, the lateral subvastus approach (LSVA) with tibial tubercle osteotomy (TTO) is considered advantageous in certain cases, such as valgus deformities or patellar tracking abnormalities. The study by Langen et al. explores the functional outcomes of LSVA with TTO compared to the standard medial parapatellar approach (MPA), focusing on TTO-related complications.

The study was conducted retrospectively using data from a local knee arthroplasty registry, including patients who underwent primary TKA at a hospital over a specified period. Patients were divided into three groups: those who received the standard MPA, those with neutral leg alignment who underwent LSVA with TTO, and those with pronounced valgus alignment who also had LSVA with TTO. All patients received a cemented LCS® complete™ prosthesis (DePuy—Synthes, Warsaw, In. USA). The LSVA involved lateral release and step-cut osteotomy to prevent proximal migration of the tibial tubercle. Rehabilitation protocols were consistent across groups, involving continuous passive motion devices and physiotherapy. Outcomes were assessed using clinical examinations, radiographs, and questionnaires like the Western Ontario and McMaster Universities Osteoarthritis Index (WOMAC) and Knee Society Score (KSS). Statistical analyses revealed no significant differences in clinical outcomes between approaches after 1 year.

The study concludes that LSVA with TTO offers comparable functional outcomes to MPA 1 year postoperatively, supporting its use as an alternative in primary TKA when technical challenges with MPA are anticipated. Despite potential complications associated with TTO, such as intraoperative fractures or wound healing issues, these did not adversely affect patient outcomes in this study. Future study could focus on longer follow-up periods to assess long-term outcomes and further refine surgical techniques to minimize complications. The findings suggest that LSVA should be reserved for cases involving significant valgus deformities or patellar alignment issues, where it can be performed safely with precise surgical technique.

Tibial Tubercle Osteotomy (TTO) in Total Knee Arthroplasty, Is It Worth It? A Review of the Literature [250]

This is a machine-generated summary of:

Divano, Stefano; Camera, Andrea; Biggi, Stefano; Tornago, Stefano; Formica, Matteo; Felli, Lamberto Tibial tubercle osteotomy (TTO) in total knee arthroplasty, is it worth it? A review of the literature [250].

Published in: Archives of Orthopaedic and Trauma Surgery (2018).

Link to original: https://doi.org/10.1007/s00402-018-2888-y

If you want to cite the papers, please refer to the original.
For technical reasons we could not place the page where the original quote is coming from.

Research Highlights

Total knee arthroplasty (TKA) is a common orthopedic procedure known for its effectiveness in alleviating pain and restoring joint function. However, the need for revision TKA is increasing, with projections indicating significant growth in the United States. Revision surgeries often yield less favorable outcomes compared to primary procedures, primarily due to complications such as bone loss and soft tissue issues. The study by Divano et al. explores the efficacy and safety of tibial tuberosity osteotomy (TTO) as a surgical approach in challenging TKA cases, particularly during revision surgeries.

The study conducted a systematic review of existing literature to assess how TTO could enhance clinical outcomes in TKA procedures and evaluate its safety profile. The researchers screened multiple databases, including PubMed and Cochrane Library, focusing on studies with substantial follow-up periods and patient cohorts. They excluded non-pertinent studies such as case reports and meta-analyses. The review process involved independent screening by two reviewers, ensuring comprehensive coverage of relevant articles. The findings revealed that TTO significantly improved clinical parameters like range of motion and functional scores in both primary and revision TKA cases. Notably, TTO was effective regardless of whether patients underwent primary or revision surgery, demonstrating comparable outcomes to other surgical approaches like quadriceps snip.

The study highlights that while TTO is not without complications—such as anterior knee pain or tibial tubercle fractures—it remains a reliable option for enhancing surgical exposure in difficult TKA cases. Future study directions could focus on refining the technique to minimize complications further and exploring its application in specific patient populations with complex knee deformities. The research underscores the importance of careful patient selection and technical precision to optimize outcomes, suggesting that TTO could be particularly beneficial in cases requiring extensive exposure or dealing with severe valgus deformities.

9.2.1.3 V-Y Turndown

V-Y Turndown Flap Augmentation for Acute Quadriceps Rupture After Total Knee Arthroplasty: A Prospective Matched Cohort Study [251]

This is a machine-generated summary of:

Miralles-Muñoz, Francisco A.; Rubio-Morales, Marta; Ruiz-Lozano, Matias; Martinez-Mendez, Daniel; Gonzalez-Parreño, Santiago; Lizaur-Utrilla, Alejandro V-Y turndown flap augmentation for acute quadriceps rupture after total knee arthroplasty: a prospective matched cohort study [251].

Published in: International Orthopaedics (2021).

Link to original: https://doi.org/10.1007/s00264-021-04939-0

If you want to cite the papers, please refer to the original.

For technical reasons we could not place the page where the original quote is coming from.

Research Highlights

Extensor mechanism rupture following total knee arthroplasty (TKA) is a rare but significant complication that severely impacts knee function, particularly when it involves the quadriceps tendon. The prevalence of quadriceps tendon rupture post-TKA is notably low, ranging between 0.1% and 1.1%, and typically necessitates surgical intervention. The study by Miralles-Muñoz et al. y prospectively assesses the outcomes of quadriceps V-Y turndown augmentation for repairing quadriceps tendon ruptures in TKA patients.

The study employed a prospective comparative cohort design involving 23 patients who experienced quadriceps tendon rupture post-TKA. These patients underwent surgical repair using the V-Y turndown technique, which involves creating a partial-thickness triangular flap from the proximal quadriceps tendon to augment the repair. The control group consisted of TKA patients without complications, matched for various factors including age and type of surgery. Over a minimum follow-up period of 3 years, outcomes were assessed using Knee Society Scores (KSS) and the Western Ontario and McMaster Universities Osteoarthritis Index (WOMAC). The results indicated significant improvements in KSS scores post-repair, although these were lower compared to the control group. Importantly, no re-ruptures were observed, and most patients reported satisfactory quality of life.

The study advances our understanding of surgical options for quadriceps tendon ruptures in TKA settings by demonstrating that the V-Y turndown technique is both effective and safe. While functional outcomes were not as high as those in uncomplicated TKA cases, patient satisfaction remained positive. Future study could explore longer-term outcomes and compare this technique with other repair methods to further refine treatment strategies for this challenging complication. The findings underscore the potential benefits of using autogenous tissue for repair augmentation, which may enhance healing through improved blood supply without introducing additional morbidity associated with synthetic materials or allografts.

9.2.2 *Ligament Balancing*

9.2.2.1 Comparison Between Ligament Balancing and Measured Resection in Robot-Assisted Total Knee Arthroplasty: A 2-Year Follow Up Cohort Study [252]

This is a machine-generated summary of:

Yu, Muyang; Yang, Xingdong; Xu, Yiming; Zhu, Wei; Peng, Huiming; Lin, Jin; Weng, Xisheng; Feng, Bin Comparison between ligament balancing and measured resection in robot-assisted total knee arthroplasty: a 2-year follow up cohort study [252].

Published in: BMC Musculoskeletal Disorders (2025).

Link to original: https://doi.org/10.1186/s12891-025-08388-3

If you want to cite the papers, please refer to the original.

For technical reasons we could not place the page where the original quote is coming from.

Research Highlights

Total knee arthroplasty (TKA) is a common surgical procedure aimed at alleviating pain and restoring function in patients with end-stage knee diseases. Key factors influencing the success of TKA include alignment, prosthesis positioning, and soft tissue balance. Image-based robotic systems have been developed to enhance the precision of these factors by predicting virtual joint gaps before bone cuts and measuring actual gaps during surgery. These systems allow for adjustments in prosthesis positioning, potentially leading to more accurate outcomes compared to manual TKA. However, there is ongoing debate regarding the optimal technique for achieving balanced gaps in TKA, with measured resection (MR) and ligament balancing (LB) being the two primary methods. The study by Yu et al. investigates the differences between MR-TKA with mechanical alignment (MA) and LB-TKA with functional alignment (FA) in robot-assisted TKA (RA-TKA).

The study was conducted using prospectively collected data from a single center, involving patients who underwent unilateral primary RA-TKA. The cohort was divided into two groups: one undergoing LB-TKA based on FA and the other MR-TKA based on MA. The procedures were performed by experienced surgeons using the MAKO robotic system (Stryker Orthopaedics, Mahwah, New Jersey, USA). The study compared intraoperative bone cut thickness, soft tissue release, prosthesis position, and clinical and radiological postoperative results between the two techniques. The LB group employed a "Ligament Balancing" workflow that involved assessing ligament tension before bone resection, while the MR group used a "measure and resection" workflow focusing on bone cuts perpendicular to mechanical axes. Outcomes such as bone cut thickness, soft tissue release rates, femoral component rotation, and postoperative inflammatory markers were analyzed.

The study found that RA-TKA guided by LB effectively reduces soft tissue release rates and bone recut requirements compared to MR-TKA. This may help alleviate early postoperative inflammatory reactions and pain. Although no significant differences in knee function were observed between the two groups after years of follow-up, the LB group exhibited lower inflammatory serum markers in the early postoperative stage. The findings suggest that adopting FA principles in LB-TKA allows for adjustments in prosthetic positioning within safe ranges to minimize soft tissue trauma while restoring joint line height and angle.

9.2.2.2 Objective Quantification of Ligament Balancing Using VERASENSE in Measured Resection and Modified Gap Balance Total Knee Arthroplasty [253]

This is a machine-generated summary of:

Cho, Kyu-Jin; Seon, Jong-Keun; Jang, Won-Young; Park, Chun-Gon; Song, Eun-Kyoo Objective quantification of ligament balancing using VERASENSE in measured resection and modified gap balance total knee arthroplasty [253].

Published in: BMC Musculoskeletal Disorders (2018).

Link to original: https://doi.org/10.1186/s12891-018-2190-8

If you want to cite the papers, please refer to the original.

For technical reasons we could not place the page where the original quote is coming from.

Research Highlights

Total knee arthroplasty (TKA) success hinges on precise surgical factors, including bone resection, component alignment, and soft tissue balancing. While technological advancements like navigation systems have improved alignment accuracy, achieving optimal soft tissue balance remains challenging, particularly for less experienced surgeons who rely on subjective judgment. This subjective approach can be influenced by various factors such as the surgeon's experience and the patient's physical characteristics. Despite TKA's generally excellent long-term outcomes, instability due to improper ligament balancing is a significant cause of revision surgeries. The study by Cho e al. introduces the VERASENSE Knee System (Zimmer-Biomet, Warsaw, In., USA), an orthosensor that provides real-time data to objectively quantify ligament balance during TKA.

The study involved patients with varus-deformed osteoarthritic knees undergoing TKA using the VERASENSE system at Chonnam National University Hwasun Hospital, Gwangji, South Korea. The research compared two surgical techniques: measured resection using the ROBODOC® system (Curexo Inc., South Korea) and modified gap balancing. The VERASENSE sensor was used intraoperatively to measure compartment pressures in the knee joint across a range of motion. If initial measurements indicated imbalance, additional soft tissue releases or bony resections were performed to achieve balance. The study recorded compartment pressures at various stages: after initial bone resection, following any additional procedures, and post-final implantation of components. Statistical analyses were conducted to evaluate the effectiveness of these procedures in achieving balanced knee pressure.

The study demonstrated that objective quantification using the VERASENSE system significantly improved soft tissue balance in both TKA techniques. Although both methods showed decreased compartment pressures post-implantation, measured resection TKAs initially exhibited higher pressure differences and required more additional procedures than modified gap balancing TKAs. Future study could explore long-term clinical outcomes of objectively balanced versus traditionally balanced TKAs. The findings suggest that regardless of surgical technique, patient-specific ligament balancing may necessitate additional procedures to ensure optimal outcomes and reduce complications associated with soft tissue imbalance.

9.2.2.3 Individualized Alignment and Ligament Balancing Technique with the ROSA® Robotic System for Total Knee Arthroplasty [254]

This is a machine-generated summary of:

Rossi, Stefano Marco Paolo; Benazzo, Francesco Individualized alignment and ligament balancing technique with the ROSA® robotic system for total knee arthroplasty [254].

Published in: International Orthopaedics (2023).

Link to original: https://doi.org/10.1007/s00264-022-05671-z

If you want to cite the papers, please refer to the original.

For technical reasons we could not place the page where the original quote is coming from.

Research Highlights

In recent years, robotic systems have gained traction in orthopaedics, particularly in total knee arthroplasty (TKA), due to their potential for improved implant positioning accuracy and reduced alignment outliers compared to traditional methods. The introduction of computer and robotic-assisted surgery has led to the development of various techniques and alignment options, such as mechanically aligned, kinematic, anatomic, and functional alignments. However, there remains a knowledge gap regarding the optimal use of these systems to balance precision with soft tissue preservation. The study by Rossi e al. explores the ROSA® Knee System (Zimmer-Biomet, Warsaw, In., USA)surgical technique, focusing on alignment options and ligament balancing while reviewing current literature on the system.

The study details the ROSA® robotic-arm system's procedure, which involves placing the patient in a supine position and using trackers on the femur and tibia to monitor leg movements. The system allows for both image-based and image-less navigation, with intra-operative planning conducted via dedicated software to determine ideal resection thickness and angles for balanced TKA. The robotic arm operates in automatic, collaborative, and static modes to assist in precise jig placement for bone cuts. Surgeons can choose from various surgical strategies—measured resection, gap balancing, functional alignment—based on their preferences. The system provides real-time feedback on resection thickness, joint gaps, and limb alignment during surgery, allowing for individualized patient alignment.

The ROSA® Knee System offers significant advances in TKA by enabling individualized alignment based on real-time intra-operative data. This approach allows surgeons to achieve precise limb alignment while minimizing soft tissue disruption. Future study directions may include expanding the limits of safe coronal alignment zones as more data becomes available. The system's versatility is highlighted by its adaptability to different surgical techniques and its potential to reduce surgeon stress and improve efficiency. While preliminary results are promising regarding accuracy and clinical outcomes, further research is needed to compare its efficacy with other robotic systems comprehensively.

9.2.2.4 Using a Patella Reduced Technique while Balancing a TKA Results in Restored Physiological Strain in the Collateral Ligaments: An Ex Vivo Kinematic Analysis [255]

This is a machine-generated summary of:

Ghijselings, Ignace; Taylan, Orcun; Delport, Hendrik Pieter; Slane, Josh; Van den Wyngaert, Hans; Demurie, Alex; Scheys, Lennart Using a patella reduced technique while balancing a TKA results in restored physiological strain in the collateral ligaments: an ex vivo kinematic analysis [255].

Published in: Archives of Orthopaedic and Trauma Surgery (2021).

Link to original: https://doi.org/10.1007/s00402-021-04010-y

If you want to cite the papers, please refer to the original.

For technical reasons we could not place the page where the original quote is coming from.

Research Highlights

Orthopedic surgeons face challenges in achieving optimal patient satisfaction following total knee arthroplasty (TKA), despite advancements in surgical techniques and instrumentation. Traditional methods often focus on mechanical alignment, potentially neglecting the critical role of soft tissue balance, which is essential for a natural knee feel post-surgery. However, improved soft tissue balancing techniques have not consistently yielded reproducible results, leaving a gap in achieving optimal outcomes. The study by Ghijselings et al. introduces the patella-in-place balancing (PIPB) technique, which aims to enhance post-operative outcomes by maintaining the patella's natural position during surgery without soft tissue releases.

The study conducted a detailed ex vivo biomechanical analysis using eight fresh-frozen cadaveric legs to compare post-TKA tibiofemoral kinematics and collateral ligament behavior with native knee conditions. The researchers employed a dynamic knee simulator system to replicate physiological movements and assess the effectiveness of the PIPB technique. By preserving the posterior cruciate ligament and avoiding collateral ligament releases, the PIPB method focuses on achieving isometry of the collateral ligaments throughout flexion. The experimental setup involved attaching calibrated axial extensometers to measure ligament strain and using motion capture technology to track kinematic changes during various functional motions such as passive flexion and squatting.

The findings indicate that the PIPB technique successfully reduces post-operative laxity in both valgus and varus compared to native conditions, achieving symmetrical medial/lateral balance and good patellar tracking throughout the range of motion. The study highlights that this novel approach effectively restores femoral rollback patterns similar to native knees while maintaining comparable collateral ligament strains. Future study directions include assessing the PIPB technique's clinical outcomes and its applicability across different TKA designs. While promising, these results underscore the need for further in vivo research to validate the technique's efficacy in improving patient satisfaction and implant longevity.

9.2.2.5 A New Method to Measure Ligament Balancing in Total Knee Arthroplasty: Laxity Measurements in 100 Knees [256]

This is a machine-generated summary of:

Aunan, Eirik; Kibsgård, Thomas; Clarke-Jenssen, John; Röhrl, Stephan M. A new method to measure ligament balancing in total knee arthroplasty: laxity measurements in 100 knees [256].

Published in: Archives of Orthopaedic and Trauma Surgery (2012).

Link to original: https://doi.org/10.1007/s00402-012-1536-1

If you want to cite the papers, please refer to the original.

For technical reasons we could not place the page where the original quote is coming from.

Research Highlights

Symmetric ligament balance is crucial for optimal function and longevity in total knee arthroplasty (TKA), as asymmetry in the flexion or extension gaps can lead to instability and poor outcomes. Despite various techniques and devices developed to assist in achieving ligament balance, the process often relies on the surgeon's subjective judgment rather than objective measurement. A significant knowledge gap exists in the literature regarding a simple, reliable method to measure ligament balance intra-operatively. The study by Aunan et al. introduces a straightforward method to measure medial and lateral condylar lift-off during TKA, aiming to improve intra-operative assessment of ligament balance.

The study involved 100 knees from patients undergoing TKA due to osteoarthritis, with strict inclusion and exclusion criteria ensuring a focused cohort. The surgeries were performed using a measured resection technique with a cruciate-retaining prosthesis. The researchers introduced a set of polyethylene spatulas to measure medial and lateral gaps in both extension and 90 degrees of flexion. Measurements were taken by stressing the ligaments until a firm endpoint was felt, with inter-observer reliability assessed through consecutive measurements by different surgeons. The study found high inter-observer agreement, indicating that the method is reliable. The researchers also compared ligament-balanced knees with non-ligament-balanced knees, finding no significant differences in medial-lateral symmetry or gap equality.

The study advances the field by providing an easy-to-use, reliable method for measuring ligament balance during TKA, potentially aiding surgeons in achieving better outcomes. While the method does not replace existing techniques, it offers an objective way to document ligament balance data, which could be valuable for future studies exploring the relationship between ligament balance and TKA outcomes. Future study could focus on validating this method against established standards and exploring its impact on long-term prosthetic function and survival.

9.2.3 Fixation

9.2.3.1 Metaphyseal Cones/Sleeves

Metaphyseal Cones Combined with Diaphyseal Impaction Grafting Provide Good Outcomes and Survival in a Complex Revision Total Knee Arthroplasty: A Matched Comparative Analysis [257]

This is a machine-generated summary of:

Dzidzishvili, Lika; Sáez, David; Calvo, Emilio Metaphyseal cones combined with diaphyseal impaction grafting provide good outcomes and survival in a complex revision total knee arthroplasty: a matched comparative analysis [257].

Published in: European Journal of Orthopaedic Surgery & Traumatology (2023).

Link to original: https://doi.org/10.1007/s00590-023-03659-y

If you want to cite the papers, please refer to the original.

For technical reasons we could not place the page where the original quote is coming from.

Research Highlights

Over the last decade, the demand for revision total knee arthroplasty (rTKA) has surged due to an aging population, presenting significant challenges for surgeons, particularly in cases with severe bone loss. Traditional methods like structural allografts have shown high complication rates, while highly porous metaphyseal cones have demonstrated improved survival rates due to their biocompatibility and osseointegration. However, rTKA often involves substantial diaphyseal bone loss, compromising future construct fixation. The study by Dzidzishvili et al. explores the efficacy of combining metaphyseal cones with diaphyseal impaction bone grafting (IBG) in addressing these complex cases.

The study conducted a comparative case-control analysis involving patients undergoing complex rTKA with hinged knee prostheses and metaphyseal cones. Some patients also received diaphyseal IBG to address extensive cancellous bone loss. Preoperative radiographic assessments were performed to evaluate bone defects, followed by intraoperative classification before grafting and cone placement. Patients were monitored through regular follow-ups with radiographic evaluations and functional assessments using the Knee Society Score. The study employed statistical analyses to compare outcomes between groups using metaphyseal cones alone versus those combined with IBG. Results indicated significant improvements in Knee Society Scores postoperatively in both groups, with no significant differences in radiolucency or implant survivorship between them.

The study's findings suggest that combining metaphyseal cones with diaphyseal IBG offers comparable clinical outcomes and survival rates to using metaphyseal cones alone in patients with severe bone loss. This approach provides a stable construct by achieving biological fixation, potentially allowing for shorter diaphyseal stems in future procedures. While the study's short follow-up period limits long-term conclusions, the results are promising for managing severe bone defects in rTKA. Future studies could focus on refining this technique and exploring its long-term efficacy to enhance clinical and radiological outcomes further.

Metaphyseal Bone Loss in Revision Knee Arthroplasty [258]

This is a machine-generated summary of:

Ponzio, Danielle Y.; Austin, Matthew S. Metaphyseal bone loss in revision knee arthroplasty [258].

Published in: Current Reviews in Musculoskeletal Medicine (2015).
Link to original: https://doi.org/10.1007/s12178-015-9291-x

If you want to cite the papers, please refer to the original.
For technical reasons we could not place the page where the original quote is coming from.

Research Highlights

Metaphyseal bone loss poses significant challenges in revision total knee arthroplasty (TKA), potentially compromising both initial and long-term fixation of components. This condition can lead to malalignment due to the loss of normal anatomical landmarks, with causes ranging from stress shielding and osteolysis to infection and mechanical abrasion. The primary goals of revision surgery include preserving viable host bone, reconstructing bone deficiencies, restoring the joint line, and achieving proper alignment and stability. However, a knowledge gap exists in determining the most effective method for managing metaphyseal bone loss during revision TKA. The study by Ponzio et al. explores various reconstructive techniques to address this issue.

The study examines several methods for reconstructing metaphyseal bone deficiencies, including impaction grafting, prosthetic augmentation, bulk structural allografts, and the use of metaphyseal cones and sleeves. Impaction grafting involves using morselized cancellous autograft or allograft bone for contained defects, while uncontained defects may require wire mesh for containment. Prosthetic augmentation utilizes modular or customized augments to restore joint line and balance the knee efficiently. Bulk structural allografts are considered for larger uncontained defects, offering potential long-term biologic integration but with risks such as nonunion and infection. Metaphyseal cones and sleeves are designed to fill large cavitary defects, providing mechanical support and potential for osseous ingrowth. Each technique has its advantages and limitations, with selection often based on defect size, location, ligamentous stability, and patient factors.

The study highlights that porous metal metaphyseal cones and sleeves represent recent advances in managing metaphyseal bone loss during revision TKA. These technologies offer potential benefits such as biologic ingrowth fixation and a mechanically sound scaffold while avoiding issues associated with traditional bone grafting methods. Future study could focus on long-term outcomes and comparisons with other reconstruction options to determine their efficacy in providing superior clinical success over time. The findings underscore the need for continued research to establish optimal strategies for addressing complex bone deficiencies in revision TKA procedures.

Unbalanced Metaphyseal Fixation Is Associated with an Increased Aseptic Loosening of Revision Total Knee Arthroplasty at Mean 4-Year Follow-Up [259]

This is a machine-generated summary of:

Russo, Antonio; Alessio-Mazzola, Mattia; Massè, Alessandro; Burastero, Giorgio Unbalanced metaphyseal fixation is associated with an increased aseptic loosening of revision total knee arthroplasty at mean 4-year follow-up [259].

Published in: Archives of Orthopaedic and Trauma Surgery (2024).

Link to original: https://doi.org/10.1007/s00402-024-05600-2

If you want to cite the papers, please refer to the original.

For technical reasons we could not place the page where the original quote is coming from.

Research Highlights

The global incidence of total knee arthroplasty (TKA) is on the rise, with projections indicating a doubling in prevalence in the coming years. This increase is attributed to advancements in TKA designs and improved clinical outcomes, which have broadened the indications for the procedure to include both younger, more active patients and older patients with multiple comorbidities. Consequently, the number of revision TKAs (rTKAs) is expected to increase significantly. Despite the generally positive outcomes of primary TKA, rTKA cases often experience higher rates of complications and failures, with lower survivorship compared to primary cases. A critical factor in rTKA success is achieving secure implant fixation, particularly following the "zonal fixation" principles. However, challenges remain in cases involving significant bone loss or septic revisions. The study by Russo et al. investigates whether unbalanced metaphyseal fixation affects implant survivorship in rTKA.

In this retrospective single-center study, Russo et al. analyzed data from patients who underwent two-stage rTKA for periprosthetic joint infection (PJI) between January 2010 and January 2020. The study included patients who received standard trabecular metal cones during reconstruction and had at least 5 years of follow-up data available. Patients were divided into two groups: those with unbalanced metaphyseal fixation (cones on either femoral or tibial side) and those with balanced fixation (cones on both sides). The researchers assessed clinical and radiographic outcomes preoperatively and at regular intervals postoperatively. The primary endpoint was the prevalence of aseptic loosening, while secondary endpoints included clinical and functional outcomes such as knee stability and range of motion. Statistical analyses were conducted to compare outcomes between the two groups.

The study found that unbalanced metaphyseal fixation was associated with a higher risk of aseptic loosening, particularly affecting the femoral component when only tibial cones were used. This suggests that achieving balanced fixation may be crucial for improving implant longevity in rTKA procedures. While functional outcomes improved significantly from baseline across all patients, no differences were observed between groups at final follow-up regarding knee scores or range of motion. Future studies could explore larger cohorts to validate these findings further and investigate potential strategies for optimizing metaphyseal fixation in complex rTKA cases. These insights could inform surgical practices and improve long-term outcomes for patients undergoing revision knee arthroplasty due to infection-related complications.

Revision Total Knee Arthroplasty: Experience with Tantalum Cones in Severe Bone Loss [260]

This is a machine-generated summary of:

Fosco, Matteo; Amendola, Luca; Fantasia, Rossana; Pipino, Gennaro; Tigani, Domenico Revision total knee arthroplasty: experience with tantalum cones in severe bone loss [260].

Published in: European Orthopaedics and Traumatology (2013).

Link to original: https://doi.org/10.1007/s12570-013-0160-z

If you want to cite the papers, please refer to the original.

For technical reasons we could not place the page where the original quote is coming from.

Research Highlights

Femoral or tibial bone loss presents a significant challenge in revision total knee arthroplasty, often necessitating complex reconstructive techniques. Traditional methods for addressing smaller bone defects include the use of cement, bone grafts, and modular metal augments, while larger defects require more extensive solutions such as structural allografts and megaprostheses. Trabecular metal cones, a novel biomaterial with favorable mechanical and biological properties, have been developed to address large metaphyseal defects. However, concerns about infection rates associated with these cones persist. The study by Fosco et al. evaluates the use of tantalum tibial and femoral metaphyseal cones in revision knee arthroplasty, focusing on infection rates.

The study retrospectively reviewed total knee revisions performed over a year, involving ten patients who received porous tantalum metal (TM) cones for significant bone defects. The cohort included both men and women with an average age of 67 years at the time of surgery. Indications for surgery varied from deep infections to aseptic loosening and malrotation of prosthetic components. The surgical protocol involved pre- and post-operative clinical assessments, including blood tests and radiographic evaluations to rule out infections. TM cones were implanted using a hybrid fixation technique with antibiotic-loaded bone cement for definitive fixation. The study found no intra-operative complications related to cone implantation and no cases of re-infection or aseptic loosening at an average follow-up of 24 months.

The findings suggest that TM cones provide effective osteointegration without increasing infection risk in revision knee arthroplasty. The study highlights the potential of TM cones to enhance implant stability while maintaining load transfer to host bone. Future studies could focus on long-term outcomes and larger patient populations to validate these results further. Despite its retrospective nature and small sample size, this study contributes valuable insights into the use of TM cones in complex knee revisions, potentially guiding future clinical practices in orthopaedic surgery.

Promising Short-Term Outcomes of Free-Hand Burring Technique to Implant Second-Generation Metaphyseal Cone in Asian Knees—A Case Series [261]

This is a machine-generated summary of:

Leung, Thomas Ka Chun; Chan, Ping Keung; Fu, Henry; Cheung, Amy; Luk, Michelle Hilda; Lau, Lawrence Chun Man; Chiu, Kwong Yuen Promising short-term outcomes of free-hand burring technique to implant second-generation metaphyseal cone in Asian knees—a case series [261].

Published in: Arthroplasty (2024).

Link to original: https://doi.org/10.1186/s42836-024-00254-2

If you want to cite the papers, please refer to the original.

For technical reasons we could not place the page where the original quote is coming from.

Research Highlights

The demand for revision total knee arthroplasty (TKA) is increasing due to an aging population, and managing bone loss in these cases presents significant challenges. The Anderson Orthopaedic Research Institute classification system is widely used to categorize bone defects, and metaphyseal cones are instrumental in addressing these defects by enhancing prosthesis fixation. Despite satisfactory outcomes with first-generation cones, their use involves technical difficulties and potential inaccuracies during bone preparation. The second-generation cone, made from porous titanium and designed using a CT-based anatomical database, offers improved precision and user-friendliness. However, data on its effectiveness in Asian populations are limited. The study by Leung et al. investigates the clinical and radiological outcomes of second-generation titanium cones in an Asian setting.

The study reviewed patients who underwent revision TKA at The University of Hong Kong, in Hong Kong, China, between April,2017, and June 2022. The Institutional Review Board approved the study, and informed consent was obtained from all participants. The inclusion criteria focused on revision TKA using tibial and/or femoral second-generation titanium metaphyseal cones, with bone preparation performed via free hand burring due to anatomical constraints that precluded the use of cannulated reamers. The study recorded demographic data, clinical outcomes such as knee range of motion and Knee Society Knee Scores, and radiological assessments for osteointegration and complications. All surgeries were conducted by a single senior surgeon using a standard medial parapatellar approach, with careful classification of bone defects intraoperatively.

The study found that using free-hand burring techniques for implanting second-generation metaphyseal cones yielded promising mid-term outcomes despite anatomical differences in Asian osteometry. Future studies incorporating computed tomography could further elucidate anatomical differences between Asian and Caucasian knees, potentially leading to modifications in implant design to better accommodate diverse osteometries. This research underscores the importance of considering ethnic variations in surgical planning and highlights the need for longer-term follow-up to assess the durability of these implants in different populations.

Medium Term Clinical Outcomes of Tibial Cones in Revision Knee Arthroplasty [262]

This is a machine-generated summary of:

Erivan, Roger; Tracey, Robert; Mulliez, Aurélien; Villatte, Guillaume; Paprosky, Wayne Medium term clinical outcomes of tibial cones in revision knee arthroplasty [262].

Published in: Archives of Orthopaedic and Trauma Surgery (2020).
Link to original: https://doi.org/10.1007/s00402-020-03532-1

If you want to cite the papers, please refer to the original.
For technical reasons we could not place the page where the original quote is coming from.

Research Highlights

Revision total knee arthroplasty (TKA) is the primary treatment for failed primary TKA, with anticipated increases in both volume and cost. However, outcomes after revision TKA are less predictable than those following primary surgery, particularly due to challenges in assessing and managing bone defects. Various treatment options exist, but none have demonstrated clear superiority. Trabecular metal cones have emerged as a promising option for reconstructing major bone defects during revision TKA, showing good primary fixation in cadaver studies. The study by Erivan et al. retrospectively assesses the medium-term results of trabecular metal tibial cones in revision TKA, hypothesizing excellent clinical and radiological outcomes.

The study involved a single-center retrospective review of all consecutive cases of tibial revision using trabecular metal cones. Conducted between January 2010 and December 2015, the study included patients with a minimum of 5 years follow-up. The inclusion criteria were patients undergoing revision TKA with tibial component revision using highly porous tantalum biomaterial cones. Clinical scores such as the Knee injury and Osteoarthritis Outcome Scores (KOOS) and SF-36 were used to evaluate outcomes, alongside radiographic assessments for cone integration and mechanical stability. The primary endpoint was tibial cone survivorship, while secondary endpoints included all-cause survivorship and patient-reported outcomes. Statistical analyses were performed using Stata software to compare pre- and post-operative data.

The study concluded that trabecular metal tibial cones provide excellent medium-term results for managing tibial bone defects in revision TKA, with high survivorship rates for aseptic loosening. These findings align with previous studies on femoral defect management using similar cones. Despite limitations such as its retrospective nature and small sample size, the study supports the use of tibial cones as a viable option in revision TKA. Future studies could focus on longer-term outcomes and larger patient populations to further validate these findings and explore potential improvements in surgical techniques or materials used for metaphyseal fixation.

Utilizing 3d-Printed Patient-Specific Porous Titanium Cones in Complex Primary and Revision Total Knee Arthroplasty [263]

This is a machine-generated summary of:

Vaziri, Arash Sharafat; Moradkhani, Ghazaleh; Farahmand, Farzam; Karimpour, Morad; Tahmasebi, Mohammad Naghi; Vosoughi, Fardis; Salimi, Maryam; Shayan-Moghadam, Ramin Utilizing 3d-printed patient-specific porous titanium cones in complex primary and revision total knee arthroplasty [263].

Published in: European Journal of Orthopaedic Surgery & Traumatology (2025).

Link to original: https://doi.org/10.1007/s00590-025-04229-0

If you want to cite the papers, please refer to the original.

For technical reasons we could not place the page where the original quote is coming from.

Research Highlights

Revision total knee arthroplasty (rTKA) aims to provide a stable prosthesis with an acceptable pain-free range of motion while preserving bone structure and reconstructing bone defects. This process is challenging due to bone defects, low bone quality, and additional bone loss through prosthesis removal. Managing these defects often involves reinforcement techniques such as structural allografts, augments, cones, and sleeves. Among these, porous cones have gained attention for their ability to reconstruct large bone defects with favorable mid- and long-term outcomes. However, off-the-shelf (OTS) cones often do not fit the anatomy of all patients, particularly those of Asian descent who generally have smaller knees than Caucasians. The study by Vaziriet al. explores the use of patient-specific 3D-printed titanium cones in complex primary and revision total knee arthroplasty to address these challenges.

The study involved patients who were candidates for complex primary TKA or complicated rTKA. The researchers used computed tomography scans to create segmented models of each patient's lower limb, which informed the design of customized porous titanium cones using additive manufacturing technology. The selective laser melting technique was employed to produce these patient-specific implants, which were tailored to fit the unique anatomy and defect size of each patient. The cones were designed with adjusted stiffness similar to bone to prevent stress shielding and promote osseointegration. During surgery, the customized cones were implanted without technical issues after minimal host bone preparation, achieving precise reconstruction of defects. Radiographic imaging confirmed that postoperative results aligned with preoperative planning.

The study's early outcomes demonstrated that patient-specific porous titanium cones provided well-fixed components with no evidence of loosening or implant migration. All patients returned to full activity with a full range of motion and no pain or instability. These findings suggest that personalized approaches can overcome the limitations of OTS cones by accommodating narrow medullary canals and massive bone defects while preserving bone stock. Future study should focus on long-term follow-up to confirm these promising early results and explore the broader applicability of this technique in diverse patient populations. Increasing the number of studied cases will also be essential for validating these findings further.

A Prospective Study on Outcome of Patient-Specific Cones in Revision Knee Arthroplasty [264]

This is a machine-generated summary of:

Cherny, Alexander A.; Kovalenko, Anton N.; Kulyaba, Taras A.; Kornilov, Nikolai N. A prospective study on outcome of patient-specific cones in revision knee arthroplasty [264].

Published in: Archives of Orthopaedic and Trauma Surgery (2021).

Link to original: https://doi.org/10.1007/s00402-021-04047-z

If you want to cite the papers, please refer to the original.

For technical reasons we could not place the page where the original quote is coming from.

Research Highlights

Total knee arthroplasty (TKA) often requires revision due to complications such as aseptic loosening, with bone loss being a significant challenge in these procedures. Current methods for managing bone defects include various grafts and implants, each with limitations, especially in cases of extensive bone loss. Accurate preoperative assessment is crucial for surgical planning yet remains challenging. The study by Cherny et al. explores the use of patient-specific 3D-printed metal cones to address extensive femoral and tibial bone loss during revision TKA (RTKA).

The study involved designing and implanting patient-specific titanium cones in patients with significant bone defects due to aseptic loosening or other complications. Using advanced imaging and computer modeling, the researchers created personalized implants tailored to each patient's anatomy. The process included creating virtual models and plastic prototypes to ensure proper fit before manufacturing the final titanium cones through 3D printing. The surgical procedure involved standard approaches for implant removal and preparation of the host bone for the new implant. Postoperative assessments showed significant improvements in functional outcomes, with no major complications or need for further revisions within the follow-up period.

This study demonstrates that patient-specific 3D-printed cones can be a viable solution for managing extensive bone loss in RTKA, offering a high level of personalization and potentially improving surgical outcomes. The authors highlight the importance of individualized implant design to preserve bone stock and enhance fixation while minimizing soft tissue adhesion issues. Future study could focus on long-term outcomes to confirm these findings and explore further refinements in implant design and manufacturing processes to optimize patient outcomes in complex orthopaedic surgeries.

Porous-Coated Metaphyseal Sleeves and MBT Implant for Severe Bone Loss in Revision Total Knee Arthroplasty: A Mean 2.4-Year Follow-Up [265]

This is a machine-generated summary of:

Wu, Yushun; Feng, Eryou; Zhang, Yiyuan; Lin, Feitai; Lin, Liqiong; Li, Zhanglai; Xiao, Lili Porous-coated metaphyseal sleeves and MBT implant for severe bone loss in revision total knee arthroplasty: a mean 2.4-year follow-up [265].

Published in: Arthroplasty (2020).

Link to original: https://doi.org/10.1186/s42836-020-00031-x

If you want to cite the papers, please refer to the original.

For technical reasons we could not place the page where the original quote is coming from.

Research Highlights

Knee arthroplasty is a well-established treatment for end-stage knee osteoarthritis, but the increasing number of revision surgeries poses challenges, particularly concerning bone loss and implant fixation. Various reconstruction techniques, such as bone cement filling and autologous bone grafting, have been employed to address these issues, yet the optimal strategy remains unclear. The study by Wu et al. evaluates the clinical and radiographic outcomes of using porous-coated metaphyseal sleeves in revision total knee arthroplasty (TKA) for severe bone loss in Chinese patients. The study hypothesizes that these sleeves could enhance bone ingrowth and reduce short-term revision rates.

The study was conducted retrospectively on patients with Anderson Orthopaedic Research Institute (AORI) II or III bone loss who underwent revision TKA using press-fit tibial and/or femoral porous-coated metaphyseal sleeves. All procedures were performed by a senior surgeon at Fuzhou Second Hospital Affiliated to Xiamen University. The researchers collected data on patient demographics, primary diagnoses leading to revision, and preoperative radiographs to classify bone loss. Surgical techniques involved assessing sleeve and stem sizes based on the contact area with host bone, ensuring proper alignment and fixation without cement when feasible. Postoperative rehabilitation included infection prophylaxis and quadriceps strength training. Patients were followed up for an average of 24 months, with assessments using Knee Society Score (KSS), Hospital for Special Surgery (HSS) score, and Visual Analog Scale (VAS) scores.

The study found significant improvements in KSS, HSS scores, and range of motion postoperatively, with no radiographic evidence of implant loosening or progressive radiolucent lines. The use of porous-coated metaphyseal sleeves demonstrated effective fixation and stability in revision TKA cases with severe bone loss. Future studies could focus on long-term outcomes to confirm these findings further. While the study's retrospective nature and lack of comparison with other methods are limitations, it provides valuable insights into the potential benefits of metaphyseal sleeve use in knee revisions.

Novel Metaphyseal Porous Titanium Cones Allow Favorable Outcomes in Revision Total Knee Arthroplasty [266]

This is a machine-generated summary of:

Shichman, Ittai; Oakley, Christian; Willems, Jore H.; van Hellemondt, Gijs G.; Heesterbeek, Petra; Rozell, Joshua; Marwin, Scott; Schwarzkopf, Ran Novel metaphyseal porous titanium cones allow favorable outcomes in revision total knee arthroplasty [266].

Published in: Archives of Orthopaedic and Trauma Surgery (2022).

Link to original: https://doi.org/10.1007/s00402-022-04645-5

Research Highlights

The increasing prevalence of revision total knee arthroplasty (rTKA) is driven by factors such as obesity and aging, which contribute to the failure of primary total knee arthroplasties (TKAs). Common causes of TKA failure include aseptic loosening, infection, and instability, often necessitating revision surgeries. A significant challenge in rTKA is managing bone loss due to implant removal and bone resection. Various techniques and implants have been developed to address this issue, but the optimal approach remains unclear due to insufficient long-term data. The study by Shichman et al., investigates the use of novel porous titanium metaphyseal cones with stems of variable length and fixation methods in rTKA, aiming to improve functional outcomes and implant survival.

The study was conducted as a retrospective analysis across two large institutions, focusing on patients who underwent rTKA with severe tibial or femoral bone defects. The researchers utilized porous titanium metaphyseal cones to augment reconstruction in these cases. The study included patients aged 18 years or older who received the Legion Cone System (Zimmer-Biomet, Warsaw, In., USA) for their revision surgeries. Data were collected from electronic medical records, including demographic information, surgical characteristics, and clinical outcomes such as operative time and hospital length of stay. Radiographic assessments were performed postoperatively at various intervals to evaluate implant stability and integration. The study employed Kaplan-Meier survival analysis and multivariable logistic regression to assess re-revision rates and the impact of different stem fixation methods on outcomes.

The findings indicate that both tibial and femoral cones demonstrated high rates of freedom from aseptic re-revisions and explantation at a minimum follow-up of 2 years. The study found no significant differences in all-cause re-revision rates between hybrid cementation and fully cemented stem groups, suggesting that both fixation methods are viable options depending on patient-specific factors. Future study could focus on comparing different cone systems and further exploring postoperative stability across various augmentation strategies. This research contributes valuable insights into the efficacy of novel porous cone designs in managing bone loss during complex rTKA procedures.

The Use of Tantalum Cones and Diaphyseal-Engaging Stems in Tibial Component Revision: A Consecutive Series [267]

This is a machine-generated summary of:

Spinello, P.; Thiele, R. A. Ruberte; Zepeda, K.; Giori, N.; Indelli, P. F. The use of tantalum cones and diaphyseal-engaging stems in tibial component revision: a consecutive series [267].

Published in: Knee Surgery & Related Research (2022).

Link to original: https://doi.org/10.1186/s43019-022-00141-7

If you want to cite the papers, please refer to the original.

For technical reasons we could not place the page where the original quote is coming from.

Research Highlights

Total knee arthroplasty (TKA) failures can arise from various causes, including instability, infection, and stiffness, as well as aseptic loosening and osteolysis. Revision knee arthroplasty poses challenges such as bone loss and ligamentous deficiency, necessitating solid fixation for early weight-bearing. Traditional methods like cemented components and metal augments have been used to address these issues, but newer techniques involving metaphyseal sleeves and porous tantalum cones are gaining attention. A knowledge gap exists in understanding the clinical outcomes of using porous tantalum metaphyseal cones combined with long uncemented diaphyseal-engaging stems in managing tibial bone loss during revision TKA. The study by Spinello et al. explores this technique's effectiveness in improving tibial fixation and alignment.

The study is a single-center retrospective analysis of aseptic revision TKA cases performed by two senior authors. It involved patients with various indications for revision, such as instability with bone loss and severe tibial osteolysis. The researchers employed a hybrid fixation technique using trabecular metal tantalum cones with long press-fit diaphyseal-engaging stems to reconstruct metaphyseal bone defects. Excluding patients with cemented stems, the study assessed clinical outcomes using the Knee Society Score and radiographic evidence of osteointegration. The surgical procedure involved meticulous preparation of the tibial canal and cone implantation to ensure proper alignment and stability. Statistical analysis compared pre- and post-intervention values to evaluate improvements in knee function.

The study demonstrated that hybrid fixation with uncemented diaphyseal-engaging stems and porous tantalum metaphyseal cones yields favorable clinical outcomes, with a survivorship rate of 95% at a mean follow-up of 36 months. The technique showed significant improvements in knee function scores and tibiofemoral alignment while ensuring osteointegration of the tantalum cones. Future study directions could include mid- to long-term follow-up to confirm the durability of these results over time. Despite limitations such as its retrospective design and small sample size, the study aligns with existing literature on hybrid fixation techniques, suggesting its potential as a reliable approach for managing complex tibial bone defects in revision TKA.

Cementless Metaphyseal Sleeves without Stem in Revision Total Knee Arthroplasty [268]

This is a machine-generated summary of:

Gøttsche, David; Lind, Thomas; Christiansen, Thorbjørn; Schrøder, Henrik M. Cementless metaphyseal sleeves without stem in revision total knee arthroplasty [268].

Published in: Archives of Orthopaedic and Trauma Surgery (2016).

Link to original: https://doi.org/10.1007/s00402-016-2583-9

If you want to cite the papers, please refer to the original.

For technical reasons we could not place the page where the original quote is coming from.

Research Highlights

Total knee arthroplasty (TKA) revisions are often necessitated by complications such as aseptic loosening, deep infection, pain without loosening, and instability. Traditionally, these revisions have involved the use of prostheses with stems to ensure stability. However, recent approaches have increasingly utilized metaphyseal sleeves and cones to address bone loss, with some studies suggesting that these components provide stability through bone ingrowth. The study by Gøttsche et al. t Gentofte Hospital, University of Copenhagen, explores the clinical outcomes of using the P.F.C.® SIGMA® Knee System (DePuy-Synthes, Warsaw, In., USA) with cementless metaphyseal sleeves without stems in revision TKA (rTKA), aiming to reduce "end-of-stem pain" while maintaining fixation and alignment.

The study involved a retrospective review of patients who underwent rTKA with cementless metaphyseal sleeves without stems at Gentofte Hospital. The researchers identified patients through X-ray reviews and included those who had femoral or tibial components implanted. The surgical technique involved extracting the failed primary TKA, preparing the tibia and femur for sleeve insertion using sequential broaching, and fixing the revision knee with cement on the baseplate while avoiding cement on the proximal coated part of the sleeve. Patients were assessed using the American Knee Society Score (AKSS) and Oxford Knee Score (OKS), with satisfaction measured on a four-stage scale. The study found that while prostheses were generally well-fixed radiologically, moderate-to-severe pain was reported by a significant number of patients.

The study concludes that using cementless metaphyseal sleeves without stems in rTKA can achieve good fixation with minimal cases of aseptic loosening. However, many patients experienced significant pain, potentially linked to non-optimal alignment or comorbid conditions. The close relationship between pain and patient satisfaction underscores the need for careful preoperative patient counseling regarding expectations. Future studies could focus on larger populations to better understand the correlation between bone loss and clinical outcomes, as well as explore potential mechanisms behind persistent pain post-surgery.

Mid-Term Clinical and Radiographic Outcomes of Porous-Coated Metaphyseal Sleeves Used in Revision Total Knee Arthroplasty [269]

This is a machine-generated summary of:

Gurel, Ron; Morgan, Samuel; Elbaz, Etay; Ashlenazi, Itay; Snir, Nimrod; Kadar, Assaf; Gold, Aviram; Warschawski, Yaniv Mid-term clinical and radiographic outcomes of porous-coated metaphyseal sleeves used in revision total knee arthroplasty [269].

Published in: Knee Surgery & Related Research (2021).

Link to original: https://doi.org/10.1186/s43019-021-00103-5

If you want to cite the papers, please refer to the original.

For technical reasons we could not place the page where the original quote is coming from.

Research Highlights

The increasing number of revision total knee arthroplasty (RTKA) procedures worldwide, coupled with rising life expectancy, has highlighted the challenge of managing bone loss in the femoral and tibial articular surfaces. Metaphyseal bone loss can compromise component fixation and lead to malalignment due to the loss of anatomical landmarks. Traditional management of large and uncontained bone defects involves structural allografts or metal filling devices like cones and sleeves, but these methods have limitations such as instability and infection risks. The study by Gurel et al. explores the mid-term outcomes of using metaphyseal sleeves in RTKA, hypothesizing that they offer a promising solution for bone defects with good mid-term survivorship.

The study was conducted as a retrospective analysis with institutional ethics approval, focusing on patients who underwent RTKA using a specific CCKMB prosthesis (Press-Fit Condylar Sigma Total Condylar 3 Rotating-Platform; DePuy, Warsaw, IN, USA) combined with osteointegrative sleeves. The researchers included cases with a minimum follow-up of 5 years, gathering data from electronic medical records on patient characteristics, implant details, and complications. Clinical outcomes were assessed using Knee Society Scores (KSS), while radiographic evaluations were performed to classify bone defects and check for signs of aseptic loosening. Statistical analyses compared preoperative and postoperative KSS scores, revealing significant improvements. The study found that metaphyseal sleeves provided stable fixation with low re-revision rates over an average follow-up period of 56 months.

The findings suggest that metaphyseal sleeves offer excellent mid-term clinical and radiographic outcomes in RTKA, with significant improvements in KSS scores and range of motion. The study's results align with previous short-term studies but extend the evidence to a longer follow-up period. However, limitations such as the lack of a control group and potential sampling bias highlight the need for further research. Future studies should focus on long-term outcomes to confirm the durability and effectiveness of metaphyseal sleeves compared to other methods. Despite these limitations, this study contributes valuable insights into the mid-term viability of metaphyseal sleeves in addressing bone loss during RTKA.

Bone Mineral Density Changes of the Proximal Tibia After Revision Total Knee Arthroplasty. A Randomised Study with the Use of Porous Tantalum Metaphyseal Cones [270]

This is a machine-generated summary of:
Jensen, Claus L.; Petersen, Michael M.; Schrøder, Henrik M.; Lund, Bjarne Bone mineral density changes of the proximal tibia after revision total knee arthroplasty. A randomised study with the use of porous tantalum metaphyseal cones [270].
Published in: International Orthopaedics (2012).
Link to original: https://doi.org/10.1007/s00264-012-1601-y

Research Highlights

Total knee arthroplasties (TKA) generally have a high 10-year survival rate, but failures can occur due to factors such as aseptic loosening, infection, and bone loss. The reconstruction of bone defects in the proximal tibia during revision TKA (rTKA) is crucial for successful outcomes. While smaller bone losses are well-managed, severe bone loss presents challenges and may require advanced solutions like metal augmentation or mega prostheses. The study by Jensen et al. explores the use of a porous Tantalum biomaterial, known as the Trabecular Metal Cone, for addressing severe bone loss in rTKA. This study aims to measure changes in bone mineral density (BMD) using dual-energy X-ray absorptiometry (DEXA) and evaluate the remodelling patterns with or without the TM Cone.

The study involved 40 patients undergoing rTKA with significant proximal tibial bone loss. Participants were randomly assigned to receive either the TM Cone or conventional treatment. DEXA scans were used to measure BMD at various intervals post-surgery, focusing on regions of interest around the tibial component. The study meticulously controlled variables such as surgical technique and patient positioning during scans to ensure reliable data. Statistical analyses were conducted using SPSS software to compare BMD changes between groups. Despite some exclusions due to complications or poor scan quality, the study provided comprehensive data on BMD changes over 2 years.

The findings revealed that both groups experienced similar patterns of BMD change, with no significant differences between those treated with the TM Cone and those without it. Notably, an increase in BMD was observed along the tibial stem in both groups after 12 months, suggesting effective load transfer and bone remodelling. This study is pioneering in its focus on BMD changes post-rTKA and suggests that while the TM Cone does not significantly alter overall BMD outcomes compared to conventional methods, it may still offer benefits in specific clinical scenarios. Future studies could further explore long-term outcomes and refine techniques for managing severe bone loss in rTKA.

Metaphyseal Cones and Sleeves in Revision Total Knee Arthroplasty: Two Sides of the Same Coin? Complications, Clinical and Radiological Results—A Systematic Review of the Literature [271]

This is a machine-generated summary of:

Zanirato, A.; Formica, M.; Cavagnaro, L.; Divano, S.; Burastero, G.; Felli, L. Metaphyseal cones and sleeves in revision total knee arthroplasty: Two sides of the same coin? Complications, clinical and radiological results—a systematic review of the literature [271].

Published in: MUSCULOSKELETAL SURGERY (2019).

Link to original: https://doi.org/10.1007/s12306-019-00598-y

If you want to cite the papers, please refer to the original.

For technical reasons we could not place the page where the original quote is coming from.

Research Highlights

The number of primary total knee arthroplasties (TKAs) has surged in recent years, leading to a projected increase in revision procedures. Revision total knee arthroplasty (rTKA) aims to address bone deficiencies and optimize joint function, but managing massive bone defects remains challenging. Various strategies have been explored, yet the optimal treatment method is still undetermined. The study by Zanirato et al. systematically reviews the use of metaphyseal porous metal devices, specifically cones and sleeves, in rTKA to address these challenges.

The study conducted a systematic review of literature from Medline through PubMed, focusing on clinical and radiological outcomes of metaphyseal cones and sleeves in rTKA. The inclusion criteria encompassed studies providing relevant data on these devices with a minimum follow-up of 1 year. Exclusion criteria ruled out studies lacking specific outcome data or focusing on complex primary TKA. The review included 22 articles, predominantly level IV evidence, with two level III case-control studies. Data extracted included patient demographics, types of bone defects, fixation methods, and clinical outcomes such as aseptic loosening rates and infection rates. The analysis revealed that both metaphyseal cones and sleeves achieved favorable short- to mid-term outcomes with good implant stability and bone ingrowth.

Metaphyseal cones and sleeves offer promising solutions for managing severe bone defects in rTKA by providing stable fixation closer to the joint line, enhancing rotational stability compared to diaphyseal fixation alone. Despite their advantages, these devices require careful consideration due to their cost and potential for increased bone removal during implantation. Future study could focus on high-quality long-term research to better understand the complications and outcomes associated with these techniques. The choice between cones and sleeves often depends on surgeon preference and defect characteristics, highlighting the need for further comparative studies to refine their use in clinical practice.

9.2.3.2 Stems Cemented/ Press Fit

Hybrid Stems Are Superior to Cemented Stems in Revision Total Knee Arthroplasty: A Systematic Review and Meta-analysis of Recent Comparative Studies [272]

This is a machine-generated summary of:

Sheridan, Gerard A.; Garbuz, Donald S.; Masri, Bassam A. Hybrid stems are superior to cemented stems in revision total knee arthroplasty: a systematic review and meta-analysis of recent comparative studies [272].

Published in: European Journal of Orthopaedic Surgery & Traumatology (2020).
Link to original: https://doi.org/10.1007/s00590-020-02752-w

If you want to cite the papers, please refer to the original.

For technical reasons we could not place the page where the original quote is coming from.

Research Highlights

The demand for revision total knee arthroplasty (TKA) has been increasing globally, with projections indicating a continued rise in these procedures. In revision TKA, femoral and tibial stems are often used to enhance the stability of primary components, especially in cases of bone loss and instability. Fixation can be achieved in three anatomical zones: the epiphysis, metaphysis, and diaphysis. However, there is ongoing debate regarding the most effective fixation method for these stems—cemented versus hybrid fixation. The study by Sheridan et al. conducted a systematic review and meta-analysis of recent comparative studies to determine the optimal fixation method for stems in revision TKA.

The study employed a rigorous methodology adhering to PRISMA (Preferred Reporting Items for *Systematic reviews* and Meta analysis) guidelines, analyzing comparative studies published within the last decade that directly compared cemented and hybrid stem outcomes in revision TKA. The researchers conducted an extensive search across multiple electronic databases using specific MeSH (Medial Subject Headings) terms to identify relevant studies. After applying strict inclusion criteria, seven comparative studies were selected for systematic review.

Data extraction was performed using an electronic form, and any disagreements were resolved through consensus among the authors. Statistical analyses were conducted using random-effects meta-analysis to account for missing data and potential inter-study heterogeneity. The primary outcome measure was "all-cause failure," which included re-revision for any reason and radiographic failure.

The findings of this study indicate that hybrid stem fixation in revision TKA is associated with a significantly lower overall failure rate compared to cemented stems across all assessed outcome measures. This suggests that hybrid stems may offer advantages such as preservation of bone stock and ease of implant removal if re-revision is necessary. The study highlights the importance of recent advancements in uncemented fixation technology and improved surgical proficiency with hybrid techniques. Future study could focus on further refining these techniques and exploring long-term outcomes to enhance the success rates of revision TKA procedures.

Does Stem Profile Have an Impact on the Failure Patterns in Revision Total Knee Arthroplasty? [273]

This is a machine-generated summary of:

Maslaris, Alexander; Tsiridis, Eleftherios; Schoeneberg, Carsten; Pass, Bastian; Spyrou, Georgios; Maris, Alexandros; Matziolis, Georg Does stem profile have an impact on the failure patterns in revision total knee arthroplasty? [273].

Published in: Archives of Orthopaedic and Trauma Surgery (2022).

Link to original: https://doi.org/10.1007/s00402-022-04683-z

Research Highlights

The increasing incidence of revision total knee arthroplasty (RTKA) worldwide presents significant challenges for healthcare systems, both currently and in the future. Despite advancements, RTKA outcomes remain unsatisfactory, with failure rates still concerningly high. A critical factor in these failures is the design of the stem used in the implants, which affects both the stability and revisability of RTKA. Conical stem designs have been suggested to offer advantages over cylindrical stems, particularly in terms of ease of removal and potentially better osteointegration. However, there is a lack of literature evaluating the impact of conical stem profiles on failure patterns in RTKA. The study by Maslaris et al. investigates this issue by comparing failure modes between conical and cylindrical stem profiles in RTKA.

The study was conducted as a single-center retrospective epidemiological analysis at an orthopaedic teaching hospital. It included all consecutive ReRTKA cases with implant removal, focusing on constrained and semi-constrained implant revisions. The researchers collected demographic data and identified RTKA failure patterns requiring implant removal. Exclusion criteria included cases with only spacer or liner exchange, isolated patella revisions, or revisions due to malignancies. The study stratified RTKA stems into conical–cylindrical or cylindrical–conical designs using preoperative planning software to measure angles. Statistical analyses were performed using IBM SPSS Statistics (Statistical Package for the Social Sciences) to compare differences between groups. The results showed no statistical differences in revision complexity between conical and cylindrical stem designs; however, a subgroup analysis revealed that aseptic loosening occurred more frequently in full-cemented cylindrical stems compared to conical ones.

The main advance from this study is the identification of an association between aseptic loosening and stem profile in failed cemented RTKA implants. While periprosthetic joint infection remains the most common cause of ReRTKA, the study highlights that cemented cylindrical stems may pose a greater risk for aseptic loosening than conical designs. This finding suggests that conical stems could offer mechanical advantages by reducing micromotions at the cement–implant interface, potentially improving long-term outcomes. Future study directions could include larger series with survival rates to further clarify these findings and explore other stem design properties that might impact failure patterns.

Isolated Zone 2 and Zone 3 Cementless Tibial Fixation Shows Early Promise in Revision Total Knee Arthroplasty [274]

This is a machine-generated summary of:

Maniar, Adit R.; Kazarian, Gregory S.; Torres-Ramirez, Ricardo J.; Ranawat, Amar S. Isolated Zone 2 and Zone 3 Cementless Tibial Fixation Shows Early Promise in Revision Total Knee Arthroplasty [274].

Published in: Indian Journal of Orthopaedics (2025).

Link to original: https://doi.org/10.1007/s43465-025-01354-0

If you want to cite the papers, please refer to the original.

For technical reasons we could not place the page where the original quote is coming from.

Research Highlights

As the incidence of primary total knee arthroplasty (TKA) has increased in recent decades, the demand for revision TKA (rTKA) has similarly risen, with expectations for further growth. rTKA presents challenges, particularly due to extensive bone loss in the tibial epiphysis. Traditional fixation methods focus on Zones 1 and 2, but Zone 3 fixation is often necessary to enhance stability. Current techniques for addressing tibial bone loss include cementation, metal augmentation, and bone grafting. The study by Maniar et al. explores the use of unsupported tibial base plates with metaphyseal sleeves and non-cemented stems in rTKA to provide adequate fixation while minimizing bone resection.

The study involved a retrospective review of patients who underwent rTKA using unsupported tibial base plates with metaphyseal sleeves and non-cemented stems. All surgeries were performed by a single surgeon at one center, focusing on complex cases with significant proximal medial bone loss. The surgical technique included removing the existing implant and cement, preparing the tibial canal for the stem and sleeve, and assembling the components without cement fixation. Postoperative radiographs assessed osteointegration and stability of the metaphyseal sleeve. The study reported a 97% survivorship free from revision for aseptic loosening or mechanical failure at an average follow-up of 2.5 years.

The findings suggest that using unsupported tibial base plates with metaphyseal sleeves can bypass extensive epiphyseal bone resection associated with traditional Zone 1 fixation, preserving bone and potentially improving outcomes in rTKA. This approach may offer advantages such as enhanced bony ingrowth due to the absence of cement, which can inhibit compression and settling of the sleeve. Future study could focus on long-term outcomes and comparisons with traditional methods to validate these early results further. The strategy may also facilitate faster surgeries with less technical complexity while maintaining implant stability, although longer follow-up is needed to confirm durability against mechanical forces over time.

Fixation Techniques and Stem Dimensions in Hinged Total Knee Arthroplasty: A Finite Element Study [275]

This is a machine-generated summary of:

El-Zayat, Bilal Farouk; Heyse, Thomas J.; Fanciullacci, Nelson; Labey, Luc; Fuchs-Winkelmann, Susanne; Innocenti, Bernardo Fixation techniques and stem dimensions in hinged total knee arthroplasty: a finite element study [275].

Published in: Archives of Orthopaedic and Trauma Surgery (2016).
Link to original: https://doi.org/10.1007/s00402-016-2571-0

If you want to cite the papers, please refer to the original.

For technical reasons we could not place the page where the original quote is coming from.

Research Highlights

Total knee arthroplasty (TKA) is increasingly common due to an aging and active population, with revision surgeries becoming necessary in a significant percentage of cases. The demand for primary TKAs in the USA is projected to grow substantially, leading to a comparable increase in revision and re-revision procedures. Despite advancements, the clinical outcomes of revision TKA often fall short of primary TKA due to factors like poor bone stock and ligament instability. The study by El-Zayat et al. explores the biomechanical effects of different fixation techniques in revision TKA using a three-dimensional numerical model.

The study employed finite element analysis (FEA) to evaluate stress distribution and micromotions in the tibial bone during lunging and squatting movements. A physiological tibial bone model was created from CT images, and four configurations were analyzed: two stem lengths with cemented and press-fit options. The models simulated surgical procedures, including reaming the intramedullary canal and positioning the stems. Material properties were assigned based on prior studies, and movements were reproduced using musculoskeletal modeling software. The analysis focused on compressive stresses along the stem and micromotions between the implant and bone.

The findings indicate that long cemented stems provide the lowest micromotion and favorable stress distribution compared to shorter or uncemented stems. Cemented stems showed reduced interface stress and micromotion, suggesting better stability. The study supports using cemented stems for improved outcomes in revision TKA, particularly where bone quality is poor. Future study could explore long-term clinical outcomes of these fixation techniques, considering factors like patient age, bone quality variations, and different loading scenarios. These insights could refine surgical decision-making processes for optimizing revision TKA procedures.

Biomechanical Analysis of Patient Specific Cone Vs Conventional Stem in Revision Total Knee Arthroplasty [276]

This is a machine-generated summary of:

Piovan, Gianluca; Bori, Edoardo; Padalino, Marika; Pianigiani, Silvia; Innocenti, Bernardo Biomechanical analysis of patient specific cone vs conventional stem in revision total knee arthroplasty [276].

Published in: Journal of Orthopaedic Surgery and Research (2024).

Link to original: https://doi.org/10.1186/s13018-024-04936-0

If you want to cite the papers, please refer to the original.

For technical reasons we could not place the page where the original quote is coming from.

Research Highlights

Primary Total Knee Arthroplasty (TKA) is a widely used orthopedic procedure aimed at restoring knee function in patients with various pathological conditions. Despite its success, complications such as pain, dissatisfaction, and implant failure can arise post-surgery, necessitating revision surgeries. Revision TKA presents significant surgical challenges due to factors like bone loss and weakened bones, especially in patients with multiple revisions or severe infections. Traditional "off-the-shelf" implants often fall short in addressing these complex cases, leading to the development of patient-specific solutions using advanced manufacturing technologies. The study by Piovan et al., explores the biomechanical benefits of custom-made porous cones compared to traditional revision techniques using finite element modeling.

The study utilized a finite element model based on a real clinical case involving a patient with severe knee conditions who underwent multiple revision surgeries. The researchers designed patient-specific cones for the femur and tibia using CT scans to match the patient's bone geometry. These custom-made cones were compared against traditional revision techniques such as cemented stems and press-fit stems. The study analyzed different configurations, including varying levels of porosity in the custom-made cones, to assess their impact on stress distribution and potential risk of fracture. Static analyses were conducted under conditions simulating daily activities to evaluate the mechanical performance of each technique.

The findings indicate that custom-made cones provide a more uniform stress distribution across the bones compared to traditional techniques, which often result in stress concentration and shielding effects. High-porosity cones demonstrated better osseointegration and reduced risk of fracture due to their ability to transmit stress more effectively to surrounding bone structures. This study highlights the potential of custom-made implants in improving prosthetic stability and reducing complications associated with revision TKA. Future studies could expand on these findings by including a broader range of patient cases and dynamic analyses to further validate the benefits of personalized implant designs in complex orthopedic scenarios.

Changes in Bone Mineral Density of the Distal Femur After Revision Total Knee Arthroplasty with Metaphyseal Press-Fit Stem [277]

This is a machine-generated summary of:

Jensen, Claus L.; Petersen, Michael M.; Schrøder, Henrik M.; Lund, Bjarne Changes in bone mineral density of the distal femur after revision total knee arthroplasty with metaphyseal press-fit stem [277].

Published in: Journal of Orthopaedics and Traumatology (2010).

Link to original: https://doi.org/10.1007/s10195-010-0098-7

If you want to cite the papers, please refer to the original.

For technical reasons we could not place the page where the original quote is coming from.

Research Highlights

Total knee arthroplasty (TKA) and its revision (rTKA) are significant surgical interventions that can lead to bone loss due to factors such as stress shielding, osteolysis, and implant loosening. While bone mineral density (BMD) changes after primary TKA have been studied, the effects of rTKA on BMD, particularly with stemmed femoral implants, remain unexplored. The study by Jensen et al. investigates BMD changes in the distal femur following cemented rTKA with a press-fit stem.

The study involved 16 patients undergoing rTKA, all of whom received NexGen® implants (Zimmer-Biomet, Warsaw, In., USA) with a consistent press-fit femoral stem length. BMD measurements were conducted using dual-energy X-ray absorptiometry (DEXA) scans at various intervals post-surgery. The scans focused on five regions of interest (ROIs) along the femoral shaft and distal femur. The analysis utilized custom software to exclude metal interference in BMD readings. Results showed a significant increase in BMD in ROIs 1–3 during the first 6–12 months post-surgery, although this increase remained significant only in ROI 1 after 1 year. No significant changes were observed in ROI 4 above the stem or in the distal tibia.

The findings suggest that adaptive bone remodeling occurs along the proximal parts of the femoral stem due to altered mechanical loading, consistent with Wolff's law. This study provides new insights into periprosthetic bone remodeling patterns following rTKA with stemmed implants. Future study could explore variations in stem length and their impact on bone remodeling patterns, as well as consider larger sample sizes to enhance result reliability. Understanding these dynamics is crucial for improving surgical outcomes and implant longevity in patients undergoing revision knee surgeries.

A Systematic Review and Meta-analysis of Hybrid vs. Cemented Stems—Which Method Is More Optimal for Revision Total Knee Arthroplasty? [278]

This is a machine-generated summary of:

Thever, Yogen; James Loh, Sir Young; Raghavan, Raghuraman; Toh, Rong Chuin; Moo, Ing How A systematic review and meta-analysis of hybrid vs. cemented stems—which method is more optimal for revision total knee arthroplasty? [278].

Published in: BMC Musculoskeletal Disorders (2024).

Link to original: https://doi.org/10.1186/s12891-024-07389-y

If you want to cite the papers, please refer to the original.

For technical reasons we could not place the page where the original quote is coming from.

Research Highlights

The increasing demand for total knee arthroplasty (TKA) and subsequent revision surgeries poses significant challenges for orthopaedic surgeons, particularly due to bone deficiencies and deformities that complicate implant stability. Intramedullary stems, either cemented or hybrid, are commonly used to enhance stability in revision TKA. However, the optimal fixation method remains controversial, with existing studies offering conflicting results. The study by Thever et al. conducts a systematic review and meta-analysis to compare the outcomes of cemented versus hybrid stem fixation in revision TKA.

The study adhered to the Preferred Reporting Items for Systematic Reviews and Meta-Analyses (PRISMA) guidelines, utilizing databases such as PubMed, Cochrane Library, Embase, and Web of Science to identify relevant studies. The authors included studies published in English that directly compared cemented and hybrid stems in revision TKA with a minimum follow-up period of 2 years. After a rigorous selection process, eight studies were included in the analysis. The meta-analysis employed a random-effects model to assess outcomes such as total re-revision rates and radiological failure. The results indicated no significant difference between the two fixation methods in terms of re-revision rates or radiological loosening, although trends slightly favored hybrid stems.

The findings suggest that both cemented, and hybrid stem fixations offer similar clinical and radiological outcomes in revision TKA. While hybrid stems may provide better alignment and bone preservation, they can also cause end-of-stem pain. Cemented stems offer initial stability but may complicate future revisions. Future study could explore other fixation techniques like metaphyseal cones for enhanced outcomes. The authors recommend considering surgeon expertise and patient-specific factors when choosing the fixation method, as both techniques have proven effective but require further investigation into functional and patient-reported outcomes post-operatively.

Bibliography

1. Della Valle CJ, Berger RA, Rosenberg AG (2006) Surgical exposures in revision total knee arthroplasty. Clin Orthop Relat Res 446:59–68
2. James A, Rand MD, Ries GH, Landis AG, Rosenberg SH (2003) Intraoperative assessment in revision total knee arthroplasty. J Bone Joint Surg Am 85-A(Suppl 1):S26–S37
3. Younger AS, Duncan CP, Masri BA (1998) Surgical exposures in revision total knee arthroplasty. J Am Acad Orthop Surg 6(1):55–64
4. Jones RE, Huo MH (2006) The infected knee: all my troubles now. J Arthroplasty 21(4 Suppl 1):50–53
5. Mendes MW, Caldwell P, Jiranek WA (2004) The results of tibial tubercle osteotomy for revision total knee arthroplasty. J Arthroplasty 19(2):167–174
6. Insall JN, Thompson FM, Brause BD (1983) Two-stage reimplantation for the salvage of infected total knee arthroplasty. J Bone Joint Surg Am 65(8):1087–1098

7. Barrack RL (1999) Specialized exposure for revision total knee arthroplasty: quadriceps snip and patellar turndown. Instr Course Lect 48:149–152
8. Clarke HD (2003) Tibial tubercle osteotomy. J Knee Surg 16(1):58–61
9. Bruni D, Iacono F, Sharma B, Zaffagnini S, Marcacci M (2013) Tibial tubercle osteotomy or quadriceps snip in Two-stage revision for prosthetic knee infection? a randomized prospective study. Clin Orthop Relat Res 471(4):1305–1318
10. Garvin KL, Scuderi G, Insall JN (1995) Evolution of the quadriceps snip. Clin Orthop Relat Res 321:131–137
11. Zanotti RM, Freiberg AA, Matthews LS (1995) Use of patellar allograft to reconstruct a patellar tendon-deficient knee after total joint arthroplasty. J Arthroplasty 10(3):271–274
12. Barrack RL, Smith P, Munn B, Engh G, Rorabeck C (1998) The ranawat award: comparison of surgical approaches in total knee arthroplasty. Clin Orthop Relat Res 356:16–21
13. Zonnenberg CB, Lisowski LA, van den Bekerom MP, Nolte PA (2010) Tuberositas osteotomy for total knee arthroplasty: a review of the literature. J Knee Surg 23(3):121–129
14. Fiddian NJ, Blakeway C, Kumar A (1998) Replacement arthroplasty of the valgus knee. A modified lateral capsular approach with repositioning of vastus lateralis. J Bone Joint Surg Br 80:859–861
15. Keblish PA (2003) The lateral approach for total knee arthroplasty. J Knee Surg 16:62–68
16. Clarke HD (2003) Tibial tubercle osteotomy. J Knee Surg 16:58–61
17. Ries MD, Richman JA (1996) Extended tibial tubercle osteotomy in total knee arthroplasty. J Arthroplasty 11:964–967
18. Piedade SR, Pinaroli A, Servien E, Neyret P (2008) Tibial tubercle osteotomy in primary total knee arthroplasty: a safe procedure or not? Knee 15:439–446
19. Bruce WJ, Rooney J, Hutabarat SR, Atkinson MC, Goldberg JA, Walsh WR (2000) Exposure in difficult total knee arthroplasty using coronal tibial tubercle osteotomy. J Orthop Surg (Hong Kong) 8:61–65
20. Chalidis BE, Ries MD (2009) Does repeat tibial tubercle osteotomy or intramedullary extension affect the union rate in revision total knee arthroplasty? A retrospective study of 74 patients. Acta Orthop 80(4):426–431
21. Deane CR, Ferran NA, Ghandour A, Morgan-Jones RL (2008) Tibial tubercle osteotomy for access during revision knee arthroplasty: Ethibond suture repair technique. BMC Musculoskelet Disord 9:98
22. Whiteside LA, Ohl MD (1990) Tibial tubercle osteotomy for exposure of the difficult total knee arthroplasty. Clin Orthop Relat Res 260:6–9
23. Maruyama M (1997) Tibial tubercle osteotomy in revision total knee arthroplasty. Arch Orthop Trauma Surg 116(6–7):400–403
24. Hirschmann MT, Hofmann M, Krause R et al (2010) Anterolateral approach with tibial tubercle osteotomy versus standard medial approach for primary total knee arthroplasty: does it matter? BMC Musculoskelet Disord 11:167

25. Arnold MP, Friederich NF, Widmer H et al (1999) Lateraler Zugang zum Kniegelenk mit Osteotomie der Tuberositas tibiae. Oper Orthop Traumatol 3(11):223–232
26. van den Broek CM, van Hellemondt GG, Jacobs WC, Wymenga AB (2006) Step-cut tibial tubercle osteotomy for access in revision total knee replacement. Knee 13:430–434
27. Arredondo J, Worland RL, Jessup DE (1998) Nonunion after a tibial shaft fracture complicating tibial tubercule osteotomy. J Arthroplasty 13(8):958–960
28. Wolff AM, Hungerford DS, Krackow KA, Jacobs MA (1989) Osteotomy of the tibial tubercle during total knee replacement. A report of 26 cases. J Bone Jt Surg Am 71(6):848–852
29. Del Pozo JL, Patel R (2009) Clinical practice. Infection associated with prosthetic joints. N Engl J Med 361:787–794. https://doi.org/10.1056/NEJMcp0905029
30. Dolin MG (1983) Osteotomy of the tibial tubercle in total knee replacement. A technical note. J Bone Joint Surg Am 65(5):704–706
31. Insall JN, Dorr LD, Scott RD, Scott WN (1989) Rationale of the Knee Society clinical rating system. Clin Orthop Relat Res 248:13–14
32. Bellamy N, Buchanan WW, Goldsmith CH, Campbell J, Stitt LW (1988) Validation study of WOMAC: a health status instrument for measuring clinically important patient relevant outcomes to antirheumatic drug therapy in patients with osteoarthritis of the hip or knee. J Rheumatol 15(12):1833–1840
33. Whiteside LA (1995) Exposure in difficult total knee arthroplasty using tibial tubercle osteotomy. Clin Orthop Relat Res 321:92–97
34. Whiteside LA, Ohl MD (1990) Tibial tubercle osteotomy for exposure of the difficult total knee arthroplasty. Clin Orthop Relat Res 260:6–9
35. Young CF, Bourne RB, Rorabeck CH (2008) Tibial tubercle osteotomy in total knee arthroplasty surgery. J Arthroplasty 23:371–375
36. Insall JN, Dorr LD, Scott RD, Scott WN: Rationale of the Knee Society clinical rating system. Clin Orthop Relat Res. 1989, 13-14. 248
37. Bach CM, Nogler M, Steingruber IE, Ogon M, Wimmer C, Gobel G, Krismer M: Scoring systems in total knee arthroplasty. Clin Orthop Relat Res. 2002, 184-196. https://doi.org/10.1097/00003086-200206000-00022.399
38. Karachalios T, Sarangi PP, Newman JH (1994) Severe varus and valgus deformities treated by total knee arthroplasty. J Bone Joint Surg 76(6):938–942
39. Stern SH, Moeckel BH, Insall JN (1991) Total knee arthroplasty in valgus knees. Clin Orthop Relat Res 273:5–8
40. Whiteside L, Ohl M (1990) Tibial tubercle osteotomy for exposure of the difficult total knee arthroplasty. Clin Orthop Relat Res 260:6–9
41. Bellamy N, Buchanan WW, Goldsmith CH, Campbell J, Stitt LW (1988) Validation study of WOMAC: a health status instrument for measuring clinically important patient relevant outcomes to antirheumatic drug therapy in patients with osteoarthritis of the hip or knee. J Rheumatol 15(12):1833–1840
42. Insall JN, Dorr LD, Scott RD, Scott WN (1989) Rationale of the knee society clinical rating system. Clin Orthop Relat Res 248:13–14

43. Hay G, Kampshoff J, Kuster M (2010) Lateral subvastus approach with osteotomy of the tibial tubercle for total knee replacement: a two-year prospective, randomised, blinded controlled trial. J Bone Joint Surg 92(6):862–866. https://doi.org/10.1302/0301-620x.92b6.24027
44. Nikolopoulos DD, Polyzois I, Apostolopoulos AP et al (2011) Total knee arthroplasty in severe valgus knee deformity: comparison of a standard medial parapatellar approach combined with tibial tubercle osteotomy. Knee Surg Sports Traumatol Arthrosc 19(11):1834–1842
45. Apostolopoulos AP, Nikolopoulos DD, Polyzois I et al (2010) Total knee arthroplasty in severe valgus deformity: interest of combining a lateral approach with a tibial tubercle osteotomy. Orthop Traumatol Surg Res 96(7):777–784
46. Chalidis BE, Ye K, Sachinis NP, Hawdon G, McMahon S (2013) Lateral parapatellar approach with tibial tubercle osteotomy for the treatment of non-correctable valgus knee osteoarthritis: a retrospective clinical study. Knee. https://doi.org/10.1016/j.knee.2013.05.008
47. Denham RA, Bishop RE (1978) Mechanics of the knee and problems in reconstructive surgery. J Bone Joint Surg Br 60-B(3):345–352
48. Dolin MG (1983) Osteotomy of the tibial tubercle in total knee replacement. A technical note. J Bone Joint Surg Am 65(5):704–706
49. Sun Z, Patil A, Song EK, Kim HT, Seon JK, (2015) Comparison of quadriceps snip and tibial tubercle osteotomy in revision for infected total knee arthroplasty International Orthopaedics (SICOT). 39:879–885 https://doi.org/10.1007/s00264-014-2546-0
50. Vajapey SP, Blackwell RE, Maki AJ, Miller TL (2019) Treatment of extensor tendon disruption after total knee arthroplasty: a systematic review. J Arthroplast 34:1279–1286. https://doi.org/10.1016/j.arth.2019.02.046
51. Shi SM, Shi GG, Laurent EM, Ninomiya JT (2019) Modified V-Y turndown flap augmentation for quadriceps tendon rupture following total knee arthroplasty: a retrospective study. J Bone Joint Surg Am 101-A:1010–1015. https://doi.org/10.2106/JBJS.18.01098
52. Chhapan J, Sankineani SR, Chiranjeevi T, Reddy MV, Reddy D, Gurava Reddy AV (2018) Early quadriceps tendon rupture after primary total knee arthroplasty. Knee 25:192–194. https://doi.org/10.1016/j.knee.2017.12.002
53. Kim TW, Kamath AF (2011) Israelite CL (2011). Suture anchor repair of quadriceps tendon rupture after total knee arthroplasty. J Arthroplast 26:817–820. https://doi.org/10.1016/j.arth.2011.01.006
54. Nodzo SR, Rachala SR (2016) Polypropylene mesh augmentation for complete quadriceps rupture after total knee arthroplasty. Knee 23:177–180. https://doi.org/10.1016/j.knee.2015.09.007
55. Fernandez-Baillo N, Garay EG, Ordonez JM (1993) Rupture of the quadriceps tendon after total knee arthroplasty: a case report. J Arthroplast 8:331–333. https://doi.org/10.1016/s0883-5403(06)80097-5
56. Daines BK, Dennis DA. Gap balancing vs. measured resection technique in total knee arthroplasty. Clin Orthop Surg. 2014;6(1):1–8. https://doi.org/10.4055/cios.2014.6.1.1

57. Hernández-Hermoso JA, Nescolarde L, Yañez-Siller F, Calle-García J, Garcia-Perdomo D, Pérez-Andres R. Combined femoral and tibial component total knee arthroplasty device rotation measurement is reliable and predicts clinical outcome. J Orthop Traumatol. 2023;24:140. https://doi.org/10.1186/s10195-023-00718-2
58. Migliorini F, Eschweiler J, Mansy YE, Quack V, Schenker H, Tingart M, Driessen A. Gap balancing versus measured resection for primary total knee arthroplasty: a meta-analysis study. Arch Orthop Trauma Surg. 2020;140(9):1245–53. https://doi.org/10.1007/s00402-020-03478-4
59. Glowalla C, Langer S, Lenze U, Lazic I, Hirschmann MT, Hinterwimmer F, et al. Postoperative full leg radiographs exhibit less residual coronal varus deformity compared to intraoperative measurements in robotic arm-assisted total knee arthroplasty with the mako™ system. Knee Surg Sports Traumatol Arthrosc. 2023;31(9):3912–8. https://doi.org/10.1007/s00167-023-07386-z
60. Nam CH, Lee SC, Kim JH, Ahn HS, Baek JH. Robot-assisted total knee arthroplasty improves mechanical alignment and accuracy of component positioning compared to the conventional technique. J Exp Orthop. 2022;9:1108. https://doi.org/10.1186/s40634-022-00546-z
61. Young SW, Zeng N, Tay ML, Fulker D, Esposito C, Carter M, et al. A prospective randomised controlled trial of mechanical axis with soft tissue release balancing vs functional alignment with bony resection balancing in total knee replacement-a study using stryker mako robotic arm-assisted technology. Trials. 2022;23:1580. https://doi.org/10.1186/s13063-022-06494-4
62. Sires JD, Craik JD, Wilson CJ. Accuracy of bone resection in mako total knee robotic-assisted surgery. J Knee Surg. 2021;34:7:745–8. https://doi.org/10.1055/s-0039-1700570
63. Oussedik S, Abdel MP, Victor J, Pagnano MW, Haddad FS. Alignment in total knee arthroplasty. Bone Joint J. 2020. https://doi.org/10.1302/0301-620X.102B3.BJJ-2019-1729. 102-B:3:276-9.
64. Lee JH, Kwon SC, Hwang JH, Lee JK, Kim JI. Functional alignment maximises advantages of robotic arm-assisted total knee arthroplasty with better patient-reported outcomes compared to mechanical alignment. Knee Surg Sports Traumatol Arthrosc. 2024;32(4):896–906. https://doi.org/10.1002/ksa.12120
65. Lee HJ, Lee JS, Jung HJ, Song KS, Yang JJ, Park CW. Comparison of joint line position changes after primary bilateral total knee arthroplasty performed using the navigation-assisted measured gap resection or gap balancing techniques. Knee Surg Sports Traumatol Arthrosc. 2011;19:122027–32. https://doi.org/10.1007/s00167-011-1468-2
66. Tapasvi SR, Shekhar A, Patil SS, Dipane MV, Chowdhry M, McPherson EJ. Comparison of gap balancing vs measured resection technique in patients undergoing simultaneous bilateral total knee arthroplasty: one technique per knee. J Arthroplasty. 2020;35:3732–40. https://doi.org/10.1016/j.arth.2019.10.002

67. Babazadeh S, Dowsey MM, Vasimalla MG, Stoney JD, Choong PFM. Gap balancing sacrifices joint-line maintenance to improve gap symmetry: 5-year follow-up of a randomized controlled trial. J Arthroplasty. 2018;33:175–8. https://doi.org/10.1016/j.arth.2017.08.021
68. Zhang Y, Zhang Y, Sun JN, An L, Chen XY, Feng S. Comparison of outcomes between gap balancing and measured resection techniques for total knee arthroplasty: a prospective, randomized, controlled trial. Acta Orthop Traumatol Turc. 2021;55:3239–45. https://doi.org/10.5152/j.aott.2021.20160
69. Tigani D, Sabbioni G, Ben Ayad R, Filanti M, Rani N, Del Piccolo N. Comparison between two computer-assisted total knee arthroplasty: gap-balancing versus measured resection technique. Knee Surg Sports Traumatol Arthrosc. 2010;18(10):1304–10. https://doi.org/10.1007/s00167-010-1124-2
70. Heesterbeek PJ, Jacobs WC, Wymenga AB. Effects of the balanced gap technique on femoral component rotation in tka. Clin Orthop Relat Res. 2009;467(4):1015–22. https://doi.org/10.1007/s11999-008-0539-2
71. Mihalko WM, Saleh KJ, Krackow KA, Whiteside LA. Soft-tissue balancing during total knee arthroplasty in the varus knee. J Am Acad Orthop Surg. 2009;17(12):766–74.
72. Lustig S, Bruderer J, Servien E, Neyret P. The bone cuts and ligament balance in total knee arthroplasty: the third way using computer assisted surgery. Knee. 2009;16(2):91.
73. Hananouchi T, Yamamoto K, AndoW FK, Ohzono K. The intraoperative gap difference (flexion gap minus extension gap) is altered by insertion of the trial femoral component. Knee. 2012;19:601–5.
74. Matsumoto T, Muratsu H, Kawakami Y, Takayama K, Ishida K, Matsushita T, et al. Soft-tissue balancing in total knee arthroplasty: cruciate-retaining versus posterior-stabilised, and measured-resection versus gap technique. Int Orthop. 2014;38(3):531–7.
75. Heesterbeek PJC, Haffner N, Wymenga AB, Stifter J, Ritschl P. Patient-related factors influence stiffness of the soft tissue complex during intraoperative gap balancing in cruciate-retaining total knee arthroplasty. Knee Surg Sports Traumatol Arthrosc. 2017;25(9):2760–8.
76. Wyss TF, Schuster AJ, Munger P, Pfluger D, Wehrli U: Does total knee joint replacement with the soft tissue balancing surgical technique maintain the natural joint line?. Arch Orthop Trauma Surg. 2006, 126 (7): 480-486. 10.1007/s00402-006-0171-0.
77. Agarwal N, To K, McDonnell S, Khan W (2020) Clinical and radiological outcomes in robotic-assisted total knee arthroplasty: a systematic review and meta-analysis. J Arthroplasty 35:3393-3409.e2. https://doi.org/10.1016/j.arth.2020.03.005
78. Chen AF, Kazarian GS, Jessop GW, Makhdom A (2018) Robotic technology in orthopaedic surgery. J Bone Joint Surg 100:1984–1992. https://doi.org/10.2106/JBJS.17.01397

79. Kayani B, Konan S, Ayuob A et al (2019) Robotic technology in total knee arthroplasty: a systematic review. EFORT Open Reviews 4:611–617. https://doi.org/10.1302/2058-5241.4.190022
80. Vanlommel L, Neven E, Anderson MB et al (2021) The initial learning curve for the ROSA® Knee System can be achieved in 6–11 cases for operative time and has similar 90-day complication rates with improved implant alignment compared to manual instrumentation in total knee arthroplasty. J Exp Ortop 8:119. https://doi.org/10.1186/s40634-021-00438-8
81. Haffar A, Krueger CA (2022) Goh, Lonner GS Total knee arthroplasty with robotic surgical assistance results in less physician stress and strain than conventional methods. J Arthroplasty 37(6S):S193–S200. https://doi.org/10.1016/j.arth.2021.11.021. (Epub 2022 Feb 17)
82. Yaffe M, Luo M, Goyal N et al (2014) Clinical, functional, and radiographic outcomes following total knee arthroplasty with patient-specific instrumentation, computer-assisted surgery, and manual instrumentation: a short-term follow-up study. Int J Comput Assist Radiol Surg 9:837–844. https://doi.org/10.1007/s11548-013-0968-6
83. Meneghini RM, Ziemba-Davis MM, Lovro LR et al (2016) Can intraoperative sensors determine the "target" ligament balance? Early outcomes in total knee arthroplasty. J Arthroplasty 31:2181–2187. https://doi.org/10.1016/j.arth.2016.03.046
84. Aunan E, Kibsgård TJ, Diep LM, Röhrl SM (2015) Intraoperative ligament laxity influences functional outcome 1 year after total knee arthroplasty. Knee Surg Sport Traumatol Arthrosc 23:1684–1692. https://doi.org/10.1007/s00167-014-3108-0
85. Azukizawa M, Kuriyama S, Nakamura S et al (2018) Intraoperative medial joint laxity in flexion decreases patient satisfaction after total knee arthroplasty. Arch Orthop Trauma Surg 138:1143–1150. https://doi.org/10.1007/s00402-018-2965-2
86. Gustke KA, Golladay GJ, Roche MW et al (2014) Increased satisfaction after total knee replacement using sensor-guided technology. Bone Jt J 96B:1333–1338. https://doi.org/10.1302/0301-620X.96B10.34068
87. Luring C, Hüfner T, Kendoff D et al (2006) Eversion or subluxation of patella in soft tissue balancing of total knee arthroplasty? Results of a cadaver experiment. Knee 13:15–18. https://doi.org/10.1016/j.knee.2004.09.007
88. Lee DS, Song EK, Seon JK, Park SJ (2011) Effect of balanced gap total knee arthroplasty on intraoperative laxities and femoral component rotation. J Arthroplasty 26(5):699–704. https://doi.org/10.1016/j.arth.2010.06.005
89. Tokuhara Y, Kadoya Y, Nakagawa S, Kobayashi A, Takaoka K (2004) The flexion gap in normal knees: an MRI study. J Bone Joint Surg Br 86(8):1133–1136
90. Whiteside LA, Saeki K, Mihalko WM (2000) Functional medial ligament balancing in total knee arthroplasty. Clin Orthop Relat Res 380:45–57

91. Lotke PA, Carolan GF, Puri N (2006) Impaction grafting for bone defects in revision total knee arthroplasty. Clin Orthop Relat Res 446:99–103. https://doi.org/10.1097/01.blo.0000214414.06464.00
92. Hilgen V, Citak M, Vettorazzi E, Haasper C, Day K, Amling M, Gehrke T, Gebauer M (2013) 10-year results following impaction bone grafting of major bone defects in 29 rotational and hinged knee revision arthroplasties: a follow-up of a previous report. Acta Orthop 84(4):387–391. https://doi.org/10.3109/17453674.2013.814012
93. Steens W, Loehr JF, Wodtke J, Katzer A (2008) Morselized bone grafting in revision arthroplasty of the knee—a retrospective analysis of 34 reconstructions after 2–9 years. Acta Orthopaedica 79(5):683–688
94. Lonner JH, Lotke PA, Kim J, Nelson C (2002) Impaction grafting and wire mesh for uncontained defects in revision knee arthroplasty. Clin Orthop Relat Res 404:145–151. https://doi.org/10.1097/00003086-200211000-00026
95. Engh GA, Ammeen DJ (1999) Bone loss with revision total knee arthroplasty: defect classification and alternatives for reconstruction. Instr Course Lect 48:167–175
96. Daines BK, Dennis DA. Management of bone defects in revision total knee arthroplasty. Instr Course Lect. 2013;62:341–8.
97. Dennis DA, Berry DJ, Engh G, et al. Revision total knee arthroplasty. J Am Acad Orthop Surg. 2008;16(8):442–54.
98. Hanna SA, Aston WJS, de Roeck NJ, Gough-Palmer A, Powles DP. Cementless revision TKA with bone grafting of osseous defects restores bone stock with a low revision rate at 4 to 10 years. Clin Orthop. 2011;469(11):3164–71. https://doi.org/10.1007/s11999-011-1938-3.
99. Vasso M, Beaufils P, Cerciello S, Schiavone PA. Bone loss following knee arthroplasty: potential treatment options. Arch Orthop Trauma Surg. 2014;134(4):543–53. https://doi.org/10.1007/s00402-014-1941-8
100. Haidukewych GJ, Hanssen A, Jones RD. Metaphyseal fixation in revision total knee arthroplasty: indications and techniques. J Am Acad Orthop Surg. 2011;19(6):311–8.
101. Huff TW, Sculco TP. Management of bone loss in revision total knee arthroplasty. J Arthroplasty. 2007;22(7, Supplement):32–6. https://doi.org/10.1016/j.arth.2007.05.022
102. Shen C, Lichstein PM, Austin MS, Sharkey PF, Parvizi J. Revision knee Arthroplasty for bone loss: choosing the right degree of constraint. J Arthroplasty. 2014;29(1):127–31. Available from: http://www.sciencedirect.com/science/article/pii/S088354031300346X. https://doi.org/10.1016/j.arth.2013.04.042.
103. Mabry TM, Hanssen AD. The role of stems and augments for bone loss in revision knee arthroplasty. J Arthroplasty. 2007;22(4, Supplement):56–60. https://doi.org/10.1016/j.arth.2007.02.008
104. Panni AS, Vasso M, Cerciello S. Modular augmentation in revision total knee arthroplasty. Knee Surg Sports Traumatol Arthrosc. 2013;21(12):2837–43. https://doi.org/10.1007/s00167-012-2258-1

105. Engh GA, Ammeen DJ (2007) Use of structural allograft in revision total knee arthroplasty in knees with severe tibial bone loss. J Bone Jt Surg Am 89(12):2640–2647. https://doi.org/10.2106/JBJS.F.00865
106. Backstein D, Safir O, Gross A. Management of bone loss: structural grafts in revision total knee arthroplasty. Clin Orthop. 2006;446:104–12. https://doi.org/10.1097/01.blo.0000214426.52206.2c .
107. Bauman RD, Lewallen DG, Hanssen AD (2009) Limitations of structural allograft in revision total knee arthroplasty. Clin Orthop Relat Res 467(3):818–824. https://doi.org/10.1007/s11999-008-0679-4
108. Long WJ, Scuderi GR. Porous tantalum cones for large metaphyseal tibial defects in revision total knee arthroplasty: a minimum 2-year follow-up. J Arthroplasty. 2009;24(7):1086–92. https://doi.org/10.1016/j.arth.2008.08.011.
109. Meneghini RM, Lewallen DG, Hanssen AD. Use of porous tantalum metaphyseal cones for severe tibial bone loss during revision total knee replacement. J Bone Joint Surg Am. 2008;90(1):78–84. https://doi.org/10.2106/JBJS.F.01495
110. Howard JL, Kudera J, Lewallen DG, Hanssen AD. Early results of the use of tantalum femoral cones for revision total knee arthroplasty. J Bone Joint Surg Am. 2011;93(5):478–84. https://doi.org/10.2106/JBJS.I.01322
111. Lachiewicz PF, Bolognesi MP, Henderson RA, Soileau ES, Vail TP. Can tantalum cones provide fixation in complex revision knee arthroplasty? Clin Orthop. 2012;470(1):199–204. https://doi.org/10.1007/s11999-011-1888-9
112. Huang R, Barrazueta G, Ong A, et al. Revision total knee arthroplasty using metaphyseal sleeves at short-term follow-up. Orthopedics. 2014;37(9):e804–9. https://doi.org/10.3928/01477447-20140825-57. *The authors provide short-term data to support the use of metaphyseal sleeves in the largest cohort studied to date and the only report on both tibial and femoral sleeves using both nonhinged and hinged designs.*
113. Schwartz AM, Farley KX, Guild GN, Bradbury TL Jr (2020) Projections and epidemiology of revision hip and knee arthroplasty in the United States to 2030. J Arthroplasty 35(6S):S79–S85. https://doi.org/10.1016/j.arth.2020.02.030
114. Russo A, Cavagnaro L, Chiarlone F, Alessio-Mazzola M, Felli L, Burastero G (2022) Predictors of failure of two-stage revision in periprosthetic knee infection: a retrospective cohort study with a minimum two-year follow-up. Arch Orthop Trauma Surg 142(3):481–490. https://doi.org/10.1007/s00402-021-04265-5
115. Morgan-Jones R, Oussedik SI, Graichen H, Haddad FS (2015) Zonal fixation in revision total knee arthroplasty. Bone Joint J 97-B(2):147–149. https://doi.org/10.1302/0301-620X.97B2.34144
116. Russo A, Clemente A, Masse A, Burastero G (2023) Medial gastrocnemius rotational flap for the reconstruction of extensor mechanism disruption in periprosthetic knee infections: a retrospective series with minimum two year

follow-up. Int Orthop 47(4):983–993. https://doi.org/10.1007/s00264-023-05716-x
117. Parvizi J, Tan TL, Goswami K, Higuera C, Della Valle C, Chen AF, Shohat N (2018) The 2018 definition of periprosthetic hip and knee infection: an evidence-based and validated criteria. J Arthroplasty 33(5):1309-1314 e2. https://doi.org/10.1016/j.arth.2018.02.078
118. Benjamin J, Engh G, Parsley B, Donaldson T, Coon T (2001) Morselized bone grafting of defects in revision total knee arthroplasty. Clin Orthop Relat Res 392:62–67
119. Ries MD (1996) Impacted cancellous autograft for contained bone defects in total knee arthroplasty. Am J Knee Surg 9:51–54
120. Engh GA, Ammeen DJ (1999) Bone loss with revision total knee arthroplasty: defect classification and alternatives for reconstruction. Instr Course Lect 48:167–175
121. Engh GA (2004) Structural femoral head allografting with revision TKA. Orthopedics 27:999–1000
122. Haidukewych GJ, Hanssen A, Jones RD (2011) Metaphyseal fixation in revision total knee arthroplasty: indications and techniques. J Am Acad Orthop Surg 19(6):311–318
123. Schildhauer TA, Peter E, Muhr G, Koller M (2009) Activation of human leukocytes on tantalum trabecular metal in comparison to commonly used orthopedic metal implant materials. J Biomed Mater Res A 88:332–341
124. Schildhauer TA, Robie B, Muhr G, Koller M (2006) Bacterial adherence to tantalum versus commonly used orthopedic metallic implant materials. J Orthop Trauma 20:476–484
125. Morgan-Jones R, Oussedik SI, Graichen H, Haddad FS. Zonal fixation in revision total knee arthroplasty. Bone Joint J. 2015;97-B(2):147-9.
126. Patel NK, Kim EG, Chughtai M, Khlopas A, Elmallah RD, Harwin SF, Delanois RE, Mont MA. Highly porous metaphyseal cones in revision total knee arthroplasty: a case series. J Knee Surg. 2016;29(8):614–20.
127. Denehy KM, Abhari S, Krebs VE, Higuera-Rueda CA, Samuel LT, Sultan AA, Mont MA, Malkani AL (2019) Metaphyseal fixation using highly porous cones in revision total knee arthroplasty: minimum two year follow up study. J Arthroplast 34(10):2439–2443. https://doi.org/10.1016/j.arth.2019.03.045
128. Tetreault MW, Perry KI, Pagnano MW, Hanssen AD, Abdel MP. Excellent two-year survivorship of 3D-printed metaphyseal cones in revision total knee arthroplasty. Bone Joint J. 2020;102-B(6_Supple_A):107-115.
129. Remily EA, Dávila Castrodad IM, Mohamed NS, Wilkie WA, Kelemen MN, Delanois RE. Short-term outcomes of 3D-printed titanium metaphyseal cones in revision total knee arthroplasty. Orthopedics. 2021;44(1):43–7.
130. Chalmers BP, Malfer CM, Mayman DJ, Westrich GH, Sculco PK, Bostrom MP, Jerabek SA. Early survivorship of newly designed highly porous metaphyseal tibial cones in revision total knee arthroplasty. Arthroplast Today. 2021;23(8):5–10.

131. Monárrez R, Bains SS, Chen Z, Sax OC, Salib CG, Mont MA, Delanois RE. Two-year survivorship and outcomes of a three-dimensional printed metaphyseal cone in the setting of revision total knee arthroplasty. J Knee Surg. 2022;35(14):1540–3.
132. Potter GD 3rd, Abdel MP, Lewallen DG, Hanssen AD (2016) Midterm results of porous tantalum femoral cones in revision total knee arthroplasty. J Bone Jt Surg Am. 98(15):1286–1291. https://doi.org/10.2106/JBJS.15.00874
133. Maslaris A, Layher F, Bungartz M et al (2019) Sagittal profile has a significant impact on the explantability of well-fixed cemented stems in revision knee arthroplasty: a biomechanical comparison study of five established knee implant models. Arch Orthop Trauma Surg 139:991–998. https://doi.org/10.1007/s00402-019-03160-4
134. Meijer MF, Boerboom AL, Stevens M et al (2017) Tibial component with and without stem extension in a trabecular metal cone construct. Knee Surg Sports Traumatol Arthrosc Off J ESSKA 25:3644–3652. https://doi.org/10.1007/s00167-016-4271-2
135. Faizan A, Bhowmik-Stoker M, Alipit V, Kirk AE, Krebs VE, Harwin SF, Meneghini RM. Development and verification of novel porous titanium metaphyseal cones for revision total knee arthroplasty. J Arthroplasty. 2017;32(6):1946–53.
136. Sandiford NA, Misur P, Garbuz DS et al (2017) No difference between trabecular metal cones and femoral head allografts in revision TKA: minimum 5-year followup. Clin Orthop 475:118–124. https://doi.org/10.1007/s11999-016-4898-9
137. Wirries N, Winnecken HJ, von Lewinski G et al (2019) Osteointegrative sleeves for metaphyseal defect augmentation in revision total knee arthroplasty: clinical and radiological 5-year follow-up. J Arthroplasty. https://doi.org/10.1016/j.arth.2019.04.024
138. Abdelaziz H, Jaramillo R, Gehrke T, Ohlmeier M, Citak M (2019) Clinical survivorship of aseptic revision total knee arthroplasty using hinged knees and tantalum cones at minimum 10-year follow-up. J Arthroplasty 34:3018–3022
139. Bohl DD, Brown NM, McDowell MA et al (2018) Do porous tantalum metaphyseal cones improve outcomes in revision total knee arthroplasty? J Arthroplasty 33:171–177. https://doi.org/10.1016/j.arth.2017.07.033
140. Burastero G, Cavagnaro L, Chiarlone F, Alessio-Mazzola M, Carrega G, Felli L (2018) The use of tantalum metaphyseal cones for the management of severe bone defects in septic knee revision. J Arthroplasty 33(12):3739–3745. https://doi.org/10.1016/j.arth.2018.08.026
141. Agarwal S, Neogi DS, Morgan-Jones R (2018) Metaphyseal sleeves in revision total knee arthroplasty: minimum seven-year follow-up study. Knee. https://doi.org/10.1016/j.knee.2018.09.010
142. Kim HJ, Lee OS, Lee SH, Lee YS. Comparative analysis between cone and sleeve in managing severe bone defect during revision total knee arthroplasty: a systematic review and meta-analysis. J Knee Surg. 2018;31(7):677–85.

143. Huten D, Pasquier G, Lambotte JC (2021) Techniques for filling tibiofemoral bone defects during revision total knee arthroplasty. Orthop Traumatol: Surg Res 107(1):102776
144. Schmitz H-CR, Klauser W, Citak M, Al-Khateeb H, Gehrke T, Kendoff D. Three-year follow up utilizing tantal cones in revision total knee arthroplasty. J Arthroplasty. 2013;28(9):1556–60. https://doi.org/10.1016/j.arth.2013.01.028
145. De Martino I, De Santis V, Sculco PK, D'Apolito R, Assini JB, Gasparini G. Tantalum Cones provide durable mid-term fixation in revision TKA. Clin Orthop Relat Res. 2015;473(10):3176–82.
146. Burastero G, Cavagnaro L, Chiarlone F, Innocenti B, Felli L (2018) A case report: custom made porous titanium implants in revision: a new option for complex issues. Open Orthop J 12(1):66
147. Cherny AA, Kovalenko AN, Kulyaba TA, Kornilov NN (2021) A prospective study on outcome of patient-specific cones in revision knee arthroplasty. Arch Orthop Trauma Surg 141(12):2277–2286. https://doi.org/10.1007/s00402-021-04047-z
148. Breer S, Hahn M, Kendoff D, Krause M, Koehne T, Haasper C, Gehrke T, Amling M, Gebauer M (2012) Histological ex vivo analysis of retrieved human tantalum augmentations. Int Orthop 36:2269–2274
149. Divano S, Cavagnaro L, Zanirato A, Basso M, Felli L, Formica M. Porous metal cones: gold standard for massive bone loss in complex revision knee arthroplasty? A systematic review of current literature. Arch Orthop Trauma Surg. 2018;138(6):851–63.
150. Zanirato A, Formica M, Cavagnaro L, Divano S, Burastero G, Felli L. Metaphyseal cones and sleeves in revision total knee arthroplasty: Two sides of the same coin? Complications, clinical and radiological results-a systematic review of the literature. Musculoskelet Surg. 2020;104(1):25–35.
151. Huten D, Pasquier G, Lambotte JC (2020) Techniques for filling tibiofemoral bone defects during revision total knee arthroplasty. Orthop Traumatol Surg Res 13:102776. https://doi.org/10.1016/j.otsr.2020.102776
152. Belt M, Smulders K, van Houten A, Wymenga A, Heesterbeek P, van Hellemondt G (2020) What is the reliability of a new classification for bone defects in revision TKA based on preoperative radiographs? Clin Orthop Relat Res 478(9):2057–2064. https://doi.org/10.1097/CORR.0000000000001084
153. Cornell CN (2020) CORR Insights®: what is the reliability of a new classification for bone defects in revision TKA based on preoperative radiographs? Clin Orthop Relat Res 478(9):2065–2066. https://doi.org/10.1097/CORR.0000000000001145
154. Sheth NP, Bonadio MB, Demange MK (2017) bone loss in revision total knee arthroplasty: evaluation and management. J Am Acad Orthop Surg 25:348–357. https://doi.org/10.5435/JAAOS-D-15-00660

155. Scuderi GR, Bourne RB, Noble PC, Benjamin JB, Lonner JH, Scott WN. The new Knee Society knee scoring system. Clin Orthop Relat Res. 2012;470(1):3–19.
156. Gonzalez Della Valle A, Sharrock N, Barlow M, Caceres L, Go G, Salvati EA. The modern, hybrid total hip arthroplasty for primary osteoarthritis at the Hospital for Special Surgery. Bone Joint J. 2016;98-B(1 Suppl A):54–9.
157. Dawson J, Fitzpatrick R, Murray D, Carr A (1998) Questionnaire on the perceptions of patients about total knee replacement. J Bone Jt Surg Br 80(1):63–69
158. Barnett SL, Mayer RR, Gondusky JS, Choi L, Patel JJ, Gorab RS. Use of stepped porous titanium metaphyseal sleeves for tibial defects in revision total knee arthroplasty: short term results. J Arthroplasty. 2014;29(6):1219–24. https://doi.org/10.1016/j.arth.2013.12.026
159. Dennis DA, Little LR. The structural allograft composite in revision total knee arthroplasty. Orthopedics. 2005;28(9):1005–7.
160. Behery OA, Shing EZ, Yu Z et al (2021) Survivorship and radiographic evaluation of metaphyseal cones with short cemented stems in revision total knee arthroplasty. J Arthroplasty 37:330–335. https://doi.org/10.1016/j.arth.2021.10.027
161. Kamath AF, Lewallen DG, Hanssen AD. Porous tantalum metaphyseal cones for severe tibial bone loss in revision knee arthroplasty: a five to nine-year follow-up. J Bone Joint Surg Am. 2015;97(3):216–23. https://doi.org/10.2106/JBJS.N.00540. *Authors and surgeon-developers of the metaphyseal cone demonstrate durable clinical results and radiographic fixation over the longest course of follow-up using this technology.*
162. Tetreault MW, Perry KI, Pagnano MW et al (2020) Excellent two-year survivorship of 3D-printed metaphyseal cones in revision total knee arthroplasty. Bone Jt J 102-B(6_Suppl A):107–115. https://doi.org/10.1302/0301-620X.102B6.BJJ-2019-1544.R1
163. Kang SG, Park CH, Song SJ (2018) Stem fixation in revision total knee arthroplasty: indications, stem dimensions, and fixation methods. Knee Surg Relat Res 30:187–192. https://doi.org/10.5792/ksrr.18.019
164. Jacquet C, Ros F, Guy S et al (2021) Trabecular metal cones combined with short cemented stem allow favorable outcomes in aseptic revision total knee arthroplasty. J Arthroplasty 36:657–663. https://doi.org/10.1016/j.arth.2020.08.058
165. Engh GA, Ammeen DJ (1998) Classification and preoperative radiographic evaluation: knee. Orthop Clin North Am 29:205–217. https://doi.org/10.1016/s0030-5898(05)70319-9
166. Pfeifer R, Sellei R, Pape HC (2010) The biology of intramedullary reaming. Injury 41:S4–S8. https://doi.org/10.1016/S0020-1383(10)70002-4
167. Haas SB, Insall JN, Montgomery W 3rd, Windsor RE (1995) Revision total knee arthroplasty with use of modular components with stems inserted without cement. J Bone Jt Surg Am 77(11):1700–1707. https://doi.org/10.2106/00004623-199511000-00009

168. Fleischman AN, Azboy I, Fuery M, Restrepo C, Shao H, Parvizi J (2017) Effect of stem size and fixation method on mechanical failure after revision total knee arthroplasty. J Arthroplasty 32:S202-S208.e201. https://doi.org/10.1016/j.arth.2017.04.055
169. Fehring TK, Odum S, Olekson C et al (2003) Stem fixation in revision total knee arthroplasty. Clin Orthop Relat Res 416:217–224. https://doi.org/10.1097/01.blo.0000093032.56370.4b
170. Jensen CL, Petersen MM, Schrøder HM, Flivik G, Lund B (2012) Revision total knee arthroplasty with the use of trabecular metal cones: a randomized radiostereometric analysis with 2 years of follow-up. J Arthroplasty 27(10):1820-1826.e2. https://doi.org/10.1016/j.arth.2012.04.036 (*Epub 2012 Jul 13 PMID: 22795879*)
171. Haidukewych GJ, Hanssen A, Jones RD (2011) Metaphyseal fixation in revision total knee arthroplasty: indications and techniques. J Am Acad Orthop Surg 19(6):311–318. https://doi.org/10.5435/00124635-201106000-00001
172. Dalury DF, Barrett WP (2016) The use of metaphyseal sleeves in revision total knee arthroplasty. Knee 23(3):545–548. https://doi.org/10.1016/j.knee.2016.02.005
173. Graichen H, Scior W, Strauch M (2015) Direct, cementless, metaphyseal fixation in knee revision arthroplasty with sleeves-short-term results. J Arthroplasty 30(12):2256–2259. https://doi.org/10.1016/j.arth.2015.06.030
174. Barrack RL (2001) Evolution of rotating hinge for complex total knee arthroplasty. Clin Orthop Relat Res 392:292–299
175. Dawson J, Fitzpatrick R, Murray D, Carr A (1998) Questionnaire on the perceptions of patients about total knee replacement. J Bone Jt Surg Brit 80(1):63–69
176. Robertsson O, Dunbar M, Pehrsson T, Knutson K, Lidgren L (2000) Patient satisfaction after knee arthroplasty: a report on 27,372 knees operated on between 1981 and 1995 in Sweden. Acta Orthop Scand 71(3):262–267. https://doi.org/10.1080/000164700317411852
177. Mancuso F, Beltrame A, Colombo E, Miani E, Bassini F (2017) Management of metaphyseal bone loss in revision knee arthroplasty. Acta Biomed 88:98–111. https://doi.org/10.23750/abm.v88i2-S.6520
178. Thorsell M, Hedström M, Wick MC, Weiss RJ (2018) Good clinical and radiographic outcome of cementless metal metaphyseal sleeves in total knee arthroplasty. Acta Orthop 89(1):84–88. https://doi.org/10.1080/17453674.2017.1398013
179. Fedorka CJ, Chen AF, Pagnotto MR, Crossett LS, Klatt BA (2018) Revision total knee arthroplasty with porous-coated metaphyseal sleeves provides radiographic ingrowth and stable fixation. Knee Surg Sports Traumatol Arthrosc 26(5):1500–1505. https://doi.org/10.1007/s00167-017-4493-y
180. Martin-Hernandez C, Floria-Arnal LJ, Muniesa-Herrero MP, Espallargas-Doñate T, Blanco-Llorca JA, Guillen-Soriano M, Ranera-Garcia M (2017) Mid-term results for metaphyseal sleeves in revision knee surgery. Knee Surg

Sports Traumatol, Arthrosc 25(12):3779–3785. https://doi.org/10.1007/s00167-016-4298-4
181. Watters TS, Martin JR, Levy DL, Yang CC, Kim RH, Dennis DA. Porous-coated metaphyseal sleeves for severe femoral and tibial bone loss in revision TKA. J Arthroplasty. 2017;32(11):3468–73.
182. Engh GA, Ammeen DJ (1999) Bone loss with revision total knee arthroplasty: defect classification and alternatives for reconstruction. Instr Course Lect 48:167–175
183. Alexander GE, Bernasek TL, Crank RL, Haidukewych GJ. Cementless metaphyseal sleeves used for large tibial defects in revision total knee arthroplasty. J Arthroplast. 2013;28(4):604–7.
184. Petersen MM, Nielsen PT, Lauritzen JB, Lund B (1995) Changes in bone mineral density of the proximal tibia following uncemented total knee arthroplasty. A 3-year follow-up of 25 knees. Acta Orthop Scand 66:513–516
185. Petersen MM, Gehrchen PM, Østgaard SE, Nielsen PK, Lund B (2005) Effect of hydroxyapatite-coated tibial components on changes in bone mineral density of the proximal tibia after uncemented total knee arthroplasty. J Arthroplasty 20:516–520
186. Morgan-Jones R, Oussedik S, Graichen H, Haddad F (2015) Zonal fixation in revision total knee arthroplasty. Bone Jt J 97-B:147–149
187. Ponzio DY, Austin MS (2015) Metaphyseal bone loss in revision knee arthroplasty. Curr Rev Musculoskelet Med 8(4):361–367
188. Mancuso F, Beltrame A, Colombo E et al (2017) Management of metaphyseal bone loss in revision knee arthroplasty. Acta Biomed 88(2-S):98–111
189. Sheth NP, Bonadio MB, Demange MK (2017) Bone loss in revision total knee arthroplasty: evaluation and management. J Am Acad Orthop Surg 25(5):348–357
190. Kurtz S, Ong K, Lau E et al (2007) Projections of primary and revision hip and knee arthroplasty in the United States from 2005 to 2030. J Bone Jt Surg Am 89(4):780
191. Divano S, Cavagnaro L, Zanirato A, Basso M, Felli L, Formica M (2018) Porous metal cones: gold standard for massive bone loss in complex revision knee arthroplasty? A systematic review of current literature. Arch Orthop Trauma Surg 138(6):851–863
192. Bonanzinga T, Gehrke T, Zahar A, Zaffagnini S, Marcacci M, Haasper C (2017) Are trabecular metal cones a valid option to treat metaphyseal bone defects in complex primary and revision knee arthroplasty? Joints 6(1):58–64
193. Zanirato A, Cavagnaro L, Basso M, Divano S, Felli L, Formica M (2018) Metaphyseal sleeves in total knee arthroplasty revision: complications, clinical and radiological results. A systematic review of the literature. Arch Orthop Trauma Surg 138(7):993–1001
194. Bohl DD, Brown NM, McDowell MA, Levine BR, Sporer SM, Paprosky WG, Della Valle CJ (2018) Do porous tantalum metaphyseal cones improve outcomes in revision total knee arthroplasty? J Arthroplasty 33(1):171–177

195. Chalmers BP, Desy NM, Pagnano MW, Trousdale RT, Taunton MJ (2017) Survivorship metaphyseal sleeves in revision total knee arthroplasty. J Arthroplasty 32(5):1565–1570
196. Cottino U, Abdel MP, Perry KI, Mara KC, Lewallen DG, Hanssen AD (2017) Long-term results after total knee arthroplasty with contemporary rotating-hinge prostheses. J Bone Jt Surg Am 99(4):324–330
197. Bottner F, Laskin R, Windsor RE, Haas SB (2006) Hybrid component fixation in revision total knee arthroplasty. Clin Orthop Relat Res 446:127–131. https://doi.org/10.1097/01.blo.0000214418.36959.c5
198. Egger M, Davey Smith G, Schneider M, Minder C (1997) Bias in meta-analysis detected by a simple, graphical test. BMJ 315(7109):629–634
199. Edwards PK, Fehring TK, Hamilton WG, Perricelli B, Beaver WB, Odum SM (2014) Are cementless stems more durable than cemented stems in two-stage revisions of infected total knee arthroplasties? Clin Orthopaedics Related Res 472(1):206–211
200. Lachiewicz PF, O'Dell JA (2020) Is there a difference between cemented and uncemented femoral stem extensions in revision knee arthroplasty? J Knee Surg 33(1):84–88. https://doi.org/10.1055/s-0038-1676567
201. Wood GC, Naudie DD, MacDonald SJ, McCalden RW, Bourne RB. Results of press-fit stems in revision knee arthroplasties. Clin Orthop Relat Res. 2009;467:810–7.
202. Heinecke M, Rathje F, Layher F, Matziolis G (2018) The proximal and distal femoral canal geometry influences cementless stem anchorage and revision hip and knee implant stability. Orthopedics 41:e369–e375. https://doi.org/10.3928/01477447-20180320-02
203. Maslaris A, Layher F, Brinkmann O et al (2018) Cemented conical stems can be removed more easily than cylindrical stems, regardless of cone angle in revision knee arthroplasty. Arch Orthop Trauma Surg 138:1747–1754. https://doi.org/10.1007/s00402-018-3053-3
204. Bedair H, Tetrault M, Choi H-R et al (2013) A comparison of modular tapered vs. modular cylindrical stems for complex femoral revisions) 71–73. J Arthroplasty 28:71–73. https://doi.org/10.1016/j.arth.2013.04.052
205. Springer BD, Sim FH, Hanssen AD, Lewallen DG (2004) The modular segmental kinematic rotating hinge for nonneoplastic limb salvage. Clin Orthop Relat Res 421:181–187
206. Efe T, Roessler PP, Heyse TJ, Hauk C, Pahrmann C, Getgood A, et al. Mid-term results after implantation of rotating-hinge knee prostheses: primary versus revision. Orthop Rev (Pavia). 2012;4(4):35 2 [cited 2018 May 5] Available from: http://www.pagepress.org/journals/index.php/or/article/view/or.2012.e35.
207. Gehrke T, Kendoff D, Haasper C. The role of hinges in primary total knee replacement. Bone Joint J. 2014;96(11):93–5.
208. Böhm P, Holy T (1998) Is there a future for hinged prostheses in primary total knee arthroplasty? A 20-year survivorship analysis of the Blauth prosthesis. J Bone Joint Surg Br 80:302–309. https://doi.org/10.1302/0301-620x.80b2.7905

209. Petrou G, Petrou H, Tilkeridis C, Stavrakis T, Kapetsis T, Kremmidas N, Gavras M (2004) Medium-term results with a primary cemented rotating-hinge total knee replacement. A 7- to 15-year follow-up. J Bone Joint Surg Br 86(6):813–817
210. Awadalla M, Al-Dirini RMA, O'Rourke D, Solomon LB, Heldreth M, Taylor M. Influence of varying stem and metaphyseal sleeve size on the primary stability of cementless revision tibial trays used to reconstruct AORI IIA defects. A simulation study. J Orthop Res. 2018;36(7):1876–86.
211. Roach RP, Clair AJ, Behery OA, Thakkar SC, Iorio R, Deshmukh AJ. Aseptic loosening of porous metaphyseal sleeves and tantalum cones in revision total knee arthroplasty: a systematic review. J Knee Surg. 2021;34(10):1033–41.
212. Byttebier, P., Dhont, T., Pintelon, S., Rajgopal, A., Burssens, A., and Victor, J. (2022). Comparison of different strategies in revision arthroplasty of the knee with severe bone loss: A systematic review and meta-analysis of clinical outcomes. *Journal Arthroplasty, 37*(6S), S371–S381. https://doi.org/10.1016/j.arth.2022.02.103
213. Vanlommel J, Luyckx JP, Labey L, Innocenti B, De Corte R, Bellemans J (2011) Cementing the tibial component in total knee arthroplasty: which technique is the best? J Arthroplasty 26(3):492–496
214. Completo A, Simões JA, Fonseca F, Oliveira M (2008) The influence of different tibial stem designs in load sharing and stability at the cement-bone interface in revision TKA. Knee 15:227–232. https://doi.org/10.1016/j.knee.2008.01.008
215. Godest AC, Beaugonin M, Haug E, Taylor M, Gregson PJ (2002) Simulation of a knee joint replacement during a gait cycle using explicit finite element analysis. J Biomech 35(2):267–275
216. Wannasri SVP, Ivanova LR, Kornienko LA, Piriyayon S (2009) Increasing wear resistance of UHMWPE by mechanical activation and chemical modification combined with addition of nanofibers. Procedia Eng 1:67–70
217. Innocenti B, Bellemans J, Catani F (2015) Deviations from optimal alignment in TKA: is there a biomechanical difference between femoral or tibial component alignment? J Arthroplasty 31(1):295–301
218. Heiner AD (2008) Structural properties of fourth-generation composite femurs and tibias. J Biomech 41(15):3282–3284
219. Shen Y, Li X, Fu X, Wang W (2015) A 3D finite element model to investigate prosthetic interface stresses of different posterior tibial slope. Knee Surg Sports Traumatol Arthrosc 23(11):3330–3336
220. Radnay CS, Scuderi GR. Management of bone loss: augments, cones, Offset stems. Clin Orthop Relat Res. May 2006;446:83–92. https://doi.org/10.1097/01.blo.0000214437.57151.41.
221. Engh GA, Ammeen DJ. Bone loss with revision total knee arthroplasty: defect classification and alternatives for reconstruction. Instr Course Lect. 1999;48:167–75. https://doi.org/10.2106/00004623-196648010-00017.

222. Huten D (2013) Femorotibial bone loss during revision total knee arthroplasty. Orthop Traumatol Surg Res 99:S22-33. https://doi.org/10.1016/j.otsr.2012.11.009
223. Seebach E, Kubatzky KF. Chronic Implant-related bone infections-can Immune Modulation be a therapeutic strategy? Front Immunol. 2019;10:1724. https://doi.org/10.3389/fimmu.2019.01724.
224. Lee J, Kang C-I, Lee JH, Joung M, Moon S, Wi YM, Chung DR, Ha C-W, Song J-H, Peck KR. Risk factors for treatment failure in patients with prosthetic joint infections. J Hosp Infect. 2010;75(4):273–6. https://doi.org/10.1016/j.jhin.2010.03.012.
225. Logoluso N, Pedrini FA, Morelli I, et al. Megaprostheses for the revision of infected hip arthroplasties with severe bone loss. BMC Surg. 2022;22(68). https://doi.org/10.1186/s12893-022-01517-y.
226. Innocenti B, Fekete G, Pianigiani S (2018) Biomechanical analysis of augments in revision total knee arthroplasty. J Biomech Eng 140(11):111006
227. Burastero G, Pianigiani S, Zanvettor C, Cavagnaro L, Chiarlone F, Innocenti B (2020) Use of porous custom-made cones for meta-diaphyseal bone defects reconstruction in knee revision surgery: a clinical and biomechanical analysis. Arch Orthop Trauma Surg 140(12):2041–2055. https://doi.org/10.1007/s00402-020-03670-6
228. Innocenti B, Pianigiani S, Ramundo G, Thienpont E. Biomechanical effects of different Varus and Valgus alignments in medial unicompartmental knee arthroplasty. J Arthroplast. 2016;31(12):2685–91. https://doi.org/10.1016/j.arth.2016.07.006.
229. Mousavian A, Sabzevari S, Ghiasi S, Shahpari O, Razi A, Ebrahimpour A, Ebrahimzadeh MH. Amputation as a complication after total knee replacement, is it a real concern to be discussed? A systematic review. Archives bone Joint Surg. 2021;9(1):9–21. https://doi.org/10.22038/abjs.2020.53892.2692.
230. Gehrchen PM, Petersen MM (2008) Evaluation of a custom-made software for measurements of bone mineral density around prostethetic implants. Improved metal exclusion facility. Nordic Ortopedic Federation 54th Congress, Amsterdam, Holland, June 11–13
231. Ghazavi MT, Stockley I, Yee G, Davis A, Gross AE (1997) Reconstruction of massive bone defects with allograft in revision total knee arthroplasty. J Bone Joint Surg Am 79(1):17–25
232. Karbowski A, Schwitalle M, Eckardt A, Heine J (1999) Periprosthetic bone remodeling after total knee arthroplasty:early assessment by dual energy X-ray absorptiometry. Arch Orthop Trauma Surg 119:324–326
233. Petersen MM, Olsen C, Lauritzen JB, Lund B (1995) Changes in bone mineral density of the distal femur following uncemented total knee arthroplasty. J Arthroplasty 10:7–11
234. Mabry TM, Vessely MB, Schleck CD et al (2007) Revision total knee arthroplasty with modular cemented stems: long-term follow-up. J Arthroplasty 22:100–105. https://doi.org/10.1016/j.arth.2007.03.025

235. Murray PB, Rand JA, Hanssen AD. Cemented long-stem revision total knee arthroplasty. Clin Orthop 1994:116–23.
236. Peters CL, Erickson J, Kloepper RG, Mohr RA. Revision total knee arthroplasty with modular components inserted with metaphyseal cement and stems without cement. J Arthroplasty. 2005;20:302–8.
237. Peters CL, Erickson JA, Gililland JM. Clinical and radiographic results of 184 consecutive revision total knee arthroplasties placed with modular Cementless stems. J Arthroplasty. 2009;24:48–53. https://doi.org/10.1016/j.arth.2009.04.033.
238. Shannon BD, Klassen JF, Rand JA, Berry DJ, Trousdale RT (2003) Revision total knee arthroplasty with cemented components and uncemented intramedullary stems. J Arthroplasty 18(7 Suppl 1):27–32
239. Sheridan GA, Garbuz DS, Masri BA (2021) Hybrid stems are superior to cemented stems in revision total knee arthroplasty: a systematic review and meta-analysis of recent comparative studies. Eur J Orthop Traumatol 31(1):131–141. https://doi.org/10.1007/s00590-020-02752-w
240. Gomez-Vallejo J, Albareda-Albareda J, Seral-Garcia B, Blanco-Rubio N, Ezquerra-Herrando L (2018) Revision total knee arthroplasty: hybrid vs standard cemented fixation. J Orthop Traumatol 19(1):9
241. Gililland JM, Gaffney CJ, Odum SM, Fehring TK, Peters CL, Beaver WB (2014) Clinical and radiographic outcomes of cemented vs. diaphyseal engaging cementless stems in aseptic revision TKA. J Arthroplasty 29(9):224–228. https://doi.org/10.1016/j.arth.2014.03.049
242. Mills K, Wymenga AB, van Hellemondt GG, Heesterbeek PJC. No difference in long-term micromotion between fully cemented and hybrid fixation in revision total knee arthroplasty: a randomized controlled trial. Bone Jt J. 2022;104–B:875–83. https://doi.org/10.1302/0301-620X.104B7.BJJ-2021-1600.R1.
243. Sun, Zhenhui; Patil, Abhishek; Song, Eun-Kyoo; Kim, Hyun-Tae; Seon, Jong-Keun Comparison of quadriceps snip and tibial tubercle osteotomy in revision for infected total knee arthroplasty. International Orthopaedics (2014). 10.1007/s00264-014-2546-0
244. Choi, Ho-Rim; Burke, Dennis; Malchau, Henrik; Kwon, Young-Min Utility of tibial tubercle osteotomy in the setting of periprosthetic infection after total knee arthroplasty. International Orthopaedics (2012). https://doi.org/10.1007/s00264-012-1541-6
245. Wishart, Marc; Arnold, Markus P.; Huegli, Rolf W.; Amsler, Felix; Friederich, Niklaus F.; Hirschmann, Michael T. Anterolateral approach using tibial tubercle osteotomy for total knee arthroplasty: can we predict failure?. International Orthopaedics (2012). https://doi.org/10.1007/s00264-012-1693-4
246. Zonnenberg, Christian B. L.; van den Bekerom, Michel P. J.; de Jong, Tjitte; Nolte, Peter A. Tibial tubercle osteotomy with absorbable suture fixation in revision total knee arthroplasty: a report of 23 cases. Archives of Orthopaedic and Trauma Surgery (2014). https://doi.org/10.1007/s00402-014-1950-7

247. Segur, Josep M.; Vilchez-Cavazos, Felix; Martinez-Pastor, Juan Carlos; Macule, Francisco; Suso, Santiago; Acosta-Olivo, Carlos Tibial tubercle osteotomy in septic revision total knee arthroplasty. Archives of Orthopaedic and Trauma Surgery (2014). https://doi.org/10.1007/s00402-014-2064-y
248. Hirschmann, Michael T; Hoffmann, Mathias; Krause, Robert; Jenabzadeh, Reza-Amir; Arnold, Markus P; Friederich, Niklaus F Anterolateral approach with tibial tubercle osteotomy versus standard medial approach for primary total knee arthroplasty: does it matter?. BMC Musculoskeletal Disorders (2010). https://doi.org/10.1186/1471-2474-11-167
249. Langen, Susanne; Gaber, Sonja; Zdravkovic, Vilijam; Giesinger, Karlmeinrad; Jost, Bernhard; Behrend, Henrik Lateral subvastus approach with tibial tubercle osteotomy for primary total knee arthroplasty: clinical outcome and complications compared to medial parapatellar approach. European Journal of Orthopaedic Surgery & Traumatology (2015). https://doi.org/10.1007/s00590-015-1718-y
250. Divano, Stefano; Camera, Andrea; Biggi, Stefano; Tornago, Stefano; Formica, Matteo; Felli, Lamberto Tibial tubercle osteotomy (TTO) in total knee arthroplasty, is it worth it? A review of the literature. Archives of Orthopaedic and Trauma Surgery (2018). https://doi.org/10.1007/s00402-018-2888-y
251. Miralles-Muñoz, Francisco A.; Rubio-Morales, Marta; Ruiz-Lozano, Matias; Martinez-Mendez, Daniel; Gonzalez-Parreño, Santiago; Lizaur-Utrilla, Alejandro V-Y turndown flap augmentation for acute quadriceps rupture after total knee arthroplasty: a prospective matched cohort study. International Orthopaedics (2021). https://doi.org/10.1007/s00264-021-04939-0
252. Yu, Muyang; Yang, Xingdong; Xu, Yiming; Zhu, Wei; Peng, Huiming; Lin, Jin; Weng, Xisheng; Feng, Bin Comparison between ligament balancing and measured resection in robot-assisted total knee arthroplasty: a 2-year follow up cohort study. BMC Musculoskeletal Disorders (2025). https://doi.org/10.1186/s12891-025-08388-3
253. Cho, Kyu-Jin; Seon, Jong-Keun; Jang, Won-Young; Park, Chun-Gon; Song, Eun-Kyoo Objective quantification of ligament balancing using VERASENSE in measured resection and modified gap balance total knee arthroplasty. BMC Musculoskeletal Disorders (2018). https://doi.org/10.1186/s12891-018-2190-8
254. Rossi, Stefano Marco Paolo; Benazzo, Francesco Individualized alignment and ligament balancing technique with the ROSA® robotic system for total knee arthroplasty. International Orthopaedics (2023). https://doi.org/10.1007/s00264-022-05671-z
255. Ghijselings, Ignace; Taylan, Orcun; Delport, Hendrik Pieter; Slane, Josh; Van den Wyngaert, Hans; Demurie, Alex; Scheys, Lennart Using a patella reduced technique while balancing a TKA results in restored physiological strain in the collateral ligaments: an ex vivo kinematic analysis. Archives of Orthopaedic and Trauma Surgery (2021). https://doi.org/10.1007/s00402-021-04010-y

256. Aunan, Eirik; Kibsgård, Thomas; Clarke-Jenssen, John; Röhrl, Stephan M. A new method to measure ligament balancing in total knee arthroplasty: laxity measurements in 100 knees. Archives of Orthopaedic and Trauma Surgery (2012). https://doi.org/10.1007/s00402-012-1536-1
257. Dzidzishvili, Lika; Sáez, David; Calvo, Emilio Metaphyseal cones combined with diaphyseal impaction grafting provide good outcomes and survival in a complex revision total knee arthroplasty: a matched comparative analysis. European Journal of Orthopaedic Surgery & Traumatology (2023). https://doi.org/10.1007/s00590-023-03659-y
258. Ponzio, Danielle Y.; Austin, Matthew S. Metaphyseal bone loss in revision knee arthroplasty. Current Reviews in Musculoskeletal Medicine (2015). https://doi.org/10.1007/s12178-015-9291-x
259. Russo, Antonio; Alessio-Mazzola, Mattia; Massè, Alessandro; Burastero, Giorgio Unbalanced metaphyseal fixation is associated with an increased aseptic loosening of revision total knee arthroplasty at mean 4-year follow-up. Archives of Orthopaedic and Trauma Surgery (2024). https://doi.org/10.1007/s00402-024-05600-2
260. Fosco, Matteo; Amendola, Luca; Fantasia, Rossana; Pipino, Gennaro; Tigani, Domenico Revision total knee arthroplasty: experience with tantalum cones in severe bone loss. European Orthopaedics and Traumatology (2013). https://doi.org/10.1007/s12570-013-0160-z
261. Leung, Thomas Ka Chun; Chan, Ping Keung; Fu, Henry; Cheung, Amy; Luk, Michelle Hilda; Lau, Lawrence Chun Man; Chiu, Kwong Yuen Promising short-term outcomes of free-hand burring technique to implant second-generation metaphyseal cone in Asian knees – a case series. Arthroplasty (2024). https://doi.org/10.1186/s42836-024-00254-2
262. Erivan, Roger; Tracey, Robert; Mulliez, Aurélien; Villatte, Guillaume; Paprosky, Wayne Medium term clinical outcomes of tibial cones in revision knee arthroplasty. Archives of Orthopaedic and Trauma Surgery (2020). https://doi.org/10.1007/s00402-020-03532-1
263. Vaziri, Arash Sharafat; Moradkhani, Ghazaleh; Farahmand, Farzam; Karimpour, Morad; Tahmasebi, Mohammad Naghi; Vosoughi, Fardis; Salimi, Maryam; Shayan-Moghadam, Ramin Utilizing 3d-printed patient-specific porous titanium cones in complex primary and revision total knee arthroplasty. European Journal of Orthopaedic Surgery & Traumatology (2025). https://doi.org/10.1007/s00590-025-04229-0
264. Cherny, Alexander A.; Kovalenko, Anton N.; Kulyaba, Taras A.; Kornilov, Nikolai N. A prospective study on outcome of patient-specific cones in revision knee arthroplasty. Archives of Orthopaedic and Trauma Surgery (2021). https://doi.org/10.1007/s00402-021-04047-z
265. Wu, Yushun; Feng, Eryou; Zhang, Yiyuan; Lin, Feitai; Lin, Liqiong; Li, Zhanglai; Xiao, Lili Porous-coated metaphyseal sleeves and MBT implant for severe bone loss in revision total knee arthroplasty: a mean 2.4-year follow-up. Arthroplasty (2020). https://doi.org/10.1186/s42836-020-00031-x

266. Shichman, Ittai; Oakley, Christian; Willems, Jore H.; van Hellemondt, Gijs G.; Heesterbeek, Petra; Rozell, Joshua; Marwin, Scott; Schwarzkopf, Ran Novel metaphyseal porous titanium cones allow favorable outcomes in revision total knee arthroplasty. Archives of Orthopaedic and Trauma Surgery (2022). https://doi.org/10.1007/s00402-022-04645-5
267. Spinello, P.; Thiele, R. A. Ruberte; Zepeda, K.; Giori, N.; Indelli, P. F. The use of tantalum cones and diaphyseal-engaging stems in tibial component revision: a consecutive series. Knee Surgery & Related Research (2022). https://doi.org/10.1186/s43019-022-00141-7
268. Gøttsche, David; Lind, Thomas; Christiansen, Thorbjørn; Schrøder, Henrik M. Cementless metaphyseal sleeves without stem in revision total knee arthroplasty. Archives of Orthopaedic and Trauma Surgery (2016). https://doi.org/10.1007/s00402-016-2583-9
269. Gurel, Ron; Morgan, Samuel; Elbaz, Etay; Ashlenazi, Itay; Snir, Nimrod; Kadar, Assaf; Gold, Aviram; Warschawski, Yaniv Mid-term clinical and radiographic outcomes of porous-coated metaphyseal sleeves used in revision total knee arthroplasty. Knee Surgery & Related Research (2021). https://doi.org/10.1186/s43019-021-00103-5
270. Jensen, Claus L.; Petersen, Michael M.; Schrøder, Henrik M.; Lund, Bjarne Bone mineral density changes of the proximal tibia after revision total knee arthroplasty. A randomised study with the use of porous tantalum metaphyseal cones. International Orthopaedics (2012). https://doi.org/10.1007/s00264-012-1601-y
271. Zanirato, A.; Formica, M.; Cavagnaro, L.; Divano, S.; Burastero, G.; Felli, L. Metaphyseal cones and sleeves in revision total knee arthroplasty: Two sides of the same coin? Complications, clinical and radiological results—a systematic review of the literature. MUSCULOSKELETAL SURGERY (2019). https://doi.org/10.1007/s12306-019-00598-y
272. Sheridan, Gerard A.; Garbuz, Donald S.; Masri, Bassam A. Hybrid stems are superior to cemented stems in revision total knee arthroplasty: a systematic review and meta-analysis of recent comparative studies. European Journal of Orthopaedic Surgery & Traumatology (2020). https://doi.org/10.1007/s00590-020-02752-w
273. Maslaris, Alexander; Tsiridis, Eleftherios; Schoeneberg, Carsten; Pass, Bastian; Spyrou, Georgios; Maris, Alexandros; Matziolis, Georg Does stem profile have an impact on the failure patterns in revision total knee arthroplasty?. Archives of Orthopaedic and Trauma Surgery (2022). https://doi.org/10.1007/s00402-022-04683-z
274. Maniar, Adit R.; Kazarian, Gregory S.; Torres-Ramirez, Ricardo J.; Ranawat, Amar S. Isolated Zone 2 and Zone 3 Cementless Tibial Fixation Shows Early Promise in Revision Total Knee Arthroplasty. Indian Journal of Orthopaedics (2025). https://doi.org/10.1007/s43465-025-01354-0

275. El-Zayat, Bilal Farouk; Heyse, Thomas J.; Fanciullacci, Nelson; Labey, Luc; Fuchs-Winkelmann, Susanne; Innocenti, Bernardo Fixation techniques and stem dimensions in hinged total knee arthroplasty: a finite element study. Archives of Orthopaedic and Trauma Surgery (2016). https://doi.org/10.1007/s00402-016-2571-0
276. Piovan, Gianluca; Bori, Edoardo; Padalino, Marika; Pianigiani, Silvia; Innocenti, Bernardo Biomechanical analysis of patient specific cone vs conventional stem in revision total knee arthroplasty. Journal of Orthopaedic Surgery and Research (2024). https://doi.org/10.1186/s13018-024-04936-0
277. Jensen, Claus L.; Petersen, Michael M.; Schrøder, Henrik M.; Lund, Bjarne Changes in bone mineral density of the distal femur after revision total knee arthroplasty with metaphyseal press-fit stem. Journal of Orthopaedics and Traumatology (2010). https://doi.org/10.1007/s10195-010-0098-7
278. Thever, Yogen; James Loh, Sir Young; Raghavan, Raghuraman; Toh, Rong Chuin; Moo, Ing How A systematic review and meta-analysis of hybrid vs. cemented stems – which method is more optimal for revision total knee arthroplasty?. BMC Musculoskeletal Disorders (2024). https://doi.org/10.1186/s12891-024-07389-y

Chapter 10
Outcomes in Primary and Revision Total Knee Arthroplasty

Alfred J. Tria Jr. and Giles R. Scuderi

Introduction by the Editors

Total knee arthroplasty (TKA) has been shown to be a durable and predictable procedure in the treatment of knee arthritis as measured by survivorship analysis and long-term clinical studies. However, it has become increasing important to measure patient satisfaction and functional activity following TKA. Following TKA, the patient's perspective of improvement and satisfaction is fundamental to assessing the outcome of the procedure. Patient reported outcome measurement (PROM) has become a basic tool to assess the ultimate success of surgery. While there are several outcome tools available, each measure patient outcome over multiple domains such as pain, function and satisfaction. While the majority of patients are satisfied with their outcome, there is a significant minority that are dissatisfied, and expectations are not met. It is important that with continued research and analysis we investigate the factors that contribute to patient dissatisfaction. While there may be numerous unanswered questions to be considered, the biggest influence on satisfaction is meeting patient expectations. While these may be unreasonable, clear communication prior to surgery helps align both the patient and surgeon.

This chapter will focus on the results of primary and revision TKA. We reviewed each of the referenced articles and provide our insights as detailed below. When you read each of the computer-generated summaries that follow in this chapter you can draw your own conclusions.

Clement et al. did a comprehensive analysis of preoperative and post operative responses to the Oxford knee score questions and developed a heatmap to explore which questions might be more relevant to patients and which ones should be more

A. J. Tria Jr. (✉)
Department of Orthopedics, Rutgers-Robert Wood Johnson Medical School, New Brunswick, NJ, USA

G. R. Scuderi
Department of Orthopedic Surgery, Northwell Health, Garden City, NY, USA

A. J. Tria Jr., G. R. Scuderi (eds.), *Total Knee Arthroplasty*,
https://doi.org/10.1007/978-3-032-00175-7_10

heavily weighted. This type of study may be valuable in the future to better understand the 15% of dissatisfied patients. It is also interesting that as the worldwide number of TKA continues to increase, there are regional and demographic trends. Worlicek et al. looked at the trends in Germany over a 10-year period and noted an increase in unicompartmental knee arthroplasty, female patients, and younger patients. In addition to trends in the patient population, implant choice and surgical technique are undergoing changes. Sidhu et al. in a registry review found an ongoing preference for cement fixation and PCL retaining TKA, but an increasing trend for cementless options and robotic surgery. With this trend towards cementless fixation, Epinette et al. looked at hydroxyapatite coatings and showed potential advantage on fixation.

Understanding that the results of TKA are influenced by multiple factors. This chapter highlights some specific parameters that potentially influence the clinical outcome. Chan et al. looked at pain catastrophizing and showed a relationship to postoperative pain, emphasizing the value of preoperative mental health evaluation. Olivecrona et al. showed that prolonged tourniquet time was associated with increased complications, but this is a multifactorial problem and requires further study. Goyal e al. reported that a prior arthroscopy led to higher complications but did not indicate the time between the two procedures. Lau et al. showed that surgeon volume influenced the clinical results, but the studies that were in the review were low volume with low-quality observations. There are many studies in the literature that do support this finding.

While there is a significant improvement in patient outcome following revision TKA, patient satisfaction remains lower than primary TKA. This is because the outcome of revision TKA is difficult to quantify, since the results are dependent upon the mode of failure. The complexity of revision TKA is dependent upon bone loss and ligament integrity that need to be assessed and incorporated in a preoperative plan. Vasso et al. addressed these issues and developed an algorithmic approach by studying revision TKA over a 10-year period. This may have further application, but further investigation is needed to evaluate the plan. To further define the surgical plan, Indelli et al. reviewed the required level of constraint in several settings. Ponzio et al. review the techniques for managing metaphyseal bone loss with good insights.

Van der Wilk et al. in their systematic review and metanalysis looked at physical activity after revision and found that there was a great deal of uncertainty in the reports emphasizing the need for better standard evaluations.

It has previously been noted that surgical volume and experience influence the ultimate outcome. Pour et al. studied surgeon trends and showed that fellowship trained surgeons performed more complicated cases but the results for both trained and non-trained were the same. High volume surgeons once again reported fewer complications.

TKA has evolved over the last 50 years, with most patients having successful outcomes. As we continue to monitor the patients, success will be measured by not only the durability of the implant but by meeting patient expectations. With further refinements in surgical technique and implant design, the PROM tools should be refined so that the domains better identify the areas for potential improvement.

10.1 Primary Knee Arthroplasty

Machine Generated Summaries

Disclaimer: The summaries in this chapter were generated from Springer Nature publications using abstractive AI auto-summarization: An abstraction-based summarizer creates new text based on deep learning. New phrases are created to summarize the content. As the constituted sentences are machine selected, they may not fully reflect the body of the work, so we strongly advise that the original content is read and cited. The auto-generated summaries were curated by the editor to meet Springer Nature publication standards.

10.1.1 Long Lasting Outcome of Hydroxyapatite-Coated Implants in Primary Knee Arthroplasty: A Continuous Series of Two Hundred and Seventy Total Knee Arthroplasties at Fifteen to Twenty-Two Years of Clinical Follow-Up [97]

This is a machine-generated summary of:

Epinette, Jean-Alain Long lasting outcome of hydroxyapatite-coated implants in primary knee arthroplasty: a continuous series of 270 total knee arthroplasties at 15 to 22 years of clinical follow-up [97].

Published in: International Orthopaedics (2014).

Link to original: https://doi.org/10.1007/s00264-013-2246-1

If you want to cite the papers, please refer to the original.

For technical reasons we could not place the page where the original quote is coming from.

10.1.1.1 Research Highlights

Achieving long-term, stable implant fixation without acrylic cement through a bioactive bond between the implant and host bone is a critical goal in knee and hip arthroplasty. Hydroxyapatite (HA) coatings have shown promise in enhancing the longevity of knee implants, as evidenced by previous studies. However, there remains a need to confirm whether these promising results can withstand the test of time. The study Epinette provides a long-term review of the Omnifit Knee Prosthesis (Corin Orthopedics, Cirencester, UK) which features either partial or full HA coatings, to evaluate their performance over an extended period.

The study involved 244 HA-coated primary posterior cruciate-retaining knee replacements implanted consecutively in patients between June 1992 and December 1995. The researchers used a consistent surgical technique across all cases, with an average patient age of 67.4 years at the time of surgery. The main diagnosis was osteoarthritis in most knees, with necrosis in a few others. The study followed up with patients using clinical assessments based on the International Knee Society score and radiological evaluations to monitor implant performance and complications. Survivorship was calculated using the Kaplan-Meier method, considering both revision for any cause and specific implant-related failures as endpoints. The study found that HA-coated implants demonstrated excellent fixation over time, with minimal mechanical loosening or osteolysis observed.

The findings suggest that HA-coated Omnifit knee implants offer comparable or superior long-term outcomes to cemented or porous-coated alternatives. Radiological assessments indicated strong bone-implant interfaces, particularly in fully coated components, supporting the efficacy of HA coatings in enhancing implant stability. While technical skills and design remain crucial factors, this study underscores the potential of bioconductive coatings like HA in knee arthroplasty. Future studies could explore new materials such as trabecular titanium or tantalum interfaces to further improve implant performance. These results provide a valuable reference for ongoing advancements in knee replacement technologies.

10.1.2 Total Knee Arthroplasty after a Prior Knee Arthroscopy Has Higher Complication Rates: A Systematic Review [98]

This is a machine-generated summary of:

Goyal, Tarun; Tripathy, Sujit Kumar; Schuh, Alexander; Paul, Souvik Total knee arthroplasty after a prior knee arthroscopy has higher complication rates: a systematic review [98].

Published in: Archives of Orthopaedic and Trauma Surgery (2021).

Link to original: https://doi.org/10.1007/s00402-021-04175-6

If you want to cite the papers, please refer to the original.

For technical reasons we could not place the page where the original quote is coming from.

10.1.2.1 Research Highlights

Knee arthroscopy's role in managing osteoarthritis remains contentious, as evidence suggests it neither alleviates pain nor delays the need for knee replacement. Despite this, arthroscopic procedures are still frequently performed worldwide for osteoarthritis patients. The study by Goyal et al. systematically reviews the outcomes and complication rates of total knee arthroplasty (TKA) in patients who previously underwent knee arthroscopy for osteoarthritis. The study hypothesizes that prior knee arthroscopy may negatively impact future TKA outcomes.

The researchers conducted a systematic review following Cochrane Collaboration and Preferred Reporting Items for Systematic Reviews and Meta-Analyse (PRISMA) guidelines, searching PubMed for relevant studies published in English before April. They included cohort, case-control, and cross-sectional studies where at least one group had undergone non-ligament knee arthroscopy before TKA. Data from seven retrospective studies were analyzed, focusing on functional outcomes, complication rates, and survivorship. The meta-analysis revealed no significant differences in functional outcomes or range of motion between patients with or without prior arthroscopy. However, higher rates of postoperative infections and revisions were noted in those with previous arthroscopic procedures.

The study highlights the increased risk of complications such as prosthetic joint infections and re-operations following TKA when preceded by knee arthroscopy. While functional outcomes appeared similar between groups, the findings suggest caution in recommending arthroscopic interventions for osteoarthritic knees due to potential adverse effects on subsequent TKA. Future study directions could explore the temporal relationship between prior arthroscopy and complications, as well as compare different types of arthroscopic procedures to better understand their specific impacts on TKA outcomes.

10.1.3 Tourniquet Time Affects Postoperative Complications After Knee Arthroplasty [99]

This is a machine-generated summary of:

Olivecrona, Charlotta; Lapidus, Lasse J.; Benson, Lina; Blomfeldt, Richard Tourniquet time affects postoperative complications after knee arthroplasty [99].

Published in: International Orthopaedics (2013).

Link to original: https://doi.org/10.1007/s00264-013-1826-4

If you want to cite the papers, please refer to the original.

For technical reasons we could not place the page where the original quote is coming from.

10.1.3.1 Research Highlights

The use of pneumatic tourniquets in knee arthroplasty surgery is common practice, as it helps create a bloodless field, facilitating the procedure. However, the use of tourniquets is not without risks, as complications such as nerve injuries and wound issues have been reported, often related to excessive tourniquet time. Despite recommendations suggesting a two-hour limit for healthy patients, there is a lack of robust clinical evidence defining safe tourniquet times, particularly for vulnerable populations like the elderly or those with peripheral vascular disease. The study by Olivecrona et al. addresses this gap by investigating the influence of tourniquet time on postoperative complications in knee arthroplasty.

The study was conducted as a prospective register study at the Department of Orthopedics at Södersjukhuset in Stockholm, Sweden. It included a consecutive series of primary and revision knee arthroplasties recorded in a clinical audit database. The researchers analyzed data from 1000 patients who underwent knee arthroplasty between 2010 and 2015, focusing on complications occurring within 6 weeks post-surgery. Tourniquet times were categorized into $\leq$120 min and > 120 min for analysis. Statistical methods included univariable and multivariable logistic regression analyses to assess associations between tourniquet time and complications such as infections, deep vein thrombosis, pulmonary embolism, and nerve injuries. The study also considered factors like age, sex, ASA (American Society of Anesthesiologists) classification, diabetes, smoking status, and cuff pressure.

The findings indicate that longer tourniquet times are associated with an increased risk of postoperative complications. Specifically, every additional 10 min of tourniquet time was linked to higher odds of complications. While cuff pressure did not show a significant association with complications in this study, ASA classification emerged as an important factor; patients with higher ASA scores had increased risks. Although women appeared more susceptible to complications with longer tourniquet times than men, this difference was not statistically significant. Future studies could explore this potential sex difference further. The study underscores the importance of minimizing tourniquet time to optimize patient outcomes and suggests that individual patient comorbidities should be considered when planning surgery.

10.1.4 Sufentanil Sublingual Tablet System for Enhanced Recovery After Total Knee Arthroplasty: A Prospective Observational Case Study [100]

This is a machine-generated summary of:

Rineau, Emmanuel; Dumartinet, Benjamin; Samson, Emmanuel; Dollfus, Apolline; Aubourg, Corentin; Lasocki, Sigismond Sufentanil sublingual tablet system for enhanced recovery after total knee arthroplasty: a prospective observational case study [100].

Published in: Perioperative Medicine (2022).

Link to original: https://doi.org/10.1186/s13741-022-00284-x

If you want to cite the papers, please refer to the original.

For technical reasons we could not place the page where the original quote is coming from.

10.1.4.1 Research Highlights

Enhanced recovery after surgery (ERAS) programs have been instrumental in reducing complications and shortening hospital stays, particularly in prosthetic knee surgeries. A critical component of these programs is effective postoperative pain management, which is essential for patient mobilization and reducing hospitalization duration. Multimodal analgesia, including regional techniques like the adductor canal block, is commonly used but often requires supplemental opioid treatments. The study by Rineau et al. evaluates the efficacy of the sufentanil sublingual tablet system (SSTS) (Talphera Pharmaceuticals, San Mateo, California, USA) in facilitating early recovery after total knee arthroplasty compared to intravenous morphine patient-controlled analgesia (PCA).

The study was conducted as a prospective observational single-center trial at Angers University Hospital(4 rue Larrey, 49,100, Angers, France), involving patients scheduled for primary unilateral knee arthroplasty within an enhanced recovery pathway. Participants were divided into two groups: those receiving SSTS and those receiving morphine PCA. The primary endpoint was the Timed Up and Go (TUG) test measured on postoperative days 1, 2, and 3. Secondary endpoints included perioperative pain levels, opioid consumption, adverse effects, knee flexion, venous cannula removal time, and hospital stay length. Statistical analyses were performed using Fisher's test and Mann-Whitney test to compare categorical and qualitative variables between groups.

The study found no significant differences in postoperative rehabilitation outcomes between the SSTS and IV-morphine groups regarding TUG scores, knee flexion, or hospital stay length. Although SSTS allowed for earlier venous cannula removal, it did not enhance mobilization or reduce hospital discharge times compared to morphine PCA. The SSTS group showed higher morphine equivalent consumption without significant differences in pain control or side effects. Future studies should focus on randomized controlled trials to further evaluate SSTS's role in enhanced recovery pathways and its potential economic benefits.

10.1.5 A Comprehensive Analysis of the Pre- and Postoperative Responses to Each of the 12 Oxford Knee Score Questions One Year Following Knee Arthroplasty [101]

This is a machine-generated summary of:

Clement, N. D.; Jones, S.; Afzal, I.; Kader, D. F. A comprehensive analysis of the pre- and postoperative responses to each of the 12 Oxford knee score questions 1 year following knee arthroplasty [101].

Published in: European Journal of Orthopaedic Surgery & Traumatology (2024).

Link to original: https://doi.org/10.1007/s00590-024-03870-5

If you want to cite the papers, please refer to the original.

For technical reasons we could not place the page where the original quote is coming from.

10.1.5.1 Research Highlights

The Oxford Knee Score (OKS) is a widely used patient-reported outcome measure for evaluating knee-specific function and pain before and after knee arthroplasty, particularly within the NHS in England and Wales. Despite its longstanding use, the OKS has limitations, such as potentially masking individual pain and functional benefits when used as a summative score. The study by Clement et al. addresses these limitations by mapping individual preoperative OKS question responses to postoperative outcomes using a heatmap, aiming to enhance shared decision-making and patient understanding of expected improvements following knee arthroplasty.

The study was conducted as a single-center retrospective cohort analysis over 12 months, involving patients who underwent primary knee arthroplasty for arthritis. Preoperative and 1-year postoperative OKS data were collected via postal questionnaires, with follow-up phone calls to complete missing responses. The researchers analyzed changes in individual OKS question responses, categorizing them as better, same, or worse compared to baseline. Statistical analyses included descriptive statistics, effect size calculations, and paired t-tests to assess significance. The study found significant improvements across all OKS questions postoperatively, with moderate to large effect sizes. However, despite these improvements, many patients remained symptomatic post-surgery.

The study highlights the potential of using heatmaps to communicate expected changes in knee-specific symptoms based on preoperative responses. This approach could facilitate more personalized patient consultations regarding knee arthroplasty outcomes. Future studies may explore which OKS questions are most relevant to patients and whether their responses should be weighted differently based on patient priorities. Additionally, addressing the postoperative ceiling effect observed in this cohort could refine the OKS's clinical utility by ensuring it captures meaningful changes in patient-reported outcomes more effectively.

10.1.6 The Influence of Pain Catastrophizing on Pain and Function After Knee Arthroplasty in Knee Osteoarthritis [102]

This is a machine-generated summary of:

Chan, Diana; Saffari, Seyed Ehsan; Wong, Steven Bak Siew; Yeo, Seng Jin; Wylde, Vikki; Thumboo, Julian; Leung, Ying-Ying The influence of pain catastrophizing on pain and function after knee arthroplasty in knee osteoarthritis [102].

Published in: Scientific Reports (2024).

Link to original: https://doi.org/10.1038/s41598-024-67561-1

If you want to cite the papers, please refer to the original.

For technical reasons we could not place the page where the original quote is coming from.

10.1.6.1 Research Highlights

Knee osteoarthritis is a prevalent condition that significantly impacts the quality of life, particularly among older adults. While knee arthroplasty is a common surgical intervention for severe cases, a substantial number of patients continue to experience chronic pain and dissatisfaction post-surgery. Identifying modifiable pre-operative factors that influence outcomes is crucial for improving patient care. The study by Chan et al. investigates the role of pain catastrophizing—a psychological factor characterized by an exaggerated negative response to pain—in predicting post-operative outcomes in knee arthroplasty patients.

The authors recruited patients with knee osteoarthritis scheduled for primary knee arthroplasty. Participants were assessed for pain catastrophizing using the Pain Catastrophizing Scale (PCS) during their preoperative visit. The study excluded individuals with cognitive impairments or those undergoing revision surgeries. Pain and functional outcomes were measured using the Western Ontario and McMaster University Index (WOMAC) at 6- and 12-months post-surgery. The researchers employed regression models to analyze the association between preoperative PCS scores and changes in WOMAC scores, adjusting for potential confounders such as age, sex, BMI, and baseline pain levels.

The study found that higher pre-operative PCS scores were modestly associated with less improvement in pain at 6- and 12-months post-arthroplasty, although the effect size was smaller compared to other factors like baseline pain severity. Functional outcomes showed inconsistent associations with PCS scores across different time points. The findings suggest that while pain catastrophizing may influence postoperative pain outcomes, its impact is relatively minor compared to other variables. Future studies could explore targeted interventions to address pain catastrophizing before surgery, potentially enhancing recovery experiences for patients undergoing knee arthroplasty.

10.1.7 Pain Relief Without Impairing Muscle Function After Local Infiltration Anaesthesia in Primary Knee Arthroplasty: A Prospective Randomized Study [103]

This is a machine-generated summary of:

Mayr, H. O.; Prall, W. C.; Haasters, F.; Baumbach, S. F.; Hube, R.; Stoehr, Amelie Pain relieve without impairing muscle function after local infiltration anaesthesia in primary knee arthroplasty: a prospective randomized study [103].

Published in: Archives of Orthopaedic and Trauma Surgery (2019).

Link to original: https://doi.org/10.1007/s00402-019-03194-8

If you want to cite the papers, please refer to the original.

For technical reasons we could not place the page where the original quote is coming from.

10.1.7.1 Research Highlights

Total knee arthroplasty (TKA) is a widely performed procedure, yet managing postoperative pain remains a significant challenge. Effective pain management is crucial for immediate rehabilitation and influences patients' perceptions of their hospital experience and functional outcomes. Current strategies include various analgesics and techniques, with local infiltration anesthesia (LIA) emerging as a promising alternative to traditional in-catheter methods, which can impair quadriceps muscle strength. The study by Mayr et al. investigates the efficacy of LIA compared to in-catheter interventions, focusing on pain relief and muscle strength preservation.

The study was conducted as a single-center, prospective, randomized controlled trial following the CONSORT (Consolidated Standards for Reporting Trials) guidelines. Patients scheduled for TKA were randomly assigned to receive either LIA or an in-catheter intervention. The LIA protocol involved administering fentanyl and ropivacaine at three stages: preoperatively, intraoperatively, and post-wound closure. In contrast, the in-catheter group received ropivacaine via electrostimulation before surgery and continued postoperative dosing as needed. Pain levels were assessed using a visual analogue scale (VAS), while quadriceps strength was measured using the British Medical Research Council scale. The Oxford Knee Score (OKS) was used to evaluate functional outcomes preoperatively and 6 months postoperatively.

The study found that both LIA and in-catheter methods provided similar levels of pain relief; however, LIA preserved quadriceps muscle strength better during the early postoperative period. Functional outcomes improved significantly in both groups without intergroup differences at 6 months. These findings suggest that LIA could be a viable alternative to traditional catheter-based approaches, offering effective pain management without compromising muscle function. Future studies should explore longer-term functional outcomes and consider preoperative expectations as potential confounding factors to further validate these results.

10.1.8 Total Knee Arthroplasty in Elderly Patients with Severe Kashin-Beck Disease of the Knee [104]

This is a machine-generated summary of:

Tang, Xin; Zhou, Zong-Ke; Shen, Bin; Kang, Peng-De; Yang, Jing; Li, Jian; Pei, Fu-Xing Total knee arthroplasty in elderly patients with severe Kashin-Beck disease of the knee [104].

Published in: International Orthopaedics (2013).

Link to original: https://doi.org/10.1007/s00264-013-2171-3

If you want to cite the papers, please refer to the original.

For technical reasons we could not place the page where the original quote is coming from.

10.1.8.1 Research Highlights

Kashin-Beck disease (KBD) is a chronic, debilitating condition prevalent in regions such as China, Siberia, and North Korea, characterized by joint pain and deformities, particularly affecting the knees. The disease poses significant treatment challenges, especially in elderly patients, due to limited clinical data and the ineffectiveness of current therapies derived from osteoarthritis treatments. The study by Tang e al. explores the efficacy of total knee arthroplasty (TKA) for treating severe knee involvement in elderly KBD patients with advanced radiographic damage.

The study was conducted at West China Hospital, Sichuan University, involving patients from Aba Prefecture, Sichuan Province. Participants underwent TKA between 2010 and 2015 and were followed for over 2 years postoperatively. Eligibility criteria included severe knee pain and Kellgren-Lawrence grade IV radiographic damage. The surgical procedure involved precise bone cuts and component placement to optimize knee function. Postoperative care included pain management and rehabilitation to enhance recovery. The study utilized various assessment tools such as the Visual Analogue Scale (VAS), Hospital for Special Surgery (HSS) scores, and a specialized Functional Score for Adult Tibetans with Kashin-Beck Disease (FSAT-KBD) to evaluate outcomes.

The findings indicate that TKA significantly alleviates knee pain and improves function in elderly KBD patients, with sustained benefits observed up to the final follow-up. Radiographic assessments showed stable prosthesis positioning without signs of loosening or fracture. The study highlights TKA as a promising intervention for severe KBD of the knee, although the limited sample size suggests caution in generalizing results. Future studies with larger cohorts are necessary to validate these findings further and explore long-term outcomes. This research contributes valuable clinical evidence supporting TKA as a viable treatment option for improving quality of life in KBD patients.

10.1.9 Role of Navigated Total Knee Arthroplasty for Acute Tibial Fractures in the Elderly [105]

This is a machine-generated summary of:

Kini, Sunil Gurpur; Sathappan, S. S. Role of navigated total knee arthroplasty for acute tibial fractures in the elderly [105].

Published in: Archives of Orthopaedic and Trauma Surgery (2013).

Link to original: https://doi.org/10.1007/s00402-013-1792-8

If you want to cite the papers, please refer to the original.

For technical reasons we could not place the page where the original quote is coming from.

10.1.9.1 Research Highlights

Peri-articular knee fractures in the elderly present significant treatment challenges due to factors such as osteoporotic bone, comminution, and pre-existing arthritis. These conditions often lead to high failure rates of primary fixation, largely attributed to poor bone quality. Total knee arthroplasty (TKA) has shown promise in providing consistent results for early weight-bearing and functional outcomes, although it is underreported in this patient subset. A critical issue is the potential for malalignment of the mechanical axis at the fracture site, which is difficult to assess with conventional techniques. The study by Kini et al. explores the use of computer-assisted navigation in TKA to improve component positioning and limb alignment in elderly patients with acute tibial fractures.

The study involved patients with acute tibial fractures who underwent navigated TKA using the Stryker eNLite Navigation System (Stryker Orthopedics, Kalamazoo, Michigan, USA). The cohort included both tibial plateau and diaphyseal fractures, primarily resulting from road traffic accidents. The surgical procedure involved a standard midline incision and medial parapatellar arthrotomy, with navigation aiding in aligning cutting blocks according to the mechanical axis. For tibial plateau fractures, navigation ensured a proximal tibial cut perpendicular to the tibial axis, while diaphyseal fractures were provisionally fixed using a reconstruction plate before proceeding with TKA. The study reported short-term outcomes such as early postoperative walking and medium-term follow-up showing fracture healing and satisfactory functional recovery.

The study advances the understanding of TKA as a viable treatment option for elderly patients with acute upper tibial fractures, particularly when combined with computer-assisted navigation. This approach facilitates immediate weight-bearing and early return to activity while avoiding complications associated with internal fixation. Future study could focus on larger sample sizes and long-term outcomes to further validate these findings. Additionally, exploring cost-effectiveness and accessibility of navigation technology could enhance its application in broader clinical settings.

10.1.10 Long-Term Results of Alpina Postero-Stabilized Total Knee Replacement: 10- to 16-Year Follow-Up [106]

This is a machine-generated summary of:

Lecuire, François; Henry, Julien; Francois, Benjamin; Rubini, Jérôme; Basso, Maurice Long-term results of Alpina Postero-stabilized total knee replacement: 10- to 16-year follow-up [106].

Published in: European Journal of Orthopaedic Surgery & Traumatology (2011).

Link to original: https://doi.org/10.1007/s00590-011-0903-x

If you want to cite the papers, please refer to the original.

For technical reasons we could not place the page where the original quote is coming from.

10.1.10.1 Research Highlights

Total knee arthroplasty (TKA) is a well-established procedure with proven long-term reliability, as evidenced by significant survival rates over extended follow-up periods. Among the various types of TKA, posterior stabilized implants and mobile bearing implants have shown favorable outcomes. However, these designs often rely on high congruence between the femoral component and tibial polyethylene, which can increase the risk of long-term loosening despite improving stability. A less common approach is the "flat on flat" design, which reduces rotational stress and enhances joint function but may increase wear due to linear contact. The study by Lecuire et al. examines the clinical outcomes of the ALPINA PS posterior stabilized prosthesis (Zimmer-Biomet, Warsaw, Indiana, USA), focusing on its cemented and non-cemented versions over a 10- to 15-year period.

The study was conducted at Hôpital René Sabran in Giens, France, where 240 primary TKAs were performed using the ALPINA PS prosthesis. The cohort consisted of patients with a mean age of 69.5 years, predominantly diagnosed with osteoarthritis. The ALPINA PS TKA features a cobalt chrome femoral component, and an ultra-high molecular weight polyethylene insert on a titanium tibial tray. The study included both cemented and non-cemented versions, with optional titanium screws for improved fixation in the latter. Clinical and radiographic assessments were conducted at multiple intervals postoperatively to evaluate implant survival and function using the Knee Society scoring system. Statistical analysis was performed using SPSS (Statistical Package for Social Sciences, IBM) software, with survival rates calculated via the Kaplan-Meier method.

The study reports satisfactory long-term outcomes for the ALPINA PS prosthesis, with a 10-year survival rate of 94% in the best-case scenario. Despite some early patellar complications and polyethylene wear observed in certain cases, no implant loosening was reported at long-term follow-up. The findings suggest that both cemented and non-cemented versions offer reliable performance; however, improvements in polyethylene material could further enhance wear resistance. Future study could focus on comparing this prosthesis with newer designs that incorporate more constrained stabilization systems to assess differences in survivorship and wear over time.

10.1.11 A Retrospective Analysis of Trends in Primary Knee Arthroplasty in Germany from 2008 to 2018 [107]

This is a machine-generated summary of:

Worlicek, Michael; Koch, Matthias; Daniel, Popp; Freigang, Viola; Angele, Peter; Alt, Volker; Kerschbaum, Maximilian; Rupp, Markus A retrospective analysis of trends in primary knee arthroplasty in Germany from 2008 to 2018 [107].

Published in: Scientific Reports (2021).

Link to original: https://doi.org/10.1038/s41598-021-84710-y

If you want to cite the papers, please refer to the original.

For technical reasons we could not place the page where the original quote is coming from.

10.1.11.1 Research Highlights

In Germany, primary total knee arthroplasty (TKA) is among the most frequently performed surgical procedures, driven by an aging population and increasing demand for improved quality of life. This trend is mirrored by a rise in younger patients undergoing these procedures, leading to significant healthcare costs and a growing number of revision surgeries. Despite existing predictions for the future of primary knee arthroplasty in Germany, recent trends in specific arthroplasty procedures remain unclear. The study by Worlicek e al. provides insights into the trends of different primary knee arthroplasty procedures over a decade, examining the influence of age and sex on these surgeries.

The study utilized data from the Federal Statistical Office of Germany, covering all annual surgical procedures from 2005 to 2015. Researchers analyzed this comprehensive dataset, which includes mandatory reporting from all German hospitals, to assess trends in primary knee arthroplasty. The analysis focused on total knee arthroplasty (TKA) and unicompartimental knee arthroplasty (UKA), excluding low-volume procedures like patellofemoral and bicompartimental arthroplasties. Subgroup analyses were conducted based on age and sex. The results revealed a slight overall increase in both partial and total knee arthroplasties over the study period, with UKA showing the most significant rise. Interestingly, while there was a temporary decrease in bicondylar TKA around 2012–2013, numbers have since rebounded.

The study highlights several key findings: a consistent increase in UKA procedures, likely due to advancements in surgical techniques and changes in health insurance regulations; a predominance of female patients undergoing TKA; and a notable rise in younger patients receiving primary knee arthroplasties. These trends suggest that future studies should explore the multifactorial reasons behind the gender disparity in TKA incidence and investigate further improvements in implant technology and surgical methods. Additionally, as the population ages, healthcare systems must prepare for increased demand for both primary and revision knee arthroplasties, posing significant economic challenges.

10.1.12 The Role of Surgeon Volume on Patient Outcome in Total Knee Arthroplasty: A Systematic Review of the Literature [108]

This is a machine-generated summary of:

Lau, Rick L; Perruccio, Anthony V; Gandhi, Rajiv; Mahomed, Nizar N The role of surgeon volume on patient outcome in total knee arthroplasty: a systematic review of the literature [108].

Published in: BMC Musculoskeletal Disorders (2012).

Link to original: https://doi.org/10.1186/1471-2474-13-250

If you want to cite the papers, please refer to the original.

For technical reasons we could not place the page where the original quote is coming from.

10.1.12.1 Research Highlights

Primary total knee arthroplasty (TKA) is a widely accepted treatment for alleviating pain and disability in patients with end-stage knee osteoarthritis. Despite its success, a notable minority of patients experience complications and poor outcomes post-surgery. This is particularly concerning given the projected increase in TKA procedures in the United States over the coming years. Various factors, including patient demographics, surgical techniques, and provider characteristics, influence TKA outcomes. While hospital volume has been linked to improved surgical outcomes, the impact of surgeon volume on TKA results remains unclear. The study by Lau et al. undertakes a systematic review to explore the association between surgeon volume and primary TKA outcomes.

The study conducted a comprehensive search of PubMed and OVID MEDLINE databases to identify relevant studies comparing TKA outcomes between low-volume and high-volume surgeons. The review included 11 non-randomized observational studies from various countries, primarily North America. These studies utilized different databases to gather patient data and varied in their definitions of surgeon volume, often categorizing them based on tertiles or quartiles of annual procedures performed. The review examined several perioperative outcomes such as surgical site infections, medical complications, length of stay (LOS), procedure length, implant survivorship, and patient-reported outcomes. Despite methodological variability across studies, some trends emerged: higher surgeon volumes were generally associated with lower infection rates and shorter LOS, although statistical significance was not consistently achieved.

The findings suggest a trend towards better outcomes for higher-volume surgeons; however, the evidence is not robust enough to support widespread regionalization policies based solely on surgeon volume. The reviewed studies were predominantly low-quality observational trials with significant variability in methodology and outcome measures. Future study should focus on standardizing definitions of surgeon volume and exploring long-term implant survivorship to better understand these associations. Additionally, examining the cost-effectiveness of regionalization strategies will be crucial before implementing policies that might restrict access for certain patient populations. As healthcare resources become more limited, optimizing patient care efficiently remains a priority.

10.1.13 International Primary Knee Arthroplasty Registry Review: Findings from Current Reports [109]

This is a machine-generated summary of:

Sidhu, Arsh; Sheridan, Gerard A.; Greidanus, Nelson V.; Neufeld, Michael E.; Howard, Lisa C.; Masri, Bassam A.; Garbuz, Donald S. International primary knee arthroplasty registry review: findings from current reports [109].

Published in: European Journal of Orthopaedic Surgery & Traumatology (2023).

Link to original: https://doi.org/10.1007/s00590-023-03521-1

If you want to cite the papers, please refer to the original.

For technical reasons we could not place the page where the original quote is coming from.

10.1.13.1 Research Highlights

International joint registries provide extensive data on the performance of total knee arthroplasty (TKA) worldwide, but synthesizing this information can be challenging due to the increasing number of registries. Key questions in TKA include the superiority of fixation types, the impact of constraint levels on clinical performance, and the outcomes of partial knee replacements. The study by Sidhu et al. aims to distill key insights from major English-speaking knee arthroplasty registries, focusing on primary TKA and addressing these critical questions.

The study conducted a comprehensive review of major English-speaking knee arthroplasty registries, including those from the UK, Australia, New Zealand, and the USA. The authors analyzed trends in fixation methods, constraint levels, and partial knee replacements. Cemented fixation remains predominant across most registries, although there is a noted increase in cementless TKA in some regions like the USA and Australia. The study also highlights that cruciate-retaining designs are favored over posterior-stabilized implants due to lower revision rates. Partial knee replacements (UKA) show higher revision rates compared to TKA across all registries. Patellar resurfacing appears to reduce revision rates in TKA, particularly in older patients.

The findings underscore the ongoing preference for cemented fixation and cruciate-retaining designs in TKA due to their lower revision rates. However, there is a growing interest in cementless options and robotic-assisted procedures that may influence future trends. Future study could focus on long-term outcomes of cementless TKA and the impact of robotic assistance on revision rates. Additionally, understanding why patellar resurfacing leads to better outcomes could refine surgical approaches further. This study provides valuable insights into current practices and potential future directions in knee arthroplasty based on registry data.

Bibliography

1. Verhaar J (1995) HA coating in knee arthroplasty: principles, importance and results. In: Cahiers d'enseignement de la SOFCOT: hydroxyapatite coated hip and knee arthroplasty. Expansion Scientifique Francaise Ed., Paris, pp 319–322
2. Epinette JA (1995) Hydroxyapatite and TKR: the HA omnifit knee prosthesis. In: Cahiers d'enseignement de la SOFCOT: hydroxyapatite coated hip and knee arthroplasty. Expansion Scientifique Francaise Ed., Paris, pp 323–332
3. Nilsson KG, Kärrholm J, Carlsson L, Dalen T (1999) Hydroxyapatite coating versus cemented fixation of the tibial component in total knee arthroplasty. J Arthroplasty 14:9–20
4. Epinette JA, Manley MT (2007) Hydroxyapatite-coated total knee replacement: clinical experience at 10 to 15 years. J Bone Surg Br 89(1):34
5. Duffy GP, Berry DJ, Rand JA (1998) Cement versus cementless fixation in total knee arthroplasty. Clin Orthop Relat Res 356:66–72
6. Regner L, Carlsson L, Karrholm J, Herberts P (2000) Tibial component fixation in porous- and hydroxyapatite-coated total knee arthroplasty: a

radiostereometric evaluation of migration and inducible displacement after 5 years. J Arthroplasty 15:681–689
7. Siparsky P, Ryzewicz M, Peterson B, Bartz R (2007) Arthroscopic treatment of osteoarthritis of the knee: are there any evidence-based indications? Clin Orthop Relat Res. 455:107–12
8. Sonesson S, Kvist J, Yakob J et al (2020) Knee arthroscopic surgery in middle-aged patients with meniscal symptoms: a 5-year follow-up of a prospective, Randomized Study. Orthop J Sport Med. https://doi.org/10.1177/2325967119893920
9. Piedade SR, Pinaroli A, Servien E, Neyret P (2013) TKA outcomes after prior bone and soft tissue knee surgery. Knee Surgery, Sport Traumatol Arthrosc 21:2737–2743. https://doi.org/10.1007/s00167-012-2139-7
10. Issa K, Naziri Q, Johnson AJ et al (2012) TKA results are not compromised by previous arthroscopic procedures. J Knee Surg 25:161–164. https://doi.org/10.1055/s-0032-1313755
11. Werner BC, Burrus MT, Novicoff WM, Browne JA (2015) Total knee arthroplasty within six months after knee arthroscopy is associated with increased postoperative complications. J Arthroplasty 30:1313–1316. https://doi.org/10.1016/j.arth.2015.02.023
12. Barton SB, McLauchlan GJ, Canty SJ (2017) The incidence and impact of arthroscopy in the year prior to total knee arthroplasty. Knee 24:396–401. https://doi.org/10.1016/j.knee.2016.12.003
13. Viste A, Abdel MP, Ollivier M et al (2017) Prior knee arthroscopy does not influence long-term total knee arthroplasty outcomes and survivorship. J Arthroplasty 32:3626–3631. https://doi.org/10.1016/j.arth.2017.06.052
14. Gu A, Malahias MA, Cohen JS et al (2020) Prior knee arthroscopy is associated with increased risk of revision after total knee arthroplasty. J Arthroplasty 35:100–104. https://doi.org/10.1016/j.arth.2019.08.043
15. Rothermich MA, Nam D, Brophy RH et al (2017) The impact of prior surgery after total knee arthroplasty. J Knee Surg 30:57–62. https://doi.org/10.1055/s-0036-1579666
16. Chaudhry ZS, Salem HS, Purtill JJ, Hammoud S (2019) Does prior anterior cruciate ligament reconstruction affect outcomes of subsequent total knee arthroplasty? A systematic review. Orthop J Sport Med. https://doi.org/10.1177/2325967119857551
17. Butt U, Ahmad R, Aspros D, Bannister GC (2011) Factors affecting wound ooze in total knee replacement. Ann R Coll Surg Engl 93:54–56
18. Tai TW, Lin CJ, Jou IM, Chang CW, Lai KA, Yang CY (2011) Tourniquet use in total knee arthroplasty: a meta-analysis. Knee Surg Sports Traumatol Arthrosc 19:1121–1130
19. Rama KR, Apsingi S, Poovali S, Jetti A (2007) Timing of tourniquet release in knee arthroplasty. Meta-analysis of randomized, controlled trials. J Bone Joint Surg Am 89:699–705
20. Noel E, Miglionico L, Leclercq M, Jennart H, Fils J-F, Van Rompaey N. Sufentanil sublingual tablet system versus oral oxycodone for management

of postoperative pain in enhanced recovery after surgery pathway for total knee arthroplasty: a randomized controlled study. J Exp Orthop. 2020;7(1):92.
21. van Veen DE, Verhelst CC, van Dellen RT, Koopman J. Sublingual sufentanil (Zalviso) patient-controlled analgesia after total knee arthroplasty: a retrospective comparison with oxycodone with or without dexamethasone. J Pain Res. 2018;11:3205–10.
22. Léger M, Campfort M, Cayla C, Lasocki S, Rineau E. Postoperative quality of recovery measurements as endpoints in comparative anaesthesia studies: a systematic review. Br J Anaesth. 2021;126(6):e210–2.
23. Yuksel E, Kalkan S, Cekmece S, Unver B, Karatosun V. Assessing Minimal detectable changes and test-retest reliability of the timed up and go test and the 2-minute walk test in patients with total knee arthroplasty. J Arthroplast. 2017;32(2):426–30.
24. Murray DW, Fitzpatrick R, Rogers K et al (2007) The use of the Oxford hip and knee scores. J Bone Jt Surg Ser B 89:1010–1014
25. Clement ND, MacDonald D, Burnett R (2013) Predicting patient satisfaction using the Oxford knee score: where do we draw the line? Arch Orthop Trauma Surg. https://doi.org/10.1007/s00402-013-1728-3
26. Tay ML, Monk AP, Frampton CM et al (2023) The strongest Oxford knee score predictors of subsequent revision are overall pain, limping when walking, and knee giving way. J Arthroplast 38:S156-S161.e3. https://doi.org/10.1016/j.arth.2023.03.001
27. Dawson J, Fitzpatrick R, Murray D, Carr A (1998) Questionnaire on the perceptions of patients about total knee replacement. J Bone Jt Surg Ser B 80:63–69. https://doi.org/10.1302/0301-620X.80B1.7859
28. Leppink J, O'Sullivan P, Winston K (2016) Effect size – large, medium, and small. Perspect Med Educ 5:347–349. https://doi.org/10.1007/s40037-016-0308-y
29. Luger M, Schopper C, Krottenthaler ES et al (2023) Not all questions are created equal: the weight of the Oxford knee scores questions in a multicentric validation study. J Orthop Traumatol. https://doi.org/10.1186/s10195-023-00722-6
30. Clement ND, Afzal I, Demetriou C et al (2020) The preoperative oxford knee score is an independent predictor of achieving a postoperative ceiling score after total knee arthroplasty. Bone Jt J 102:1519–1526. https://doi.org/10.1302/0301-620X.102B11.BJJ-2019-1327.R1
31. Rice, D. *et al.* Persistent postoperative pain after total knee arthroplasty: A prospective cohort study of potential risk factors. *Br. J. Anaesth. 121*, 804–812 (2018).
32. Judge A, Arden NK, Cooper C et al (2012) Predictors of outcomes of total knee replacement surgery. Rheumatol (United Kingdom) 51:1804–1813. https://doi.org/10.1093/rheumatology/kes075
33. Lingard, E. A. and Riddle, D. L. Impact of psychological distress on pain and function following knee arthroplasty. *J. Bone Joint Surg. Am. 89*, 1161–1169. https://doi.org/10.2106/jbjs.F.00914 (2007).

34. Witvrouw, E. *et al.* Catastrophic thinking about pain as a predictor of length of hospital stay after total knee arthroplasty: A prospective study. *Knee Surg. Sports Traumatol. Arthrosc. 17*, 1189–1194. https://doi.org/10.1007/s00167-009-0817-x (2009).
35. Edwards, R. R., Haythornthwaite, J. A., Smith, M. T., Klick, B. and Katz, J. N. Catastrophizing and depressive symptoms as prospective predictors of outcomes following total knee replacement. *Pain Res. Manag. 14*, 307–311. https://doi.org/10.1155/2009/273783 (2009).
36. Sullivan, M. *et al.* The role of presurgical expectancies in predicting pain and function one year following total knee arthroplasty. *Pain 152*, 2287–2293 (2011).
37. Dave, A. J. *et al.* The association of pre-operative body pain diagram scores with pain outcomes following total knee arthroplasty. *Osteoarthr. Cartil. 25*, 667–675. https://doi.org/10.1016/j.joca.2016.12.013 (2017).
38. Burns, L. C. *et al.* Pain catastrophizing as a risk factor for chronic pain after total knee arthroplasty: A systematic review. *J. Pain Res. 8*, 21–32. https://doi.org/10.2147/jpr.S64730 (2015).
39. Lewis, G. N., Rice, D. A., McNair, P. J. and Kluger, M. Predictors of persistent pain after total knee arthroplasty: A systematic review and meta-analysis. *Br. J. Anaesth. 114*, 551–561. https://doi.org/10.1093/bja/aeu441 (2015).
40. Hernández, C. *et al.* Pre-operative predictive factors of post-operative pain in patients with hip or knee arthroplasty: A systematic review. *Reumatol. Clín. (Engl. Ed.) 11*, 361–380. https://doi.org/10.1016/j.reumae.2014.12.011 (2015).
41. Baert, I. A. C. *et al.* Does pre-surgical central modulation of pain influence outcome after total knee replacement? A systematic review. *Osteoarthr. Cartil. 24*, 213–223. https://doi.org/10.1016/j.joca.2015.09.002 (2016).
42. Olsen, U. *et al.* Factors correlated with pain after total knee arthroplasty: A systematic review and meta-analysis. *PLoS One 18*, e0283446. https://doi.org/10.1371/journal.pone.0283446 (2023).
43. Bierke, S. and Petersen, W. Influence of anxiety and pain catastrophizing on the course of pain within the first year after uncomplicated total knee replacement: A prospective study. *Arch. Orthop. Trauma Surg. 137*, 1735–1742 (2017).
44. Sullivan, M. *et al.* Psychological determinants of problematic outcomes following Total Knee Arthroplasty. *Pain 143*, 123–129. https://doi.org/10.1016/j.pain.2009.02.011 (2009).
45. Riddle, D. L., Wade, J. B., Jiranek, W. A. and Kong, X. Preoperative pain catastrophizing predicts pain outcome after knee arthroplasty. *Clin. Orthop. Relat. Res. 468*, 798–806. https://doi.org/10.1007/s11999-009-0963-y (2010).
46. Yakobov, E. *et al.* The role of perceived injustice in the prediction of pain and function after total knee arthroplasty. *Pain 155*, 2040–2046. https://doi.org/10.1016/j.pain.2014.07.007 (2014).
47. Bellamy, N., Buchanan, W. W., Goldsmith, C. H., Campbell, J. and Stitt, L. W. Validation study of WOMAC: A health status instrument for measuring clinically important patient relevant outcomes to antirheumatic drug therapy

in patients with osteoarthritis of the hip or knee. *J. Rheumatol. 15*, 1833–1840 (1988).
48. Leung, Y.-Y., Thumboo, J., Yeo, S.-J., Wylde, V. and Tannant, A. Validation and interval scale transformation of the Western Ontario and McMaster Universities Osteoarthritis Index (WOMAC) in patients undergoing knee arthroplasty, using the Rasch model. *Osteoarthr. Cartil. Open* https://doi.org/10.1016/j.ocarto.2022.100322 (2022).
49. Albrecht E, Guyen O, Jacot-Guillarmod A, Kirkham KR (2016) The analgesic efficacy of local infiltration analgesia vs femoral nerve block after total knee arthroplasty: a systematic review and meta-analysis. Br J Anaesth 116:597–609
50. Matsumoto S, Matsumoto K, Lida H (2015) Transdermal fentanyl patch improves post-operative pain relief and promotes early functional recovery in patients undergoing primary total knee arthroplasty: a prospective, randomised, controlled trial. Arch Orthop Trauma Surg. 135(9):1291–1297
51. Wiesmann T, Piechowiak K, Duderstadt S, Haupt D, Schmitt J, Eschbach D, Feldmann C, Wulf H, Zoremba M, Steinfeldt T (2016) Continuous adductor canal block versus continuous femoral nerve block after total knee arthroplasty for mobilisation capability and pain treatment: a randomised and blinded clinical trial. Arch Orthop Trauma Surg. 136(3):397–406
52. Fu H, Wang J, Zhang W, Cheng T, Zhang X (2017) Potential superiority of periarticular injection in analgesic effect and early mobilization ability over femoral nerve block following total knee arthroplasty. Knee Surg Sports Traumatol Arthrosc 25:291–298
53. Zhang LK, Ma JX, Kuang MJ, Ma XL (2018) Comparison of periarticular local infiltration analgesia with femoral nerve block for total knee arthroplasty: a meta-analysis of randomized controlled trials. J Arthroplasty 33(6):1972–1978 (*review*
54. Zhou Z, Shen B, Pei F et al (2009) Relation between affected big joints and classification of Kashin–Beck disease in adult of Tibet (Article in Chinese). Chin J Bone Joint Surg 2:352–356
55. Luo R, Liu G, Liu W et al (2011) Efficacy of celecoxib, meloxicam and paracetamol in elderly Kashin-Beck disease (KBD) patients. Int Orthop 35:1409–1414
56. Bjordal JM, Ljunggren AE, Klovning A et al (2004) Non-steroidal anti-inflammatory drugs, including cyclo-oxygenase-2 inhibitors, in osteoarthritic knee pain: meta-analysis of randomised placebo controlled trials. BMJ 329:1317
57. Mathieu F, Suetens C, Begaux F et al (2001) Effects of physical therapy on patients with Kashin-Beck disease in Tibet. Int Orthop 5:191–193
58. Guo X (2001) Diagnostic, clinical and radiological characteristics of Kashin Beck disease in Shaanxi Province, PR China. Int Orthop 25:147–150
59. Mathieu F, Begaux F, Lan ZY et al (1997) Clinical manifestations of Kashin–Beck disease in Nyemo Valley, Tibet. Int Orthop 21:151–156
60. Ali AM, El-Shafie M, Willett KM (2002) Failure of fixation of tibial plateau fractures. J Orthop Trauma 16–5:323–329

61. Larsen JE, Chao EY, Fitzgerald RH (1991) Bypassing femoral cortical defects with cemented intramedullary stems. J Orthop Res 9:414–421
62. Insall JN, Lachiewicz PF, Burstein AH (1982) The posterior stabilized condylar prosthesis: a modification of the total condylar design. J Bone Jt Surg A 64:1317–1323
63. Rodriguez JA (1997) The press-fit condylar modular total knee system with a posterior cruciate-substituting design. J Bone Jt Surg A 79:342–348
64. Ritter MA (2009) The anatomical graduated component total knee replacement: a long-term evaluation with 20 years survival analysis. J Bone Jt Surg 91-B:745–749
65. Berger RA, Rosenberg AG, Barden RM, Sheinkop MB, Jacob JJ, Galante JO (2001) Long term follow up of the Miller-Galante total knee replacement. Clin Orthop Relat Res 338:58–67
66. Hon-Ming M, Yung-Chang L, Fang-Yuan H, Chun-Hsiung H (2005) Long term results of total condylar knee arthroplasty. J Arthroplasty 20(5):580–584
67. Ranawat CS, Flynn WF Jr, Saddler S (1993) Long-term results of the total condylar knee arthroplasty. A 15-year survivorship study. Clin Orthop Relat Res 286:94–102
68. Buechel FF Sr (2002) Long term follow-up after mobile-bearing total knee replacement. Clin Orthop Relat Res 404:40–50
69. Ewald FC (1989) The knee society total knee arthroplasty roentgenographic evaluation and scoring system. Clin Orthop Relat Res 248:9–12
70. Gademan, M. G., Hofstede, S. N., Vliet Vlieland, T. P., Nelissen, R. G. and Marang-van de Mheen, P. J. Indication criteria for total hip or knee arthroplasty in osteoarthritis: a state-of-the-science overview. *BMC Musculoskelet. Disord. 17*, 463. https://doi.org/10.1186/s12891-016-1325-z (2016).
71. Robertsson, O. *et al.* Knee arthroplasty in Denmark, Norway and Sweden. A pilot study from the Nordic Arthroplasty Register Association. *Acta Orthop. 81*, 82–89. https://doi.org/10.3109/17453671003685442 (2010).
72. Slover, J. and Zuckerman, J. D. Increasing use of total knee replacement and revision surgery. *JAMA 308*, 1266–1268. https://doi.org/10.1001/jama.2012.12644 (2012).
73. Kurtz, S. M. *et al.* Future young patient demand for primary and revision joint replacement: national projections from 2010 to 2030. *Clin. Orthop. Relat. Res. 467*, 2606–2612. https://doi.org/10.1007/s11999-009-0834-6 (2009).
74. Kurtz, S. *et al.* Prevalence of primary and revision total hip and knee arthroplasty in the United States from 1990 through 2002. *J. Bone Joint Surg. Am. 87*, 1487–1497. https://doi.org/10.2106/JBJS.D.02441 (2005).
75. Cram, P. *et al.* Long-term trends in hip arthroplasty use and volume. *J. Arthroplasty 27*, 278–285. https://doi.org/10.1016/j.arth.2011.04.043 (2012) (*e72*).
76. Kurtz, S., Ong, K., Lau, E., Mowat, F. and Halpern, M. Projections of primary and revision hip and knee arthroplasty in the United States from 2005 to 2030. *J. Bone Joint Surg. Am. 89*, 780–785. https://doi.org/10.2106/JBJS.F.00222 (2007).

77. Culliford, D. *et al.* Future projections of total hip and knee arthroplasty in the UK: results from the UK Clinical Practice Research Datalink. *Osteoarthr. Cartil. 23*, 594–600. https://doi.org/10.1016/j.joca.2014.12.022 (2015).
78. Romanini, E. *et al.* Total knee arthroplasty in Italy: reflections from the last fifteen years and projections for the next thirty. *Int. Orthop. 43*, 133–138. https://doi.org/10.1007/s00264-018-4165-7 (2019).
79. Aujla, R. S. and Esler, C. N. Total knee arthroplasty for osteoarthritis in patients less than fifty-five years of age: a systematic review. *J. Arthroplasty 32*, 2598–2603. https://doi.org/10.1016/j.arth.2017.02.069 (2017) (*e2591*).
80. Losina, E., Thornhill, T. S., Rome, B. N., Wright, J. and Katz, J. N. The dramatic increase in total knee replacement utilization rates in the United States cannot be fully explained by growth in population size and the obesity epidemic. *J. Bone Joint Surg. Am. 94*, 201–207. https://doi.org/10.2106/JBJS.J.01958 (2012).
81. Maradit Kremers, H. *et al.* Prevalence of total hip and knee replacement in the United States. *J. Bone Joint Surg. Am. 97*, 1386–1397. https://doi.org/10.2106/JBJS.N.01141 (2015).
82. Bourne RB, McCalden RW, MacDonald SJ, Mokete L, Guerin J: Influence of patient factors on TKA outcomes at 5 to 11 years followup. Clin Orthop Relat Res. 2007, 464: 27-31.
83. Rolfson O, Dahlberg LE, Nilsson J-A, Malchau H, Garellick G: Variables determining outcome in total hip replacement surgery. J Bone Joint Surg Br. 2009, 91: 157-161. https://doi.org/10.1302/0301-620X.91B2.20765 .
84. Barrack RL, Schrader T, Bertot AJ, Wolfe MW, Myers L: Component rotation and anterior knee pain after total knee arthroplasty. Clin Orthop Relat Res. 2001, 392: 46-55.
85. Katz JN, Barrett J, Mahomed NN, Baron JA, Wright RJ, Losina E: Association between hospital and surgeon procedure volume and the outcomes of total knee replacement. J Bone Joint Surg Am. 2004, 86-A: 1909-1916.
86. Hervey SL, Purves HR, Guller U, Toth AP, Vail TP, Pietrobon R: Provider Volume of Total Knee Arthroplasties and Patient Outcomes in the HCUP-Nationwide Inpatient Sample. J Bone Joint Surg Am. 2003, 85-A: 1775-1783.
87. Baker P, Dowen D, McMurtry I: The effect of surgeon volume on the need for transfusion following primary unilateral hip and knee arthroplasty. Surgeon. 2011, 9: 13-17. https://doi.org/10.1016/j.surge.2010.08.011 .
88. Katz JN, Mahomed NN, Baron JA, Barrett JA, Fossel AH, Creel AH, Wright J, Wright EA, Losina E: Association of hospital and surgeon procedure volume with patient-centered outcomes of total knee replacement in a population-based cohort of patients age 65 years and older. Arthritis Rheum. 2007, 56: 568-574. https://doi.org/10.1002/art.22333 .
89. Wei M-H, Lin Y-L, Shi H-Y, Chiu H-C: Effects of provider patient volume and comorbidity on clinical and economic outcomes for total knee arthroplasty: a population-based study. J Arthroplasty. 2010, 25: 906-912. 10.1016/j.arth.2009.06.033. e1

90. Muilwijk J, van den Hof S, Wille JC: Associations between surgical site infection risk and hospital operation volume and surgeon operation volume among hospitals in the Dutch nosocomial infection surveillance network. Infect Control Hosp Epidemiol. 2007, 28: 557-563. https://doi.org/10.1086/513613 .
91. Yasunaga H, Tsuchiya K, Matsuyama Y, Ohe K: Analysis of factors affecting operating time, postoperative complications, and length of stay for total knee arthroplasty: nationwide web-based survey. J Orthop Sci. 2009, 14: 10-16. https://doi.org/10.1007/s00776-008-1294-7 .
92. Kreder HJ, Grosso P, Williams JI, Jaglal S, Axcell T, Wal EK, Stephen DJG: Provider volume and other predictors of outcome after total knee arthroplasty: a population study in Ontario. Can J Surg. 2003, 46: 15-22.
93. Styron JF, Koroukian SM, Klika AK, Barsoum WK: Patient vs Provider Characteristics Impacting Hospital Lengths of Stay After Total Knee or Hip Arthroplasty. J Arthroplasty. 2011, 26: 1418-1426. https://doi.org/10.1016/j.arth.2010.11.008.e2
94. Paterson JM, Williams JI, Kreder HJ, Mahomed NN, Gunraj N, Wang X, Laupacis A: Provider volumes and early outcomes of primary total joint replacement in Ontario. Can J Surg. 2010, 53: 175-183.
95. Garcia RM, Messerschmitt PJ, Furey CG, Bohlman HH, Cassinelli EH: Weight Loss in Overweight and Obese Patigents Following Successful Lumbar Decompression. The Journal of Bone and Joint Surgery. 2008, 90: 742-747. https://doi.org/10.2106/JBJS.G.00724 .
96. Marlow NE, Barraclough B, Collier NA, Dickinson IC, Fawcett J, Graham JC, Maddern GJ: Centralization and the relationship between volume and outcome in knee arthroplasty procedures. ANZ journal of surgery. 2010, 80: 234-241. https://doi.org/10.1111/j.1445-2197.2010.05243.x .
97. Epinette, Jean-Alain Long lasting outcome of hydroxyapatite-coated implants in primary knee arthroplasty: a continuous series of two hundred and seventy total knee arthroplasties at fifteen to twenty two years of clinical follow-up. International Orthopaedics (2014). https://doi.org/10.1007/s00264-013-2246-1
98. Goyal, Tarun; Tripathy, Sujit Kumar; Schuh, Alexander; Paul, Souvik Total knee arthroplasty after a prior knee arthroscopy has higher complication rates: a systematic review. Archives of Orthopaedic and Trauma Surgery (2021). https://doi.org/10.1007/s00402-021-04175-6
99. [99] Olivecrona, Charlotta; Lapidus, Lasse J.; Benson, Lina; Blomfeldt, Richard Tourniquet time affects postoperative complications after knee arthroplasty. International Orthopaedics (2013). https://doi.org/10.1007/s00264-013-1826-4
100. Rineau, Emmanuel; Dumartinet, Benjamin; Samson, Emmanuel; Dollfus, Apolline; Aubourg, Corentin; Lasocki, Sigismond Sufentanil sublingual tablet system for enhanced recovery after total knee arthroplasty: a prospective observational case study. Perioperative Medicine (2022). https://doi.org/10.1186/s13741-022-00284-x
101. Clement, N. D.; Jones, S.; Afzal, I.; Kader, D. F. A comprehensive analysis of the pre- and postoperative responses to each of the 12 Oxford knee score ques-

tions one year following knee arthroplasty. European Journal of Orthopaedic Surgery & Traumatology (2024). https://doi.org/10.1007/s00590-024-03870-5
102. Chan, Diana; Saffari, Seyed Ehsan; Wong, Steven Bak Siew; Yeo, Seng Jin; Wylde, Vikki; Thumboo, Julian; Leung, Ying-Ying The influence of pain catastrophizing on pain and function after knee arthroplasty in knee osteoarthritis. Scientific Reports (2024). https://doi.org/10.1038/s41598-024-67561-1
103. Mayr, H. O.; Prall, W. C.; Haasters, F.; Baumbach, S. F.; Hube, R.; Stoehr, Amelie Pain relieve without impairing muscle function after local infiltration anaesthesia in primary knee arthroplasty: a prospective randomized study. Archives of Orthopaedic and Trauma Surgery (2019). https://doi.org/10.1007/s00402-019-03194-8
104. Tang, Xin; Zhou, Zong-Ke; Shen, Bin; Kang, Peng-De; Yang, Jing; Li, Jian; Pei, Fu-Xing Total knee arthroplasty in elderly patients with severe Kashin-Beck disease of the knee. International Orthopaedics (2013). https://doi.org/10.1007/s00264-013-2171-3
105. Kini, Sunil Gurpur; Sathappan, S. S. Role of navigated total knee arthroplasty for acute tibial fractures in the elderly. Archives of Orthopaedic and Trauma Surgery (2013). https://doi.org/10.1007/s00402-013-1792-8
106. Lecuire, François; Henry, Julien; Francois, Benjamin; Rubini, Jérôme; Basso, Maurice Long-term results of Alpina Postero-stabilized total knee replacement: 10- to 16-year follow-up. European Journal of Orthopaedic Surgery & Traumatology (2011). https://doi.org/10.1007/s00590-011-0903-x
107. Worlicek, Michael; Koch, Matthias; Daniel, Popp; Freigang, Viola; Angele, Peter; Alt, Volker; Kerschbaum, Maximilian; Rupp, Markus A retrospective analysis of trends in primary knee arthroplasty in Germany from 2008 to 2018. Scientific Reports (2021). https://doi.org/10.1038/s41598-021-84710-y
108. Lau, Rick L; Perruccio, Anthony V; Gandhi, Rajiv; Mahomed, Nizar N The role of surgeon volume on patient outcome in total knee arthroplasty: a systematic review of the literature. BMC Musculoskeletal Disorders (2012). https://doi.org/10.1186/1471-2474-13-250
109. Sidhu, Arsh; Sheridan, Gerard A.; Greidanus, Nelson V.; Neufeld, Michael E.; Howard, Lisa C.; Masri, Bassam A.; Garbuz, Donald S. International primary knee arthroplasty registry review: findings from current reports. European Journal of Orthopaedic Surgery & Traumatology (2023). https://doi.org/10.1007/s00590-023-03521-1

10.2 Revision Knee Arthroplasty

Machine Generated Summaries

Disclaimer: The summaries in this chapter were generated from Springer Nature publications using abstractive AI auto-summarization: An abstraction-based summarizer creates new text based on deep learning. New phrases are created to summarize the content. As the constituted sentences are machine selected, they may not fully reflect the body of the work, so we strongly advise that the original content is read and cited. The auto-generated summaries were curated by the editor to meet Springer Nature publication standards.

10.2.1 The Effect of Time Spent with a Dynamic Spacer on Clinical and Functional Outcomes in Two-Stage Revision Knee Arthroplasty [113]

This is a machine-generated summary of:

Golgelioglu, Fatih; Oguzkaya, Sinan; Misir, Abdulhamit; Guney, Ahmet The Effect of Time Spent with a Dynamic Spacer on Clinical and Functional Outcomes in Two-Stage Revision Knee Arthroplasty [113].

Published in: Indian Journal of Orthopaedics (2020).

Link to original: https://doi.org/10.1007/s43465-020-00247-8

If you want to cite the papers, please refer to the original.

For technical reasons we could not place the page where the original quote is coming from.

10.2.1.1 Research Highlights

Periprosthetic joint infection (PJI) is a severe complication following total knee arthroplasty (TKA), often necessitating revision surgeries. With the increasing number of TKA procedures performed annually in the USA, the incidence of infections and subsequent revisions is expected to rise. Single- and two-stage revisions are primary treatments for chronic infected TKA, with two-stage revision being the preferred method. Dynamic spacers are favored over static ones due to better functional outcomes. However, the impact of time spent with a spacer on knee range of motion (ROM), functional outcomes, quality of life, and treatment costs remains unexplored. The study by Golgelioglu et al. investigates these effects, hypothesizing that shorter spacer duration leads to improved outcomes.

The study retrospectively evaluated patients who underwent two-stage revision TKA due to chronic PJI between 2010 and 2020, with a minimum follow-up of 1 year. Patients were divided into two groups based on spacer duration: less than 3 months (Group 1) and more than 3 months (Group 2). The Musculoskeletal Infection Society criteria were used for diagnosing PJI, followed by implant removal, debridement, and insertion of an antibiotic-loaded dynamic spacer. The second stage was performed based on clinical resolution indicators. Functional outcomes were assessed using Knee Society Scores (KSS) and quality of life via the

Short Form-36 survey. Treatment costs were also analyzed. Statistical analyses included t-tests, chi-square tests, and Kaplan-Meier survival analysis.

The study found that patients with shorter spacer durations had significantly better postoperative KSS-Knee and KSS-Function scores, as well as higher quality of life scores in general health domains. Treatment costs were notably lower for this group due to reduced hospital stays and antibiotic use. Importantly, there was no significant difference in reinfection rates between groups. These findings suggest that minimizing spacer duration can enhance clinical outcomes without increasing reinfection risk. Future studies could further explore these relationships in larger cohorts and consider additional factors influencing spacer duration decisions.

10.2.2 Sagittal Profile Has a Significant Impact on the Explantability of Well-Fixed Cemented Stems in Revision Knee Arthroplasty: A Biomechanical Comparison Study of Five Established Knee Implant Models [114]

This is a machine-generated summary of:

Maslaris, Alexander; Layher, Frank; Bungartz, Matthias; Zippelius, Timo; Liodakis, Emmanouil; Brinkmann, Olaf; Matziolis, Georg Sagittal profile has a significant impact on the explantability of well-fixed cemented stems in revision knee arthroplasty: a biomechanical comparison study of five established knee implant models [114].

Published in: Archives of Orthopaedic and Trauma Surgery (2019).

Link to original: https://doi.org/10.1007/s00402-019-03160-4

If you want to cite the papers, please refer to the original.

For technical reasons we could not place the page where the original quote is coming from.

10.2.2.1 Research Highlights

Primary knee arthroplasty (TKA) remains the gold standard for treating gonarthrosis but revision knee arthroplasty (TKR) is becoming increasingly common due to rising complication rates. Despite advancements in implant technology and surgical techniques, TKR outcomes are limited by high complication rates, including periprosthetic infections and re-revision needs. The study by Maslaris et al. investigates the explantability of five well-fixed cemented revision knee prostheses, focusing on how design properties like sagittal profile, cross-sectional design, and surface roughness affect the debonding process of the implant-cement interface.

The study involved biomechanical testing of five shaft extensions from different TKR models to assess their explantation energy (EE) requirements. Each stem was cemented into a metal tube and subjected to axial pull forces using a slotted weight system. The team conducted multiple tests for each stem design to ensure statistical significance. Results showed that stems with a purely conical profile required significantly less EE for removal compared to cylindrical designs. Regression analysis revealed a strong negative correlation between the conicity proportion of the sagittal stem profile and EE, indicating that conical designs facilitate easier explantation. Surface roughness and cross-sectional design had minimal impact on EE compared to conicity.

The study advances our understanding of implant design's role in TKR procedures, highlighting that conical stem profiles significantly ease explantation compared to cylindrical ones. This finding suggests that selecting implants with favorable design characteristics could reduce surgical morbidity associated with TKR revisions. Future study could explore clinical trials to further assess how sagittal stem profiles influence revision outcomes and implant longevity. These insights can guide surgeons in choosing appropriate implants and removal techniques, potentially improving patient outcomes in revision knee arthroplasty.

10.2.3 Constraint Choice in Revision Knee Arthroplasty [115]

This is a machine-generated summary of:

Vasso, Michele; Beaufils, Philippe; Schiavone Panni, Alfredo Constraint choice in revision knee arthroplasty [115].

Published in: International Orthopaedics (2013).

Link to original: https://doi.org/10.1007/s00264-013-1929-y

If you want to cite the papers, please refer to the original.

For technical reasons we could not place the page where the original quote is coming from.

10.2.3.1 Research Highlights

The increasing number of total knee arthroplasties (TKAs) performed annually has led to a rise in revision surgeries, which are more complex and often result in poorer outcomes compared to primary procedures. Factors such as host bone stock deficiency, extensor mechanism problems, and ligamentous instability contribute to these challenges. A significant issue in revision TKA is managing ligamentous instability, which affects the function and longevity of knee joint reconstructions. The study by Vasso et al. presents a modern algorithm for selecting implant constraints based on the state of peripheral ligaments and bone defects classified by the Anderson Orthopaedic Research Institute (AORI) system, aiming to improve stability and long-term success in knee revisions.

The study involved consecutive revision TKAs performed between 2005 and 2015, with patients assessed preoperatively and at regular intervals post-revision. The researchers categorized ligament conditions as intact, insufficient, or absent, and bone loss according to the AORI classification. They used different prosthetic designs based on these assessments: primary postero-stabilized (PS) implants for intact ligaments with minimal bone loss, condylar constrained knee (CCK) implants for ligament insufficiency with moderate bone defects and rotating hinged prostheses for cases with severe ligament disruption and significant bone loss. The study collected data prospectively, evaluating clinical outcomes using the International Knee Society scores and radiographic assessments over a median follow-up of 9 years.

The study's findings suggest that using an algorithm to select implant constraints based on ligament condition and bone loss can lead to stable knee reconstructions with improved long-term outcomes. The results showed significant improvements in knee function scores and range of motion (ROM), particularly with PS designs showing higher ROM values. Future study could focus on refining this algorithm further or exploring its application in different patient populations. This approach provides a structured method for surgeons to address the complexities of revision TKA, potentially reducing failure rates associated with mechanical factors like instability and aseptic loosening.

10.2.4 Trends in Primary and Revision Knee Arthroplasty among Orthopaedic Surgeons Who Take the American Board of Orthopaedics Part II Exam [116]

This is a machine-generated summary of:

Pour, Aidin Eslam; Bradbury, Thomas L.; Horst, Patrick; Harrast, John J.; Erens, Greg A.; Roberson, James R. Trends in primary and revision knee arthroplasty among orthopaedic surgeons who take the American Board of Orthopaedics part II exam [116].

Published in: International Orthopaedics (2016).

Link to original: https://doi.org/10.1007/s00264-016-3137-z

If you want to cite the papers, please refer to the original.

For technical reasons we could not place the page where the original quote is coming from.

10.2.4.1 Research Highlights

Total knee arthroplasty (TKA) is a highly effective surgical procedure that significantly improves knee pain and function for individuals with knee joint arthrosis. As the demand for TKA increases, it is projected that over three million procedures will be performed annually in the United States. While many of these surgeries are conducted by surgeons with specialized fellowship training in adult reconstruction, a substantial number are performed by those without such training. The impact of fellowship training on surgical outcomes and case complexity remains unclear. The study by Pour et al. investigates the influence of adult reconstruction fellowship training on the practice patterns and outcomes of surgeons undergoing the American Board of Orthopaedic Surgery (ABOS) Part II examination.

The study utilized data from the ABOS database, which includes self-reported surgical cases from candidates for board certification. The researchers analyzed procedural volumes, complication rates, and practice trends among surgeons with and without fellowship training in adult reconstruction. The dataset comprised cases submitted between 2003 and 2013, focusing on primary and revision knee arthroplasty procedures. Statistical analyses were conducted to compare outcomes between fellowship-trained and non-fellowship-trained surgeons, as well as high-volume versus low-volume surgeons. The findings revealed that while fellowship-trained surgeons performed more complex knee surgeries, there was no significant difference in early complication rates for primary TKA between the two groups. However, high-volume surgeons reported fewer complications overall, highlighting the importance of surgical experience.

The study advances our understanding of how fellowship training influences knee arthroplasty outcomes. It suggests that while specialized training is beneficial for handling complex cases, surgical volume plays a more critical role in reducing complications. Future study could explore long-term outcomes and patient-reported measures to further assess the impact of fellowship training on TKA results. Additionally, as the density of fellowship-trained surgeons increases across the United States, understanding their role in meeting rising demand for TKA will be crucial for healthcare planning and policy development.

10.2.5 Management of a Tibial Periprosthetic Fracture Following Revision Knee Arthroplasty Using a Pulsed Electromagnetic Field Stimulation Device: A Case Report [117]

This is a machine-generated summary of:

Doorgakant, Ashtin; Bhutta, Mohammed A; Marynissen, Hans Management of a tibial periprosthetic fracture following revision knee arthroplasty using a pulsed electromagnetic field stimulation device: a case report [117].

Published in: Cases Journal (2009).

Link to original: https://doi.org/10.4076/1757-1626-2-8706

10.2.5.1 Research Highlights

Osteoarthritis is a common degenerative joint disease that often leads to the need for total knee arthroplasty (TKA), a surgical procedure to replace the knee joint. While TKA is generally successful, complications such as periprosthetic fractures can occur, particularly in revision surgeries. These fractures are challenging to manage due to their rarity and the compromised bone quality in affected patients. The study by Doorgakant et al. presents a case of a complex Type-IIA tibial periprosthetic fracture following TKA, highlighting the successful use of a pulsed electromagnetic field device (PEMFD) for non-operative management.

The study details the case of a Caucasian woman who underwent TKA for osteoarthritis with valgus deformity. Following initial surgery and subsequent complications, including medial collateral ligament failure and periprosthetic fracture, the patient was managed non-operatively due to the complexity of her fracture pattern. The team applied a PEMFD to promote bone healing, given its potential to enhance proteoglycan and collagen synthesis and encourage mineralization. The device was used consistently for several hours daily over an extended period. Despite the fracture's complexity and initial concerns about non-union or delayed union, complete bony union was achieved 8 months after sustaining the fracture.

This case represents a significant advancement in managing complex tibial periprosthetic fractures using PEMFDs, which have traditionally been underutilized in such scenarios. The successful outcome suggests that PEMFDs could be considered more broadly for similar cases, potentially expanding treatment options for an aging population with compromised bone health. Future study could explore larger cohorts to validate these findings and refine treatment protocols, potentially leading to improved outcomes for patients with challenging periprosthetic fractures.

10.2.6 Physical Activity After Revision Knee Arthroplasty Including Return to Sport and Work: A Systematic Review and Meta-analysis Including GRADE [118]

This is a machine-generated summary of:

van der Wilk, Sten; Hoorntje, Alexander; Blankevoort, Leendert; van Geenen, Rutger; Kerkhoffs, Gino M. M. J.; Kuijer, P. Paul F. M. Physical activity after revision knee arthroplasty including return to sport and work: a systematic review and meta-analysis including GRADE [118].

Published in: BMC Musculoskeletal Disorders (2023).

Link to original: https://doi.org/10.1186/s12891-023-06458-y

If you want to cite the papers, please refer to the original.

For technical reasons we could not place the page where the original quote is coming from.

10.2.6.1 Research Highlights

Osteoarthritis (OA) is a degenerative joint disease that significantly impacts the adult population worldwide, often leading to disability. Factors such as genetic predisposition, injuries, obesity, and aging contribute to the risk of developing OA. When conservative treatments fail, surgical interventions like knee arthroplasty (TKA) are considered to alleviate pain and improve joint function. However, with the increasing prevalence of knee OA, particularly among younger patients, there is a growing demand for primary knee arthroplasty (TKA), which subsequently raises the likelihood of revision surgeries due to factors like an active lifestyle and implant lifespan limitations. The study by Wilk et al. aims to address the knowledge gap regarding physical activity levels and return to sport (RTS) and work (RTW) after revision knee arthroplasty (TKR).

The study conducted a systematic review following PRISMA (Preferred Reporting Items for Systematic Reviews and Meta-Analyses) guidelines to assess physical activity post-TKR. A clinical librarian developed a search strategy in collaboration with the authors, using databases like Medline and Embase to identify relevant literature up until February 2023. The inclusion criteria focused on patients undergoing TKR or revision UKA after primary procedures, with studies reporting on physical activity measures or RTS/RTW rates. Data extraction was performed independently by two authors using a standardized form, while study quality was assessed using the Newcastle–Ottawa Scale. The review included 16 studies with varying methodological quality, primarily reporting patient-reported outcome measures (PROMs) such as the University of California Los Angeles (UCLA) activity scale and Knee injury and Osteoarthritis Outcome Scores (KOOS) scores. Meta-analyses were conducted to evaluate pre- and postoperative PROMs, revealing an overall improvement in self-reported physical activity levels post-TKR.

The study highlights that while patients generally report improved activity levels after TKR, there remains substantial uncertainty due to methodological limitations in existing research. Future study could benefit from incorporating objective physical activity measurements to provide more reliable estimates of RTS and RTW outcomes. Additionally, exploring non-surgical treatments or alternative techniques for younger patients may help delay the need for TKA or TKR. Rehabilitation programs tailored to individual goals could enhance patient satisfaction and outcomes post-TKR. As the demand for TKR increases among younger populations globally, further research is essential to better inform patients about realistic postoperative expectations and guide clinical decision-making.

10.2.7 Management of the Bone Loss by Metaphyseal Sleeves in Primary and Revision Knee Arthroplasty: Clinical Experience and Outcome after Forty Three Cases [119]

This is a machine-generated summary of:

Gill, Usman Nazir; Ahmed, Nasir; Noor, Syed Shahid; Memon, Iftikhar Ahmed; Memon, Zulfiqar Ali Management of the bone loss by metaphyseal sleeves in primary and revision knee arthroplasty: clinical experience and outcome after forty three cases [119].

Published in: International Orthopaedics (2020).

Link to original: https://doi.org/10.1007/s00264-020-04663-1

If you want to cite the papers, please refer to the original.

For technical reasons we could not place the page where the original quote is coming from.

10.2.7.1 Research Highlights

Knee arthroplasties are increasingly performed worldwide, with improvements in implant design leading to enhanced patient satisfaction and outcomes. However, the rise in knee arthroplasties has also led to an increase in revision surgeries, particularly in cases involving complex deformities and significant bone loss. Managing bone defects remains a challenge for arthroplasty surgeons, who seek reliable implants that provide immediate stability and improve long-term survival. The study by Gil et al. investigates the use of metaphyseal sleeves in managing bone defects during complex primary and revision total knee arthroplasties (TKA) at Liaqat National Hospital, Karachi.

The study retrospectively analyzed cases involving Anderson Orthopaedic Research Institute (AORI) type IIB and III bone defects. Excluding patients with conditions affecting outcomes, the research included both primary and revision arthroplasties performed by a single experienced surgeon. The team utilized DePuy Synthes® Metaphyseal sleeves (DePuy Orthopedics, Warsaw, Indiana, USA) alongside press-fit stemmed PFC® SIGMA® systems or S-ROM® Noiles™ Rotating Knee Hinge Systems. In cases with Anderson Orthopaedic Research Institute (AORI) type III defects, hinged implants were used to address compromised collateral ligaments. The study reported successful outcomes with no aseptic loosening observed during follow-ups. Patients were mobilized early post-surgery, and continuous passive motion was employed to aid recovery. The study also noted minimal complications, such as iatrogenic fractures managed without instrumentation.

The findings suggest that metaphyseal sleeves are a viable option for addressing bone metaphyseal defects in complex TKA cases, offering excellent short- to mid-term survivorship. The porous coating of these sleeves promotes bone ingrowth, enhancing biological fixation and avoiding stress shielding. Future studies could explore long-term outcomes and further refine techniques to minimize intra-operative complications like iatrogenic fractures. This research contributes valuable insights into improving surgical strategies for managing challenging knee arthroplasty cases with significant bone loss.

10.2.8 Midterm Results of Modular Hinge Total Knee Arthroplasty Using Cementless Osseointegrating Stems: Low Fixation Associated Complications and Good Functional Outcome in Primary and Revision Knee Arthroplasty [120]

This is a machine-generated summary of:

Schnetz, M.; Hofmann, L.; Ewald, L.; Klug, A.; Hoffmann, R.; Gramlich, Y. Midterm results of modular hinge total knee arthroplasty using cementless osseointegrating stems: low fixation associated complications and good functional outcome in primary and revision knee arthroplasty [120].

Published in: Archives of Orthopaedic and Trauma Surgery (2023).

Link to original: https://doi.org/10.1007/s00402-023-05148-7

If you want to cite the papers, please refer to the original.

For technical reasons we could not place the page where the original quote is coming from.

10.2.8.1 Research Highlights

Hinged total knee arthroplasty (H-TKA) is often employed in cases of severe bone or soft tissue damage, particularly in revision surgeries where traditional implants fail. The demand for revision total knee arthroplasty (TKR) is expected to rise significantly in the coming years, driven by issues such as aseptic loosening, infection, and implant failure. Despite advancements in implant design and improved survival rates of up to 95% for third-generation hinged TKA, there remains no international consensus on the optimal choice between cemented and cementless fixation techniques. The study by Schnetz et al. investigates the functional outcomes and complication rates associated with a hybrid modular rotating hinge implant using cementless osseointegrating stems.

The study was conducted as a prospective monocentre trial at a primary academic referral centre for arthroplasty. It included patients who underwent H-TKA with the MUTARS® GenuX® MK System (Implantcast GmbH.Buxtehude, Germany) between 2015 and 2020. The hybrid implantation approach involved cemented femoral and tibial components with cementless stems and modular components like augments, sleeves, or cones. Surgeries were performed by experienced surgeons using preoperative planning software, and patients were followed up for a minimum of 24 months. The study assessed functional outcomes using the Knee Society Score (KSS) and Western Ontario McMasters Universities Osteoarthritis Index (WOMAC), alongside radiological evaluations to monitor implant survival and complications.

The study found significant improvements in KSS scores postoperatively, indicating enhanced functional outcomes and reduced pain levels. Implant survivorship was reported at 92% after an average follow-up of 36 months, with complications related to cementless stem fixation occurring in only 5% of cases. While the overall complication rate was relatively high due to the complex nature of cases involved, fixation-associated complications were low compared to existing literature. Future study directions could focus on long-term outcomes beyond the midterm results presented here, as well as comparisons between hybrid and fully cemented fixation methods to further refine surgical approaches in complex primary and revision arthroplasty cases.

10.2.9 Medium Term Clinical Outcomes of Tibial Cones in Revision Knee Arthroplasty [121]

This is a machine-generated summary of:

Erivan, Roger; Tracey, Robert; Mulliez, Aurélien; Villatte, Guillaume; Paprosky, Wayne Medium term clinical outcomes of tibial cones in revision knee arthroplasty [121].

Published in: Archives of Orthopaedic and Trauma Surgery (2020).

Link to original: https://doi.org/10.1007/s00402-020-03532-1

If you want to cite the papers, please refer to the original.

For technical reasons we could not place the page where the original quote is coming from.

10.2.9.1 Research Highlights

Revision total knee arthroplasty (TKA) is the primary treatment for failed primary TKA, with anticipated increases in both volume and cost. However, outcomes after revision TKA are less predictable than those following primary surgery, particularly due to challenges in assessing and managing bone defects. Various treatment options exist, but none have demonstrated clear superiority. Trabecular metal cones have emerged as a promising option for reconstructing major bone defects during revision TKA, showing good primary fixation in cadaver studies. The study by Erivan et al. retrospectively assesses the medium-term results of trabecular metal tibial cones in revision TKA, hypothesizing excellent clinical and radiological outcomes.

The study involved a single-center retrospective review of all consecutive cases of tibial revision using trabecular metal cones. Conducted between January 2010 and December 2015, the study included patients with a minimum of 5 years follow-up. The inclusion criteria were patients undergoing revision TKA with tibial component revision using highly porous tantalum biomaterial cones. Clinical scores such as the Knee injury and Osteoarthritis Outcome Scores (KOOS) and SF-36 were used to evaluate outcomes, alongside radiographic assessments for cone integration and mechanical stability. The primary endpoint was tibial cone survivorship, while secondary endpoints included all-cause survivorship and patient-reported outcomes. Statistical analyses were performed using Stata software to compare pre- and post-operative data.

The study concluded that trabecular metal tibial cones provide excellent medium-term results for managing tibial bone defects in revision TKA, with high survivorship rates for aseptic loosening. These findings align with previous studies on femoral defect management using similar cones. Despite limitations such as its retrospective nature and small sample size, the study supports the use of tibial cones as a viable option in revision TKA. Future studies could focus on longer-term outcomes and larger patient populations to further validate these findings and explore potential improvements in surgical techniques or materials used for metaphyseal fixation.

10.2.10 Level of Constraint in Revision Knee Arthroplasty [122]

This is a machine-generated summary of:

Indelli, Pier Francesco; Giori, Nick; Maloney, William Level of constraint in revision knee arthroplasty [122].

Published in: Current Reviews in Musculoskeletal Medicine (2015).

Link to original: https://doi.org/10.1007/s12178-015-9295-6

If you want to cite the papers, please refer to the original.

For technical reasons we could not place the page where the original quote is coming from.

10.2.10.1 Research Highlights

The increasing number of patients undergoing primary total knee arthroplasty (TKA) has led to a rise in revision surgeries, with instability being a leading cause of late revisions. Early instability after TKA is often due to issues such as flexion/extension gap mismatch and improper component alignment, while late instability is linked to factors like bone loss and polyethylene wear. The study by Indelli et al. reviews recent reports on the functional outcomes of different prosthetic designs—posterior stabilized, unlinked constrained, or fully constrained—in managing bone loss and instability during revision TKA.

The study involved evaluating different modes of instability, such as flexion/extension gap mismatch, component malpositioning, and ligament insufficiency. The authors emphasized the importance of thorough preoperative assessment, including radiographic and laboratory evaluations, to identify the underlying causes of instability. They also discussed surgical strategies for managing these issues, ranging from isolated polyethylene exchange to full component revision and hinged arthroplasty. The review highlighted the need for selecting the appropriate level of prosthetic constraint based on the specific type and severity of instability encountered during revision surgery.

The study provides insights into the selection of prosthetic designs based on specific instability patterns. The authors suggest that future studies should focus on refining surgical techniques and developing new prosthetic designs that offer better stability while minimizing complications. Additionally, they highlight the potential benefits of using rotating hinge designs in certain cases to reduce stress at the bone-implant interface. These findings underscore the importance of personalized treatment approaches in improving outcomes for patients undergoing revision TKA due to instability.

10.2.11 Preliminary Clinical Results of Coated Porous Tibia Cones in Septic and Aseptic Revision Knee Arthroplasty [123]

This is a machine-generated summary of:

Ohlmeier, Malte; Lausmann, Christian; Wolff, Matthias; Abdelaziz, Hussein; Gehrke, Thorsten; Citak, Mustafa Preliminary clinical results of coated porous tibia cones in septic and aseptic revision knee arthroplasty [123].

Published in: Archives of Orthopaedic and Trauma Surgery (2020).
Link to original: https://doi.org/10.1007/s00402-020-03434-2

If you want to cite the papers, please refer to the original.
For technical reasons we could not place the page where the original quote is coming from.

10.2.11.1 Research Highlights

Tibial bone loss in revision knee arthroplasty (RKA) presents significant challenges, particularly in septic cases where massive femoral and tibial bone stock loss complicates joint reconstruction. Traditional methods for addressing bone loss have evolved from structural grafts to the use of metal cones, such as trabecular tantalum cones, which have shown lower loosening rates. However, the integration and stability of these implants remain areas of active research. The study by Ohlmeier et al. investigates the use of coated porous titanium cones, specifically TrabecuLink®-CaP cones (Waldemar LINK, Hamburg, Germany), in both septic and aseptic RKA cases to evaluate their effectiveness in enhancing osteointegration and implant stability.

The study was conducted at a single center with patients who underwent revision knee arthroplasty using TrabecuLink®-CaP tibia cones between January 2016 to December 2017. The researchers excluded patients without cone implantation or with insufficient follow-up data, resulting in a final cohort of 52 patients. These custom-made titanium alloy cones are coated with calcium-phosphate to promote faster integration and are designed for press-fit fixation due to their elastic properties. The surgical procedure involved standard preparation protocols, debridement of affected tissues, trial cone insertion for defect assessment, and final implantation using bone cement for fixation. The study primarily measured implant survival rates and causes of re-revision while also assessing patient satisfaction through the Oxford Knee Score.

The findings suggest that TrabecuLink®-CaP tibia cones offer promising results for structural bone defects in both septic and aseptic revisions, with an overall revision rate of 7.7%. The study highlights the potential antimicrobial effects of calcium-phosphate-coated implants and suggests that cementless fixation might be reconsidered given recent advancements in implant technology. Future studies should focus on long-term outcomes to further validate these initial findings and explore the broader application of 3D-printed titanium implants in orthopaedic surgery. Despite limitations such as low follow-up radiograph availability and lack of preoperative functional scores, this research provides valuable insights into improving RKA outcomes with innovative implant designs.

10.2.12 The Role of Offset Stems in Revision Knee Arthroplasty [124]

This is a machine-generated summary of:

Baldini, Andrea; Balato, Giovanni; Franceschini, Vincenzo The role of offset stems in revision knee arthroplasty [124].

Published in: Current Reviews in Musculoskeletal Medicine (2015).

Link to original: https://doi.org/10.1007/s12178-015-9294-7

If you want to cite the papers, please refer to the original.

For technical reasons we could not place the page where the original quote is coming from.

10.2.12.1 Research Highlights

Revision total knee arthroplasty (TKA) is a complex procedure often necessitated by septic or aseptic failures, presenting challenges in achieving stable, well-balanced, and well-fixed implants. The primary goals of revision TKA include restoring bone stock, ensuring long-term implant stability, and enabling immediate weight-bearing and functional activity. However, the removal of a previously well-fixed prosthesis can lead to significant bone loss in the distal femur and proximal tibia, complicating reconstruction efforts. The Anderson Orthopaedic Research Institute classification is commonly used to assess bone defects in revision TKA, but it falls short in guiding successful outcomes when bone quality and defect location are critical. The study by Baldini et al. highlights the importance of offset stems in addressing these challenges, focusing on their classification, indications, surgical techniques, and outcomes.

The study explores the concept of zonal fixation in revision TKA, emphasizing the need for preoperative planning to determine available fixation zones and appropriate methods. Stemmed implants are highlighted as a valuable option for providing stability by distributing load away from damaged areas and reducing stress on critical interfaces. The research delves into the types of stems available—cemented and uncemented—and their respective advantages. Cemented stems offer versatility across various geometries due to their excellent fixation capabilities, while uncemented press-fit stems are suitable for patients with favorable canal geometry or periprosthetic fractures. The study also discusses modular stem designs that allow for personalized fixation strategies. Offset stems are particularly beneficial in cases where anatomical mismatches exist between the metaphysis and diaphysis, aiding in proper implant alignment and gap balancing during surgery.

The study concludes that offset stems play a crucial role in the surgeon's toolkit for revision TKA by allowing personalized fixation strategies tailored to individual anatomical features or surgical goals. Mid-term results demonstrate good outcomes with no specific complications associated with their use. Future study directions may focus on design refinements and enhancing proximal fixation at the metaphyseal level to further improve diaphyseal expansions. This research underscores the importance of offset stems in achieving successful revision TKA outcomes by addressing anatomical challenges and optimizing implant positioning.

10.2.13 Revision Knee Arthroplasty with Rotating Hinge Systems in Patients with Gross Ligament Instability [125]

This is a machine-generated summary of:

Boelch, Sebastian P.; Arnholdt, Joerg; Holzapfel, Boris M.; Jakuscheit, Axel; Rudert, Maximilian; Hoberg, Maik Revision knee arthroplasty with rotating hinge systems in patients with gross ligament instability [125].

Published in: International Orthopaedics (2018).

Link to original: https://doi.org/10.1007/s00264-018-3982-z

If you want to cite the papers, please refer to the original.

For technical reasons we could not place the page where the original quote is coming from.

10.2.13.1 Research Highlights

Primary total knee arthroplasty (TKA) is a widely used treatment for end-stage osteoarthritis, with patient satisfaction and implant survivorship improving over recent decades. However, as the population ages and the number of TKAs increases, the absolute number of TKA revisions is also rising, with instability being a major cause. Addressing this issue, hinged knee prostheses have been developed to manage instability after TKA, but fixed hinged designs have shown high failure rates due to increased rotational forces. The study by Belch et al. compares two rotating hinge knee (RHK) designs—the Link Endo-Model SL™ (Waldemar Link GmbH & Co. KG, Hamburg, Germany) and the EnduRo RHK (Aesculap AG, Tuttlingen, Germany) — a randomized prospective study to evaluate their effectiveness in revision TKA for instability.

The study included patients undergoing TKA revision for gross ligament insufficiency, excluding those with other indications such as infection or implant failure. Patients were randomized into two groups to receive either the EnduRo or Endo-Model RHK. Surgical procedures involved standard medial arthrotomy and cemented stem extensions where necessary. Postoperative care included partial weight-bearing mobilization and unrestricted range of motion. Clinical scores, patient function, and radiographic evaluations were conducted preoperatively and at several postoperative intervals up to 1 year. Statistical analyses revealed no significant differences in patient demographics or surgical outcomes between the two groups. Both RHK designs showed significant improvements in function and patient-reported outcomes, with no intraoperative complications or postoperative implant failures reported.

The study concludes that both RHK designs are reliable options for TKA revision due to instability, providing good clinical results in terms of knee function and pain reduction. However, despite improvements in overall status, revision remains a salvage procedure with potential for persistent impairment in daily activities and unsatisfactory physical health perception. The authors note that infection remains a significant threat post-revision. Future studies should focus on mid- and long-term outcomes to better understand the clinical relevance of observed radiolucency lines and further explore differences between RHK designs in larger patient cohorts.

10.2.14 Metaphyseal Bone Loss in Revision Knee Arthroplasty [126]

This is a machine-generated summary of:

Ponzio, Danielle Y.; Austin, Matthew S. Metaphyseal bone loss in revision knee arthroplasty [126].

Published in: Current Reviews in Musculoskeletal Medicine (2015).

Link to original: https://doi.org/10.1007/s12178-015-9291-x

If you want to cite the papers, please refer to the original.

For technical reasons we could not place the page where the original quote is coming from.

10.2.14.1 Research Highlights

Metaphyseal bone loss poses significant challenges in revision total knee arthroplasty (TKA), potentially compromising both initial and long-term fixation of components. This condition can lead to malalignment due to the loss of normal anatomical landmarks, with causes ranging from stress shielding and osteolysis to infection and mechanical abrasion. The primary goals of revision surgery include preserving viable host bone, reconstructing bone deficiencies, restoring the joint line, and achieving proper alignment and stability. However, a knowledge gap exists in determining the most effective method for managing metaphyseal bone loss during revision TKA. The study by Ponzio e al. explores various reconstructive techniques to address this issue.

The study examines impaction grafting, prosthetic augmentation, bulk structural allografts, and the use of metaphyseal cones and sleeves. Impaction grafting involves using morselized cancellous autograft or allograft bone for contained defects, while uncontained defects may require wire mesh for containment. Prosthetic augmentation utilizes modular or customized augments to restore joint line and balance the knee efficiently. Bulk structural allografts are considered for larger uncontained defects, offering potential long-term biologic integration but with risks such as nonunion and infection. Metaphyseal cones and sleeves are designed to fill large cavitary defects, providing mechanical support and potential for osseous ingrowth. Each technique has its advantages and limitations, with selection often based on defect size, location, ligamentous stability, and patient factors.

The study highlights that porous metal metaphyseal cones and sleeves represent recent advances in managing metaphyseal bone loss during revision TKA. These technologies offer potential benefits such as biologic ingrowth fixation and a mechanically sound scaffold while avoiding issues associated with traditional bone grafting methods. Future study could focus on long-term outcomes and comparisons with other reconstruction options to determine their efficacy in providing superior clinical success over time. The findings underscore the need for continued research to establish optimal strategies for addressing complex bone deficiencies in revision TKA procedures.

10.2.15 Modular Knee Arthrodesis Secures Limb, Mobility, Improves Quality of Life, and Leads to High Infection Control in Periprosthetic Knee Infection, When Revision Knee Arthroplasty Is Not an Option [127]

This is a machine-generated summary of:

Gramlich, Y.; Steinkohl, D.; Kremer, M.; Kemmerer, M.; Hoffmann, R.; Klug, A. Modular knee arthrodesis secures limb, mobility, improves quality of life, and leads to high infection control in periprosthetic knee infection, when revision knee arthroplasty is not an option [127].

Published in: Archives of Orthopaedic and Trauma Surgery (2021).

Link to original: https://doi.org/10.1007/s00402-021-03907-y

If you want to cite the papers, please refer to the original.

For technical reasons we could not place the page where the original quote is coming from.

10.2.15.1 Research Highlights

Chronic and difficult-to-treat periprosthetic joint infections (PJI) following total knee arthroplasty (TKA) present significant challenges in orthopedic surgery. Two-stage exchange procedures are often employed in these cases due to their high remission rates; despite the complexity and financial burden they impose. However, when faced with severe bone loss and compromised soft tissues, traditional revision TKA may not be feasible, necessitating alternative approaches such as knee arthrodesis. The study by Gramlich et al., investigates the outcomes of hinged TKA versus knee arthrodesis using a stem-guided module in patients with failed infected TKA treated with two-stage revision.

The study was conducted at an EndoCert® certified primary academic referral center for arthroplasty, involving patients with chronic recurrent periprosthetic joint infection (PJI) who did not meet criteria for single-step exchange. Patients were retrospectively selected and divided into two groups: those receiving a Rotating Hinge Knee (RHK) prosthesis and those treated with a Knee Arthrodesis Module (KAM) (Peter Brehm GmbH, Weisendorf Germany). The surgical procedure involved multiple stages of debridement and systemic antibiotic therapy tailored to microbiological findings. The decision between RHK and KAM was based on the quality of the extensor mechanism and soft tissue status. Outcomes were assessed using various scores, including the Knee Society Score (KSS), Western Ontario McMasters Universities Osteoarthritis Index (WOMAC), and SF-36 health survey.

The study found that both treatment options led to significant pain reduction post-reimplantation, with comparable PJI remission rates between groups. However, patients in the KAM group experienced reduced walking distances and lower functional scores compared to those in the RHK group. Despite these limitations, patient satisfaction remained high due to successful limb salvage and pain management. Future study could explore optimizing rehabilitation protocols for KAM patients to enhance mobility outcomes further. This research underscores the viability of knee arthrodesis as a limb-preserving alternative when revision TKA is not possible, highlighting its role in maintaining quality of life despite reduced physical function.

10.2.16 A Prospective Study on Outcome of Patient-Specific Cones in Revision Knee Arthroplasty [128]

This is a machine-generated summary of:

Cherny, Alexander A.; Kovalenko, Anton N.; Kulyaba, Taras A.; Kornilov, Nikolai N. A prospective study on outcome of patient-specific cones in revision knee arthroplasty [128].

Published in: Archives of Orthopaedic and Trauma Surgery (2021).

Link to original: https://doi.org/10.1007/s00402-021-04047-z

If you want to cite the papers, please refer to the original.

For technical reasons we could not place the page where the original quote is coming from.

10.2.16.1 Research Highlights

Total knee arthroplasty (TKA) often requires revision due to complications such as aseptic loosening, with bone loss being a significant challenge in these procedures. Current methods for managing bone defects include various grafts and implants, each with limitations, especially in cases of extensive bone loss. Accurate preoperative assessment is crucial for surgical planning yet remains challenging. The study by Cherny et al. explores the use of patient-specific 3D-printed metal cones to address extensive femoral and tibial bone loss during revision TKA (RTKA).

The study involved designing and implanting patient-specific titanium cones in patients with significant bone defects due to aseptic loosening or other complications. Using advanced imaging and computer modeling, the researchers created personalized implants tailored to each patient's anatomy. The process included creating virtual models and plastic prototypes to ensure proper fit before manufacturing the final titanium cones through 3D printing. The surgical procedure involved standard approaches for implant removal and preparation of the host bone for the new implant. Postoperative assessments showed significant improvements in functional outcomes, with no major complications or need for further revisions within the follow-up period.

This study demonstrates that patient-specific 3D-printed cones can be a viable solution for managing extensive bone loss in RTKA, offering a high level of personalization and potentially improving surgical outcomes. The authors highlight the importance of individualized implant design to preserve bone stock and enhance fixation while minimizing soft tissue adhesion issues. Future study could focus on long-term outcomes to confirm these findings and explore further refinements in implant design and manufacturing processes to optimize patient outcomes in complex orthopaedic surgeries.

Bibliography

1. Wingert, N. C., Gotoff, J., Parrilla, E., Gotoff, R., Hou, L., and Ghanem, E. (2016). The ACS NSQIP risk calculator is a fair predictor of acute periprosthetic joint infection. *Clinical Orthopaedics and Related Research, 474*(7), 1643–1648. https://doi.org/10.1007/s11999-016-4717-3. *(Epub 2016/02/26, PMID: 26911971).*
2. Warth, L. C., Hadley, C. J., and Grossman, E. L. (2020). Two-stage treatment for total knee arthroplasty infection utilizing an articulating prefabricated antibiotic spacer. *J Arthroplast, 35*(3s), S57–s62. https://doi.org/10.1016/j.arth.2019.10.049. *(Epub 2020/02/13, PMID: 32046834).*
3. Pangaud, C., Ollivier, M., and Argenson, J.-N. (2019). Outcome of single-stage versus two-stage exchange for revision knee arthroplasty for chronic periprosthetic infection. *EFORT Open Rev., 4*(8), 495–502. https://doi.org/10.1302/2058-5241.4.190003. *PMID: 31537999.*
4. Lizaur-Utrilla, A., Gonzalez-Parreño, S., Martinez-Mendez, D., Miralles-Muñoz, F. A., and Lopez-Prats, F. A. (2020). Minimal clinically important differences and substantial clinical benefits for knee society scores. *Knee Surgery, Sports Traumatology, Arthroscopy, 28*(5), 1473–1478. https://doi.org/10.1007/s00167-019-05543-x. *(Epub 2019/05/22, PMID: 31111184).*
5. Bini SA, Chan PH, Inacio MCSS et al (2016) Antibiotic cement was associated with half the risk of re-revision in 1154 aseptic revision total knee arthroplasties. Acta Orthop 87:55–59. https://doi.org/10.3109/17453674.2015.1103568
6. Maslaris A, Layher F, Brinkmann O et al (2018) Cemented conical stems can be removed more easily than cylindrical stems, regardless of cone angle in revision knee arthroplasty. Arch Orthop Trauma Surg 138:1747–1754. https://doi.org/10.1007/s00402-018-3053-3
7. Engh GA (1997) Bone loss classification. In: Engh GA, Rorabeck CH (eds) Revision total knee arthroplasty. Williams and Wilkins, Baltimore, pp 63–120
8. Mahomed NN, Barrett J, Katz JN, Baron JA, Wright J, Losina E (2005) Epidemiology of total knee replacement in the United States medicare population. J Bone Joint Surg Am 87:1222–1228
9. Johnson AJ, Sayeed SA, Naziri Q, Khanuja HS, Mont MA (2012) Minimizing dynamic knee spacer complications in infected revision arthroplasty. Clin Orthop Relat Res 470:220–227
10. Hwang SC, Kong JY, Nam DC, Kim DH, Park HB, Jeong ST, Cho SH (2010) Revision total knee arthroplasty with a cemented posterior stabilized, condylar constrained or fully constrained prosthesis: a minimum 2-year follow-up analysis. Clin Orthop Surg 2:112–120
11. Kim Y, Kim J (2009) Revision total knee arthroplasty with use of a constrained condylar knee prothesis. J Bone Jt Surg 91:1440–1447. https://doi.org/10.2106/JBJS.H.00425
12. Meijer MF, Reininga IH, Boerboom AL, Stevens M, Bulstra SK (2013) Poorer survival after a primary implant during revision total knee arthroplasty. Int Orthop 37:415–419

13. Radnay CS, Scuderi GR (2006) Management of bone loss. Augments, cones, offset stems. Clin Orthop Relat Res 446:83–92
14. Murray PB, Rand JA, Hanssen AD (1994) Cemented long-stem revision total knee arthroplasty. Clin Orthop Relat Res 309:116–123
15. Ethgen O, Bruyerè O, Richy F, Dardennes C, Reginster JY. Health-Related Quality of Life in Total Hip and Total Knee Arthroplasty: A Qualitative and Systematic Review of the Literature. J Bone Joint Surg Ser A. 2004;86(5):963–74.
16. Lingard EA, Sledge CB, Learmonth ID. Patient expectations regarding total knee arthroplasty: Differences among the United States, United Kingdom, and Australia. J Bone Joint Surg Ser A. 2006;88(6):1201–7.
17. Page MJ, McKenzie JE, Bossuyt PM, Boutron I, Hoffmann TC, Mulrow CD, The PRISMA, et al. statement: An updated guideline for reporting systematic reviews. BMJ. 2020;2021:372.
18. Piuzzi NS. Patient-Reported Outcome Measures (Pain, Function, and Quality of Life) After Aseptic Revision Total Knee Arthroplasty. J Bone Joint Surg Am. 2020;102(20):e114.
19. Carr AJ, Robertsson O, Graves S et al (2012) Knee replacement. Lancet 379:1331–1340
20. Kurtz, S., Ong, K., Lau, E., Mowat, F. and Halpern, M. Projections of primary and revision hip and knee arthroplasty in the United States from 2005 to 2030. *JBJS 89*, 780–785 (2007).
21. Kurtz SM, Ong KL, Lau E, Widmer M, Maravic M, Gómez-Barrena E, et al. International survey of primary and revision total knee replacement. Int Orthop. 2011;35(12):1783–9.
22. Hamilton DF, Howie CR, Burnett R, Simpson AHRW, Patton JT. Dealing with the predicted increase in demand for revision total knee arthroplasty: Challenges, risks and opportunities. Bone Joint J. 2015;97-B(6):723–8.
23. Klug A, Gramlich Y, Rudert M, Drees P, Hoffmann R, Weißenberger M, et al. The projected volume of primary and revision total knee arthroplasty will place an immense burden on future heath care systems over the next 30 years. Knee Surg Sports Traumatol Arthrosc. 2020;(0123456789). https://doi.org/10.1007/s00167-020-06154-7.
24. Walker-Santiago R, Tegethoff JD, Ralston WM, Keeney JA. Revision Total Knee Arthroplasty in Young Patients: Higher Early Reoperation and Rerevision. J Arthroplasty. 2021;36(2):653–6. https://doi.org/10.1016/j.arth.2020.08.052.
25. Bayliss LE, Culliford D, Monk AP, Glyn-Jones S, Prieto-Alhambra D, Judge A, et al. The effect of patient age at intervention on risk of implant revision after total replacement of the hip or knee: a population-based cohort study. Lancet. 2017;389(10077):1424–30.
26. Pitta M, Esposito CI, Li Z, Lee Y yu, Wright TM, Padgett DE. Failure After Modern Total Knee Arthroplasty: A Prospective Study of 18,065 Knees. J Arthroplasty. 2018;33(2):407–14.

27. Houfani F, Mainard D, Rubens-Duval B, Papin PE, Pasquier G, Ehlinger M. Rotating-hinge prosthesis for aseptic revision knee arthroplasty: A multicentre retrospective study of 127 cases with a mean follow-up of five years. Orthop Traumatol Surg Res. 2021;107(3):102855.
28. Erivan R, Tracey R, Mulliez A, Villatte G, Paprosky W. Medium term clinical outcomes of tibial cones in revision knee arthroplasty. Arch Orthop Trauma Surg. 2021;141(1):113–8. https://doi.org/10.1007/s00402-020-03532-1.
29. Dahm DL, Barnes SA, Harrington JR, Berry DJ. Patient Reported Activity After Revision Total Knee Arthroplasty. J Arthroplasty. 2007;22(6 SUPPL.):106–10.
30. Turnbull GS, Scott CEH, MacDonald DJ, Breusch SJ. Gender and Preoperative Function Predict Physical Activity Levels After Revision Total Knee Arthroplasty. J Arthroplasty. 2019;34(5):939–46. https://doi.org/10.1016/j.arth.2019.01.040.
31. Crawford DA, Adams JB, Hobbs GR, Berend KR, Lombardi AV. Higher Activity Level Following Total Knee Arthroplasty Is Not Deleterious to Mid-Term Implant Survivorship. J Arthroplasty. 2020;35(1):116–20. https://doi.org/10.1016/j.arth.2019.07.044.
32. Ponzio DY, Austin MS (2015) Metaphyseal bone loss in revision knee arthroplasty. Curr Rev Musculoskelet Med 8:361–367
33. Chun CH, Kim JW, Kim SH, Kim BG, Chun KC, Kim KM (2014) Clinical and radiological results of femoral head structural allograft for severe bone defects in revision TKA—a minimum 8-year follow-up. Knee 21:420–423
34. Graichen H, Scior W, Strauch M (2015) Direct, Cementless, Metaphyseal fixation in knee revision Arthroplasty with sleeves-short-term results. J Arthroplasty 30:2256–2259
35. Tarazi JM, Chen Z, Scuderi GR, Mont MA (2021) The epidemiology of revision total knee arthroplasty. J Knee Surg 34(13):1396–1401
36. Sadoghi P, Liebensteiner M, Agreiter M, Leithner A, Böhler N, Labek G (2013) Revision surgery after total joint arthroplasty: a complication-based analysis using worldwide arthroplasty registers. J Arthroplasty 28(8):1329–1332
37. Wignadasan W, Chang JS, Kayani B, Kontoghiorghe C, Haddad FS (2021) Long-term results of revision total knee arthroplasty using a rotating hinge implant. Knee 28:72–80
38. Kang SG, Park CH, Song SJ (2018) Stem fixation in revision total knee arthroplasty: indications, stem dimensions, and fixation methods. Knee Surg Relat Res 30(3):187–192
39. Bingham JS, Bukowski BR, Wyles CC, Pareek A, Berry DJ, Abdel MP (2019) Rotating-hinge revision total knee arthroplasty for treatment of severe arthrofibrosis. J Arthroplasty 34(7s):S271-s276
40. Houfani F, Mainard D, Rubens-Duval B, Papin PE, Pasquier G, Ehlinger M (2021) Rotating-hinge prosthesis for aseptic revision knee arthroplasty: a multicentre retrospective study of 127 cases with a mean follow-up of five years. Orthop Traumatol Surg Res 107(3):102855

41. Theil C, Schmidt-Braekling T, Gosheger G et al (2020) Acceptable mid- to long-term survival rates and functional outcomes following a single design rotating hinge total knee arthroplasty. Knee Surg Sports Traumatol Arthrosc 28(6):1868–1875
42. Potter GD 3rd, Abdel MP, Lewallen DG, Hanssen AD (2016) Midterm results of porous tantalum femoral cones in revision Total knee Arthroplasty. J Bone Joint Surg 98:1286–1291
43. Maslaris A, Layher F, Bungartz M et al (2019) Sagittal profile has a significant impact on the explantability of well-fixed cemented stems in revision knee arthroplasty: a biomechanical comparison study of five established knee implant models. Arch Orthop Trauma Surg 139:991–998. https://doi.org/10.1007/s00402-019-03160-4
44. Meijer MF, Boerboom AL, Stevens M et al (2017) Tibial component with and without stem extension in a trabecular metal cone construct. Knee Surg Sports Traumatol Arthrosc Off J ESSKA 25:3644–3652. https://doi.org/10.1007/s00167-016-4271-2
45. Faizan A, Bhowmik-Stoker M, Alipit V et al (2017) Development and verification of novel porous titanium metaphyseal cones for revision total knee arthroplasty. J Arthroplasty 32:1946–1953. https://doi.org/10.1016/j.arth.2017.01.013
46. Sandiford NA, Misur P, Garbuz DS, Greidanus NV, Masri BA. No Difference Between Trabecular Metal Cones and Femoral Head Allografts in Revision TKA: Minimum 5-year Followup. Clin Orthop Relat Res. 2017;475(1):118–24.
47. Wirries N, Winnecken HJ, von Lewinski G et al (2019) Osteointegrative sleeves for metaphyseal defect augmentation in revision total knee arthroplasty: clinical and radiological 5-year follow-up. J Arthroplasty. https://doi.org/10.1016/j.arth.2019.04.024
48. Denehy KM, Abhari S, Krebs VE et al (2019) Excellent metaphyseal fixation using highly porous cones in revision total knee arthroplasty. J Arthroplasty. https://doi.org/10.1016/j.arth.2019.03.045
49. Abdelaziz H, Jaramillo R, Gehrke T et al (2019) Clinical survivorship of aseptic revision total knee arthroplasty using hinged knees and tantalum cones at minimum 10-year follow-up. J Arthroplasty 34:3018–3022. https://doi.org/10.1016/j.arth.2019.06.057
50. Bohl DD, Brown NM, McDowell MA et al (2018) Do porous tantalum metaphyseal cones improve outcomes in revision total knee arthroplasty? J Arthroplasty 33:171–177. https://doi.org/10.1016/j.arth.2017.07.033
51. Burastero G, Cavagnaro L, Chiarlone F et al (2018) The use of tantalum metaphyseal cones for the management of severe bone defects in septic knee revision. J Arthroplasty 33:3739–3745. https://doi.org/10.1016/j.arth.2018.08.026
52. Agarwal S, Neogi DS, Morgan-Jones R (2018) Metaphyseal sleeves in revision total knee arthroplasty: minimum seven-year follow-up study. Knee. https://doi.org/10.1016/j.knee.2018.09.010

53. Kim HJ, Lee O-S, Lee SH, Lee YS (2018) Comparative analysis between cone and sleeve in managing severe bone defect during revision total knee arthroplasty: a systematic review and meta-analysis. J Knee Surg 31:677–685. https://doi.org/10.1055/s-0037-1606564
54. Sharkey PF, Hozack WJ, Rothman RH, Shastri S, Jacoby SM. Insall award paper: why are total knee arthroplasty failing today? Clin Orthop Relat Res. 2002;404:7–13. *This study reviews current mechanisms of failure of total knee arthroplasties. The reasons for failure listed in order of prevalence among the patients in this study include polyethylene wear, aseptic loosening, instability, infection, arthrofibrosis, malalignment or malposition, deficient extensor mechanism, avascular necrosis in the patella, periprosthetic fracture, and isolated patellar resurfacing.*
55. Rodriguez-Merchan EC. Instability following total knee arthroplasty. HSS J. 2011;7:273–8.
56. Vince KG, Abdeen A, Sugimori T. The unstable total knee arthroplasty: causes and cures. J Arthroplasty. 2006;21(4 Suppl 1):44–9.
57. Gonzalez MH, Mekhail AO. The failed total knee arthroplasty: evaluation and etiology. J Am Acad Orthop Surg. 2004;12:436–46.
58. Berend ME, Bertrand T. The role of implant constraint: not too little, not too much. Orthopedics. 2007;30(9):793.
59. Azzam K, Parvizi J, Kaufman D, Purtill JJ, Sharkey PF, Austin MS. Revision of the unstable total knee arthroplasty: outcome predictors. J Arthroplasty. 2011;26(8):1139–44. https://doi.org/10.1016/j.arth.2011.02.028 .
60. Babis GC, Trousdale RT, Morrey BF. The effectiveness of isolated tibial insert exchange in revision total knee arthroplasty. J Bone Joint Surg Am. 2002;84-A(1):64.
61. Lachiewicz PF, Watters TS (2014) Porous metal metaphyseal cones for severe bone loss: when only metal will do. Bone Joint J 96-B(11 Suppl A):118–121. https://doi.org/10.1302/0301-620X.96B11.34197
62. Bonanzinga T, Gehrke T, Zahar A et al (2018) Are trabecular metal cones a valid option to treat metaphyseal bone defects in complex primary and revision knee arthroplasty? Joints 6(1):58–64. https://doi.org/10.1055/s-0037-1608950
63. Levine B, Sporer S, Della Valle CJ et al (2007) Porous tantalum in reconstructive surgery of the knee: a review. J Knee Surg 20(3):185–194
64. Beckmann NA, Mueller S, Gondan M et al (2015) Treatment of severe bone defects during revision total knee arthroplasty with structural allografts and porous metal cones-a systematic review, vol 2, United States
65. Fedorka CJ, Chen AF, Pagnotto MR, Crossett LS, Klatt BA (2017) Revision total knee arthroplasty with porous-coated metaphyseal sleeves provides radiographic ingrowth and stable fixation. Knee Surg Sports Traumatol Arthrosc 26(5):1500–1505
66. Henricson A, Linder L, Nilsson KG (2008) A trabecular metal tibial component in total knee replacement in patients younger than 60 years: a two-year radiostereophotogrammetric analysis. J Bone Joint Surg Br 90(12):1585–1593. https://doi.org/10.1302/0301-620X.90B12.20797

67. Heinl P, Muller L, Korner C et al (2008) Cellular Ti-6Al-4V structures with interconnected macro porosity for bone implants fabricated by selective electron beam melting. Acta Biomater 4(5):1536–1544. https://doi.org/10.1016/j.actbio.2008.03.013
68. Wang H, Zhao B, Liu C et al (2016) A comparison of biocompatibility of a titanium alloy fabricated by electron beam melting and selective laser melting. PLoS ONE 11(7):e0158513. https://doi.org/10.1371/journal.pone.0158513
69. de Martino I, de Santis V, Sculco PK et al (2015) Tantalum cones provide durable mid-term fixation in revision TKA. Clin Orthop Relat Res 473(10):3176–3182. https://doi.org/10.1007/s11999-015-4338-2
70. Papas PV, Congiusta D, Cushner FD (2019) Cementless versus cemented fixation in total knee arthroplasty. J Knee Surg 32(07):596–599. https://doi.org/10.1055/s-0039-1678687
71. Mancuso F, Beltrame A, Colombo E et al (2017) Management of metaphyseal bone loss in revision knee arthroplasty. Acta Biomed 88(2S):98–111. https://doi.org/10.23750/abm.v88i2
72. Bugbee WD, Ammeen DJ, Engh GA. Does implant selection affect outcome of revision knee arthroplasty? J Arthroplasty. 2001;16:581–5.
73. Hanssen AD. Cemented stems are requisite in revision knee replacement. Orthopedics. 2004;27(9):990–1003.
74. Nelson CL, Lonner JH, Rand JA, Lotke PA. Strategies of stem fixation and the role of supplemental bone graft in revision total knee arthroplasty. J Bone Joint Surg Am. 2003;85A:S52–7.
75. Abraham R, Malkani AL, Lewis J, Beck D. An anatomical study of tibial metaphyseal/diaphyseal mismatch during revision total knee arthroplasty. J Arthroplasty. 2007;22(2):241–4.
76. Brilhault JM, Ries MD. Influence of offset stem couplers in femoral revision knee arthroplasty: a radiographic study. Knee. 2012;19(2):112–5. *Highlights the importance of an offset femoral stem extension in balancing the flexion gap and improving the alignment of the stem.*
77. Brilhault JM, Ries MD. Posteriorly offset femoral component to restore anteroposterior position of the distal femur in revision total knee arthroplasty. J Arthroplasty. 2011;26(2):214–7.
78. Nakasone CK, Abdeen A, Khachatourians AG, Sugimori T, Vince KG. Component alignment in revision total knee arthroplasty using diaphyseal engaging modular offset press-fit stems. J Arthroplasty. 2008;23(8):1178–81.
79. Innocenti M, Matassi F, Carulli C, Soderi S, Villano M, Civinini R. Joint line position in revision total knee arthroplasty: the role of posterior femoral offset stems. Knee. 2013;20(6):447–50.
80. Guenoun B, Latargez L, Freslon M, Defossez G, Salas N, Gayet LE (2009) Complications following rotating hinge Endo-Modell (Link) knee arthroplasty. Orthop Traumatol Surg Res 95(7):529–536. https://doi.org/10.1016/j.otsr.2009.07.013

81. Whittaker JP, Dharmarajan R, Toms AD. The management of bone loss in revision total knee replacement. J Bone Joint Surg (Br). 2008;90(8):981–7.
82. Ochs BG, Schreiner AJ, de Zwart PM, Stockle U, Gonser CE (2016) Computer-assisted navigation is beneficial both in primary and revision surgery with modular rotating-hinge knee arthroplasty. Knee Surg Sports Traumatol Arthrosc 24(1):64–73. https://doi.org/10.1007/s00167-014-3316-7
83. Efe T, Roessler PP, Heyse TJ, Hauk C, Pahrmann C, Getgood A, Schmitt J (2012) Mid-term results after implantation of rotating-hinge knee prostheses: primary versus revision. Orthop Rev (Pavia) 4(4):e35. https://doi.org/10.4081/or.2012.e35
84. Daines BK, Dennis DA. Management of bone defects in revision total knee arthroplasty. Instr Course Lect. 2013;62:341–8.
85. Dennis DA, Berry DJ, Engh G, et al. Revision total knee arthroplasty. J Am Acad Orthop Surg. 2008;16(8):442–54.
86. Hanna SA, Aston WJ, de Roeck NJ, Gough-Palmer A, Powles DP (2011) Cementless revision TKA with bone grafting of osseous defects restores bone stock with a low revision rate at 4 to 10 years. Clin Orthop Relat Res 469:3164–3171
87. Vasso M, Beaufils P, Cerciello S, Schiavone PA. Bone loss following knee arthroplasty: potential treatment options. Arch Orthop Trauma Surg. 2014;134(4):543–53. https://doi.org/10.1007/s00402-014-1941-8.
88. Haidukewych GJ, Hanssen A, Jones RD. Metaphyseal fixation in revision total knee arthroplasty: indications and techniques. J Am Acad Orthop Surg. 2011;19(6):311–8.
89. Huff TW, Sculco TP. Management of bone loss in revision total knee arthroplasty. J Arthroplasty. 2007;22(7, Supplement):32–6. https://doi.org/10.1016/j.arth.2007.05.022.
90. Shen C, Lichstein PM, Austin MS, Sharkey PF, Parvizi J (2014) Revision knee arthroplasty for bone loss: choosing the right degree of constraint. J Arthroplasty 29(1):127–131
91. Lonner JH, Lotke PA, Kim J, Nelson C. Impaction grafting and wire mesh for uncontained defects in revision knee arthroplasty. Clin Orthop. 2002;404:145–51.
92. Mabry TM, Hanssen AD. The role of stems and augments for bone loss in revision knee arthroplasty. J Arthroplasty. 2007;22(4 Suppl 1):56–60.
93. Panni AS, Vasso M, Cerciello S (2012) Modular augmentation in revision total knee arthroplasty. Knee Surg Sports Traumatol Arthrosc. https://doi.org/10.1007/s00167-012-2258-1
94. Engh GA, Ammeen DJ. Use of structural allograft in revision total knee arthroplasty in knees with severe tibial bone loss. J Bone Joint Surg Am. 2007;89(12):2640–7. https://doi.org/10.2106/JBJS.F.00865 .
95. Backstein D, Safir O, Gross A (2006) Management of bone loss: structural grafts in revision total knee arthroplasty. Clin Orthop Relat Res 446:104. https://doi.org/10.1097/01.blo.0000214426.52206.2c

96. Bauman RD, Lewallen DG, Hanssen AD. Limitations of structural allograft in revision total knee arthroplasty. Clin Orthop. 2009;467(3):818–24. https://doi.org/10.1007/s11999-008-0679-4 .
97. Long WJ, Scuderi GR. Porous tantalum cones for large metaphyseal tibial defects in revision total knee arthroplasty: a minimum 2-year follow-up. J Arthroplasty. 2009;24(7):1086–92. https://doi.org/10.1016/j.arth.2008.08.011.
98. Meneghini RM, Lewallen DG, Hanssen AD (2008) Use of porous tantalum metaphyseal cones for severe tibial bone loss during revision total knee replacement. J Bone Joint Surg Am 90(1):78–84. https://doi.org/10.2106/JBJS.F.01495
99. Howard JL, Kudera J, Lewallen DG, Hanssen AD. Early results of the use of tantalum femoral cones for revision total knee arthroplasty. J Bone Joint Surg Am. 2011;93(5):478–84. https://doi.org/10.2106/JBJS.I.01322 .
100. Lachiewicz PF, Bolognesi MP, Henderson RA, Soileau ES, Vail TP. Can tantalum cones provide fixation in complex revision knee arthroplasty? Clin Orthop. 2012;470(1):199–204. https://doi.org/10.1007/s11999-011-1888-9 .
101. Huang R, Barrazueta G, Ong A, et al. Revision total knee arthroplasty using metaphyseal sleeves at short-term follow-up. Orthopedics. 2014;37(9):e804–9. https://doi.org/10.3928/01477447-20140825-57 . *The authors provide short-term data to support the use of metaphyseal sleeves in the largest cohort studied to date and the only report on both tibial and femoral sleeves using both nonhinged and hinged designs.*
102. Fröschen FS, Friedrich MJ, Randau TM, Gravius S, Gravius N (2019) Conversion of cemented revision total knee prostheses to arthrodesis using custom-made arthrodesis modules that preserve the cemented stem anchorage in patients with long-established extensor mechanism insufficiency: a case series. Knee 26(5):1117–1124
103. Dohmae Y, Bechtold J, Sherman R, Puno R, Gustilo R (1988) Reduction in cement-bone interface shear strength between primary and revision arthroplasty. Clin Orthop Relat Res 236:214–220
104. Osmon D, Berbari E, Berendt A, Lew D, Zimmerli W, Steckelberg J, Rao N, Hanssen A, Wilson W (2013) Infectious diseases society of a: diagnosis and management of prosthetic joint infection: clinical practice guidelines by the infectious diseases society of America. Clin Infect Dis 56(1):e1–e25
105. Tande AJ, Gomez-Urena EO, Berbari EF, Osmon DR (2017) Management of prosthetic joint infection. Infect Dis Clin North Am 31(2):237–252
106. Bejon P, Berendt A, Atkins B, Green N, Parry H, Masters S, McLardy-Smith P, Gundle R, Byren I (2010) Two-stage revision for prosthetic joint infection: predictors of outcome and the role of reimplantation microbiology. J Antimicrob Chemother 65(3):569–575
107. Hurst N, Ruta D, Kind P (1998) Comparison of the MOS short form-12 (SF12) health status questionnaire with the SF36 in patients with rheumatoid arthritis. Br J Rheumatol 37(8):862–869

108. Huten D, Pasquier G, Lambotte JC (2020) Techniques for filling tibiofemoral bone defects during revision total knee arthroplasty. Orthop Traumatol Surg Res 13:102776. https://doi.org/10.1016/j.otsr.2020.102776
109. Belt M, Smulders K, van Houten A, Wymenga A, Heesterbeek P, van Hellemondt G (2020) What is the reliability of a new classification for bone defects in revision TKA based on preoperative radiographs? Clin Orthop Relat Res 478(9):2057–2064. https://doi.org/10.1097/CORR.0000000000001084
110. Cornell CN (2020) CORR Insights®: what is the reliability of a new classification for bone defects in revision TKA based on preoperative radiographs? Clin Orthop Relat Res 478(9):2065–2066. https://doi.org/10.1097/CORR.0000000000001145
111. Sheth NP, Bonadio MB, Demange MK (2017) bone loss in revision total knee arthroplasty: evaluation and management. J Am Acad Orthop Surg 25:348–357. https://doi.org/10.5435/JAAOS-D-15-00660
112. Zanirato A, Formica M, Cavagnaro L, Divano S, Burastero G, Felli L (2020) Metaphyseal cones and sleeves in revision total knee arthroplasty: two sides of the same coin? Complications, clinical and radiological results-a systematic review of the literature. Musculoskelet Surg 104(1):25–35. https://doi.org/10.1007/s12306-019-00598-y
113. Golgelioglu, Fatih; Oguzkaya, Sinan; Misir, Abdulhamit; Guney, Ahmet The Effect of Time Spent with a Dynamic Spacer on Clinical and Functional Outcomes in Two-Stage Revision Knee Arthroplasty. Indian Journal of Orthopaedics (2020). https://doi.org/10.1007/s43465-020-00247-8
114. Maslaris, Alexander; Layher, Frank; Bungartz, Matthias; Zippelius, Timo; Liodakis, Emmanouil; Brinkmann, Olaf; Matziolis, Georg Sagittal profile has a significant impact on the explantability of well-fixed cemented stems in revision knee arthroplasty: a biomechanical comparison study of five established knee implant models. Archives of Orthopaedic and Trauma Surgery (2019). https://doi.org/10.1007/s00402-019-03160-4
115. Vasso, Michele; Beaufils, Philippe; Schiavone Panni, Alfredo Constraint choice in revision knee arthroplasty. International Orthopaedics (2013). https://doi.org/10.1007/s00264-013-1929-y
116. Pour, Aidin Eslam; Bradbury, Thomas L.; Horst, Patrick; Harrast, John J.; Erens, Greg A.; Roberson, James R. Trends in primary and revision knee arthroplasty among orthopaedic surgeons who take the American Board of Orthopaedics part II exam. International Orthopaedics (2016). https://doi.org/10.1007/s00264-016-3137-z
117. Doorgakant, Ashtin; Bhutta, Mohammed A; Marynissen, Hans Management of a tibial periprosthetic fracture following revision knee arthroplasty using a pulsed electromagnetic field stimulation device: a case report. Cases Journal (2009). https://doi.org/10.4076/1757-1626-2-8706
118. van der Wilk, Sten; Hoorntje, Alexander; Blankevoort, Leendert; van Geenen, Rutger; Kerkhoffs, Gino M. M. J.; Kuijer, P. Paul F. M. Physical activity after revision knee arthroplasty including return to sport and work: a systematic

review and meta-analysis including GRADE. BMC Musculoskeletal Disorders (2023). https://doi.org/10.1186/s12891-023-06458-y
119. Gill, Usman Nazir; Ahmed, Nasir; Noor, Syed Shahid; Memon, Iftikhar Ahmed; Memon, Zulfiqar Ali Management of the bone loss by metaphyseal sleeves in primary and revision knee arthroplasty: clinical experience and outcome after forty three cases. International Orthopaedics (2020). https://doi.org/10.1007/s00264-020-04663-1
120. Schnetz, M.; Hofmann, L.; Ewald, L.; Klug, A.; Hoffmann, R.; Gramlich, Y. Midterm results of modular hinge total knee arthroplasty using cementless osseointegrating stems: low fixation associated complications and good functional outcome in primary and revision knee arthroplasty. Archives of Orthopaedic and Trauma Surgery (2023). https://doi.org/10.1007/s00402-023-05148-7
121. Erivan, Roger; Tracey, Robert; Mulliez, Aurélien; Villatte, Guillaume; Paprosky, Wayne Medium term clinical outcomes of tibial cones in revision knee arthroplasty. Archives of Orthopaedic and Trauma Surgery (2020). https://doi.org/10.1007/s00402-020-03532-1
122. Indelli, Pier Francesco; Giori, Nick; Maloney, William Level of constraint in revision knee arthroplasty. Current Reviews in Musculoskeletal Medicine (2015). https://doi.org/10.1007/s12178-015-9295-6
123. Ohlmeier, Malte; Lausmann, Christian; Wolff, Matthias; Abdelaziz, Hussein; Gehrke, Thorsten; Citak, Mustafa Preliminary clinical results of coated porous tibia cones in septic and aseptic revision knee arthroplasty. Archives of Orthopaedic and Trauma Surgery (2020). https://doi.org/10.1007/s00402-020-03434-2
124. Baldini, Andrea; Balato, Giovanni; Franceschini, Vincenzo The role of offset stems in revision knee arthroplasty. Current Reviews in Musculoskeletal Medicine (2015). https://doi.org/10.1007/s12178-015-9294-7
125. Boelch, Sebastian P.; Arnholdt, Joerg; Holzapfel, Boris M.; Jakuscheit, Axel; Rudert, Maximilian; Hoberg, Maik Revision knee arthroplasty with rotating hinge systems in patients with gross ligament instability. International Orthopaedics (2018). https://doi.org/10.1007/s00264-018-3982-z
126. Ponzio, Danielle Y.; Austin, Matthew S. Metaphyseal bone loss in revision knee arthroplasty. Current Reviews in Musculoskeletal Medicine (2015). https://doi.org/10.1007/s12178-015-9291-x
127. Gramlich, Y.; Steinkohl, D.; Kremer, M.; Kemmerer, M.; Hoffmann, R.; Klug, A. Modular knee arthrodesis secures limb, mobility, improves quality of life, and leads to high infection control in periprosthetic knee infection, when revision knee arthroplasty is not an option. Archives of Orthopaedic and Trauma Surgery (2021). https://doi.org/10.1007/s00402-021-03907-y
128. Cherny, Alexander A.; Kovalenko, Anton N.; Kulyaba, Taras A.; Kornilov, Nikolai N. A prospective study on outcome of patient-specific cones in revision knee arthroplasty. Archives of Orthopaedic and Trauma Surgery (2021). https://doi.org/10.1007/s00402-021-04047-z

Conclusion

Alfred J. Tria Jr. and Giles R. Scuderi

In the evolving field of total knee arthroplasty (TKA), staying updated with the current trends in implant designs and surgical techniques are essential. Textbooks provide a reliable source of information that surgeons can consult to increase their knowledge. Libraries and medical publishers have vast resources that allow for deep exploration of specific topics. As the editors of this textbook, we explored the Springer Nature library, defined specific TKA topics and refined the AI generated content trying to ensure accuracy and relevance. Using keywords to gather references from the Springer Nature library, the highlighted content on implant design, kinematics, surgical technique, fixation, and revision TKA was reviewed and presented to the readership. It was a challenging process to ensure accuracy. There is no doubt that this is the early days of AI generated textbooks and that it is learning process. With that in mind, we felt obligated to provide you an editorial summary on current trends in TKA based upon our decades of surgical experience.

It is well known that TKA is the most common treatment for knee osteoarthritis. Given the success of modern TKA, the volume of TKA has risen over the past decades in the United States, making it one of the most performed orthopedic procedures. The most recent 2040 projections for primary TKA are over 1.2 million cases per year and over 2.9 million in 2060 [1]. This is an estimated increase of 139% in 2040 and 469% in 2060. TKA has proven to be a predictable and durable procedure, returning patients to both activities of daily living and recreational activities with overall good survivorship. With improved life expectancy and increasing preference to leading an active life, TKA is being performed in younger and more active patients. This shift to a younger population results in greater demands

A. J. Tria Jr.
Department of Orthopedics, Rutgers-Robert Wood Johnson Medical School, New Brunswick, NJ, USA

G. R. Scuderi
Department of Orthopedic Surgery, Northwell Health, Garden City, NY, USA

A. J. Tria Jr., G. R. Scuderi (eds.), *Total Knee Arthroplasty*,
https://doi.org/10.1007/978-3-032-00175-7

durability with higher expectations. Satisfying patient expectations is the goal. Despite advances in implant design and surgical technique over the years, there is a 10 to 20% rate of dissatisfaction [2–4]. To further improve patient satisfaction, improvements in implant design, instrumentation, and surgical technique are evolving and are directed towards a more personalized approach, which is expected to be assisted by innovative technology.

The issue of patient dissatisfaction may be reduced by a more individualized patient specific approach to TKA with more personalized designs and surgical technique. The current inventory of modern implants is providing a wide range of shapes and sizes with more anatomically shaped components. The main direction of newer TKA design is to optimize component fit without compromise, improve knee kinematics by restoring the radii of femoral curvature, improve patella tracking with a patella friendly trochlea and restore limb alignment.

There is currently a trend away from the historical designs and towards more guided motion knee designs that replicate knee kinematics by the geometry of the femoral tibial articular surface. The American Joint Replacement Registry [5] reports that while PCL substituting (PS) knee designs had been the most popular implant design, PCL retaining (CR) implants are gaining popularity and are the most implanted design. However, the recent AJRR report also noted that there is an increased interest in guided motion knee implant designs, such as the ultracongruent, medial congruent and medial pivot. These newer implant designs may continue to erode on both the PS and CR market share. It appears that the guided motion surface geometries, with differential medial and lateral conformities, influences knee kinematics without the need for the cruciate ligaments or cam-post mechanism. What may be driving the increased interest in guided motion knee designs is that it appears to be coupled with the new interest in alternative alignments in TKA, such as kinematic alignment in contrast to mechanical alignment.

Although mechanical alignment has been considered the "gold standard", alternative alignments are being considered to improve patient satisfaction. The advent of modern components and advanced technologies has fueled the debate on whether mechanical alignment can be justified in all knees. Currently, a personalized approach to TKA has numerous novel schemes and techniques such as anatomic alignment, unrestricted kinematic alignment, restricted kinematic alignment, inverse restricted kinematic alignment, adjusted mechanical alignment, and functional alignment. With each of these personalized alignments, the nuances are differing with varying resection targets and boundaries. The range of variability in targets for the hip knee angle (HKA); femoral and tibial coronal alignment; femoral and tibial sagittal alignment; and femoral axial alignment is wide and varying. There has yet to be an agreed upon personalized technique that has been widely accepted as mechanical alignment [6]. Further research is needed to assess the relevance of these alternative alignments to see if they are worth the change and which ones are the most relevant for which patients, diagnoses, and degrees of coronal deformity [7].

Currently, the most common surgical technique for TKA is conventional manual instrumentation. However, there has been a shift to innovative technologies to assist in surgical accuracy. Studies have shown that patient anatomy in 3 dimensions (3D) varies from patient to patient that can be better defined with advanced imaging and related technologies. While computer navigation introduced the concept of a more individualized approach, robotic systems now create a 3-dimensional (3D) plan based upon intraoperativc bonc morphology mapping or a preoperative MRI or CT scan. Based upon the 3D data, the personalized preoperative plan for each patient is created. The robotic assisted surgery also allows an assessment of ligament balancing based upon the bone cuts and implant position. This has the potential to be further enhanced by collecting all the information into a large database and allow artificial intelligence (AI) and machine learning (ML) analysis of the alignment and outcome [8]. With the best aggregated clinical results determined by ML, the computer can be programmed to learn how to make the best recommendation for alignment of each patient that is then incorporated into the robotic surgical plan. The role of AI will continue to expand with ongoing advances, pushing the boundaries of its capabilities. Incorporating ML has the potential to elevate patient care by identifying the best preoperative patient parameters and postoperative pathways to help drive higher patient satisfaction.

One of the challenges of achieving a satisfactory TKA is ligament balancing, which has historically been a qualitative "feel" rather than a quantitative measurement. This "feel" is based upon surgeon experience but is influenced by many patient factors including degree of deformity, ligament laxity, joint stiffness, obesity, and sex. The introduction of intraoperative sensors with the surgical instrumentation facilitates decision-making regarding implant position and soft tissue releases to improve balance and stability through the arc of motion [9]. Further development of real time intraoperative sensors incorporated robotic surgical systems will need to define the normal pressures, as well as the normal ligament tension, within the joint to achieve a well-balanced TKA. This information, along with ML analysis, has the potential to provide a personalized approach to ligament balance for each patient.

The knowledge and technology from our current experience in TKA is setting the stage for future developments [10]. Enhancements in our understanding of knee anatomy and biomechanics are suggesting ways of improving outcomes and potentially patient satisfaction. Applying this knowledge to implant designs and instrumentation along with innovative technology for a personalized approach will be the future of TKA. Sharing this knowledge with AI generated resources can be a valuable tool in disseminating information, but should not be a substitute for human knowledge and expertise.

References

1. Shichman I, Roof M, Askew N, Nherera L, Rozell JC, Seyler TM, Schwarzkopf R. Projections and epidemiology of primary hip and knee arthroplasty in Medicare patients to 2040-260. J Bone Joint Surg Open Acess. 2023;e22.00112 https://doi.org/10.2106/JBJS.OA22.00112.
2. Noble PC, Conditt MA, Cook KF, Mathis KB. The John Insall award: patient expectations affect satisfaction with total knee arthroplasty. Clin Orthop Relat Res. 2006;452:35–43.
3. Bourne RB, Chesworth BM, Davis AM, Mahomed NN, Charron KDJ. Patient satisfaction after total knee arthroplasty: who is satisfied and who is not? Clin Orthop Relat Res. 2010;468:57–63.
4. DeFrance MJ, Scuderi GR. Are 20% of patients actually dissatisfied following total knee arthroplasty? A systematic review of the literature. J Arthroplast. 2023;38:594–9.
5. American Joint Replacement Registry Annual Report 2024.
6. MacDessi SJ, Oussedik S, Abdel MP, Victor J, Pagnano MW, Haddad FS. The language of knee alignment. Updated definitions and considerations for reporting outcomes in total knee arthroplasty. Bone Joint J. 2023;105B(2):102–8.
7. MacDessi SJ, Griffiths-Jones W, Harris IA, Bellemans J, Chen DB. Coronal Plane Alignment of the Knee (CPAK) classification. Bone Joint J. 2021;103-B(2):329–37.
8. Myers TG, Ramkumar PN, Ricciardi BF, Urish KL, Kioper J, Ketonis C. Artificial intelligence and orthopedics: an introduction for clinicians. J Bone Joint Surg Am. 2020;102(9):830–40.
9. Batailler C, Swan J, Marinier ES, Servien LS. New technologies in knee arthroplasty: current concepts. J Clin Med. 2021;10:47. https://doi.org/10.3390/jcm10010047.
10. Scuderi GR, Tria AJ. Future considerations in the cruciate ligaments in total knee Arthroplasty ed. By AJ Tria and GR Scuderi, Springer Nature, Switzerland; 2024; pp. 213–218.

A. J. Tria Jr., G. R. Scuderi (eds.), *Total Knee Arthroplasty*,
https://doi.org/10.1007/978-3-032-00175-7